Compliments of Solvay Pharmaceuticals, Inc.
makers of

CREON®
MINIMICROSPHERES®
5·10·20*(Pancrelipase Delayed-Release Capsules, USP)
★ Numbers indicate 5,000/10,000/20,000 units of lipase

Clinical Pancreatology
for Practising Gastroenterologists and Surgeons

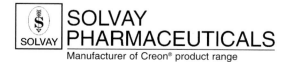

Clinical Pancreatology
for Practising Gastroenterologists and Surgeons

Edited by

J. Enrique Domínguez-Muñoz MD PhD

Associate Professor of Medicine
Department of Gastroenterology
University Hospital of Santiago de Compostela
Santiago de Compostela
Spain

With a foreword by

Peter Malfertheiner MD

Professor and Head of the Department of Gastroenterology,
 Hepatology, and Infectious Diseases
Otto-von-Guericke University
Magdeburg
Germany

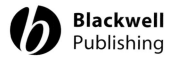

Blackwell
Publishing

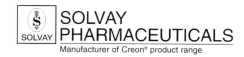

SOLVAY
PHARMACEUTICALS
Manufacturer of Creon® product range

First published 2005
2   2006

Library of Congress Cataloging-in-Publication Data
Clinical pancreatology for practising gastroenterologists and surgeons / edited by J. Enrique Domínguez-Muñoz ; with foreword by Peter Malfertheiner.
    p. ; cm.
  Includes index.
  ISBN-13: 978-1-4051-2276-4
  ISBN-10: 1-4051-2276-5
  1. Pancreas-Diseases.
  [DNLM: 1. Pancreatitis–diagnosis.   2. Pancreatitis–therapy.
3. Gastroenterology–methods.   WI 805 C641 2004]   I. Domínguez-Muñoz, J. Enrique.

  RC857.C556 2004
  616.3'7–dc22

                                                            2004023744

ISBN-13: 978-1-4051-2276-4
ISBN-10: 1-4051-2276-5

A catalogue record for this title is available from the British Library

Set in Sabon/Stone Sans by SNP Best-set Typesetter Ltd, Hong Kong
Printed and bound by Replika Press Pvt. Ltd, India

Commissioning Editor: Alison Brown
Development Editor: Mirjana Misina
Production Controller: Kate Charman

For further information on Blackwell Publishing, visit our website:
http://www.blackwellpublishing.com

The publisher's policy is to use permanent paper from mills that operate a sustainable forestry policy, and which has been manufactured from pulp processed using acid-free and elementary chlorine-free practices. Furthermore, the publisher ensures that the text paper and cover board used have met acceptable environmental accreditation standards.

Contents

Part II Chronic pancreatitis and cystic fibrosis

Contributors

Guido Adler MD
Professor of Internal Medicine
Chief, Department of Internal Medicine I
University of Ulm
Ulm
Germany

Åke Andrén-Sandberg MD PhD
Professor of Surgery
University of Bergen and Stavangar Hospital Trust
Stavanger
Sweden

Emiliano Astudillo MD
University of Barcelona
Hospital Clinic
Barcelona
Spain

Costas Avgerinos MD
Consultant Surgeon
Agia Olga Hospital
Athens
Greece

Emil J. Balthazar MD
Professor Emeritus of Radiology
New York University
New York, NY
USA

Peter A. Banks MD
Professor of Medicine
Harvard Medical School;
Director, Center for Pancreatic Disease
Brigham and Women's Hospital
Boston, MA
USA

Jennifer Barro MD
Senior Fellow in Gastroenterology

Stanford University School of Medicine
Stanford University Hospital
Stanford, CA
USA

Claudio Bassi MD
Professor of Surgery
University of Verona
Hospital G.B. Rossi
Verona
Italy

Marchelle J. Bean MD
Instructor
Johns Hopkins University Outpatient Center
Baltimore, MD
USA

Hans G. Beger MD FACS
Professor of Surgery
University of Ulm
Ulm
Germany

Dale E. Bockman PhD
Professor and Chairman Emeritus
Department of Cellular Biology and Anatomy
The Medical College of Georgia
Augusta, GA
USA

Edward L. Bradley III MD
Professor of Clinical Sciences (Surgery)
Florida State University College of Medicine
Tallahassee, FL
USA

William R. Brugge MD
Gastrointestinal Unit
Massachusetts General Hospital
Boston, MA
USA

Markus W. Büchler MD FRCS
Professor and Chairman
Department of General Surgery
University of Heidelberg
Heidelberg
Germany

Giovanni Butturini MD
University of Verona
Hospital G.B. Rossi
Verona
Italy

Julio Calvete-Chornet MD PhD
Department of Surgery
University Hospital Clinic
Valencia
Spain

David L. Carr-Locke MD FRCP
Director of Endoscopy
Harvard Medical School and Brigham and Women's
    Hospital
Boston, MA
USA

Gregorio Castellanos MD PhD
Department of Surgery
Virgen de la Arrixaca University Hospital
Murcia
Spain

Gleydson Cesar-Borges MD
University of Barcelona
Hospital Clinic
Barcelona
Spain

Guido Costamagna MD FACG
Full Professor of Surgery
Digestive Endoscopy Unit
Catholic University
Rome
Italy

Harry Cuppens PhD
Center for Human Genetics
Leuven
Belgium

Christos Dervenis MD
Department of Surgery
Agia Olga Hospital
Athens
Greece

Pierluigi Di Sebastiano MD
Consultant Surgeon
Department of General Surgery
University of Heidelberg
Heidelberg
Germany

J. Enrique Domínguez-Muñoz MD PhD
Associate Professor of Medicine
Department of Gastroenterology
University Hospital of Santiago de Compostela
Santiago de Compostela
Spain

Massimo Falconi MD
Consultant Surgeon
University of Verona
Hospital G.B. Rossi
Verona
Italy

Antonio Farré MD PhD
Senior Consultant in Gastroenterology
Hospital de la Santa Creu i Sant Pau
Barcelona
Spain

Laureano Fernández-Cruz MD FRCS (Ed)
Professor of Surgery
University of Barcelona
Hospital Clinic
Barcelona
Spain

Carlos Fernández-del Castillo MD
Associate Professor of Surgery
Harvard Medical School and Massachusetts General
    Hospital
Boston, MA
USA

Elliot K. Fishman MD FACR
Professor of Radiology and Oncology
Director, Diagnostic Imaging and Body Computed
  Tomography
Johns Hopkins University Outpatient Center
Baltimore, MD
USA

Ulrich R. Fölsch MD
Director, Department of Internal Medicine
University of Kiel
Kiel
Germany

Helmut Friess MD
Vice-Chairman, Department of General Surgery
University of Heidelberg
Heidelberg
Germany

Isabella Frigerio MD
General Surgeon
University of Verona
Hospital G.B. Rossi
Verona
Italy

Rosa Gelabert MD
University of Barcelona
Hospital Clinic
Barcelona
Spain

Paula Ghaneh MB ChB MD FRCS
Senior Lecturer in Surgery
University of Liverpool
Liverpool
UK

Marc Giovannini MD
Chief of Endoscopic Unit
Paoli-Calmettes Institute
Marseille
France

Luisa Guarner MD
Consultant Gastroenterologist
Vall d'Hebrón University Hospital
Barcelona
Spain

Lucio Gullo MD
Professor of Internal Medicine
University of Bologna;
Director, St. Orsola Hospital
Bologna
Italy

Werner Hartwig MD
Consultant Surgeon
Department of General Surgery
University of Heidelberg
Heidelberg
Germany

Naoki Hiki MD
Department of General Surgery
University of Ulm
Ulm
Germany

Oscar Joe Hines MD
Associate Professor of Surgery
University College of Los Angeles School of Medicine
Los Angeles, CA
USA

Karen M. Horton MD
Associate Professor
Johns Hopkins University Outpatient Center
Baltimore, MD
USA

Tomas Hucl MD
Department of Medicine II
University of Heidelberg Hospital at Mannheim
Mannheim
Germany

Matthew M. Hutter MD
Instructor in Surgery
Harvard Medical School;
Assistant in Surgery
Massachusetts General Hospital

Boston, MA
USA

Julio Iglesias-García MD
Department of Gastroenterology
University Hospital of Santiago de Compostela
Santiago de Compostela
Spain

Clement W. Imrie BSc MB ChB FRCS
Consultant Surgeon and Professor of Pancreatobiliary
    Surgery
Glasgow Royal Infirmary
Glasgow
UK

Ramon E. Jimenez MD
Assistant Professor of Surgery
University of Connecticut Medical School and
    Hartford Hospital
Hartford, CT
USA

Stefan Kahl MD
Consultant Gastroenterologist
Otto-von-Guericke University
University Hospital of Magdeburg
Magdeburg
Germany

Karlheinz Kiehne MD PhD
Department of Internal Medicine
University of Kiel
Kiel
Germany

Günter Klöppel MD
Professor of Pathology and Head of Pathology
    Department
University of Kiel
Kiel
Germany

Jörg Köninger MD
Consultant Surgeon
Department of General Surgery
University of Heidelberg
Heidelberg
Germany

Markus Kosmahl MD
Consultant Pathologist
University of Kiel
Kiel
Germany

Richard A. Kozarek MD
Chief of Gastroenterology and Director of the
    Gastrointestinal Unit
Virginia Mason Medical Center
Seattle, WA
USA

Glenn Krinsky MD
Associate Professor of Radiology
New York University
New York, NY
USA

Beat M. Künzli MD
Department of General Surgery
University of Heidelberg
Heidelberg
Germany

Richard S. Kwon MD
Gastroenterology Fellow
Center for Pancreatic Disease
Brigham and Women's Hospital
Harvard Medical School
Boston, MA
USA

Paul G. Lankisch MD FRCP FACG
Department of Internal Medicine
University Hospital of Lüneburg
Lüneburg
Germany

René Laugier MD
Department of Gastroenterology
Hospital La Timone
Marseille
France

Peter Layer MD PhD
Professor of Medicine

Chairman and Director, Department of Medicine
Israelitic Hospital
Hamburg
Germany

Bernhard Lembcke MD
Department of Medicine
St. Barbara Hospital
Gladbeck
Germany

Nicholas R. Lemoine MD PhD FRCPath
Director, Institute of Cancer and Cancer Research UK
    Clinical Centre
Barts and the London School of Medicine
London
UK

Markus M. Lerch MD FRCP
Professor and Chair
Department of Gastroenterology, Endocrinology, and
    Nutrition
University of Greifswald
Greifswald
Germany

Zhanbing Liu MD
Department of General Surgery
University of Ulm
Ulm
Germany

Salvador Lledo-Matoses MD PhD
Department of Surgery
University Hospital Clinic
Valencia
Spain

Félix Lluis MD PhD
Chairman, Department of General and Digestive
    Surgery
University General Hospital
Alicante
Spain

Matthias Löhr MD
Professor of Medicine and Molecular
    Gastroenterology
University of Heidelberg Hospital at Mannheim
Mannheim
Germany

Colin J. McKay MD FRCS
Senior Lecturer in Surgery
West of Scotland Pancreatic Unit
Glasgow Royal Infirmary
Glasgow
UK

Peter Malfertheiner MD
Professor and Head of the Department of
    Gastroenterology, Hepatology, and Infectious
    Diseases
Otto-von-Guericke University
Magdeburg
Germany

Isidro Martínez MD
University of Barcelona
Hospital Clinic
Barcelona
Spain

Juan Martínez PhD
Department of Gastroenterology
University Hospital of Alicante
Alicante
Spain

Ulrike Melle MD
Department of Medicine
Israelitic Hospital
Hamburg
Germany

Fabio F. di Mola MD
Department of General Surgery
University of Heidelberg
Heidelberg
Germany

Joachim Mössner MD
Professor of Medicine
Head of Department of Internal Medicine II
University Hospital of Leipzig
Leipzig
Germany

Bernd Mühling MD
Department of General Surgery
University of Ulm
Ulm
Germany

Salvador Navarro MD
Consultant, Department of Gastroenterology
Hospital Clinic
Barcelona
Spain

John P. Neoptolemos MA MB BChir MD FRCS
Professor of Surgery
Head of Division of Surgery and Oncology
University of Liverpool
Liverpool
UK

Joanne Nyarangi
Department of General Surgery
University of Heidelberg
Heidelberg
Germany

Georgios I. Papachristou MD
Gastroenterology Fellow
University of Pittsburgh Medical Center
Pittsburgh, PA
USA

Konstantina Paraskeva MD
Consultant Gastroenterologist
Agia Olga Hospital
Athens
Greece

Pascual Parrilla MD PhD
Department of Surgery
Virgen de la Arrixaca University Hospital
Murcia
Spain

Paolo Pederzoli MD
Professor of General Surgery
University of Verona
Hospital G.B. Rossi
Verona
Italy

Miguel Pérez-Mateo PhD
Professor of Medicine
Head of Department of Gastroenterology
University Hospital of Alicante
Alicante
Spain

George Perides PhD
Assistant Professor of Surgery
Tufts University School of Medicine
Boston, MA
USA

Raffaele Pezzilli MD
Department of Gastroenterology
St. Orsola Hospital
Bologna
Italy

Antonio Piñero MD PhD
Department of Surgery
Virgen de la Arrixaca University Hospital
Murcia
Spain

Bertram Poch MD
Department of General Surgery
University of Ulm
Ulm
Germany

Parviz M. Pour MD
Professor of Pathology
University of Nebraska Medical Center
Omaha, NE
USA

Michael G.T. Raraty MB BS PhD FRCS
Lecturer in Surgery
University of Liverpool
Liverpool
UK

Howard A. Reber MD
Professor of Surgery
Chief, Gastrointestinal Surgery
University College of Los Angeles School of Medicine
Los Angeles, CA
USA

Luis Sabater-Ortí MD PhD
Department of Surgery
University Hospital Clinic
Valencia
Spain

Roberto Salvia MD PhD
Consultant Surgeon
University of Verona
Hospital G.B. Rossi
Verona
Italy

Nora Sartori MD
University of Verona
Hospital G.B. Rossi
Verona
Italy

Alexander Schneider MD
Attending Physician
Department of Medicine II
University of Heidelberg Hospital at Mannheim
Mannheim
Germany

Thomas Seufferlein MD
Consultant, Department of Internal Medicine I
University of Ulm
Ulm
Germany

Manfred V. Singer MD
Professor of Medicine and Chairman
Department of Medicine II
University of Heidelberg Hospital at Mannheim
Mannheim
Germany

Roy M. Soetikno MD
Associate Professor of Medicine
Stanford University School of Medicine
Stanford, CA
USA

Antonio Soriano MD
Medical Researcher, Department of Gastroenterology
Hospital Clinic
Barcelona
Spain

Michael L. Steer MD PhD
Professor of Surgery, Anatomy, and Cellular Biology
Tufts University School of Medicine
Boston, MA
USA

Andrea Tringali MD
Consultant Gastroenterologist
Digestive Endoscopy Unit
Catholic University
Rome
Italy

Waldemar Uhl MD FRCS
Professor of Surgery and Chairman
Ruhr University and St. Josef Hospital
Bochum
Germany

Enrique Vazquez-Sequeiros MD PhD
Consultant Gastroenterologist
Ramón y Cajal University Hospital
Madrid
Spain

Carmen Villalba-Martín MD
Abdominal Radiologist
University of Santiago de Compostela
Conxo Hospital

Santiago de Compostela
Spain

Andrew L. Warshaw MD
W. Gerald Austen Professor of Surgery
Harvard Medical School;
Surgeon-in-Chief and Chairman
Department of Surgery
Massachusetts General Hospital
Boston, MA
USA

Markus A. Weigand MD
Department of General Surgery
University of Heidelberg
Heidelberg
Germany

Frank Ulrich Weiss PhD
Head of the Laboratory of Molecular
    Gastroenterology
University of Greifswald
Greifswald
Germany

Jens Werner MB
Senior Surgeon
Department of General Surgery
University of Heidelberg

Heidelberg
Germany

Frederik Wenz MD
University of Heidelberg Hospital at Mannheim
Mannheim
Germany

David C. Whitcomb MD PhD
Professor of Medicine, Cell Biology, Physiology, and
    Human Genetics
Chief, Division of Gastroenterology, Hepatology, and
    Nutrition
University of Pittsburgh
Pittsburgh, PA
USA

Martin Wirtz MD
Surgical Resident
Department of General Surgery
University of Heidelberg
Heidelberg
Germany

Zhengfei Zhou MD
Department of General Surgery
University of Ulm
Ulm
Germany

Foreword

Our knowledge in the field of pancreatology is continually accumulating. Relevant basic and clinical research studies, published in recent years, have provided new information that has changed our view of and approach to the diagnosis and therapy of pancreatic diseases. The challenge now is to disseminate these advances among all practicing gastroenterologists and surgeons treating pancreatic diseases, so that they will, in turn, benefit our patients.

This book, edited by Enrique Domínguez-Muñoz, is indeed a comprehensive treatise on clinical pancreatology. The carefully selected contributors are all dedicated pancreatologists of many years' experience who have greatly contributed to where we stand today in the clinical management of pancreatic diseases.

The chapters on inflammatory and neoplastic diseases of the pancreas provide a complete and comprehensive insight into all clinical problems and offer solutions to everyday clinical needs in the management of pancreatic diseases. The individual aspects of diagnostic options, sometimes conflicting or even redundant, are presented in a very balanced and objective way. Clinical concepts are well illustrated and the reader can follow clear diagrams and excellent algorithms. The therapeutic sections, too, are very nicely developed and the necessary emphasis is given to the importance of an interdisciplinary approach. This is a particular requirement for all those who aim to operate successfully in this clinical field. The arguments put forward in several chapters go even beyond our state of the art knowledge and raise important considerations that will stimulate further clinical research.

Enrique Domínguez-Muñoz is to be congratulated for having thoughtfully selected topics corresponding to the sequence of decisions we need to consider when faced with the challenging problems of patients affected by an acute or chronic morbid condition of the pancreas. In my judgment this book is a must for specialists but also a gift to all clinicians who at times have to take responsibility for the care of patients with pancreatic pathologies.

Peter Malfertheiner

Preface

The pancreas continues to be, to some extent, the hidden organ for many gastroenterologists and surgeons. The diseases of the pancreas are frequently difficult to diagnose and/or treat, and the results of the treatment are usually disappointing. Mortality of acute pancreatitis remains high, diagnosis of chronic pancreatitis in its early stages is still a challenge, therapy of cystic fibrosis is far from satisfactory, and pancreatic cancer continues to be a devastating disease.

The exploration of the pancreas and its inherent difficulties has, over the last few decades, stimulated gastroenterologists, surgeons, radiologists, pathologists, and scientists to delve deep into their knowledge of molecular biology, genetics, physiology, pathophysiology, diagnosis, and therapeutic approaches to pancreatic diseases. Societies devoted to the study of the pancreas and its diseases have emerged all over the world and there is a demand for specific journals and books.

Many important advances have been made in pancreatology in recent years, many of them changing the approach to the patient with pancreatic diseases in clinical practice. Nevertheless, practicing gastroenterologists and surgeons, who face patients with pancreatic diseases daily, but who are not especially devoted to the field of pancreatology, can hardly apply these recent research advances to the management of their patients. In fact, pancreatology books and journals are highly specialized. Most of the knowledge contained therein has no direct clinical application and/or is difficult to comprehend for non-pancreatologists. Therefore, general gastroenterologists and surgeons have difficulty accessing the most recent and relevant advances in pancreatic diseases.

The goal of *Clinical Pancreatology* is to provide practicing gastroenterologists and surgeons with clear information regarding the current diagnostic and therapeutic approaches to pancreatic diseases. The book consists of short and concise chapters providing clear, evidence-based, but also experience-based, information, immediately relevant to clinical practice. Chapters have been written by internationally recognized gastroenterologists, surgeons, radiologists, and pathologists, specially dedicated to the study of the pancreas. This is, therefore, a book from expert pancreatologists for practicing medical doctors, in which controversies have been avoided as far as possible. Each chapter concludes with a list of the most relevant literature as "recommended reading" to provide readers with easy access to more detailed information.

As editor, I am deeply grateful and indebted to all authors for their dedication and efforts in contributing to this book. It is they who are really responsible for the high quality of this work. I also thank the team at Blackwell Science for their support, patience, and skill. Finally, my special thanks to Friederike Henniges, Global Medical Affairs Director of Solvay Pharmaceuticals, Germany, for her enthusiasm and support for this work.

J. Enrique Domínguez-Muñoz

Dedication

I would like to dedicate this book to all the friends who have supported me throughout my professional life and who have helped me to grow, not only as a clinician but also as a person. Among all of them, I would especially like to thank Professor Peter Malfertheiner and Professor Fernando Carballo, who were, and still are, my teachers and friends.

The editing of this book has required dedication and a major effort. This has been possible thanks to the love, understanding, and support of my wife, Victoria, and my children, Irene and Enrique.

Finally, I would like to dedicate this book to my parents, Enrique and Concepción.

1 Acute pancreatitis: definition and classification for clinical practice

Edward L. Bradley III

Overview

Acute pancreatitis is a protean disease, capable of resulting in pathologic findings ranging from mild pancreatic edema to total organ necrosis, and from regional retroperitoneal inflammation to systemic multiorgan failure. Depending upon the severity and scope of the underlying pathologic processes, acute pancreatitis may present anywhere on the spectrum of clinical severity, from mild abdominal discomfort to apocalyptic prostration.

Perhaps due to this very breadth in pathology and presentation, considerable clinical confusion has existed regarding acute pancreatitis. For much of the past century, standards did not exist to measure severity, nor were there any clinically useful definitions of acute pancreatitis and its complications. These deficiencies not only caused both researchers and clinicians to experience great difficulty in attempting to communicate with each other, but also resulted in idiosyncratic, and frequently conflicting, recommendations for therapy. As a case in point, during a personal 1980s literature search for articles restricted to "pancreatic abscess" a total of 45 reports were found, but only 11 had actually offered any definition of "pancreatic abscess," the topic of their paper. Most troubling, however, was the observation that no two of these eleven definitions for "pancreatic abscess" were the same! Apparently, each of the authors had assumed that their working definition of "pancreatic abscess" was the same one used by everyone else, much as did Humpty Dumpty in Lewis Carroll's *Alice's Adventures in Wonderland* when he said, "When I use a word, it means just what I choose it to mean—neither more nor less!"

A further analysis of those disparate definitions of "pancreatic abscess" revealed that a variety of post-pancreatitic infections, such as infected fluid collections, infected pseudocysts, peripancreatic abscesses, and infected pancreatic necrosis, had been included under the single rubric of "pancreatic abscess." This taxonomic confusion necessarily led to wide variations in proposals for diagnosis and therapy: proposed management for an infected pancreatic pseudocyst could hardly be expected to be successful if mistakenly applied to infected pancreatic necrosis. Clinical management for other complications of acute pancreatitis was similarly afflicted by confusing, and often conflicting, definitions.

Heterogeneous definitions of acute pancreatitis and its complications existed until relatively recently, being principally the result of the difficulty attendant upon attempting to study the natural history and variations of acute pancreatitis with the inadequate technology available at the time. Given the remote anatomic location of the pancreas, and the limitations of early noninvasive imaging, much of what was known (or thought to be known) about the pathology of acute pancreatitis was the result of autopsy or surgical studies. Clearly, material obtained from such studies could not be representative of those cases from the less severe spectrum of pathology. Inability to measure severity and the absence of precise disease definitions were therefore two of the major factors responsible for the prolonged delay in the development of a useful clinical approach to acute pancreatitis. From a historical standpoint, the first of these two problems to be addressed was the stratification of severity.

Stratification of severity

In 1974, John Ranson published his seminal paper on the stratification of severity of clinical acute pancreatitis. Using statistical manipulation of 43 clinical and laboratory variables obtained from a consecutive series of 100 patients with acute pancreatitis, he was able to identify 11 "prognostic signs" that proved to be significantly associated with clinical severity, as measured by the development of morbidity or mortality. For many subsequent years, these Ranson Criteria were all that were available to assign severity to an individual episode of acute pancreatitis. The necessity for severity assignment was nevertheless clear; in a disease process capable of wide variations in clinical severity, specific stratification of severity is necessary not only to compare the results of clinical investigations but also to predict patient prognosis. Today, we would add a third reason for determination of severity: selection among therapeutic options.

Despite the usefulness of the Ranson Criteria in comparing large patient populations, their ability to predict the severity of an episode of acute pancreatitis in individual patients was ultimately shown to be limited, being subject to error in as many as one patient out of every three. In addition to the recognized limitation in assigning severity to individual patients, the Criteria were also restricted by the often overlooked requirement that full assignment of severity was withheld until 48 hours following admission. Furthermore, it is equally important to point out that the Criteria have never been validated for any periods *later* than 48 hours. Even today, one can hear such incorrect statements as "there were four Ranson Criteria present at three days, five days." Given these practical limitations in individual clinical application, and restriction to the initial 48 hours of the hospital course, it is not surprising that use of the Ranson Criteria has become decidedly less frequent today.

Over the succeeding years, a number of different approaches to the assignment of severity in an individual episode of acute pancreatitis have been proposed. These proposals have ranged from those based upon physical signs, to various predictive laboratory findings, to imaging features, to the results of clinical procedures, or to permutations and combinations of these approaches. An ideal system for assigning severity to an episode of acute pancreatitis would be consistently accurate, capable of being determined at any point in the episode, free of risk, simple and quick to perform, and inexpensive. To cut to the chase, at present no determinant of either the severity or the prognosis of an episode of acute pancreatitis has been identified that satisfies all of these optimal requirements.

The Acute Physiology and Chronic Health Evaluation (APACHE) II is perhaps the best system for stratifying the severity of an individual episode of acute pancreatitis available today. The reliability of the APACHE II system in the setting of acute pancreatitis has been validated in numerous clinical reports, a value of 8 points or more signifying a severe episode. Recent clinical studies have established an overall clinical accuracy of 80% for APACHE II in predicting the severity of acute pancreatitis. Moreover, the APACHE II system can also be used at any time during the patient's course, i.e., at onset, day 2, day 5, etc. Finally, by comparing serial determinations of APACHE II, and noting whether the values are increasing or decreasing over time, the efficacy of therapy can also be determined (Fig. 1.1). Despite these obvious clinical advantages over the Ranson Criteria, the principal disadvantage of the APACHE II system is that it is cumbersome, as it requires 15 separate entries (each entry with multiple grades) in order to summate a score. Because of this unavoidable complexity in recording, this system is much better suited to electronic entry in an intensive care environment, or to large-scale clinical investigations, than it is for use in other circumstances.

More recently, other measures of severity have been proposed. Within the past generation, surgical investigators have advanced the proposition that the development of necrotizing pancreatitis is the most significant determinant of the clinical severity of an episode of acute pancreatitis and, indeed, of the prognosis for overall patient survival. These clinicopathologic observations arose from several European surgical clinics, where programmatic surgical resection or débridement was advocated for clinically severe acute pancreatitis. As a result of subsequent worldwide validation of these clinicopathologic observations, methods for the determination of the presence of pancreatic necrosis have received considerable attention as predictors of severity and prognosis (Table 1.1).

The majority of these approaches to the detection of pancreatic necrosis have been biochemical in origin. Despite initial promise, most have proved less reliable than necessary, difficult to perform, time-consuming, or expensive. An exception to this generalization has

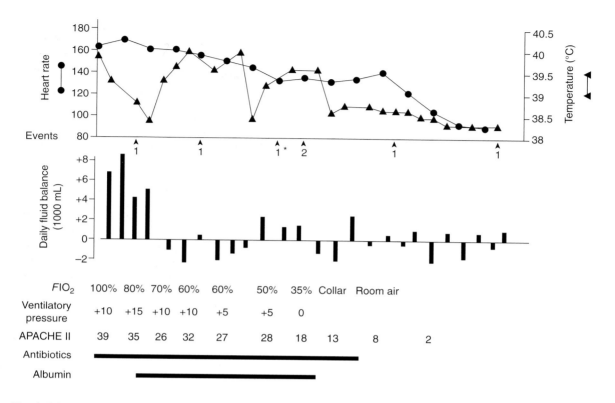

FIO$_2$	100%	80%	70%	60%	60%	50%	35%	Collar	Room air
Ventilatory pressure	+10	+15	+10	+10	+5	+5	0		
APACHE II	39	35	26	32	27	28	18	13	8	2

Antibiotics

Albumin

Hospital day   0 1 2 3 4 5 6 7 8 9 10 11 12 13 14 15 16 17 18 19 20 21 22 23 24 25 26 27 28 29 30 32

Figure 1.1 Graphical course of a 57-year-old male patient with severe acute pancreatitis due to sterile pancreatic necrosis. Note that serial APACHE II determinations did not deteriorate after intensive supportive therapy was begun.

Event numbers: 1, contrast-enhanced computed tomography; 2, tracheostomy; *, fine-needle aspiration for bacteriology.

been C-reactive protein (CRP). When associated with the finding of hyperamylasemia in the appropriate clinical setting, a value of 120 mg/dL permits a reasonably secure diagnosis of necrotizing pancreatitis. Although inexpensive to perform, since the CRP test will not normally become positive until 48 hours after the onset of necrotizing pancreatitis, it cannot often be used to make initial clinical decisions.

Today, the test that is widely regarded as the most reliable for the determination of the presence or absence of pancreatic necrosis is contrast-enhanced computed tomography (CECT) (Fig. 1.2). Whenever the nonenhancing segment(s) of the pancreatic parenchyma exceed 30% of the area of the gland, the accuracy of CECT in establishing the presence of pancreatic necrosis exceeds 95%. In the absence of nonenhancement of the gland, however, the true negative value for CECT has not been established. Clinically, this means that a patient could have a "negative" CT and still have pancreatic necrosis, but its extent would be less than 30% of the gland. This observation fits with modern knowledge regarding histopathology in acute pancreatitis, as microfoci of pancreatic necrosis are the rule in clinical acute pancreatitis, even when coalescence of scattered foci of parenchymal necrosis is insufficient to result in clinical necrotizing pancreatitis.

In addition to the detection of necrosis, tomography-based clinical severity scoring systems using the images obtained from CECT have also been proposed. Although these image-based severity scoring systems are quite useful when comparing groups of patients with necrotizing pancreatitis, they add little to individual

Table 1.1 Proposed clinical determinants of necrotizing pancreatitis.

Serum factors
Methemalbumin
Fibrinogen
Pa_{O_2}
Lactate dehydrogenase*
Hypocalcemia
Ribonuclease I
Deoxyribonuclease
α_1-Antitrypsin
α_2-Macroglobulin
Complement C3 and C4
C-reactive protein*
Pancreas-specific protein
Phospholipase A_2
Trypsinogen activation peptide
Free fatty acids
Carbolic ester hydrolase
Fibronectin
Absolute lymphocyte count
Interleukin 6
Polymorphonuclear elastase

Clinical observations
Grey Turner's sign; Cullen's sign
Fat necrosis
Diagnostic peritoneal lavage

Imaging techniques
Contrast-enhanced computed tomography*
Magnetic resonance imaging*

* Author's choice for easily available and clinically dependable determinants of pancreatic necrosis.

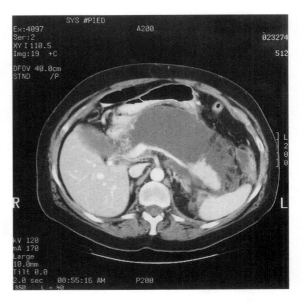

Figure 1.2 Contrast-enhanced computed tomography in a patient with necrotizing pancreatitis. Observe that only the tail of the pancreas enhances with intravenous contrast, indicating the presence of necrosis in the head and body of the pancreas. Since the normal pancreas enhances to the same degree as the liver and spleen, comparison of pancreatic enhancement with these other organs is often helpful in the diagnosis of necrosis.

patient management. From a clinical standpoint, it is often sufficient to know that pancreatic necrosis is present in a patient with clinically severe pancreatitis, without the necessity for grading the radiologic appearance. Although CECT scanning is quite accurate for detecting necrosis, it is unfortunately neither inexpensive nor completely risk-free, and is therefore reserved for situations in which it is necessary to definitively establish the presence of necrotizing pancreatitis.

In what circumstances would it be necessary for us to know that a particular episode of clinically severe acute pancreatitis was due to necrotizing pancreatitis? Aside from clinical research requirements or assignment of prognosis, the principal reason is to identify those patients requiring therapy specific for necrotizing pancre-

atitis. Since as many as 10% of cases of nonnecrotizing acute pancreatitis (interstitial, or edematous, pancreatitis) can also be clinically "severe," distinction between the two pathologic forms may be necessary. Currently, there are two, perhaps three, major clinical therapeutic decisions which must initially be made in a patient with clinically severe acute pancreatitis: (i) should the patient be admitted to the intensive care unit, (ii) should prophylactic antibiotics be started, and (iii) should an urgent endoscopic sphincterotomy be done? With regard to the first and second questions, knowledge of whether a clinically severe episode of acute pancreatitis is due to pancreatic necrosis is useful for decision-making. Acute interstitial (edematous) pancreatitis never requires prophylactic antibiotics, and less frequently requires intensive care management. Knowledge of the existence of necrotizing pancreatitis is less critical for addressing the question regarding endoscopic sphincterotomy, as this issue revolves principally around demonstrating the existence of gallstones associated with cholangitis or biliary obstruction. However, some endoscopists may hesitate to perform sphincterotomy using endoscopic retrograde cholangiopancreatography in patients with documented pancreatic necrosis, fearing that iatrogenic introduction of bacteria might lead to conversion of sterile to infected necrosis.

Furthermore, we can anticipate that, like the ill-fated platelet antagonist factor lexipafant, another agent will be proposed in the not too distant future purporting to ameliorate the clinical course of acute pancreatitis. Since edematous acute pancreatitis resolves with appropriate supportive therapy in the vast majority of cases, employment of an expensive putative therapeutic agent will require prior substantiation of the diagnosis of necrosis before the agent can be given. We can conclude that the more definitive treatments for necrotizing pancreatitis become available in the future, the greater will be the need for establishing severity and detecting necrosis.

Definitions of acute pancreatitis and its complications

Beginning with the Edwin Smith Papyrus (and possibly considerably before), it has been axiomatic in medicine that correct therapy must be preceded by a correct diagnosis. Although other logical combinations exist, such as wrong diagnosis–wrong therapy and correct diagnosis–wrong therapy, patients can only improve with either the serendipitous combination of wrong diagnosis–correct therapy or the more desirable possibility of correct diagnosis–correct therapy. Given the primacy of diagnosis to effective therapy, the necessity for accuracy in diagnosis is clear.

Accuracy in clinical diagnosis, in turn, depends upon a precise and consistent definition for the particular disease process. Without precise definitions, differentiation between closely related disease processes becomes difficult if not impossible. Finally, not only is precision in disease definition required for accurate diagnosis, but in order for the proposed definition to be useful in the clinical situation, a clinical definition must be created that is capable of being determined by clinical means.

We have already noted the clinical difficulties created by an imprecise definition of "pancreatic abscess." Another case in point is that of "pancreatic phlegmon."

Originally coined in 1973 to describe a sterile mass of inflammatory tissue, subsequent authors embraced the term to describe other forms of pancreatic masses in patients with acute pancreatitis, i.e., necrotic masses, and even infected collections. As a result, "phlegmon" was no longer a specific term used to describe sterile inflammation, but could now improperly refer to any one of four possible combinations (sterile or infected, edema or necrosis), depending upon the views of the author. The persistent use of similarly imprecise definitions resulted in a pancreatic Tower of "Babble."

For almost 100 years, from the time of the initial pathologic description of acute pancreatitis and its complications by Fitz in 1889 until the advent of noninvasive imaging in the 1980s, progress in the diagnosis and management of pancreatic inflammatory diseases was glacially slow. Not until the technology for noninvasive monitoring became available could the full spectrum of acute pancreatitis and its complications be appreciated in real time, and in the clinical situation. With the new technologies, it was no longer necessary for clinicopathologic correlation to require tissue confirmation from surgical or autopsy specimens; noninvasive data could provide similar information. Indeed, these imaging breakthroughs in the 1980s led to an unmasking of the scope of retroperitoneal mischief caused by pancreatic inflammation, and resulted in a pancreatic renaissance.

In appreciation of the wealth of natural history and clinical information then becoming available, and in recognition of the imprecise and often conflicting definitions in use at that time for acute pancreatitis, an International Symposium on Acute Pancreatitis was convened in Atlanta in 1992. In attendance were 40 internationally recognized experts in acute pancreatitis from 15 countries and six disciplines (pathology, anatomy, radiology, gastroenterology, medicine, and surgery). Their assigned tasks were to provide a series of consensus clinical definitions for acute pancreatitis and its complications, and, where possible, to provide an evidence-based approach to therapy. The clinical definitions proposed, and subsequently adopted by the worldwide medical community, are outlined in Table 1.2 and more fully discussed below.

Acute pancreatitis

Definition

Acute pancreatitis is an acute inflammatory process

Table 1.2 Summary of the Atlanta clinical definitions for acute pancreatitis and its complications.

Acute pancreatitis
    Mild
    Severe
Organ failure
Interstitial (edematous) pancreatitis
Necrotizing pancreatitis
    Sterile
    Infected
Acute fluid collections
Acute pseudocysts
Pancreatic abscesses
Loculated fat necrosis

---

of the pancreas, with variable involvement of other regional tissues or remote organ systems.

Clinical manifestations
Most often, acute pancreatitis has a rapid onset, is accompanied by upper abdominal pain, and is associated with variable abdominal findings ranging from mild tenderness to rebound. Acute pancreatitis is often accompanied by vomiting, fever, tachycardia, leukocytosis, and elevated pancreatic enzymes in the blood and/or urine.

Pathology
Findings range from microscopic interstitial edema and fat necrosis of the pancreatic parenchyma to macroscopic areas of pancreatic and peripancreatic necrosis and hemorrhage. These pathologic changes in acute pancreatitis therefore represent a continuum; interstitial edema and minimal histologic evidence of necrosis are at the minor end of the scale, and confluent macroscopic necrosis at the other extreme.

Clinical discussion
Despite all attempts at objectivity, in a small number of patients acute pancreatitis remains a *clinical* diagnosis. Other causes of hyperamylasemia must be excluded, since significant surgical conditions presenting with hyperamylasemia may clinically masquerade as acute pancreatitis. If clinical doubt exists about whether the abdominal findings are due to acute pancreatitis or are being caused by a correctable intraabdominal catastrophe, CT findings of pancreatic/peripancreatic edema or necrosis are pathognomonic for acute pancreatitis. In the absence of pancreatic/peripancreatic edema, acute pancreatitis is unlikely, and other causes of intra-abdominal disease should be sought.

Severe acute pancreatitis

Definition
Severe acute pancreatitis is associated with organ failure and/or local complications, such as necrosis, abscess, or pseudocyst.

Clinical manifestations
Abdominal findings are of increased tenderness, rebound, distension, and hypoactive or absent bowel sounds. An epigastric mass may be present. Rarely, flank ecchymosis (Grey Turner's sign) or periumbilical ecchymosis (Cullen's sign) may be seen. Severe acute pancreatitis is further characterized by either three or more Ranson criteria or eight or more APACHE II criteria. Organ failure is defined as shock (systolic blood pressure <90 mmHg), pulmonary insufficiency (P_{AO_2} <60 mmHg), renal failure (creatinine >2 mg/dL after rehydration), or gastrointestinal bleeding (>500 mL per 24 hours). Systemic complications, such as disseminated intravascular coagulation (platelets <100 000/mm^3, fibrinogen <100 mg/dL, fibrin split products >80 μg/mL), or severe metabolic disturbances (calcium <7.5 mg/dL) may also be seen. Local complications, such as necrosis, abscess, and pseudocyst, are described below.

Pathology
Most often, severe acute pancreatitis is a clinical expression of the development of pancreatic necrosis (see below). Less commonly, however, patients with interstitial (edematous) pancreatitis can also develop clinically severe acute pancreatitis.

Clinical discussion
Severe acute pancreatitis usually declares itself shortly after onset. A delayed progression from mild acute pancreatitis to severe acute pancreatitis is rare. The APACHE II system may be used to quantify severity at any time during the course of acute pancreatitis, while Ranson Criteria have not been validated for time periods longer than 48 hours after onset. Severe acute pancreatitis requires continuous monitoring in an intensive care environment.

Mild acute pancreatitis

Definition

Mild acute pancreatitis is associated with minimal organ dysfunction and an uneventful recovery, and lacks the described features of severe acute pancreatitis.

Clinical manifestations

Patients with mild acute pancreatitis respond to appropriate fluid administration with prompt normalization of physical signs and laboratory values. Failure to improve within 48–72 hours after treatment begins should prompt additional investigations for the presence of complications of pancreatitis. Contrast enhancement of pancreatic parenchyma does not demonstrate necrosis if dynamic computed tomography is performed (see below).

Pathology

The predominant macroscopic and histologic feature of mild acute pancreatitis is interstitial edema, although microscopic areas of parenchymal necrosis may also be found. Peripancreatic fat necrosis may or may not be present.

Clinical discussion

Since the clinical course of acute pancreatitis is uncomplicated in approximately 75% of cases, uneventful recovery with appropriate supportive management can be anticipated. Investigations into the possibility of biliary calculi being the cause of the episode should also be carried out, in order to prevent recurrent acute pancreatitis.

Acute fluid collections

Definition

Acute fluid collections occur early in the course of acute pancreatitis (within the first 2 weeks), are located in or near the pancreas, and always lack a wall of granulation or fibrous tissue.

Clinical manifestations

Acute fluid collections are common in patients with severe pancreatitis, occurring in 30–50% of cases. However, more than half of these lesions regress spontaneously. They are rarely demonstrable by physical findings and are usually discovered by imaging techniques. Imaging techniques do not demonstrate a defined wall surrounding an acute fluid collection, and the collections often have an irregular shape.

Pathology

The precise composition of these acute fluid collections is unknown. Bacteria are variably present. The clinical distinction between an acute fluid collection and a pseudocyst (or a pancreatic abscess) is the lack of a defined wall on imaging studies.

Clinical discussion

Acute fluid collections have the potential to develop into acute pseudocysts or pancreatic abscesses. Why the majority of acute fluid collections regress, while others persist to become pseudocysts or abscesses, is not known. The important point is that continued observation is necessary to determine the direction a fluid collection will take over time.

Pancreatic necrosis

Definition

Pancreatic necrosis is a focal or diffuse area of nonviable pancreatic parenchyma that is typically associated with peripancreatic fat necrosis.

Clinical manifestations

While the likelihood of pancreatic necrosis increases with increasing clinical severity, objective verification is necessary. Dynamic CECT is the current gold standard for the clinical diagnosis of pancreatic necrosis. Focal or diffuse, well-marginated zones of nonenhanced pancreatic parenchyma (>3 cm in size or >30% of the area of the pancreas) are requisite criteria for the CT diagnosis of necrosis. Contrast density fails to exceed 50 Hounsfield units (HU) in areas of necrosis after intravenous administration (normal enhancement 50–150 HU). A semiquantitative measure of pancreatic enhancement can be obtained by visually comparing pancreatic density to splenic density, since in the absence of necrosis the densities of the two organs are similar. Heterogeneous densities demonstrated in the peripancreatic fat represent a combination of fat necrosis, fluid collections, and hemorrhage. As a result, the extent of peripancreatic fat necrosis cannot be reliably determined by CT. Although the overall accuracy of dynamic CT in demonstrating parenchymal pancreatic necrosis is 95%, this technique should not be considered infallible. Pancreatic necrosis may also be reliably determined by magnetic resonance imaging, although at a considerable increase in cost.

Pathology

Macroscopically, focal or diffuse areas of devitalized pancreatic parenchyma and peripancreatic fat necrosis are evident. Fat necrosis may be superficial and patchy, or deep and confluent. Hemorrhage in the pancreatic or peripancreatic tissues is variably present. Microscopically, extensive interstitial fat necrosis with vessel damage is found, along with necrosis that affects acinar cells, islet cells, and the pancreatic ductal system. Pancreatic parenchymal necrosis rarely involves the entire gland, however. Usually, pancreatic necrosis is confined to the periphery, and the central core of the gland is preserved. Uncommonly, peripancreatic fat necrosis may become loculated, and is often misdiagnosed as a pseudocyst or a sterile abscess. Loculated fat necrosis can be differentiated from a pancreatic pseudocyst by the demonstration of thick viscous contents without pancreatic enzymes, and from a pancreatic abscess by the absence of bacteria.

Clinical discussion

The clinical distinction between sterile pancreatic necrosis and infected pancreatic necrosis is critical, since development of infection in the necrotic tissues results in a trebling of mortality risk. Furthermore, while selected patients with documented *sterile* pancreatic necrosis can usually be managed without surgical intervention, infected necrosis is uniformly fatal without surgical drainage. Because clinical and laboratory findings are often similar in patients with either sterile or infected necrosis, this important distinction is best made by transcutaneous needle aspiration bacteriology. This technique is safe and accurate, and a positive result is regarded as an indication for surgery.

Acute pseudocyst

Definition

A pseudocyst is a collection of pancreatic juice enclosed by a nonepithelialized wall, which arises as a consequence of acute pancreatitis, pancreatic trauma, or chronic pancreatitis.

Clinical manifestations

Pseudocysts in patients with acute pancreatitis are rarely palpable, and are most often discovered by imaging techniques. It is important to note that they are round or ovoid in shape, in contrast to acute fluid collections, and have a well-defined wall, as demonstrated by CT or sonography.

Pathology

The presence of a well-defined wall composed of granulation or fibrous tissue distinguishes a pseudocyst from an acute fluid collection. A pseudocyst is usually rich in pancreatic enzymes, and is most often sterile.

Clinical discussion

Formation of a pseudocyst requires 4 weeks or more from the onset of acute pancreatitis. In this regard, an acute pseudocyst is a fluid collection that arises in association with an episode of acute pancreatitis, is of more than 4 weeks' duration, and is surrounded by a defined wall. Fluid collections less than this age that lack a defined wall are more properly termed acute fluid collections. In contrast, chronic pseudocysts have a well-defined wall, but arise in patients with chronic pancreatitis and lack an antecedent episode of acute pancreatitis. Bacteria may be present in a pseudocyst, but often are of no clinical significance, since they represent contamination and not clinical infection. If purulent material is present, the lesion is more correctly termed a pancreatic abscess.

Pancreatic abscess

Definition

A pancreatic abscess is a circumscribed intra-abdominal collection of pus in proximity to the pancreas, containing little or no pancreatic necrosis, which arises as a consequence of acute pancreatitis or pancreatic trauma.

Clinical manifestations

Clinical presentation is variable. Most commonly, however, the clinical picture is that of infection. Pancreatic abscesses occur later in the course of severe acute pancreatitis, often 4 weeks or more after onset.

Pathology

The presence of pus and a positive culture for bacteria or fungi, but little or no pancreatic necrosis, serves to differentiate a pancreatic or peripancreatic abscess from infected necrosis. Pancreatic abscesses probably arise as a consequence of *limited* necrosis with subsequent liquification and secondary infection. Accordingly, pancreatic abscess and infected necrosis differ in clinical expression and extent of associated necrosis.

Clinical discussion

In the past, the term "pancreatic abscess" has been improperly used for all forms of pancreatic infection. The distinction between pancreatic abscess and infected necrosis is critical for two reasons: the mortality risk for infected necrosis is double that for pancreatic abscess, and specific therapy for each condition is different. Abscesses that arise as a consequence of elective pancreatic surgery are not properly termed pancreatic abscesses, but are more accurately classified as postoperative abscesses.

Summary

Since their original proposal over 10 years ago, numerous investigators have confirmed the validity and clinical utility of the Atlanta definitions. As a result, these clinical definitions have received worldwide acceptance. In one sense, it might be considered remarkable that the Atlanta definitions have survived relatively intact over this period of time. On the other hand, there can be little doubt that some changes in these clinical definitions will be necessary in the future as new concepts are developed and more clinical information becomes available.

However, the search for a clinically friendly method to stratify the severity of an episode of acute pancreatitis is continuing. A number of potential approaches are being actively investigated. Until such time as one proves to be superior, the APACHE II system, despite its limitations, offers considerable clinical value.

Recommended reading

Balthazar EJ, Robinson DL, Megibow AJ. Acute pancreatitis: value of CT scanning in establishing prognosis. *Radiology* 1990;174:331–336.

Bradley EL III. A clinically based classification system for acute pancreatitis: summary of the International Symposium on Acute Pancreatitis, Atlanta, Georgia, September 11–13, 1992. *Arch Surg* 1993;128:586–590.

Bradley EL III (ed.) *Acute Pancreatitis: Principles and Practice.* New York: Raven Press, 1994.

Kloppel G, von Gerkan R, Dreyer T. Pathomorphology of acute pancreatitis. In: KE Gyr, MV Singer, H Sarles (eds) *Pancreatitis: Concepts and Classifications.* Amsterdam: Elsevier, 1984.

Ranson JHC, Rifkind KM, Roses DF, Fink SD, Eng K, Spencer FC. Prognostic signs and the role of operative management in acute pancreatitis. *Surg Gynecol Obstet* 1974;139: 69–81.

2

Pathogenesis: how does acute pancreatitis develop?

Michael L. Steer and George Perides

Introduction

Acute pancreatitis is an inflammatory disease of the pancreas that may be either acute or chronic, severe or mild. Severe pancreatitis is usually associated with systemic derangements, the most common of which is an acute lung injury that can clinically present as adult respiratory distress syndrome (ARDS), or with local complications including abscesses and pseudocysts. Most of the current concepts regarding the mechanisms responsible for acute pancreatitis are based on the results of experiments performed using models in which pancreatitis has been induced in experimental animals. This chapter reviews some of those concepts, as well as the experimental studies upon which those concepts are based. This review will be highly selective, primarily focused on work done in the authors' laboratory. It should be recognized, however, that a number of other laboratories and investigators have made important contributions to our understanding of the pathogenesis of acute pancreatitis. Some, but not all, of their work is discussed as well.

Pathology of acute and chronic pancreatitis

The pathologic picture of acute pancreatitis is dominated by an acute inflammatory process involving the parenchyma of the pancreas either diffusely or in a patchy manner. Necrosis of cellular elements, including acinar cells, duct cells, and islet cells, may be extensive in severe forms of acute pancreatitis but necrosis is usually absent or relatively limited in mild forms. Pancreatic and peripancreatic edema as well as fat necrosis are commonly observed in both mild and severe acute pancreati-

tis but, in the severe form of pancreatitis, there may also be hemorrhage within the pancreas. Ductal disruptions can occur leading to extravasation of pancreatic juice and the formation of pancreatic pseudocysts.

In contrast to the changes observed in acute pancreatitis, the pathologic picture in chronic pancreatitis is dominated by fibrosis and the presence of a chronic inflammatory process. To a varying degree, both exocrine and endocrine elements may be lost and enlargement of nerves as well as perineural inflammation have also been observed. Other changes observed in acute pancreatitis, including necrosis and pseudocyst formation, can also occur in chronic pancreatitis.

The relationship between acute pancreatitis and chronic pancreatitis has been controversial in the past and, to a considerable degree, controversy persists. Historically, most observers have tended to think of acute pancreatitis and chronic pancreatitis as being different diseases from their outset, characterized by different pathologic changes and the result of different triggering events. More recently, however, opinion has changed and many currently believe that the pathologic and functional changes of chronic pancreatitis merely reflect the effects of repeated episodes of acute pancreatitis. According to this *necrosis–fibrosis* hypothesis, repeated episodes of acute inflammation and necrosis lead to the chronic inflammation and fibrosis which characterize chronic pancreatitis. If valid, this hypothesis would suggest that the earliest cellular events responsible for chronic pancreatitis may be similar, or even identical, to those which trigger acute pancreatitis. Thus, later events, including those leading to pancreatic fibrosis and chronic inflammation, may underlie the evolution of chronic pancreatitis while the absence of those events may permit the morphologic and functional recovery of the pancreas that characterizes acute pancreatitis.

Pathology of pancreatitis-associated lung injury

Extrapancreatic manifestations of severe acute pancreatitis include injury to the lungs, kidney, liver, and other organs. Most of the studies evaluating extrapancreatic complications of severe pancreatitis have focused on the associated lung injury since it is an important clinical entity that is the cause of death for 60% of the patients who die within the first 2 weeks of an acute pancreatitis attack. The lung injury associated with severe pancreatitis is very similar, and even possibly identical, to the lung injury associated with sepsis, shock, severe burns, and ischemia/reperfusion. Clinically, it is usually manifested as ARDS. The pathologic changes of pancreatitis-associated lung injury include neutrophil sequestration within the pulmonary microvasculature, necrosis of type 2 pneumocytes, alveolar membrane thickening, and increased alveolar/endothelial membrane permeability leading to a pulmonary capillary leak phenomenon and the transudation of intravascular fluid into the bronchoalveolar space.

Etiologies of acute pancreatitis

Most patients with acute pancreatitis develop their disease in association with any one of a number of other disease processes. Collectively, these associated diseases are referred to as the etiologies of acute pancreatitis (Table 2.1). Roughly 80% of patients with acute pancreatitis develop their pancreatitis in association with either prolonged alcohol abuse or the passage of biliary tract stones. Alcohol abuse is more commonly a cause of chronic pancreatitis than a cause of acute pancreatitis. However, the earliest events in alcohol-induced chronic pancreatitis may closely resemble those responsible for acute pancreatitis (see above).

In addition to biliary tract stones and alcohol abuse, acute pancreatitis can be related to a number of miscellaneous etiologies which, taken together, account for roughly 10–15% of patients with acute pancreatitis. These miscellaneous causes of acute pancreatitis include exposure to a large number of drugs or infectious agents, trauma to the pancreas, hyperlipoproteinemias, hypercalcemia, pancreatic ischemia, retrograde injection of the pancreatic duct or manipulation of the

Table 2.1 Etiologies of acute pancreatitis.

Biliary tract stones
Ethanol abuse
Drugs
Scorpion sting
Endoscopic retrograde cholangiopancreatography
Trauma
Infections
Parasites
Idiopathic
Hyperlipidemia
Hypercalcemia
Ischemia
Postoperative

sphincter of Oddi (as in endoscopic retrograde cholangiopancreatography). Pancreatitis can also be triggered by pancreatic duct obstruction caused by either a mass lesion or inflammatory process involving the pancreas or periampullary region of the duodenum. Dysfunction of the sphincter of Oddi or the dorsal pancreatic ductal hypertension that can occur in patients with pancreas divisum have been considered to be the cause of pancreatitis in some patients. Finally, recent studies have drawn attention to the small but still significant number of patients who develop acute pancreatitis on a genetic basis, either because they carry mutations associated with hereditary pancreatitis or because they express mutations of the cystic fibrosis transmembrane conductance regulator (*CFTR*) gene.

In spite of a diligent search for an underlying cause or etiology, roughly 10–15% of patients with acute pancreatitis develop their disease in association with no identifiable etiology. These individuals are said to have idiopathic acute pancreatitis although, with time and further investigation, an etiology may eventually become apparent. Recent reports have suggested that some of these individuals have overlooked biliary tract disease and that their pancreatitis is triggered by passage of microcrystals or biliary sludge. Other patients in this "idiopathic pancreatitis" group may have developed their pancreatitis on an autoimmune basis.

Theoretical considerations

The design of therapies to prevent pancreatitis or

reduce its severity depends upon an understanding of the mechanisms by which the "etiology" of pancreatitis initiates the disease and the cellular events that couple this initiating event to the injury and inflammation which characterize acute pancreatitis. In a general sense, the etiologies of pancreatitis have been considered to trigger pancreatitis by one or more of the following mechanisms: (i) toxic/metabolic; (ii) genetic; and (iii) mechanical.

Toxic/metabolic

The earliest changes of acute pancreatitis appear to involve pancreatic acinar cells (see below) and these initial acinar cell changes may reflect either a toxic or a metabolic insult triggered by the underlying etiology. This is particularly likely to be the case in pancreatitis caused by alcohol abuse and also when pancreatitis is caused by exposure to various drugs. However, the actual mechanisms by which alcohol or drugs might bring about toxic or metabolic injury of acinar cells is not known. Hypercalcemia and scorpion bites may also be linked to pancreatitis by a toxic/metabolic mechanism. Hypercalcemia could cause intracellular ionized calcium levels to rise and that, at least theoretically, could trigger intracellular digestive enzyme activation leading to cellular injury and pancreatitis. Scorpion toxin contains a potent pancreatic secretagogue that is believed to act by opening sodium channels and this might be the mechanism by which it triggers pancreatitis. Most of the other identified etiologies of pancreatitis probably trigger the disease via genetic or mechanical mechanisms rather than by causing a toxic or metabolic change in the pancreas.

Genetic

There has been much recent interest in the possibility that genetic events may contribute to the pathogenesis of acute pancreatitis. Many kindreds with high rates of acute pancreatitis have been identified and, in many instances, the affected individuals experience their first attacks of acute pancreatitis at a young age. Patients with hereditary pancreatitis have been shown to be at increased risk of developing pancreatic cancer, particularly if the pedigree demonstrates a male pattern of inheritance. In many instances, hereditary pancreatitis has been shown to result from mutations of the cationic trypsinogen gene, resulting in expression of a

trypsinogen that, once activated, is resistant to inactivation by trypsin inhibitors or, alternatively, is more sensitive to autoactivation. These gain-of-function mutations could therefore potentially result in elevated intraacinar cell levels of activated trypsin. Kindreds of individuals with genetic mutations of the secretory trypsin inhibitor SPINK1 have also been identified. These patients presumably have loss-of-function mutations resulting in expression of defective trypsin inhibitors and, as a result, their acinar cells are susceptible to injury caused by trypsinogen that is activated, but not inhibited, within the cell.

Increased risk of developing acute pancreatitis has also been noted in patients carrying mutations of the cystic fibrosis gene *CFTR*. Some have suggested that these mutations may be more common among alcoholics who develop pancreatitis than among alcoholics who do not develop pancreatitis. *CFTR* mutations may also be more common among patients with presumed idiopathic pancreatitis than among the general population. The mechanisms by which *CFTR* mutations might sensitize the pancreas to injury, either spontaneous or alcohol induced, are not clear but it is conceivable that similar mechanisms might explain why only a small fraction of patients who abuse alcohol eventually develop pancreatitis. It is also possible that these or other as yet unidentified mutations may sensitize the pancreas to other forms of injury, including that which follows passage of a biliary tract stone. This could explain the observation that only a fraction of individuals passing biliary tract stones go on to develop gallstone pancreatitis.

Mechanical

Passage of biliary tract stones into or through the terminal biliopancreatic ductal system and into the duodenum has been repeatedly shown to be the event that triggers so-called gallstone pancreatitis but the mechanism(s) by which stone passage is related to pancreatic injury is not entirely clear. In a general sense, three mechanical theories have been proposed to explain this relationship. The first was suggested by Opie in 1901 when he described a patient who died of gallstone pancreatitis and who, at the time of autopsy, was found to have a gallstone impacted in the distal bile duct. In addition, bile-stained fluid was found in the pancreatic duct suggesting, to Opie, that bile had refluxed retrogradely from the bile duct into the pancreatic duct through a "common" bile/pancreatic duct channel. This so-called *common channel theory of Opie* has been widely cited but its validity has been repeatedly questioned by a number of studies demonstrating that (i) most patients with gallstone pancreatitis lack a common channel long enough to allow a distally obstructing stone to cause bile reflux into the pancreatic duct; (ii) pancreatic duct pressure normally exceeds bile duct pressure and therefore rather than bile refluxing into the pancreatic duct, a distal obstruction would cause pancreatic juice to reflux into the bile duct; and (iii) perfusion of the pancreatic duct with bile or a bile–intestinal juice mixture, under normal pressures, does not cause pancreatic injury unless pressure in the pancreatic duct is also increased. Because of these concerns, support for Opie's common channel theory has been limited and, currently, most observers do not accept it as the likely explanation for gallstone-induced pancreatitis.

Another theory attempting to explain the relationship between stone passage and pancreatitis is the *duodenal reflux theory*. According to this theory, the offending stone passes through the sphincter of Oddi into the duodenum and, in the process of being passed, the stone stretches the sphincter making it incompetent and thus permitting duodenal juice containing activated pancreatic digestive enzymes to reflux backward into the pancreatic ductal system. This theory has been, to a great degree, invalidated by the observation that patients undergoing either endoscopic or surgical division of the sphincter of Oddi, and who therefore have acquired sphincter of Oddi incompetence, do not experience repeated episodes of pancreatitis.

The final mechanical theory proposed as an explanation for gallstone-induced pancreatitis has been called the *ductal hypertension theory*. Interestingly, this theory was also proposed by Opie in 1901 when he performed an autopsy on another patient dying of pancreatitis. That patient was also found to have a biliary stone obstructing the pancreatic duct but, in this case, the stone had not caused bile reflux into the pancreatic duct. He suggested that the stone might have created a closed pancreatic ductal space and that, with continued secretion into the obstructed pancreatic duct, ductal hypertension would develop. Ductal hypertension was presumed to lead to rupture of the pancreatic duct and subsequently to extravasation of pancreatic juice, containing digestive enzymes, into the gland parenchyma. The ductal hypertension theory is a widely accepted explanation for the mechanism by which a bile duct stone might trigger acute pancreatitis but, at best, it is an incomplete explanation because, for the most part, pancreatic secretions within the pancreatic duct contain inactive precursor or zymogen forms of the potentially harmful pancreatic digestive enzymes. Therefore, even with rupture of the duct and extravasation of secretions into the parenchyma of the gland, it is not clear how ductal hypertension would trigger pancreatic parenchymal injury and pancreatitis. On the other hand, it is likely that obstruction of the duct and/or ductal hypertension has other effects on the pancreas and, if those effects included intrapancreatic activation of digestive enzymes, they might explain the relationship between duct obstruction and pancreatic cell injury.

Where does acute pancreatitis begin?

Until relatively recently, the site at which acute pancreatitis begins was not known. There existed three schools of thought: that pancreatitis begins in the periductal area of the pancreas as a result of duct disruption; that pancreatitis begins in peripheral, perilobular areas as a result of ischemia; and that pancreatitis begins within the acinar cells of the pancreas.

Clearly, studies designed to identify the location of the earliest changes in pancreatitis could not be performed using patients because most patients with pancreatitis are not identified within the initial minutes of the disease. Rather, the diagnosis of pancreatitis is usually made 24 hours or more after the onset of an attack and at a time when this initial pancreatic injury has already occurred. Furthermore, access to pancreatic tissue in patients with early acute pancreatitis is generally not possible. For this reason, most investigators have recognized the necessity for experimental models of pancreatitis in animals for studies designed to examine early events in pancreatitis. To complicate matters further, however, most experimental animals do not develop severe pancreatitis when their pancreatic duct is obstructed; rather, they develop mild changes of inflammation, acinar cell apoptosis, and pancreatic atrophy. The American opossum is an exception to this generalization. Ligation of the opossum pancreatic duct, or the common bile/pancreatic duct segment, results in severe necrotizing pancreatitis. The pancreatitis evolves and increases in severity over the 5–7 days following duct ligation. Interestingly, in this model, ligation of the pancreatic duct, the combined common channel segment, or the pancreatic and bile ducts separately results in pancreatitis with similar severity and time of progression. The three types of ligation share the feature of pancreatic duct obstruction but only animals with ligation of the common channel segment could, even theoretically, experience reflux of bile into the pancreatic duct. The finding that pancreatitis is similar in all three groups argues strongly against the common channel theory and in favor of the duct obstruction/hypertension theory.

We used the American opossum in a series of studies designed to determine the location of the earliest pathologic changes when pancreatitis was induced by ligating the biliopancreatic duct. In our studies, animals were sacrificed at planned intervals during the initial 24 hours after duct ligation and the pancreas was examined by light microscopy. The earliest changes were noted to occur within acinar cells. Within 3 hours of duct ligation, the acinar cells lost their basal–apical polarity, developed altered staining characteristics, and demonstrated changes suggestive of early acinar cell necrosis. These changes increased with time, and by 6 hours after duct ligation larger groups of acinar cells were noted to be necrotic. By 12 hours after duct ligation, entire lobules were necrotic and areas of hemorrhage as well as neutrophil infiltration were seen. By 24 hours after the biliopancreatic duct had been ligated, there was massive necrosis and an intense inflammatory reaction. We concluded from these studies that, at least in the opossum model, acute pancreatitis begins within acinar cells.

Acinar cell biology

The observation that acute pancreatitis might begin within the acinar cells of the pancreas, if valid when applied to the clinical disease, suggests that an understanding of the cellular events leading to pancreatitis might be achieved by studies examining pancreatic acinar cell biology during the early stages of experimental pancreatitis. A number of such studies have been performed but, before examining their results, it would be appropriate to briefly review the normal features of acinar cell biology. Acinar cell biology is, clearly, an enormous subject and a comprehensive review would be beyond the scope of this chapter. Thus, this review focuses only on those areas which are currently believed to play an important role in the pathophysiology of pancreatitis.

Pancreatic protein synthesis, transport, and secretion (Fig. 2.1)

The pancreatic acinar cell is the most active protein-synthesizing cell in the body and roughly 90% of newly synthesized proteins are digestive enzymes and digestive enzyme zymogens. These proteins are destined for secretion into the pancreatic ductal space and for discharge into the duodenum. These secretory proteins, as well as structural proteins and other proteins that are targeted for transport to sites within acinar cells, are assembled within the cisternae of the rough endoplasmic reticulum where they fold and assume their tertiary structure. They are then transported in small transport vesicles to the Golgi complex.

Digestive enzymes and their zymogens pass through the Golgi stacks and, at the trans surface, they are packaged in membrane-bound condensing vacuoles that migrate toward the luminal surface of the cell. During this migration, they evolve into zymogen granules that contain an electron-dense core of concentrated digestive enzymes. At the luminal pole of the cell, the zymogen granule limiting membrane fuses with the plasmalemma and, by fission, a pore (i.e., a fusion pore) develops within that fused segment of membrane, thus permitting egress of granule contents (i.e., digestive enzymes and zymogens) into the acinar/ductal space. The subapical filamentous actin cytoskeleton is believed to play a critical role in facilitating this process of fusion–fission and exocytosis. Interventions that disrupt the subapical F-actin web have been shown to prevent acinar cell secretion of digestive enzymes.

As they pass through the Golgi complex, newly sythesized enzymes destined for inclusion within lysosomes (i.e., lysosomal hydrolases) are posttranslationally modified by glycosylation and 6-mannose phosphorylation. They are then bound to mannose 6-phosphate-specific receptors that segregate the lysosomal hydrolases from other newly synthesized proteins. Subsequent to this segregation event, the lysosomal hydrolases, bound to their receptors, are transported in small vesicles that bud from the Golgi to the prelysosomes, where the acid environment causes the lysosomal hydrolases to dissociate from their receptors. Following dissociation from the mannose 6-phosphate

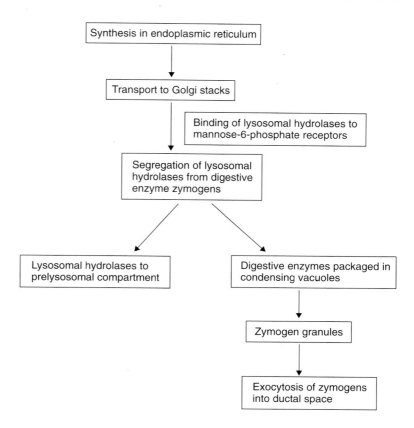

Figure 2.1 Normal protein trafficking and the colocalization phenomenon.

receptors, the hydrolases remain within the lysosomal compartment while the transport vesicles, containing the unliganded mannose 6-phosphate receptors, shuttle back to the Golgi where they are available for binding of additional mannose 6-phosphate-labeled lysosomal hydrolases.

Protective mechanisms

In an overall sense, this scheme of synthesis, intracellular transport, and secretion of enzymes by pancreatic acinar cells has two characteristics that may be of major importance to the problem of acute pancreatitis, particularly if the disease is considered to be the result of acinar cell autodigestion by its own secretory product. The first is the fact that, from their point of assembly in the endoplasmic reticulum to their site of discharge at the luminal cell surface, the newly synthesized digestive enzymes and their zymogens are continually sequestered from the cytoplasmic space by being con-tained within membrane-bound organelles. It is likely that a fraction of those zymogens becomes prematurely activated during intracellular transport but proteolytic enzyme inhibitors, synthesized and cotransported along with the zymogens, protect the acinar cells from injury when this occurs. Furthermore, confinement of the digestive enzymes and their zymogens within membrane-bound organelles prevents activated enzymes from reaching intracellular targets that could potentially be injured. The second characteristic of the intracellular transport scheme that may be relevant to pancreatitis is the fact that it involves the segregation of lysosomal hydrolases from digestive enzymes and their zymogens. Several studies have shown that cathepsin B, a lysosomal hydrolase, can activate trypsinogen and it is well known that trypsin can activate the other zymogens. The segregation of lysosomal hydrolases (including cathepsin B) from digestive enzyme zymogens (including trypsinogen) could reduce the risk and extent of intracellular zymogen activation.

15

Table 2.2 Experimental models of acute pancreatitis.

Retrograde injection of the pancreatic duct
Administration of a choline-deficient ethionine-
  supplemented diet
Supramaximal secretagogue stimulation with
  cholecystokinin or its analog cerulein
Ligation of the opossum pancreatic duct

Altered acinar cell biology in pancreatitis

Experimental models (Table 2.2)

Studies designed to evaluate acinar cell biological events during the evolution of acute pancreatitis can only be performed using experimental models of pancreatitis since, almost without exception, it is not possible to obtain tissue from patients with pancreatitis for such studies. Until the mid-1970s, most investigators exploring issues related to pancreatitis utilized models in which the disease was induced by retrogradely injecting the pancreatic duct with some noxious fluid (e.g., bile, bile plus trypsin, bile plus blood plus trypsin, bile salts, etc.). Unfortunately, the severity of the resulting pancreatitis was difficult to control and tissue destruction was usually too extensive to permit studies evaluating subtle cell biological events. More recently, however, methods of producing submassive pancreatic injury by duct injection have been developed and, in some cases, pancreatitis that is amenable to cell biological studies can be induced using this approach. Perhaps of even greater importance has been the development of at least three models of experimental pancreatitis that do not involve duct injection but which result in pancreatitis that can be readily used for studies of cell biological events during the evolution of the disease.

In 1975, Lombardi and his coworkers reported that young female mice, fed a choline-deficient diet supplemented with 0.5% ethionine, developed massive hemorrhagic pancreatic necrosis and that all of the mice died of pancreatitis if the diet was administered continually for 5 days. Because of its relatively slow development and noninvasive nature, this diet-induced model has proven to be quite useful for studies designed to examine acinar cell events during the evolution of pancreatitis, the coupling of pancreatitis to generation of inflammatory mediators, and the relationship between pancreatitis and lung injury. The morphologic changes of diet-induced pancreatitis closely resemble those of severe clinical pancreatitis. This, and the fact that the mortality rate associated with diet-induced pancreatitis can be adjusted downward by reducing the amount of administered ethionine, have made this model attractive for studies of severe pancreatitis. However, the major criticism of this model is the obvious concern about clinical relevance since few, if any, patients develop pancreatitis because of exposure to an ethionine-containing diet.

In the early 1970s Solcia and colleagues noted that animals given high doses of cholecystokinin (CCK) or its decapeptide analog cerulein developed evidence of pancreatitis. This observation was largely overlooked until 1977 when Lampel and Kern showed that rats developed acute interstitial (edematous) pancreatitis when they were infused with a dose of cerulein that was in excess of that which stimulated a maximal rate of digestive enzyme secretion from the pancreas. Since then, this model of pancreatitis, induced by supraphysiologic (supramaximal) secretagogue stimulation has been extensively employed. The observed morphologic changes include extensive pancreatic edema, acinar cell vacuolization, and pancreatic inflammation. Pancreatitis develops rapidly and reproducibly in this secretagogue-induced model and the pancreatitis is associated with clear evidence of acute lung injury. When applied to mice instead of rats, the resulting pancreatitis is more severe but, for the most part, it is still transient and nonfatal. In mice, cerulein-induced pancreatitis is associated with less edema than in the rat but there is extensive acinar cell necrosis, hemorrhage, and considerable inflammation. Furthermore, lung injury is more severe in mice than in rats. The mouse and rat secretagogue-induced models of acute pancreatitis are the most widely employed models of acute pancreatitis, perhaps because they are easily induced in relatively cheap experimental animals and because they evolve in a consistent and reproducible fashion. Induction of pancreatitis and pancreatitis-associated lung injury requires only 3–12 hours of exposure to supramaximally stimulating doses of cerulein. Attraction to these models is also increased by the fact that many of the events that characterize secretagogue-induced pancreatitis can be replicated when mouse or rat pancreatic acini are incubated *in vitro* with a supramaximally stimulating concentration of CCK or cerulein. On the other hand, the secretagogue-induced models are subject to the same criticisms that have been raised about the diet model with regard to clinical relevance, since few if any patients develop pancreatitis as a result of supramaximal secretagogue stimulation.

Responding to the concern regarding clinical relevance, Senninger and Moody developed a model of pancreatitis that could be induced by obstructing the biliopancreatic duct. Although in most animals this leads to exocrine pancreatic atrophy and relatively little acute pancreatic injury, these investigators found that extensive pancreatic necrosis and hemorrhage occurred when the biliopancreatic duct of the American opossum was obstructed. This opossum model of pancreatitis is attractive for its clinical relevance and because the morphologic changes within the pancreas resemble those of severe gallstone pancreatitis. In addition, cell biological studies with this model are possible because the lesion develops relatively slowly over hours to days. The major problems with this model, however, are those presented by the animal itself. Opossums are trapped in the wild, difficult to handle, infested with parasites, and not inbred. Thus, there exists considerable animal-to-animal variation and studies must involve large numbers of animals to compensate for these variations. For these reasons, the opossum model, although perhaps the most clinically relevant, has not been widely employed by investigators studying acute pancreatitis.

Protein synthesis and enzyme secretion

Protein synthesis by pancreatic acinar cells during the evolution of pancreatitis has been studied using both the secretagogue- and the diet-induced models, but the results of these studies have varied somewhat. Protein synthesis and the synthesis of digestive enzymes appear to be unaltered during evolution of diet-induced pancreatitis. In secretagogue-induced pancreatitis, however, some studies have suggested that synthesis may be unaltered but more recent studies have indicated that supramaximal stimulation with cerulein reduces acinar cell protein synthesis.

Pancreatic digestive enzyme secretion has been evaluated during evolution of diet-induced pancreatitis, rat cerulein-induced pancreatitis, mouse cerulein-induced pancreatitis, duct injection-induced pancreatitis, and opossum pancreatitis. It has also been studied under conditions in which pancreatic acini are exposed to supramaximally stimulating concentrations of either cerulein or CCK in vitro. In each of these cases, a profound inhibition of pancreatic enzyme secretion has been observed. The consistency of this observation, regardless of the model used, suggests that it may be a characteristic of clinical pancreatitis as well and several groups have suggested that inhibition of acinar cell digestive enzyme secretion may be one of the essential early events that underlie development of pancreatitis.

Intracellular trafficking

The diet-induced model of pancreatitis and both the rat and mouse models of secretagogue-induced pancreatitis have been used to examine intracellular transport of newly synthesized protein (i.e., digestive enzymes, digestive enzyme zymogens, and lysosomal hydrolases) during the evolution of pancreatitis. Surprisingly, the changes noted in each of these models is similar. In each, the expected intracellular segregation of lysosomal hydrolases from digestive enzyme zymogens is perturbed and, in each model, both types of enzymes are colocalized within cytoplasmic vacuoles. The mechanism by which this colocalization occurs appears to be different with each of the models (Fig. 2.2). In the diet model of pancreatitis, this colocalization occurs because zymogen granules and lysosomes fuse by crinophagy. In the secretagogue models, colocalization is caused by both crinophagic fusion of zymogen granules with lysosomes and defective sorting of lysosomal hydrolases from digestive enzymes as they traverse the Golgi stacks. In vitro exposure of rat or mouse pancreatic acini with a supramaximally stimulating dose of cerulein leads to the colocalization of digestive enzyme zymogens with lysosomal hydrolases inside cytoplasmic vacuoles and this phenomenon is assumed to occur as a result of perturbed intracellular trafficking of these enzymes.

Colocalization of digestive enzymes with lysosomal hydrolases also occurs in the opossum model of duct ligation-induced pancreatitis but, in this model, the colocalization phenomenon does not appear to be caused by perturbed intracellular trafficking. Rather, it is caused by cellular reuptake, into the lysosomal compartment, of secreted digestive enzymes and their zymogens.

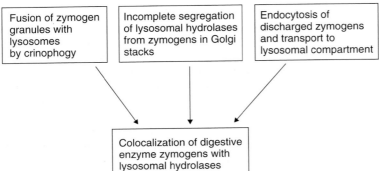

Fusion of zymogen granules with lysosomes by crinophogy	Incomplete segregation of lysosomal hydrolases from zymogens in Golgi stacks	Endocytosis of discharged zymogens and transport to lysosomal compartment

Colocalization of digestive enzyme zymogens with lysosomal hydrolases

Figure 2.2 Mechanisms of colocalization.

Colocalization and digestive enzyme activation

Digestive enzyme activation within acinar cells has been noted in each of the experimental models of pancreatitis and has also been observed in pancreatic samples taken from patients with acute pancreatitis. It is generally believed that intraacinar cell activation of digestive enzyme zymogens is a critical event in the pathogenesis of pancreatitis, leading to acinar cell injury and eventually to pancreatitis. We have suggested that the colocalization of digestive enzyme zymogens with lysosomal hydrolases is the initial event and that this colocalization phenomenon leads to zymogen activation because it permits the lysosomal hydrolase cathepsin B to catalytically activate trypsinogen and trypsin to activate the remaining zymogens. Indeed, it is well known that cathepsin B can catalytically activate trypsinogen, that trypsin can activate the other zymogens, and that, at least in the experimental models of pancreatitis, zymogen activation occurs at the site in which lysosomal hydrolases are colocalized with digestive enzyme zymogens. Furthermore, in virtually all the experimental models examined to date, colocalization of digestive enzyme zymogens with lysosomal hydrolases has been observed to occur and that colocalization can be detected prior to the appearance of demonstrable cell injury.

In spite of these findings, the importance of the colocalization phenomenon to intraacinar cell zymogen activation and the initiation of pancreatitis has been the subject of considerable controversy. Some of the objections to the colocalization hypothesis include the following.

1 The colocalization of digestive zymogens with lysosomal hydrolases occurs, to some extent, even under physiologic conditions because sorting is incomplete during normal intracellular trafficking. Thus, by itself, the colocalization phenomenon may not be of pathologic significance.

2 Similarly, since colocalization can be induced by various agents and interventions that do not, by themselves, cause either intracellular zymogen activation or pancreatitis, the colocalization phenomenon may not be of pathologic significance.

3 The extent of colocalization is not related to the severity of pancreatitis and, therefore, colocalization may not be of pathologic significance.

4 Although digestive enzyme zymogens and lysosomal hydrolases may become colocalized, the microenvironment within the colocalization compartment may not be ideal for either cathepsin B activation of trypsinogen or trypsin activation of the other zymogens. Indeed, the cytoplasmic vacuoles in which digestive zymogens and lysosomal hydrolases are colocalized are believed to have an internal pH of around 5.5–6.0 and this may be too high for optimal cathepsin B activity and too low for optimal trypsin activity.

Taken together, these concerns have led some to suggest that the colocalization phenomenon may in fact be an epiphenomenon and not an event which is critical to the evolution of acute pancreatitis. Some have even suggested that the colocalization phenomenon may be the result, rather than the cause, of acute pancreatitis. These concerns have stimulated a series of studies designed to determine if in fact the colocalization phenomenon is an early and critical event in the evolution of pancreatitis. These studies have shown that:

1 the colocalization phenomenon precedes the onset of zymogen activation during pancreatitis and zymogen activation can be detected prior to the appearance of cell injury in pancreatitis;

2 zymogen activation occurs at the site of colocalization;

3 prevention of colocalization prevents zymogen activation and cell injury;

4 neither preventing zymogen activation nor inhibiting activated zymogens prevents colocalization;

5 inhibition or deletion of lysosomal hydrolases prevents zymogen activation and cell injury and it reduces the severity of pancreatitis.

Taken together, these findings have provided strong arguments for the validity of the colocalization hypotheses and, at present, the concept that colocalization of digestive enzyme zymogens with lysosomal hydrolases plays an important role in triggering pancreatitis is generally accepted. However, it is clear that the colocalization phenomenon is not, by itself, sufficient to induce acinar cell injury and/or pancreatitis since colocalization can occur without causing pancreatitis. It would appear, therefore, that in addition to the colocalization phenomenon, other acinar cell events are also required for the induction of pancreatitis. One likely candidate for the other required event(s) would be inhibition of acinar cell digestive enzyme secretion. This inhibition of secretion has been noted to occur in each of the models of acute pancreatitis.

Acinar cell injury

Acinar cell injury is an early event in each of the experimental models of pancreatitis and, as noted above, the earliest morphologic changes in the opossum model of pancreatitis involve acinar cells. The mechanisms responsible for acinar cell injury in pancreatitis are not entirely clear. *In vitro* studies, using acini exposed to supramaximally stimulating concentrations of cerulein, have shown that inhibition of pancreatic proteases such as trypsin protects acinar cells from cerulein-induced injury. Furthermore, overexpression of trypsin inhibitors in acinar cells has also been found to reduce the severity of cerulein-induced pancreatitis. These observations suggest that acinar cell injury, at least during the earliest stages of pancreatitis, may be caused by intracellularly activated zymogens including trypsinogen. It is likely that the progression of injury at later times is also mediated by these activated enzymes and in addition by other factors, including oxygen-derived free radicals, released from inflammatory cells that have been activated and chemoattracted to the pancreas during the early phases of the disease.

Intraacinar cell mediators

Many studies have been designed to examine the intracellular mediators and intracellular pathways that might play important roles in the initiation of acute pancreatitis (Fig. 2.3). Most of these studies have employed the secretagogue (i.e., cerulein)-induced models of pancreatitis in rodents (i.e., mice or rats) or, alternatively, *in vitro* systems in which rodent pancreatic acini are exposed to a supramaximally stimulating concentration of cerulein.

Physiologic or maximally-stimulating concentrations of cerulein, which do not induce pancreatitis, are known to interact with high-affinity CCK-A receptors on the acinar cell surface and to activate phospholipase C in the cell membrane. This activation is known to result in hydrolysis of phosphatidylinositol 4,5-bisphosphate (PIP_2) yielding inositol 1,4,5-trisphosphate (IP_3) and diacylglycerol. Diacylglycerol activates protein kinase C while IP_3 binds to receptors on the endoplasmic reticulum, triggering release of calcium from intracellular stores and an oscillatory rise in cytoplasmic calcium concentrations. The supramaximally stimulating concentrations of cerulein that induce pancreatitis bind to lower-affinity CCK-A receptors and, by unclear mechanisms, cause a sustained rise in cytoplasmic calcium concentrations. This sustained rise is believed to reflect the combined effects of releasing calcium from intracellular storage pools and accelerating influx of extracellular calcium into the cell. Supramaximally stimulating concentrations of cerulein also cause activation of protein kinase C, activation of adenylate cyclase, a rise in acinar cell cyclic AMP (cAMP) levels, and activation of protein kinase A. In addition, supramaximally stimulating concentrations of cerulein trigger activation of many other downstream events that may play roles in initiating pancreatitis. Included among these downstream events are activation of tyrosine kinases, activation of proinflammatory transcription factors, induction of cytoskeletal changes, and possible activation of phosphoinositide 3-kinase (PI3K).

Calcium

The sustained rise in cytoplasmic calcium levels that follows exposure of acini to a supramaximally stimulating concentration of cerulein appears to play a critical role in coupling supramaximal cerulein stimulation with intracellular zymogen activation and acinar cell

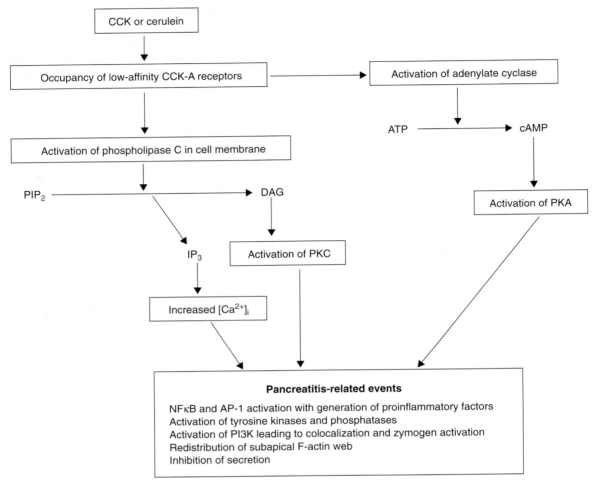

Figure 2.3 Intracellular mediators and pathways in acute pancreatitis. cAMP, cyclic AMP; CCK, cholecystokinin; DAG, diacylglycerol; IP$_3$, inositol 1,4,5-trisphosphate; PI3K, phosphoinositide 3-kinase; PIP$_2$, phosphatidylinositol 4,5-bisphosphate; PKA, protein kinase A; PKC, protein kinase C.

injury. Aborting this sustained calcium rise, either by removing calcium from the suspending medium or by preloading the acini with the calcium chelator BAPTA, can prevent both zymogen activation and cell injury. Ward and coworkers have hypothesized that this rise in calcium is, by itself, sufficient to cause zymogen activation and cell injury in the cerulein model of pancreatitis and they have suggested that a pathologic rise in cytosolic calcium may be responsible for pancreatitis in the other models as well as clinically. They argue that sustained elevations of cytoplasmic calcium could result from ductal hypertension, alcohol ingestion, hypoxia, hypercalcemia, hyperlipidemia, viral infection, and exposure to various drugs and that these elevations of calcium could directly cause zymogen activation as well as cell injury. However, their hypothesis is quite controversial and most workers, including ourselves, believe that while a change in calcium is necessary for induction of pancreatitis, this is not by itself sufficient to cause the alterations of pancreatitis.

Protein kinase C and tyrosine kinases

Protein kinase C is the downstream target of the diacylglycerol generated in response to cerulein-induced phospholipase C activation and hydrolysis of PIP_2 in the cell membrane. Protein kinase C is, under resting conditions, a cytosolic protein but during activation it is recruited to membrane sites. Subsequent to its activation, protein kinase C functions to phosphorylate proteins that regulate a large number of metabolic pathways. The tyrosine kinases are another group of receptor-coupled kinases that regulate metabolic pathways by phosphorylating downstream proteins. Some of the pathways regulated by protein kinase C and receptor-coupled tyrosine kinases undoubtedly control cellular processes critical to maintenance of the cytoskeleton, facilitation of secretion, and generation of proinflammatory mediators. *In vitro* studies, evaluating intracellular activation of digestive enzyme zymogens in acinar cells exposed to a supramaximally stimulating concentration of cerulein, have indicated that inhibition of protein kinase C or inhibition of tyrosine kinases interferes with cerulein-induced intraacinar cell activation of trypsinogen. These findings suggest that protein kinase C and tyrosine kinases play a critical role in mediating intraacinar cell zymogen activation but, as yet, the actual events mediated by these kinases have not been identified.

Phosphoinositide 3-kinase

PI3K is an important phospholipid kinase discovered by Cantley and coworkers in 1988. It catalyzes phosphorylation of membrane phosphoinositides in the 3′ OH position and, as a result, it regulates a vast number of downstream metabolic pathways. Three classes of PI3K have been identified. Class I PI3Ks signal downstream to G protein-coupled receptors or tyrosine kinase-coupled receptors. They yield phosphatidylinositol 3,4-bisphosphate, phosphatidylinositol 3,5-bisphosphate, or phosphatidylinositol 3,4,5-trisphosphate as their products, and cause downstream activation of the key regulatory protein Akt/PKB. Class II PI3Ks signal downstream to growth factor receptors and generate the same products as class I PI3Ks. Class III PI3Ks are constitutively active enzymes that phosphorylate only phosphatidylinositol and yield only phosphatidylinositol 3-phosphate as their product. In yeast, class III PI3Ks regulate trafficking to the vacuole, which is analogous to mammalian lysosomes; according to recent reports, class III PI3Ks function in mammalian cells to regulate trafficking to lysosomes.

In recently reported studies, we have found that inhibition of PI3K reduces the severity of secretagogue-induced and duct infusion-induced pancreatitis. Under *in vitro* conditions, inhibition of PI3K was also found to prevent supramaximal cerulein-induced intraacinar cell zymogen activation and the colocalization phenomenon but not to alter supramaximal secretagogue-induced NF-κB activation or cytoskeletal changes. We suggested that this phenomenon might be mediated by a class III PI3K and that this PI3K might play an important role in facilitating the colocalization of digestive enzyme zymogens with lysosomal hydrolases. Subsequent reports by Pandol and coworkers have confirmed our observation that inhibition of PI3K prevents cerulein-induced intrapancreatic digestive enzyme activation and reduces the severity of secretagogue-induced pancreatitis, although these studies suggested that the relevant PI3K might belong to the class I group and that it might function by activating Akt/PKB. Thus, at present, the identity of the relevant PI3K remains to be determined with certainty, but in either case these recent studies suggest that PI3K inhibition might be of therapeutic or prophylactic value in the management of patients with pancreatitis.

Protein kinase A

Supramaximal stimulation of pancreatic acinar cells with CCK or cerulein results in activation of adenylate cyclase and the generation of cAMP from ATP. This key second messenger has at least three downstream targets but the most well characterized is protein kinase A. Acinar cell adenylate cyclase can also be activated by other hormones including secretin. Recently reported studies by Gorelick and his coworkers have indicated that secretin stimulation of acinar cells sensitizes them to stimulation with cerulein and that, in the presence of secretin, submaximally stimulating concentrations of cerulein can cause intraacinar cell activation of digestive enzyme zymogens. Their studies have indicated that this effect of secretin is mediated by cAMP and that the sensitizing effect of secretin is itself mediated by activation of protein kinase A. In preliminary studies, we have confirmed these observations and found that secretin stimulation, and cAMP generation, also sensitizes acinar cells to other cerulein-induced changes including the cytoskeletal changes that would otherwise require supramaximally stimulating concentrations of cerulein. Whether cAMP and protein kinase A play an important role in other models of pancreatitis or in clinical pancreatitis remains to be established.

Severity determinants

Clinically, acute pancreatitis is a disease of variable severity. The vast majority of patients with acute pancreatitis have a mild disease that resolves spontanenously and is associated with little morbidity and virtually no mortality. On the other hand, approximately 20% of patients with acute pancreatitis have a severe disease and in most of these patients their attack of pancreatitis is accompanied by systemic changes, including an acute lung injury that presents clinically as ARDS.

The very early events that characterize the evolution of pancreatitis, including intraacinar cell zymogen activation and acinar cell injury, appear to be similar regardless of whether the disease is mild or severe and, for the most part, these early events have been completed prior to the time the diagnosis of pancreatitis is made. For these reasons, it is generally believed that while treatments designed to alter early events might be of prophylactic value, these treatments are unlikely to be therapeutically useful in the management of patients with established severe pancreatitis. In contrast to the initiation of pancreatitis, however, most observers believe that the ultimate severity of a pancreatitis attack is determined by proinflammatory events that are superimposed on the initiating events (Table 2.3). It is generally thought that a lag phase, perhaps ranging from hours to several days, occurs between the initiating events and the secondary "severity-determining" events and that this lag phase could present the clinician with a window of therapeutic opportunity, during which antiinflammatory interventions that moderate the severity-determining events might result in a reduction in pancreatitis severity. This belief has prompted many to search for the factors that regulate the severity of a pancreatitis attack and, to date, a number of metabolic pathways and important mediators have been identified.

Proinflammatory transcription factors

One of the earliest changes following supramaximal stimulation of acinar cells with cerulein, either *in vivo* or *in vitro*, is the activation of proinflammatory tran-

Table 2.3 Severity determinants for acute pancreatitis.

Proinflammatory
Transcription factors: NF-κB, AP-1
Stress-activated kinases: MAPK, ERK, JUNK
Platelet-activating factor
Tumor necrosis factor-α
Ligands acting on CCR-1 receptors
Substance P
Adhesion molecules: intercellular adhesion molecule-1, P-selectin, E-selectin
Neutrophils
Products of cyclooxygenase-2
Interleukins: IL-1, IL-6, IL-8
CXC-ELR chemokines
Reactive oxygen species

Antiinflammatory
Complement factor C5a
Heat-shock proteins
Interleukins: IL-10, IL-11
Apoptosis

scription factors (NF-κB, AP-1, and others), stress-activated kinases (MAPK, ERK, and others), and oncogenes (c-*fos*, c-*jun*, c-*myc*, and others). Activation of these factors during the early stages of other experimental pancreatitis models and during the early stages of clinical pancreatitis may also occur but studies aimed at documenting such changes have not been as extensively pursued. It appears that activation of these proinflammatory transcription factors and downstream kinases reflects binding to low-affinity CCK receptors in the secretagogue-induced models and that their activation is not dependent upon prior intraacinar cell activation of digestive enzyme zymogens. In fact, activation of these transcription factors occurs so quickly after the onset of supramaximal stimulation that activation of proinflammatory cascades may actually precede intraacinar cell activation of the digestive enzyme zymogens.

NF-κB is perhaps the most well studied of the transcription factors that are activated during the early stages of experimental pancreatitis. The role of PI3K in NF-κB activation is uncertain, with one study suggesting that PI3K plays no role in this process and another claiming that PI3K plays a critical role in mediating NF-κB activation during experimental pancreatitis. Subsequent to its activation, NF-κB translocates to the nucleus where it regulates expression of many proinflammatory and antiinflammatory factors. The overall effect of NF-κB in pancreatitis has been controversial, with some studies indicating that, on balance, it is proinflammatory and others suggesting that it may function to reduce the severity of pancreatitis. However, the prevailing opinion is that NF-κB activation mediates the worsening of pancreatitis severity and that the severity of pancreatitis can be reduced by preventing NF-κB activation.

Generation of inflammatory factors

Activation of transcription factors such as NF-κB and AP-1 results in the altered expression of many downstream proteins that regulate inflammatory processes, and there is a growing list of those regulatory proteins and inflammatory processes that play a role in pancreatitis. For the most part, studies evaluating the cytokines, chemokines, and other inflammatory factors that might regulate the severity of pancreatitis have employed (i) drugs or antibodies to abort the actions of these factors or (ii) genetically manipulated mouse strains that either do not express certain factors or lack the relevant receptors for those factors. As a result of these studies, a number of factors are now known to regulate the severity of pancreatitis and/or to couple pancreatic injury with lung injury. The proinflammatory factors for pancreatitis include platelet-activating factor (PAF), tumor necrosis factor-α, chemokines acting via the CCR-1 receptor, the neurotransmitter substance P, the adhesion molecules P- and E-selectin as well as intercellular adhesion molecule (ICAM)-1, and a number of interleukins including IL-1, IL-6, and IL-8. It is likely that most or all of these factors play critical roles in activating inflammatory cells and mediating their chemoattraction to the pancreas but they may also function to directly regulate the extent of acinar cell injury. IL-10, IL-11, and complement factor C5a have been found to reduce the severity of acute pancreatitis.

Activation and recruitment of inflammatory cells

Recruitment of inflammatory cells to areas of pancreatic injury as well as the activation of these inflammatory cells is an early and critical event in the inflammatory process of pancreatitis. A number of the factors elaborated by the injured pancreas, including interleukins, chemokines, and cytokines, are known to play an important role in these processes. Many act directly on resident macrophages within the pancreas and/or on circulating inflammatory cells, including neutrophils, lymphocytes, and macrophages. Many of the elaborated factors also act by increasing endothelial cell expression of adhesion molecules within the pancreatic (and pulmonary) microcirculation. Taken together, these various events result in a number of changes including (i) activation and priming of inflammatory cells for subsequent participation in the inflammatory reaction, (ii) chemoattraction of activated inflammatory cells to the pancreatic (and pulmonary) microcirculation, (iii) adhesion of inflammatory cells to the endothelial lining of the pancreatic (and pulmonary) microvasculature, and (iv) transmigration of activated and chemoattracted inflammatory cells across the microvascular barrier and into areas of inflammation.

Factors such as PAF and substance P, as well as many of the prostaglandins, appear to act primarily by increasing vascular endothelial permeability and in this way they promote transudation of intravascular fluid into the areas of pancreatic injury. They also promote fluid transudation across the pulmonary microvascular lining and, as a result, contribute to generation of the acute lung injury associated with severe pancreatitis.

A number of experimental studies have shown that the severity of pancreatitis, and of pancreatitis-associated lung injury, is directly related to the magnitude of these inflammation-related events and that interruption of these events can alter the severity of pancreatitis and/or pancreatitis-associated lung injury. Thus, genetic deletion or pharmacologic inhibition of PAF, cyclooxygenase-2, CCR-1 receptors, substance P, as well as various interleukins, chemokines, and cytokines has been shown to reduce the severity of pancreatitis and its associated lung injury. Neutrophil depletion, as well as genetic deletion or pharmacologic inhibition of adhesion molecules, have also been shown to reduce the severity of pancreatitis and pancreatitis-associated lung injury. Some of the inflammation-related factors have been found to exert an antiinflammatory effect: genetic deletion or pharmacologic inhibition of these factors increases the severity of pancreatitis and/or pancreatitis-associated lung injury. This has been reported to be the case for complement factor C5a (and the C5a receptor) and for IL-10 and IL-11.

Reactive oxygen species

Considerable evidence has been presented indicating that reactive oxygen species, generated and released by injured acinar cells or by inflammatory cells that have been activated and recruited to the injured pancreas, can dramatically alter the inflammatory reaction in pancreatitis. Some investigators have suggested that the initial acinar cell injury may itself reflect the deleterious effects of reactive oxygen species generated in response to the inciting event, although most investigators believe that the initiating events in pancreatitis are not mediated by reactive oxygen species. Rather, reactive oxygen species appear to primarily regulate the extent of acinar cell necrosis, the development of pancreatic edema, the sequestration of inflammatory cells within the pancreas, and the generation of inflammatory mediators by acinar and nonacinar cells of the pancreas and lung.

Expression of heat-shock proteins

Heat-shock proteins, including HSP27, HSP60, and HSP70, have been implicated as regulators of pancreatitis severity. The most well studied have been the proteins of the HSP70 superfamily. HSP70 expression in the pancreas is upregulated during pancreatitis and this upregulated expression appears to dampen the severity of pancreatitis. Induction of HSP70, by prior thermal stress, adrenergic stimulation, or exposure to agents such as arsenic, has been shown to reduce the severity of pancreatitis. The mechanisms by which HSP70, and other heat-shock proteins, ameliorate the severity of pancreatitis are not known but this issue is of considerable interest since there exists the potential for preventing or reducing the severity of pancreatitis by interventions that promote HSP70 expression.

Balance between apoptosis and necrosis

Severe pancreatitis is characterized by extensive necrosis but relatively little apoptosis of pancreatic acinar cells. Several studies have suggested that interventions which alter the balance between necrosis and apoptosis can affect the severity of pancreatitis: those that favor cell death by apoptosis reduce the severity of pancreatitis, whereas those that favor cell death by necrosis lead to an increase in the severity of pancreatitis. The mechanisms by which pancreatitis severity might by regulated by the mode of cell death have not been explored and they are currently unknown.

Prophylaxis versus treatment

As demonstrated by the above discussion, many factors that regulate the severity of pancreatitis have been identified and interventions which interfere with the expression or action of those that are proinflammatory have been shown to reduce the severity of pancreatitis. Unfortunately, the vast majority of the studies demonstrating that interfering with these factors is beneficial have involved interventions that are begun prior to, or coincident with, the initiation of pancreatitis and the beneficial effect has not been noted when the intervention is delayed until after the pancreatitis has become established. Similarly, in clinical practice interventions that have been shown to reduce the severity of experimental pancreatitis when begun prior to the onset of the disease have failed to benefit patients with established pancreatitis.

Chronic pancreatitis

According to the prevailing wisdom, chronic pancreatitis is the end product of repeated attacks of acute pancreatitis yet chronic pancreatitis differs from acute pancreatitis by the appearance of irreversible fibrosis, along with exocrine and/or endocrine insufficiency in the chronic disease. The mechanisms responsible for the changes of chronic pancreatitis and the reasons why only a subset of patients with acute inflammation progress to chronic pancreatitis are not known. Recent studies have demonstrated that the evolution of chronic pancreatitis depends upon activation and stimulation of pancreatic stellate cells, which contain smooth muscle α-actin, secrete collagen, and are responsible for the development of fibrosis. Some investigators have suggested that stellate cell activation and deposition of collagen might also occur in acute pancreatitis but that matrix metalloproteinases may promote collagen degradation and, by this means, prevent acute pancreatitis from evolving into chronic pancreatitis. Presumably, a defect in matrix metalloproteinase function (either genetic or acquired by exposure to factors such as ethanol that cause chronic pancreatitis) could interrupt this remodeling process and result in the development of chronic pancreatitis.

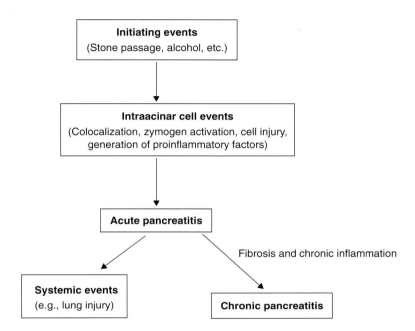

Figure 2.4 The phases of pancreatitis.

Summary and overview

Pancreatitis is a disease which is believed to evolve in phases (Fig. 2.4). The initial phase is triggered by an inciting event such as passage of a biliary tract stone, exposure to a pancreatico-toxic drug, or abuse of ethanol. This brings about intracellular changes within the acinar cells of the pancreas that cause inhibition of digestive enzyme secretion, along with the colocalization of digestive enzyme zymogens with lysosomal hydrolases within intracellular organelles. This colocalization phenomenon results in digestive zymogen activation within acinar cells and acinar cell injury. In addition, intracellular zymogen activation leads to the elaboration of a number of proinflammatory factors that serve to regulate the severity of pancreatitis as well as to couple pancreatic injury with systemic events, including acute lung injury and ARDS. Repeated bouts of acute pancreatic injury associated with pancreatic necrosis triggers intrapancreatic fibrogenesis and a chronic inflammatory reaction that eventually leads to the development of chronic pancreatitis.

This concept about the pathogenesis of pancreatitis may have important implications with regard to the prevention and/or treatment of the disease. An understanding of the early pathogenetic events that underlie the triggering of acute pancreatitis may suggest methods of preventing the disease. The recognition that a number of proinflammatory and antiinflammatory factors regulate the severity of an attack of pancreatitis may suggest methods of minimizing the severity of an attack and preventing the development of systemic complications including acute lung injury. Finally, the observation that there may be a window of therapeutic opportunity between the onset of pancreatitis and the commitment of events governing the severity of an attack may identify the optimal timing for initiation of treatment designed to minimize pancreatitis severity.

Recommended reading

Bhagat L, Singh V, Hiertaranta A, Agrawal S, Steer M, Saluja A. Heat shock protein 70 presents secretagogue-induced cell injury in pancreas by preventing intracellular trypsinogen activation. *J Clin Invest* 2000;106:81–89.

Bhatia M, Saluja A, Singh V *et al.* Complement factor C5a exerts an anti-inflammatory effect in acute pancreatitis and pancreatitis-associated lung injury. *Am J Physiol* 2001; 280:G974–G978.

Frossard JL, Saluja AK, Bhagat L *et al.* The role of intracellular adhesion molecule 1 and neutrophils in acute pancreatitis and pancreatitis-associated lung injury. *Gastroenterology* 1999;116:694–701.

Gukovskaya AS, Gukovsky I, Zasnninovic V *et al.* Pancreatic acinar cells produce, release, and respond to tumor necrosis factor-alpha. Role in regulating cell death and pancreatitis. *J Clin Invest* 1997;100:1853–1862.

Haber PS, Keogh GW, Apte MV *et al.* Activation of pancreatic stellate cells in human and experimental pancreatic fibrosis. *Am J Pathol* 1999;155:1087–1095.

Halangk W, Lerch MM, Brandt-Nedelev B *et al.* Role of cathepsin B in intracellular trypsinogen activation and the onset of acute pancreatitis. *J Clin Invest* 2000;106:773–781.

Hofbauer B, Saluja AK, Lerch M *et al.* Intra-acinar cell activation of trypsinogen during caerulein-induced pancreatitis in rats. *Am J Physiol* 1998;275:G352–G362.

Kaiser A, Saluja A, Sengupta A, Saluja M, Steer ML. Relationship between severity, necrosis and apoptosis in five models of experimental acute pancreatitis. *Am J Physiol* 1995;38: C1295–C1304.

Kloppel G, Maillet B. The morphological basis for the evolution of acute pancreatitis into chronic pancreatitis. *Virchows Arch A* 1992;420:1–4.

Lerch MM, Saluja AK, Dawra R, Ramarao P, Saluja M, Steer ML. Acute necrotizing pancreatitis in the opossum: earliest morphologic changes involve acinar cells. *Gastroenterology* 1992;103:205–213.

Lerch MM, Saluja A, Runzi M, Dawra R, Saluja M, Steer ML. Pancreatic duct obstruction triggers acute necrotizing pancreatitis in the opossum. *Gastroenterology* 1993;104: 853–861.

Norman J, Franz M, Messina J *et al.* Interleukin-1 receptor antagonist decreases severity of experimental acute pancreatitis. *Surgery* 1995;117:648–655.

Phillips PA, McCarroll JA, Park S *et al.* Rat pancreatic stellate cells secrete matrix metalloproteinases: implications for extracellular matrix turnover. *Gut* 2003;52:275–282.

Rongione AJ, Kusske AM, Kwan K, Ashley SW, Reber HA, McFadden DW. Interleukin 10 reduces the severity of acute pancreatitis in rats. *Gastroenterology* 1997;112:960–967.

Saluja AK, Saito I, Saluja M *et al.* In-vivo rat pancreatic acinar cell function during supramaximal stimulation with caerulein. *Am J Physiol* 1985;249:G702–G710.

Saluja AK, Bhagat L, Lee HS, Bhatia M, Frossard JL, Steer ML. Secretagogue-induced digestive enzyme activation and cell injury in rat pancreatic acini. *Am J Physiol* 1999;276:G835–G842.

Sans MD, DiMagno MJ, D'Alecy LG, Williams JA. Cerulein-induced acute pancreatitis inhibits protein synthesis in mouse pancreas through effects on eucaryotic initiation factors 2B and 4F. *Am J Physiol* 2003;285:G517–G528.

Singh VP, Saluja AK, Bhagat L *et al.* Phosphatidylinositol 3-kinase-dependent activation of trypsinogen modulates the severity of acute pancreatitis. *J Clin Invest* 2001;108: 1387–1395.

Song AM, Bhagat L, Singh V, Van Acker GJD, Steer ML, Saluja AK. Inhibition of cyclooxygenase-2 ameliorates the severity of pancreatitis and associated lung injury. *Am J Physiol* 2001;283:G1166–G1174.

Steer ML. Frank Brooks memorial Lecture: The early intra-acinar cell events which occur during acute pancreatitis. *Pancreas* 1998;17:31–37.

van Acker GJD, Saluja AK, Bhagat B, Singh VP, Song AM, Steer ML. Cathepsin B inhibition prevents trypsinogen activation and reduces pancreatitis severity. *Am J Physiol* 2001;283:G794–G800.

Whitcomb DC, Gorry MC, Preston RA *et al.* Hereditary pancreatitis is caused by a mutation in the cationic trypsinogen gene. *Nat Genet* 1996;14:141–145.

3

Pathophysiology of acute pancreatitis: which events are clinically relevant?

Miguel Pérez-Mateo and Juan Martínez

Once acute pancreatitis has developed (see Chapter 1) and regardless of the etiologic factor involved, several pathophysiologic events are clinically relevant. Among these, circulatory changes within the pancreas, the local and systemic inflammatory response, and the role of gut permeability should be emphasized.

Circulatory changes in the pancreas

Microcirculatory changes, including vasoconstriction, capillary stasis, decreased oxygen saturation, and progressive ischemia, occur early in experimental models of acute pancreatitis. These changes cause increased vascular permeability and swelling of the gland (edematous or interstitial pancreatitis). Vascular injury could lead to local microcirculatory failure and amplification of the pancreatic injury. A recent clinical study in patients with acute pancreatitis has shown a decrease in the superior mesenteric arterial pulsatility index (measured using Doppler sonography) during the early stage of severe acute pancreatitis.

There is also speculation about the role of ischemia/reperfusion injury in the pancreas. Hypoxia resulting from the vasoconstriction is followed by vasodilation during reoxygenation. The reintroduction of molecular oxygen during reperfusion/vasodilation transforms hypoxanthine to xanthine and initiates the release of oxygen radicals. The potential candidates mediating vasoconstriction/vasodilation are endothelin (vasoconstriction) and NO (vasodilation). An imbalance between endothelin and NO may be the major

determinant that regulates regional hemodynamics and local perfusion. In fact, extremely high plasma endothelin-1 concentrations have been reported in patients with pancreatic and diffuse intestinal necrosis, and the pancreatic origin of endothelin has been demonstrated in experimental models of acute pancreatitis. On the other hand, the urinary excretion of nitrites, as stable metabolites of NO, has been shown to be increased in patients with severe acute pancreatitis, probably as a consequence of endotoxin-mediated upregulation of inducible NO synthase (iNOs) activity. However, it is not clearly delimited if pharmacologic inhibition of iNOs could be beneficial or detrimental in the course of acute pancreatitis.

Another vasoactive mediator possibly implicated in the pathophysiology of acute pancreatitis is amylin. This 37-amino-acid polypeptide secreted by islet β cells produces a selective exocrine hypoperfusion. Amyline plasma levels are significantly higher in severe acute pancreatitis than in mild cases.

Finally it has been demonstrated recently that many tissues and organs, including the pancreas, have their own renin–angiotensin system. Some experimental data show that acute pancreatitis could markedly upregulate the expression of the renin–angiotensin system. In this respect, recent findings in experimental pancreatitis have further demonstrated that the administration of renin–angiotensin inhibitors, such as angiotensin II receptor antagonists, could protect against the severity of pancreatic injury by ameliorating the oxidative stress. Such a protective effect may open up a new strategy in the treatment of pancreatitis through the use of angiotensin II receptor antagonists.

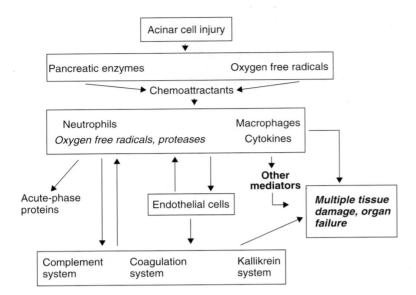

Figure 3.1 Pathophysiologic events in acute pancreatitis.

Leukocyte chemoattraction, release of cytokines, and oxidative stress

Inflammation is a complex and dynamic process that begins when cells are damaged by a noxious agent (Fig. 3.1). Injured cells then generate reactive oxygen species that attack the membranes of other cells and stimulate the release of chemoattractants. Moreover, several studies have shown decreased plasma levels of antioxidants (i.e., total ascorbic acid) and increased release of products derived from lipid peroxidation in patients with acute pancreatitis. Similarly, patients with mild cases of acute pancreatitis show significantly higher serum levels of antioxidants (retinol and β-carotene) than patients with severe acute pancreatitis and a close inverse relationship has been reported between C-reactive protein (CRP) and levels of antioxidants.

The migration of leukocytes into the injured tissue is the consequence of a complex cascade of biochemical events in which adhesion molecules play a major role. In experimental studies using two different models of acute pancreatitis, increased levels of intercellular adhesion molecule (ICAM)-1 have been demonstrated in pancreas, lung, and serum. On the other hand, neutrophil sequestration within the pancreas, evaluated by tissue myeloperoxidase activity, is significantly blunted in ICAM-deficient knockout mice, to the same extent as mice given antineutrophil serum. The effects of both

maneuvers combined are no different from those noted with either approach alone, indicating that ICAM-1-independent and neutrophil-independent events also contribute to the evolution of pancreatitis. In the same line of research, a recent clinical study suggests that the time course of elevated plasma soluble ICAM-1 concentrations reflects the risk of developing necrosis and clinical complications in human acute pancreatitis.

Additionally, plasma levels of different CXC chemokines, such as interleukin (IL)-8, growth-related oncogene (GRO)-α, and epithelial neutrophil-activating protein (ENA)-78, are significantly higher in patients with severe acute pancreatitis than in those with mild cases of the disease. Another factor responsible for recruitment of specific leukocyte subpopulations to the site of the inflammatory reaction is E-selectin. Patients with severe acute pancreatitis exhibit significantly higher plasma levels of E-selectin than patients with mild cases of pancreatitis throughout the clinical course of the disease.

The damaged tissue is invaded by neutrophils, which constitute the first line of defence, being followed by macrophages, monocytes, and lymphocytes. Several studies, including our own, have shown that the peak plasma level of polymorphonuclear (PMN) elastase, which indicates the degree of PMN activation, appears early in the course of acute pancreatitis and is significantly increased in severe forms compared with mild forms. Neopterin, a macrophage activation marker, shows similar behavior but with a later peak. On the other hand, patients with severe acute pancreatitis become immunosuppressed, highlighted in several studies that show a decrease in circulating CD3, CD4, and CD8 lymphocytes, impaired neutrophil and monocyte phagocytosis, and lower expression of human leukocyte antigen (HLA)-DR on peripheral monocytes.

Cytokines are a family of low-molecular-mass proteins (16–25 kDa) that are secreted by a myriad of cells. They are usually not found in normal tissue but are produced in response to stimuli via receptor-induced pathways. Cytokine secretion is a very closely regulated process and the expression of most cytokines is modulated by transcription factors such as NF-κB. All cytokines induce the activation of highly specific cell surface receptors. Most cytokines have pleiotropic activity and show multiple functional effects on a variety of target cells. There is a large redundancy within the system such that many cytokines can share similar biological effects, and in the absence of any one cytokine others fill the gap. This is important for the potential use of cytokine antagonist therapy and partially explains why single-cytokine antagonism has not proven to be of clinical benefit in trials.

Plasma levels of proinflammatory cytokines rise early in the course of acute pancreatitis. Related to this finding is the recent report of high expression of NF-κB in peripheral blood mononuclear cells of patients with severe acute pancreatitis. Regarding specific cytokines, the largest studies have focused on tumor necrosis factor (TNF)-α, IL-1β and IL-1 receptor antagonist (IL-1ra), IL-6, and IL-10. Most of these studies show higher plasma levels of TNF-α in patients with severe forms of acute pancreatitis compared with mild forms. However, circulating levels of TNF-α do not constitute a reliable indicator of disease severity, since its pattern of secretion is irregular and the liver rapidly clears TNF-α before it reaches the general circulation. The presence of soluble TNF-α receptors in the circulation may provide a better indicator of disease severity. Increased levels of circulating receptor predict organ failure in patients with acute pancreatitis even when TNF-α levels are not detectable.

IL-1β is another potent proinflammatory cytokine. Production of IL-1β is accompanied by induction of its receptors as well as IL-1 converting enzyme, now renamed caspase-1, which is responsible for cleaving pro-IL-1β to the active form. There is a correlation between the production of IL-1β and its specific receptor antagonist (IL-1ra) and the severity of acute pancreatitis. However, although IL-1β and TNF-α are both involved in the inflammatory cascade subsequent to acinar cell damage, they do not appear to play an initial causal role.

IL-6 is produced by a wide range of cells, including monocytes/macrophages, endothelial cells, and smooth muscle cells, in response to stimulation by endotoxin, IL-1β, and TNF-α. Several reports, including our own, have shown significantly higher levels of IL-6 within the first few days of hospitalization in patients with severe forms of acute pancreatitis compared with those with mild forms of the disease. The time course in individual cases demonstrated a dynamic parallel profile between CRP and phospholipase A (PLA) together with persistently raised concentrations of IL-6, suggesting a common source for the plasma levels of IL-6 and PLA. On the other hand, IL-6 is the main stimulus for the hepatic production of acute-phase proteins. We studied the serum levels of CRP in 80 patients with acute pancreatitis (40 with mild and 40 with severe forms). CRP (the single variable with highest predictive value of severity) peaked within days 2–4, with levels considerably higher in the group with severe acute pancreatitis.

IL-10 is an antiinflammatory cytokine and is thought to exert a protective role in acute pancreatitis. Serum levels are markedly raised within the first 24 hours of an attack followed by a steady decline. During the first 24 hours, serum IL-10 levels are higher in those with mild as opposed to severe acute pancreatitis.

Hepatocyte growth factor (HGF) is a potent mitogen for a wide variety of cells and is considered to be a cytokine with a critical role in tissue repair. High levels of plasma HGF have been reported in patients with acute pancreatitis. Experimentally, HGF prevents apoptotic cell death in liver, kidney, and lung, suggesting that it might function as an organotrophic factor against organ injuries in acute pancreatitis.

Other mediators not related to the cytokine cascade, such as platelet-activating factor (PAF), play an important role in the complex inflammatory process. PLA_2 released by activated neutrophils catalyzes the production of PAF from phospholipids in the cellular membrane. PAF activates platelets, neutrophils and, more importantly, increases endothelial permeability. The generalized leakage leads to hypovolemia, hypotension, hypoxemia, and ischemia of several organs. This is why PAF has been used as the target for a new thera-

Table 3.1 Inflammatory mediators in acute pancreatitis.

Inflammatory mediators	Function
TNF-α	Proinflammatory, neutrophil activation, shock
IL-1β	Proinflammatory, neutrophil activation, shock
IL-6	Leukocyte growth/activation, acute-phase response, pyrexia
IL-8, GRO-α, ENA-78	Neutrophil activation and chemotaxis
PAF	Platelet activation, neutrophil activation, increased endothelial permeability
IL-10	Antiinflammatory, inhibits release of proinflammatory cytokines
PMN elastase	Protease
ICAM-1, E-selectin	Neutrophil adhesion
MMP-1	Extracellular matrix degradation

ENA-78, epithelial neutrophil-activating protein-78; ICAM-1, intercellular adhesion molecule-1; IL, interleukin; GRO-α, growth-related oncogene-α; MMP-1, matrix metalloproteinase-1; PAF, platelet-activating factor; PMN, polymorphonuclear; TNF-α, tumor necrosis factor-α.

peutic approach, but unfortunately the results of the clinical trials have been once more disappointing.

The relationship between proinflammatory hypercytokinemia and multiple organ dysfunction syndrome (MODS) seems to be clearly established in several studies reporting similar results. In agreement with this finding, higher serum levels of matrix metalloproteinase (MMP)-1, which show a significant direct relationship with TNF-α, have been described in patients with acute pancreatitis and MODS, compared with less severe clinical cases. MMP-1 plays a central role in the degradation of the extracellular matrix. Therefore, this enzyme must be closely involved in the pathogenesis of MODS in cases of acute pancreatitis.

Table 3.1 summarizes the major inflammatory mediators implicated in acute pancreatitis.

The gut in acute pancreatitis

Increase in intestinal permeability

The bowel plays a pivotal role in the physiopathology

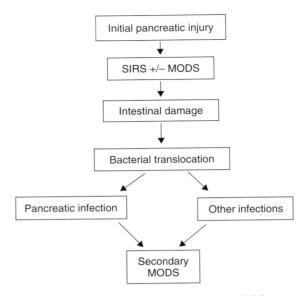

Figure 3.2 Role of the gut in acute pancreatitis. MODS, multiple organ dysfunction syndrome; SIRS, systemic inflammatory response syndrome.

of acute pancreatitis (Fig. 3.2). Increased intestinal permeability in both animal models and patients with acute pancreatitis has been reported to occur within 72 hours from the onset of symptoms. It correlates strongly with clinical outcome and persists throughout hospitalization. The mechanisms causing this bowel wall disruption are controversial. The significant fall in intramucosal pH, which is related to the intensity of the inflammatory process, suggests that intestinal ischemia contributes to the observed damage in the mucosal barrier. Moreover, other factors that may collaborate in intestinal ischemia include endothelin-1, ICAM-1, ischemia/reperfusion, malnutrition, and parenteral nutrition. On the other hand, a significant correlation has been observed between the serum concentration of endotoxin and the increase in intestinal permeability. In contrast, serum levels of IgM antibodies to endotoxin are significantly lower in patients with severe attacks of acute pancreatitis than in those with mild forms. This may be explained because antibodies to endotoxin core bind to circulating endotoxin to form complexes that are subsequently eliminated from the circulation. In addition, endotoxin is thought to be responsible for the derangements of immune function described in patients with severe acute pancreatitis, such as depletion of circulating T-helper lymphocytes, impairment of mononuclear phagocyte function, derangement of reticuloendothelial system clearance of α_2-macroglobulin–protease complexes, and reduction in delayed-type skin hypersensitivity.

From the morphologic point of view, a significant reduction in villous height, villous height/crypt ratio, and mast cell index has been observed in the small intestine of patients with necrotizing acute pancreatitis compared with controls.

Clinical consequences of changes in intestinal permeability

It is generally accepted that derangements in intestinal permeability facilitate bacterial translocation, a process of migration of bacteria and bacterial fragments from the intestinal lumen to extraintestinal sites. However, it is important to point out that the majority of probes used to study intestinal permeability cross the intestinal barrier via the paracellular route, whereas bacteria are thought to traverse it transcellularly. Bacterial translocation occurs very early in animal models of acute pancreatitis. In this phase, enteric bacteria have been found in mesenteric lymph nodes, liver, spleen, lungs, as well as pancreas. Although the hypothesis of bacterial translocation in humans remains unproven, there is supportive circumstantial evidence. In patients with necrotizing pancreatitis, Gram-negative enteric-type organisms are the agents responsible in most pancreatic and peripancreatic infections and the time course of bacterial infections of pancreatic necrosis run parallel to the changes described in intestinal permeability. On the other hand, a controlled trial of selective digestive decontamination showed that all pancreatic infections due to Gram-negative microorganisms were preceded by intestinal colonization with the same bacteria.

Despite the clear evidence of systemic endotoxin translocation, some authors propose that the process of bacterial translocation might be a phenomenon that occurs locally in humans to infect the necrotic pancreas rather than systemically, because they were unable to detect bacterial DNA in peripheral blood of patients with acute pancreatitis. The results observed by our group disagree with these findings since we have been able to detect bacterial DNA in 20% of samples obtained during the first week of hospitalization in patients with acute pancreatitis.

Systemic inflammatory response

It is clearly established that the systemic manifestations of necrotizing pancreatitis are not only produced by the acinar cell damage and the local inflammatory response but also by spillover of inflammatory mediators into the general circulation. This notion was based on the observation that patients with acute necrotizing pancreatitis, like those with multiple injuries, burns, tissue insult/injury, and major surgery, fulfil the criteria for systemic inflammatory response syndrome (SIRS) and often progress to MODS and sepsis (Table 3.2). Accordingly, tissue insult/injury triggers a triad of systems encompassing macrophages, cytokines, and endothelial cells. The consequence of this is SIRS/compensatory antiinflammatory response syndrome (CARS)/mixed antagonist response syndrome, which can progress to MODS, particularly when aggravated by a second hit (SIRS predominates), or can move toward resolution when second hits are avoided (CARS and SIRS balanced).

Patients who die from acute pancreatitis can be considered in two groups. About 50% of deaths occur within the first week. These patients suffer a severe initial attack and develop an exaggerated SIRS with the development of MODS and death. In contrast, patients with a severe attack who survive beyond this period often go on to develop extensive pancreatic necrosis. Infection in necrotic tissue leads to sepsis, a persistent systemic inflammatory response, and MODS and accounts for patients who die late.

Table 3.2 Criteria for systemic inflammatory response syndrome (SIRS), sepsis, and multiple organ dysfunction syndrome (MODS).

SIRS*	Rectal temperature > 38°C or < 36°C
	Heart rate > 90 bpm
	Respiratory rate > 20 breaths/min or $P\text{aco}_2$ < 32 mmHg
	White blood cell count > 12 000/mm³, or < 4000/mm³, or 10% immature (bands) forms
Sepsis	SIRS + documented infection
Severe sepsis	Sepsis + hemodynamic compromise
MODS	Organ failure not capable of maintaining homeostasis

* Two or more criteria required.

Different organs are damaged in patients with MODS. In the case of the lung, acute respiratory distress syndrome is typical. The lung becomes edematous and congested, leading to collapse of the smaller airways, with decreased lung compliance and respiratory failure. As a consequence of the SIRS response, the leukocytes become activated within the general circulation and some then lodge within the pulmonary microcirculation. As the process persists, leukocytes migrate into the pulmonary interstitium inducing increased endothelial permeability and tissue edema. Myocardial depression and shock are thought to be secondary to vasoactive peptides and a myocardial depressant factor. Acute renal failure has been explained on the basis of hypovolemia and hypotension. Metabolic complications include hypocalcemia, hyperlipidemia, hyperglycemia, and diabetic ketoacidosis. The pathogenesis of hypocalcemia is multifactorial and includes calcium-soap formation, hormonal imbalances (e.g., parathyroid hormone, calcitonin, glucagon), binding of calcium by free fatty acid–albumin complexes, and intracellular translocation of calcium.

These systemic complications are relatively infrequent in interstitial forms of acute pancreatitis, in contrast with necrotizing forms. However, only 50% of the cases with necrotizing pancreatitis develop organ failure and this event cannot be predicted by the extent of the necrosis or the presence of infected necrosis.

Factors conditioning severity

It has been suggested that the clinical course of an acute inflammatory illness such as acute pancreatitis may have a genetic basis, because certain genetic cytokine polymorphisms may produce functional differences and hence affect the outcome of the inflammatory process. In fact, the receptor for IgG (CD16) is constitutively expressed by neutrophils as a glycan-linked glycoprotein, which binds complexed IgG. Activated PMNs shedding CD16 might locally interfere with normal opsonization and phagocytosis. Genetic polymorphisms of CD16 are known, and an increased risk of sepsis after surgery has been demonstrated in preoperative "high expressors" in contrast with "low expressors."

Release of CD16 is mediated by TNF-α. This factor and IL-1 levels are, in turn, determined by the expression of a genetically encoded polymorphism of the major histocompatibility complex (MHC) class II (HLA-DR). Heterozygotes are higher secretors of these cytokines than homozygotes and therefore may be at greater risk of developing posttraumatic sepsis.

On the other hand, HLA-DR-bearing monocytes are of paramount importance to the immune response. This MHC class II expression is genetically regulated. It has been reported that HLA-DR expression increased after surgery in patients with uneventful recovery whereas no such increase was seen in patients who developed sepsis.

Although these observations might be applied to acute pancreatitis, functional genetic polymorphisms of IL-1, TNF-α, and IL-10 have been explored as a possible determinant of severity of pancreatitis, with no convincing results; however, an association between IL-1ra gene polymorphisms and acute pancreatitis has been demonstrated.

From pathophysiology to clinical practice: directions for the future

Recent advances in the understanding of the pathophysiology of acute pancreatitis have clarified the sequence of events taking place in these patients. Importantly, it has been shown that the process initiated in the pancreatic gland in patients with severe acute pancreatitis is associated with a marked systemic inflammatory response, and that a parallel exists between this response and prognosis. As a consequence, plasma and/or urinary measurement of some of the mediators of the inflammatory cascade or products of enzymatic activation, such as PMN elastase, IL-6, trypsinogen activation peptide, and procarboxypeptidase activation peptide, are commonly used in the early prediction of the severity of the process.

Therefore, it has been important to identify those cytokines or agents of the inflammatory process with a preeminent role in the development of SIRS and MODS. Unfortunately, therapeutic approaches employing blockade of some of these mediators (PAF antagonists, antiproteases) in the hope of constraining the inflammatory process in patients with acute pancreatitis have been disappointing, although evidence shows that blockade of IL-1 or TNF-α markedly modifies the evolution of experimental pancreatitis. It is likely that one of the main reasons for these differences is the time of application of the drug. The synthesis of cytokines in patients with acute pancreatitis takes place in the first hours of the disease but does not peak until 36–48 hours after the beginning of symptoms, and patients with severe acute pancreatitis may develop multiorgan failure 2–4 days after the onset of the disease. This temporal pattern allows a window of 2–3 days in which to antagonize those inflammatory mediators likely involved in patients with acute pancreatitis in an attempt to control the inflammatory process.

The fact that different cytokines act simultaneously in a complex and only partially understood way in patients with severe acute pancreatitis may explain why the blockade of only one of these agents has not been associated with therapeutic success, and suggests the use of a combination of different antagonists or modulators in future investigations. Furthermore, the previous negative results with the use of different drugs in patients with septic shock (anti-TNF-α, soluble TNF-α receptors, IL-1ra, soluble IL-1 receptors) may have decreased the enthusiasm for this innovative therapeutic approach. We consider, however, that some of the agents may have a place in therapeutic attempts to control the severity of acute pancreatitis since, in contrast to patients with septic shock, the diagnosis of acute pancreatitis and the precise onset of symptoms is a simple process, the patient population is usually homogeneous, and the presence of severe underlying diseases is an infrequent event.

Other future therapeutic approaches might be considered in these patients, such as the administration of the antiinflammatory cytokine IL-10, given the promising results obtained in the prevention of acute pancreatitis after endoscopic retrograde cholangiopancreatography. Following a different line of investigation, the intestine, as a "motor of organ failure," merits special attention, and the use of endothelin or ICAM-1 antagonists, relevant agents in the pathogenesis of intestinal damage in patients with acute pancreatitis, may be justified.

The initial promising results of intestinal decontamination should lead to well-designed therapeutic trials, possibly including colonic lavage. Lastly, glutamine-enriched enteric feeding has shown promising results and should also be widely investigated.

Recommended reading

Ammori BJ. Role of the gut in the course of severe acute pancreatitis. *Pancreas* 2003;26:122–129.

Bathia M, Brady M, Shokuchi S, Christmas S, Neoptolemos J, Slavin J. Inflammatory mediators in acute pancreatitis. *J Pathol* 2000;190:117–125.

Makhija R, Kingsnorth AN. Cytokine storm in acute pancreatitis. *J Hepatobiliary Pancreat Surg* 2002;9:401–410.

Norman J. The role of cytokines in the pathogenesis of acute pancreatitis. *Am J Surg* 1998;175:76–83.

Weber CK, Adler G. From acinar cell damage to systemic inflammatory response: current concepts in pancreatitis. *Pancreatology* 2001;1:356–362.

How should acute pancreatitis be diagnosed in clinical practice?

Richard S. Kwon and Peter A. Banks

Acute pancreatitis is a clinical syndrome characterized by abdominal pain and elevated pancreatic enzymes. The clinical and pathologic findings were first described in 1889. However, the diagnosis still remains quite elusive despite the availability of numerous laboratory and radiographic tests. The fact that autopsy studies continue to show a 30–42% incidence of undiagnosed pancreatitis underscores the complexity in the diagnosis of acute pancreatitis.

History and physical examination

Abdominal pain is the most prominent feature of acute pancreatitis, occurring in approximately 95% of patients. Pancreatitis has been documented without pain in association with Legionnaires' disease, insecticide, postoperative states, and dialysis. The pain is usually in the epigastric and periumbilical area of the abdomen, with radiation to the back in 50% of cases. Occasionally, the pain is diffuse or radiates to the lower abdomen. Rarely, the pain radiates to the chest. The onset is frequently acute and reaches maximum intensity within 30–60 min. The pain is often very severe, boring in character, and constant in duration. Patients often describe an inability to get comfortable and consequently may appear restless. Rarely, the pain is ameliorated by hunching forward, which frees the retroperitoneal space. Significant doses of narcotics are usually required for adequate pain control. Nausea and vomiting occurs in a majority of patients and may require the insertion of a nasogastric tube for relief.

Other diseases to consider in the differential diagnosis of acute pancreatitis include inferior wall myocardial infarction, peptic ulcer disease (including gastric or duodenal perforation), intestinal ischemia or infarction, intestinal strangulation or obstruction, biliary colic, cholecystitis, appendicitis, diverticulitis, dissecting aortic aneurysm, ovarian torsion, or ectopic pregnancy. Many of these diseases are surgical or medical emergencies and need to be ruled out quickly. Perforations often result in acute diffuse abdominal pain and peritoneal signs, such as a rigid abdomen and rebound tenderness. Pain associated with pancreatitis is usually localized to the upper abdomen and associated with less abdominal rigidity. Pain due to biliary colic and acute cholecystitis can be localized to the right upper quadrant of the abdomen but often is centered in the epigastric area similar to pain of pancreatitis. An abdominal ultrasound can identify choledocholithiasis and cholecystitis. Intestinal obstruction may cause crescendo–decrescendo pain with significant abdominal distension and, occasionally, feculent vomiting as well. Intestinal ischemia and infarction have variable degrees of pain, but often it is out of proportion to the physical examination and more gradual in onset than pancreatitis pain. Appendicitis can usually be distinguished by its history and location of pain.

In cases of mild pancreatitis, patients may appear uncomfortable but not seriously ill, and the vital signs may be normal. However, in cases of severe pancreatitis, patients may appear toxic and quite ill. In these patients, hypotension and tachycardia may be present due to dehydration and severe pain. Low-grade fever is present in up to 60% of patients with pancreatitis. At the time of admission, high-grade fevers may be an indicator of cholangitis in the appropriate clinical setting.

Tachypnea may be evident due to pain, fever, or pulmonary involvement.

Findings on physical examination can be variable as well. Jaundice may be evident in those patients with acute biliary pancreatitis. Cardiac examination may reveal tachycardia. Pulmonary examination may reveal shallow breathing due to diaphragmatic irritation from pancreatic inflammatory exudate and abdominal pain. Auscultation and percussion of the lungs may reveal signs of a pleural effusion, which is usually on the left pleural space or bilateral, and only rarely confined to the right. Abdominal examination generally reveals distension and tenderness, particularly in the epigastrium. Patients with mild pancreatitis describe pain that is moderate but strong enough to require evaluation. However, patients with severe pancreatitis may have exquisite tenderness and even a rigid abdomen that appears to be a surgical abdomen. Bowel sounds are often hypoactive due to ileus. Ecchymosis in the flanks (Grey Turner's sign) or near the umbilicus (Cullen's sign) can arise from local extravasation of pancreatic exudate. These two physical findings, while present in only 3% of cases of acute pancreatitis, are associated with 35% mortality.

Other findings on physical examintion can be quite useful. For instance, a general eye examination can be occasionally helpful in determining the etiology of pancreatitis. An arcus lipoides implicates hypertrigylceridemia. Band keratopathy suggests hypercalcemia. Rarely, Purtscher's retinopathy causes visual disturbances. Skin examination may reveal subcutaneous fat necrosis (panniculitis) over the distal extremities and rarely the trunk, buttock, or scalp. Polyarthritis has been described as well.

Laboratory evaluation

Serum and urinary tests can support the diagnosis of acute pancreatitis and may also help in the determination of its etiology. Radiologic findings can confirm the diagnosis.

Amylase

Pancreatic amylase (1,4-α-D-glucan glucanohydrolase) is an enzyme derived from acinar cells that hydrolyzes internal α-1,4 linkages in complex carbohydrates. In acute pancreatitis, amylase secretion into pancreatic juice is impaired, resulting in extravasation from the gland and reabsorption into the systemic circulation via venules or lymphatics. Serum levels rise within 2 hours, peak in the first 48 hours, and can return to normal in 3–5 days via renal and extrarenal mechanisms. Its rapid clearance and short half-life underscore the importance of determining the amylase concentration early in the course of the disease before the serum levels return to normal. Of note, the serum concentration does not correlate with either etiology or severity.

Total serum amylase concentration is generally considered the gold standard for diagnosing acute pancreatitis; however, there are several limitations to this test. In an analysis of studies determining the diagnostic accuracy of serum amylase, the sensitivity was found to be only 83% and to be particularly limited in three situations.

1 If it is determined several days after the onset of symptoms, the serum amylase concentration may have already normalized.

2 Concomitant hypertriglyceridemia can result in a normal amylase level possibly via an inhibitor, which can be negated by serial dilution.

3 In chronic acinar cell damage, for example as a result of chronic alcoholic pancreatitis, the pancreas may not be able to produce sufficient amylase during a bout of pancreatitis to be elevated.

Ultimately, if the serum amylase is normal and there is sufficient clinical suspicion of acute pancreatitis, a serum lipase level or computed tomography (CT) should be obtained to confirm the diagnosis.

An elevated amylase level does not always indicate pancreatitis (Table 4.1). There are numerous nonpancreatic sources of amylasemia, including salivary glands (which produce the most prevalent amylase isoform), ovaries, and fallopian tubes. Diseases of these organs may cause hyperamylasemia in the absence of pancreatitis. The most common intraabdominal diseases that can result in hyperamylasemia include intestinal diseases such as perforated peptic ulcer, intestinal obstruction, or mesenteric infarction (likely from leakage of intraluminal amylase and subsequent peritoneal reabsorption), and biliary diseases such as cholecystitis. Other conditions that can cause nonpancreatic hyperamylasemia include renal insufficiency (due to impaired clearance), acute alcohol intoxication (usually salivary amylase), diabetic ketoacidosis, liver metastases, head trauma, and lung cancer.

An additional cause of hyperamylasemia is

Table 4.1 Causes of hyperamylasemia. (Adapted from Banks 1985.)

Pancreatic disease
  Acute pancreatitis
  Complications of pancreatitis, e.g., pseudocyst, pancreatic
    ascites
  Pancreatic carcinoma
  Endoscopic retrograde cholangiopancreatography
Gastrointestinal disease
  Biliary disease, e.g., cholecystitis
  Hepatitis/cirrhosis
  Intestinal perforation or trauma
  Intestinal ischemia or infarction
  Intestinal obstruction
  Acute appendicitis
  Acute diverticulitis
  Aortic aneurysm
  Acute gynecologic disease, e.g., salpingitis, ruptured
    ectopic pregnancy
  Ovarian cysts
Salivary gland disease
  Mumps
  Calculous obstruction of salivary ducts
  Scorpion sting
  Effects of alcohol
Tumors
  Papillary cystadenocarcinoma of ovary
  Carcinoma of lung
Macroamylasemia
Renal insufficiency
Metabolic
  Diabetic ketoacidosis
  Anorexia nervosa
Others
  Pneumonia
  Intracranial hemorrhage
  Prostate hypertrophy
  Drugs, including opiates

macroamylasemia, an entity characterized by macromolecular immunocomplexes of amylase bound to immunoglobulins (usually IgA or IgG). These complexes are too large for glomerular filtration and result in chronically elevated levels of amylase. This benign condition may account for up to 28% of chronic unexplained hyperamylasemia and should be considered when elevated serum amylase concentrations are found in conjunction with negligible urinary amylase levels.

Because there are many nonpancreatic sources of hyperamylasemia, the specificity of serum amylase for diagnosing pancreatitis is only 88%. The specificity increases to greater than 90% when the cutoff for diagnosis is two to three times normal.

Measurement of amylase isoenzymes has been proposed as a way to clarify the significance of hyperamylasemia. Pancreatic amylase (p-isoamylase) normally comprises nearly 40% of total serum amylase, while salivary amylase makes up the remainder. In acute pancreatitis, p-isoamylase rises to over three times normal. The sensitivity and specificity of p-isoamylase in diagnosing acute pancreatitis was reported to be as high as 90 and 92%, respectively. However, elevated levels of p-isoamylase have been noted in renal insufficiency, intestinal disorders such as perforation or ischemia, diabetic ketoacidosis, and intracranial hemorrhage, and after endoscopic retrograde cholangiopancreatography (ERCP) or morphine administration. As a consequence, pancreatic isoenzymes are no more useful than total amylase and have no role in the diagnosis of acute pancreatitis.

Amylase concentrations in urine are also elevated in acute pancreatitis due to enhanced renal clearance. A normal amylase/creatinine clearance ratio is approximately 3% and rises to 6–10% or greater in acute pancreatitis. However, there have been case reports of acute pancreatitis with normal urinary clearances. The specificity of the test is limited by a number of nonpancreatic conditions that can elevate urinary clearance. These include severe burns, diabetic ketoacidosis, march hemoglobinuria, anorexia nervosa, and postoperative states. Furthermore, renal insufficiency tends to decrease creatinine clearance out of proportion to amylase clearance, which falsely elevates the ratio. Therefore, urinary clearance has no benefit over serum amylase levels in the diagnosis of acute pancreatitis. The role of the amylase/creatinine clearance ratio is to confirm the diagnosis of macroamylasemia, which is characterized by a negligible concentration of urinary amylase and consequently a very low ratio.

Lipase

Pancreatic lipase (triacylglycerol acylhydrolase) is produced by acinar cells and hydrolyzes glycerol esters of long-chain fatty acids. In acute pancreatitis, serum lipase levels rise via the same mechanism as for amylase.

Serum lipase rises 4–8 hours after the onset of symptoms and peaks at 24 hours. Its half-life is longer than that of amylase and consequently lipase levels normalize more slowly (8–14 days). Thus, the principal advantage of lipase is its increased sensitivity in cases where there is a delay between the onset of symptoms and laboratory evaluation, at which time amylase levels may have normalized. Serum lipase that is two to three times normal is generally thought to be more specific and sensitive (95% and 96% respectively) and to be more accurate than amylase, particularly at later dates in the course of the pancreatitis.

Similar to hyperamylasemia, hyperlipasemia may not always signify pancreatitis. There are alternative sources of lipase, though fewer than for amylase. These include gastric lipase and a nonspecific hepatic triacylglyceride lipase. There are an increasing number of conditions associated with hyperlipasemia. Such intraabdominal diseases include intestinal pathology such as inflammatory bowel disorders, peptic ulcer disease, bowel perforation, small bowel obstruction or infarction, or abdominal trauma (all via the same mechanism as amylase), and hepatobiliary pathology such as hepatitis, biliary obstruction, and cholecystitis. Extraabdominal diseases include hypertriglyceridemia, diabetic ketoacidosis, and renal insufficiency. In these cases, the lipase elevations are usually less than three times normal. Similar to macroamylasemia, macrolipasemia also appears to be a clinical entity, albeit rarer, and has been reported in association with Hodgkin's lymphoma, Crohn's disease, and sarcoidosis.

Amylase and lipase

Amylase has traditionally been the test of choice for diagnosing acute pancreatitis, but given its higher sensitivity and specificity, lipase may actually be more valuable. However, many clinicians often check both serum amylase and lipase in the work-up of abdominal pain. The combination does not appear to improve accuracy. A diagnostic challenge arises when only one of the two levels is elevated. For example, amylase levels have been normal in up to 32% of patients with radiographically confirmed acute pancreatitis. These patients were more likely to have alcoholic and/or chronic pancreatitis, a history of more frequent previous attacks, and a longer duration of symptoms before laboratory evaluation. In this situation, accurate diagnosis of acute pancreatitis can be made by elevated serum lipase concentrations or with radiologic tests.

The lipase/amylase ratio has been proposed as a tool for establishing alcohol as the etiology of pancreatitis. Although some studies indicate that a ratio greater than 3 may be useful in distinguishing alcoholic pancreatitis from nonalcoholic pancreatitis, the ratio lacks sensitivity and only identifies two-thirds of cases of alcoholic pancreatitis.

Liver function tests

Transaminases are used primarily to distinguish biliary pancreatitis from other causes of pancreatitis. A recent metaanalysis determined that a threefold or greater elevation of alanine aminotransferase (ALT) in the presence of acute pancreatitis had a 95% positive predictive value for gallstone pancreatitis. However, it should be noted that only half of all patients with gallstone pancreatitis have significant elevations of serum ALT, and therefore an ALT less than three times normal should not exclude the diagnosis.

Other diagnostic tests

Trypsinogen is a 25-kDa pancreatic protease that is secreted in pancreatic juice in two isoforms (trypsinogen-1 and trypsinogen-2). In acute pancreatitis, trypsinogen-2 levels rise in both serum and urine over 10-fold. In two trials of approximately 500 patients, the sensitivity and specificity of a dipstick urine test to detect trypsinogen-2 were found to be 92–94% and 95–96%, respectively. The negative predictive value was 99%; therefore, a negative test ruled out pancreatitis with high probability. The authors suggest that a negative test can quickly rule out pancreatitis but a positive test merits further evaluation. Further validation of this test is needed. A test for serum trypsinogen-2 has also shown encouraging preliminary results.

Serum immunoreactive trypsin, chymotrypsin, elastase, phospholipase A_2, α_2-macroglobulin, pancreatic activated protein, methemalbumin, carboxypeptidases, and carboxyl ester hydrolase levels have been proposed for diagnosis of pancreatitis. They have been proven to be neither more accurate nor more beneficial than serum amylase or lipase and tests are not commercially available.

Radiology

The primary role of radiology is to confirm the diagnosis, to identify the possible cause of pancreatitis, and to assess the extent and complications.

Ultrasound

Abdominal ultrasound is generally not used to diagnose pancreatitis. Its primary role is to rule out gallstones as the etiology of pancreatitis and can also be used to preclude other diseases such as acute cholecystitis or hepatic abscesses. Visualization of the pancreas is often hindered by overlying bowel gas. Findings consistent with pancreatitis include diffuse glandular enlargement, hypoechoic texture of the pancreas indicating interstitial edema, focal areas of hemorrhage or necrosis within the pancreas, and free intraperitoneal fluid.

Computed tomography

Thin-section multidetector-row CT with intravenous contrast is the most important radiographic modality used to diagnose acute pancreatitis and to exclude other conditions causing abdominal pain, including mesenteric infarction and perforated duodenal ulcer. CT can also be used to determine severity of disease and to identify complications related to pancreatitis.

Findings on CT that support the diagnosis of acute pancreatitis include diffuse edema and enlargement of the pancreas, heterogeneity of pancreatic parenchyma, peripancreatic stranding, obliteration of the peripancreatic fat planes, and peripancreatic fluid collections. Pancreatic necrosis is defined as a focal or diffuse area of the nonenhanced pancreatic parenchyma following examination with intravenous contrast. In mild cases of pancreatitis, CT may be normal.

Magnetic resonance imaging

With evolving technology, particularly the development of magnetic resonance cholangiopancreatography (MRCP), magnetic resonance imaging has been increasingly used in the care of patients with pancreatitis. MRCP can detect pancreatic necrosis and determine severity as accurately as CT, and is superior in delineating pancreatic duct anatomy and detecting choledocholithiasis. In addition, potential nephrotoxicity is minimized by the use of gadolinium contrast.

Nonetheless, despite these benefits, CT can be obtained in a much more timely and cost-effective manner than MRCP in most hospitals and therefore remains the preferable radiologic test.

Endoscopic retrograde cholangiopancreatography

ERCP has no role in the diagnosis of acute pancreatitis. Its role is to treat choledocholithiasis and cholangitis and to delineate pancreatic ductal anatomy in cases of recurrent or unresolved pancreatitis.

Endoscopic ultrasound

Endoscopic ultrasound is an emerging technology in the care of pancreatic disease. However, its role in establishing the diagnosis of acute pancreatitis has not been established. Endoscopic ultrasound may serve as an alternate modality for detecting choledocholithiasis.

Summary

At present, a serum lipase level greater than three times normal appears to be the most accurate test for diagnosing acute pancreatitis. Urinary trypsinogen-2 levels also accurately diagnose acute pancreatitis but a test is not yet commercially available. Thin-section multidetector-row CT with intravenous contrast is the study of choice to confirm the diagnosis.

Recommended reading

Balthazar EJ, Freeny PC, van Sonnenberg E. Imaging and intervention in acute pancreatitis. *Radiology* 1994;193: 297–306.

Banks PA. Tests related to the pancreas. In: JE Berk (ed.) *Bockus Gastronterology*, 4th edn. Philadelphia: WB Saunders, 1985:427–444.

Banks PA. Practice guidelines in acute pancreatitis. *Am J Gastroenterol* 1994;92:377–386.

Chase CW, Barker DE, Russell WL *et al.* Serum amylase and lipase in the evaluation of acute abdominal pain. *Ann Surg* 1996;62:1028–1033.

Dervenis C, Johnson CD, Bassi C *et al.* Diagnosis, objective assessment of severity and management of acute pancreatitis (Santorini Consensus Conference). *Int J Pancreatol* 1999; 25:195–210.

Dominguez-Muñoz JE. Diagnosis of acute pancreatitis: any news or still amylase? In: M Buchler, E Uhl, H Friess, P Malfertheiner (eds) *Acute Pancreatitis: Novel Concepts in Biology and Therapy*. Oxford: Blackwell Science, 1999: 171–179.

Elmas N. The role of diagnostic radiology in pancreatitis. *Eur J Radiol* 2001;38:120–132.

Frank B, Gottlieb K. Amylase normal, lipase elevated: is it pancreatitis? A case series and review of the literature. *Am J Gastroenterol* 1999;94:463–469.

Gullo L. Chronic nonpathological hyperamylasemia of pancreatic origin. *Gastroenterology* 1996;110:1905–1908.

Hedstrom J, Kemppainen E, Andersen J *et al*. A comparison of serum trypsinogen-2 and trypsin-2–α_1-antitrypsin complex with lipase and amylase in the diagnosis and assessment of serverity in the early phase of acute pancreatitis. *Am J Gastroenterol* 2001;96:424–430.

Keim V, Teich N, Fiedler F *et al*. A comparison of lipase and amylase in the diagnosis of acute pancreatitis in patients with abdominal pain. *Pancreas* 1998;16:45–49.

Kemppainen EA, Hedstrom JI, Puolakkainen PA *et al*. Rapid measurement of urinary trypsinogen-2 as a screening test for acute pancreatitis. *N Engl J Med* 1997;336:1788–1793.

Lankisch PG, Banks PA (eds) *Pancreatitis*. Berlin: Springer-Verlag, 1998.

Lescesne R, Tourel P, Bret PM *et al*. Acute pancreatitis: interobserver agreement and correlation of CT and MR cholangiopancreatography with outcome. *Radiology* 1999;211: 727–735.

Tenner S, Dubner H, Steinberg W. Predicting gallstone pancreatitis with laboratory parameters: a meta-analysis. *Am J Gastroenterol* 1994;89:1863–1866.

Toouli J, Brooke-Smith M, Bassi C *et al*. Working party report: guidelines for the management of acute pancreatitis. *J Gastroenterol Hepatol* 2002;17(Suppl):S15–S39.

Treacy J, Williams A, Bais R *et al*. Evaluation of amylase and lipase in the diagnosis of acute pancreatitis. *Aust NZ J Surg* 2001;71:577–582.

Yadav D, Nair S, Norkus EP *et al*. Nonspecific hyperamylasemia and hyperlipasemia in diabetic ketoacidosis: incidence and correlation with biochemical abnormalities. *Am J Gastroenterol* 2000;95:2123–2128.

Yadav D, Agarwal N, Pitchumoni CS. A critical evaluation of laboratory tests in acute pancreatitis. *Am J Gastroenterol* 2002;97:1309–1318.

5

Guidelines for the detection of the etiologic factor of acute pancreatitis

J. Enrique Domínguez-Muñoz

Acute pancreatitis is a frequent disease and one of the most frequent digestive disorders leading to hospitalization in developed countries. The incidence of acute pancreatitis varies widely among different series, ranging from 5.4 to 79.8 cases per 100 000 inhabitants per year. Although it may be accepted that the incidence of the disease is to some extent lower in countries such as the UK and the Netherlands compared with the USA, Finland, or Spain, this geographic variability explains only partly the reported differences among series. The major difference is probably explained by the study design, since the incidence of acute pancreatitis is much higher in prospective than in retrospective series. Different criteria applied for the diagnosis of acute pancreatitis most probably also play a role. Considering only prospective studies specifically designed to calculate the incidence of acute pancreatitis and that define the disease by the presence of acute abdominal pain and elevation of serum and/or urine levels of pancreatic enzymes at least twice the upper limit of normal, the incidence of acute pancreatitis ranges from 20 to 40 cases per 100 000 inhabitants per year. There is a peak of incidence between the fourth and sixth decades of life and no definite difference between males and females.

Etiology of acute pancreatitis

Several conditions are generally accepted as potential causes of acute pancreatitis (Table 5.1). Among these, gallstones and alcohol are responsible for more than 80% of episodes of the disease. Other causes are clearly less frequent, but their correct identification is highly relevant in order to apply the appropriate therapeutic measures to avoid relapses.

Gallstones

Common bile duct stones and sludge are well-known causes of acute pancreatitis. This is the most frequent etiologic factor associated with the disease in most countries. In addition, up to 75% of cases considered as idiopathic are related to biliary microlithiasis. Cholecystectomy and extraction of common bile duct stones prevent relapses of the disease, confirming the cause–effect relationship.

Despite the close association between gallstones and acute pancreatitis, only a small percentage of patients with gallstones develop pancreatitis. In fact, the prevalence of gallstones is as much as 12% in the general population. Thus, in an American study the risk of acute pancreatitis in the presence of gallstones has been estimated to be 12–35 times higher than in the general population. Two different studies in Spain provide a consistent odds ratio of 6.7 (95% confidence interval, 3.8–11.8) for acute pancreatitis in the presence of gallstones.

The mechanism by which gallstones induce acute pancreatitis is unknown. Most probably, transpapillary passage of a stone causes transient obstruction of both bile duct and pancreatic duct and this leads to acute pancreatitis. Consistent with this, small stones (diameter < 5 mm), which are more likely to pass from the gallbladder through the cystic duct, are more frequently associated with pancreatitis than large stones. Similarly, passage of microlithiasis through the papilla may cause pancreatitis by inducing ampullary edema and secondary obstruction.

Table 5.1 Causes of acute pancreatitis.

Toxic and metabolic
Alcohol
Hyperlipidemia
Hypercalcemia
Drugs
Scorpion venom

Mechanical
Gallstones, biliary sludge
Ampullary obstruction
Pancreatic obstruction
Sphincter of Oddi dysfunction
Pancreas divisum
Trauma
Congenital malformations

Others
Ischemia
Iatrogenic injury
Infection
Hereditary
Autoimmune
Cystic fibrosis
Tropical

Alcohol

Alcohol consumption is the second most frequent cause of acute pancreatitis in most countries. Although a direct relationship between the amount of alcohol intake and the risk of acute pancreatitis most probably exists, individual susceptibility to alcohol is variable. Thus, an alcohol consumption that may be considered socially normal is able to cause acute pancreatitis. It has been calculated that a mean daily consumption of 90 g alcohol is required to match the risk of pancreatitis induced by gallstones. Acute excessive alcohol intake may cause acute pancreatitis in some patients, whereas chronic alcohol consumption is most frequently associated with acute relapses of chronic pancreatitis. The diagnosis of underlying chronic pancreatitis in patients with acute alcoholic pancreatitis is often difficult. Endoscopic ultrasonography, because of its high sensitivity in the detection of early changes of chronic pancreatitis, may be of help in these situations.

The exact mechanism of alcohol-induced acute pancreatic injury is unknown, although genetic and environmental factors are most probably involved. In addition, alcohol may act by increasing the synthesis of enzymes by acinar cells or by oversensitizing acini to cholecystokinin.

Metabolic disorders

Hypertriglyceridemia is a well-known cause of acute pancreatitis. Patients with hyperlipidemic pancreatitis often present with serum triglyceride levels above 1000 mg/dL. The serum is macroscopically opalescent due to increased chylomicron concentration.

Hypertriglyceridemic pancreatitis may occur in patients with types I and V hyperlipidemia as well as in alcoholics. Alcohol intake is one of the major factors inducing elevation of serum triglycerides. In fact, it is occasionally difficult to evaluate the potential role of hypertriglyceridemia in the origin of alcohol-related acute pancreatitis.

Clinically, acute hyperlipidemic pancreatitis tends to be severe and up to 50% of patients present with necrotizing pancreatitis. Therefore, adequate dietetic and pharmacologic treatments of the lipoprotein metabolic disorder as well as alcohol abstinence are highly important in preventing relapses of pancreatitis.

The role of hypercalcemia as a cause of acute pancreatitis, although classically accepted, should be nowadays reevaluated. Although the association between hyperparathyroidism and pancreatitis has been repeatedly reported, other potential causes of pancreatitis are also frequently present in these patients. The reported incidence of pancreatitis in patients with hyperparathyroidism is very low. In addition, some series have shown that the risk of pancreatitis in these patients is similar to that observed in the general hospital population. In summary, hypercalcemia should be considered as the potential cause of acute pancreatitis only after exclusion of any other potential cause of the disease.

Drugs

A large variety of drugs have been related to acute pancreatitis, most of which have been published only as case reports. Based mainly on the repeated report of a drug as associated with acute pancreatitis and the relapse of the disease with reintroduction of the drug, the strength of association between drugs and pancreatitis has been classified as definite, probable, or possible (Table 5.2).

Table 5.2 Drugs associated with acute pancreatitis.

Definite association
Valproic acid
Azathioprine
Didanosine
Estrogen
Furosemide (frusemide)
6-Mercaptopurine
Pentamidine
Sulfonamides
Tetracycline
Tamoxifen

Probable association
L-Asparaginase
Steroids
Metronidazole
Aminosalicylates
Thiazides

Possible association
Amphetamine (amfetamine)
Cimetidine
Cyproheptadine
Cholestyramine (colestyramine)
Diazoxide
Histamine
Indomethacin (indometacin)
Isoniazid
Propoxyphene
Rifampicin
Opiates

Although some drugs such as diuretics, sulfonamides, and steroids are able to cause acute pancreatitis through a direct toxic effect, most cases of drug-related pancreatitis are probably due to individual hypersensitivity. In fact, potentially pancreatotoxic drugs are not independent risk factors for acute pancreatitis in large epidemiologic studies. The interval from the beginning of drug intake to the development of pancreatitis is highly variable, ranging from a few weeks in drug-induced immunologic reaction to many months when accumulation of toxic metabolites is required (e.g., valproic acid, pentamidine, didanosine).

Obstruction to the flow of pancreatic juice

The presence of pancreas divisum, defined as the ab-
sence of fusion of the ventral and dorsal pancreatic ducts during fetal development, is an accepted risk factor for acute pancreatitis. The mechanism by which pancreas divisum may cause pancreatitis is the obstruction of flow of pancreatic juice through the minor papilla. The relative risk of pancreatitis in subjects with this anatomic variant ranges from 2.7 to 10 times higher than in the general population. This means that 2–12 patients with pancreas divisum should be treated (e.g., by sphincterotomy of the minor papilla with or without stent insertion) to prevent one episode of acute pancreatitis. It should be noted that, despite endoscopic treatment, 10–24% of patients with pancreas divisum relapse within the following 2 years.

Acute pancreatitis secondary to sphincter of Oddi dysfunction usually presents as relapsing attacks in patients with a dilated Wirsung duct and intrapapillary stenosis (type I dysfunction) or in patients with normal-appearing Wirsung duct but a basal sphincter of Oddi pressure higher than 40 mmHg (type II dysfunction). The pathogenesis of pancreatitis secondary to sphincter of Oddi dysfunction is based on the obstruction of flow of pancreatic juice through the papilla. Because of this, endoscopic sphincterotomy is the treatment of choice in these patients and the best results have been obtained by cutting both the pancreatic and biliary sphincters.

Any other condition causing obstruction of the papilla is potentially able to cause acute pancreatitis, including periampullary diverticula and periampullary tumors.

Other potential etiologic factors

The hereditary basis of pancreatitis has received great attention over the last few years. This is mainly due to the finding of frequent genetic mutations predisposing to pancreatitis in patients with no other potential etiologic factor of the disease. In addition, some mutations may be necessary for the development of acute pancreatitis in the presence of other etiologic factors. Cationic trypsinogen gene mutations are found in up to 50% of patients with a positive family history of pancreatic diseases compared with only 0–15% of those without family history. Some mutations of the cationic trypsinogen gene are associated with a high penetrance and seem to play a key role in the development of inherited pancreatitis. Conversely, mutations in the serine protease inhibitor Kazal type 1 (*SPINK1*) gene proba-

Table 5.3 Infectious agents associated with acute pancreatitis.

Viruses
Mumps
Coxsackievirus
Hepatitis B
Cytomegalovirus
Varicella-zoster
Herpes simplex
Human immunodeficiency virus

Bacteria
Mycoplasma
Legionella
Leptospira
Salmonella

Fungi and parasites
Aspergillus
Toxoplasma
Cryptosporidium
Ascaris

---

bly act as disease modifiers. Nevertheless, the role of most described pancreatitis-associated gene mutations is still poorly understood and many other gene mutations are as yet unidentified.

A wide variety of infectious agents have been associated with acute pancreatitis. Although the scientific literature in this field is mainly based on case reports, a definite association with acute pancreatitis is accepted for some microorganisms (Table 5.3). Because of doubtful therapeutic consequences during the acute attack, as well as to prevent relapses, the routine search for an infectious agent in patients with otherwise idiopathic pancreatitis is not recommended.

Pancreatic ischemia is an accepted cause of acute pancreatitis. Diagnosis of pancreatitis may be difficult in these patients, mainly in severe cases under intensive care such as after intraoperative hypotension or hemorrhagic shock. Ischemia-related relapsing pancreatitis has been described in patients with systemic lupus erythematosus and polyarteritis nodosa.

Finally, acute iatrogenic pancreatitis may develop after invasive maneuvers on the pancreas. The prototype of this is the pancreatitis occurring after endoscopic retrograde cholangiopancreatography (ERCP). Acute pancreatitis develops in up to 5% of patients undergoing ERCP. Since abdominal discomfort or even pain in the absence of pancreatitis is not unusual after ERCP and since hyperamylasemia occurs in up to 70% of patients after ERCP, diagnosis of post-ERCP pancreatitis requires the presence of persistent severe abdominal pain and increased serum levels of pancreatic enzymes greater than five times the upper limit of normal.

Recommendations for etiologic diagnosis of acute pancreatitis in clinical practice

Considering the high morbidity and the risk of mortality secondary to acute pancreatitis, etiologic diagnosis of the disease is highly desirable in order to apply therapeutic measures to prevent relapses. Up to 80% of acute pancreatitis episodes may be explained by gallstones or alcohol consumption. Thus, etiologic diagnosis may be easy in most cases by clinical history (history of biliary disease or alcohol consumption), standard hematologic and biochemical analysis (macrocytosis as a sign of chronic alcohol abuse; liver enzymes, mainly alanine aminotransferase (ALT) for biliary etiology, aspartate aminotransferase and γ-glutamyltransferase for alcoholic pancreatitis), and abdominal ultrasound (presence of direct or indirect signs of gallstones). Biochemical analysis at admission should include serum triglyceride and calcium levels to support or exclude the potential role of serum lipids and hypercalcemia in the development of acute pancreatitis. Finally, history should include family history of pancreatitis (inherited disease?), a careful questionnaire about medications (drug-induced pancreatitis?), and associated autoimmune disorders (autoimmune pancreatitis?) (Fig. 5.1).

Because of the important role of gallstones in the etiopathogenesis of acute pancreatitis, any finding supporting the presence of gallstone disease is sufficient to classify an attack of acute pancreatitis as biliary-related. All patients with acute pancreatitis should undergo abdominal ultrasound, searching for cholecystolithiasis, common bile duct stones, or signs of biliary obstruction (biliary tract dilatation). A close relationship has been described between circulating levels of ALT at admission and acute biliary pancreatitis. In this sense, a serum ALT level greater than two or three times the upper limit of normal has a positive predictive value of 95% for the diagnosis of gallstone

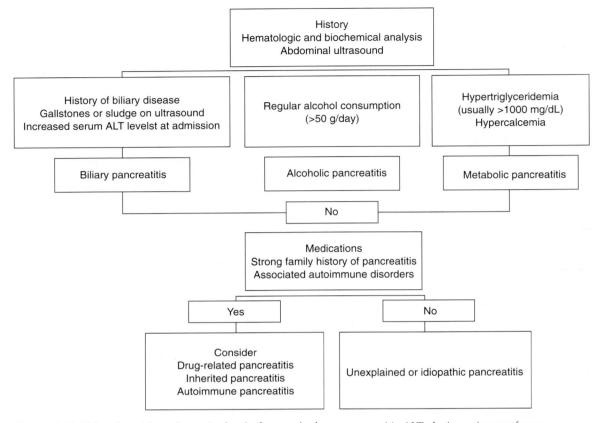

Figure 5.1 Guidelines for etiologic diagnosis after the first attack of acute pancreatitis. ALT, alanine aminotransferase.

pancreatitis. Circulating levels of bilirubin or alkaline phosphatase have less impact.

The development of pancreatitis during pharmacologic treatment in patients without any other etiologic factor is the basis for the diagnosis of drug-related pancreatitis. In these cases, pancreatitis should resolve on discontinuation of the drug and usually recurs upon its readministration.

A first episode of acute pancreatitis that cannot be explained by history, laboratory tests, and abdominal ultrasound should be classified as idiopathic or unexplained pancreatitis (Fig. 5.1). If chronic pancreatitis or pancreatic tumors are not suspected, further investigations are not required. Any alcohol consumption should be completely avoided and the presence of mild to moderate hyperlipidemia should be treated accordingly. By doing so, the risk of recurrence of acute pancreatitis is low, probably below 5% within the following 3–5 years.

Further investigations should be limited to relapsing attacks of previous unexplained pancreatitis. If this occurs, chronic pancreatitis, pancreatic tumor, and any cause of obstructive pancreatitis (pancreas divisum, sphincter of Oddi dysfunction, ampullary or periampullary disorders) should be excluded. This can be done using magnetic resonance imaging (MRI) and magnetic resonance cholangiopancreatography with intravenous gadolinium and secretin administration respectively. This exploration, which can be performed as a single procedure, provides highly accurate imaging of both pancreatic parenchyma and ducts as well as dynamic information on blood supply and pancreatic secretion. Depending on local availability, endoscopic ultrasound and dynamic computed tomography (CT) may be reserved for patients with doubtful or inconclusive findings on MRI (Fig. 5.2). This approach can be also applied to patients after the first attack of severe necrotizing pancreatitis,

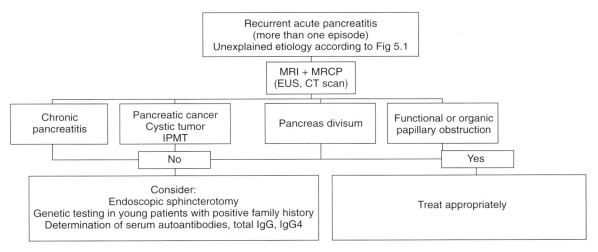

Figure 5.2 Guidelines for etiologic diagnosis in patients with recurrent unexplained or idiopathic pancreatitis. CT, computed tomography; EUS, endoscopic ultrasound; IPMT, intraductal papillary mucinous tumor; MRCP, magnetic resonance cholangiopancreatography; MRI, magnetic resonance imaging.

in whom recurrence of the disease is likely to be severe.

Any of the above-mentioned abnormalities demonstrated by MRI, endoscopic ultrasound, or CT should be managed accordingly. The presence of pancreas divisum may be considered as the cause of acute pancreatitis if a relative obstruction to the flow of pancreatic juice through the minor papilla is demonstrated. This occurs mainly in patients with relapsing pancreatitis and a dilated Santorini duct with normal-appearing Wirsung duct. Pancreas divisum is most probably not the cause of pancreatitis if the Santorini duct is normal appearing and therefore no invasive therapy should be performed in these cases.

Microlithiasis is a frequent cause of acute relapsing pancreatitis in patients with unexplained disease. Bile microscopy may be performed, but empirical treatment with ursodeoxycholic acid is an acceptable alternative. Performance of endoscopic sphincterotomy is usually preferred in these cases of unexplained acute relapsing pancreatitis (Fig. 5.2). This endoscopic approach will be successful not only in cases of microlithiasis but also in cases of sphincter of Oddi dysfunction or papillary stenosis. Because of the risk of pancreatitis, sphincter of Oddi manometry is not performed routinely. Therefore, endoscopic sphincterotomy is a valid option if sphincter dysfunction is suspected.

Finally, acute pancreatitis may be considered as

potentially inherited in young patients with a strong positive family history of pancreatic diseases. A genetic study is indicated in these cases to confirm the etiology of the disease, although appropriate genetic counseling is mandatory before and after performing any genetic test. Laboratory tests for autoimmunity (serum autoantibodies, total IgG, and IgG subtypes, mainly IgG4) should also be performed even in the absence of any other autoimmune disorder if no other potential cause of acute relapsing pancreatitis is detected (Fig. 5.2).

Recommended reading

Carballo F, Domínguez-Muñoz JE, Martínez-Pancorbo C, de la Morena J. Epidemiology of acute pancreatitis. In: HG Beger, M Büchler, P Malfertheiner (eds) *Standards in Pancreatic Surgery*. Berlin: Springer-Verlag, 1993: 25–33.

Domínguez-Muñoz JE, Malfertheiner P, Ditschuneit HH *et al.* Hyperlipidemia in acute pancreatitis: relationship with etiology, onset and severity of the disease. *Int J Pancreatol* 1991;10:261–267.

Domínguez-Muñoz JE, Junemann F, Malfertheiner P. Hyperlipidemia in acute pancreatitis: cause or epiphenomenon? *Int J Pancreatol* 1995;18:101–106.

Fortson MR, Freedman SN, Webster PD III. Clinical assessment of hyperlipidaemic pancreatitis. *Am J Gastroenterol* 1995;90:2134–2139.

Hanck C, Singer MV. Does acute alcoholic pancreatitis exist without pre-existing chronic pancreatitis? *Scand J Gastroenterol* 1997;32:625–626.

Kaw M, Brodmerkel GJ Jr. ERCP, biliary crystal analysis and sphincter of Oddi manometry in idiopathic recurrent pancreatitis. *Gastrointest Endosc* 2002;55:157–162.

Lankisch PG, Droge M, Gottesleben F. Drug-induced pancreatitis: incidence and severity. *Gut* 1995;37:565–567.

Lee SP, Nichols JF, Park HZ. Biliary sludge as a cause of acute pancreatitis. *N Engl J Med* 1992;326:589–593.

Lehman GA, Sherman S. Pancreas divisum: diagnosis, clinical significance, and management alternatives. *Gastrointest Endosc Clin North Am* 1995;5:145–170.

Lerch MM, Weidenbach H, Hernandez CA, Preclick G, Adler G. Pancreatic outflow obstruction as the critical event for human gallstone-induced pancreatitis. *Gut* 1994;35:1501–1503.

McArthur KE. Drug-induced pancreatitis. *Aliment Pharmacol Ther* 1996;10:23–38.

Moreau JA, Zinsmeister AR, Melton LJ, DiMagno EP. Gallstone pancreatitis and the effect of cholecystectomy: a population-based cohort study. *Mayo Clin Proc* 1988;63:466–473.

Parenti DM, Steinberg W, King P. Infectious causes of pancreatitis. *Pancreas* 1996;13:356–371.

Ros E, Navarro S, Bru C *et al.* Occult microlithiasis in "idiopathic" acute pancreatitis: prevention of relapses by cholecystectomy or ursodeoxycholic acid therapy. *Gastroenterology* 1991;101:1701–1709.

Singh M. Etiology and epidemiology of alcohol-induced pancreatitis. In: HG Beger, AL Warshaw, MW Büchler *et al.* (eds) *The Pancreas*. Oxford: Blackwell Science, 1998: 275–282.

Steinberg WM, Geenen JE, Bradley EL III, Barkin JS. Controversies in clinical pancreatology. Recurrent "idiopathic" acute pancreatitis: should a laparoscopic cholecystectomy be the first procedure of choice? *Pancreas* 1996;13:329–334.

Tenner S, Dubner H, Steinberg W. Predicting gallstone pancreatitis with laboratory parameters: a meta-analysis. *Am J Gastroenterol* 1994;89:1863–1866.

Testoni PA, Caporuscio S, Bagnolo F, Lella F. Idiopathic recurrent pancreatitis: long-term results alter ERCP, endoscopic sphicterotomy, or ursodeoxycholic acid treatment. *Am J Gastroenterol* 2000;95:1702–1707.

Toouli J, Brooke-Smith M, Bassi C *et al.* Working party report. Guidelines for the management of acute pancreatitis. *J Gastroenterol Hepatol* 2002;17(Suppl 1):15–39.

Warshaw AL. Pancreas divisum and pancreatitis. In: HG Beger, AL Warshaw, MW Büchler *et al.* (eds) *The Pancreas*. Oxford: Blackwell Science, 1998: 364–374.

6

Early prognostic evaluation of acute pancreatitis: why and how should severity be predicted?

J. Enrique Domínguez-Muñoz

One of the most relevant features of acute pancreatitis is the great variability in clinical severity. Most patients with acute pancreatitis (80–85% in most series) present with a mild and self-limiting disease. These patients require just general supportive therapy consisting of fasting, analgesics, and intravenous fluids for a few days. Conversely, 15–20% of patients with acute pancreatitis develop some major local and/or systemic complications of the disease, frequently leading to multiple organ failure and death. Severe acute pancreatitis was clearly defined in 1992 by a wide group of experts in the so-called Atlanta classification as a disease associated with the failure of one or more organs and/or with the development of local complications such as necrosis, abscess, or pseudocysts (see Chapter 1 for details). These severe cases require early intensive monitoring and treatment, including appropriate nutrition, prevention of infection of the pancreatic necrosis, and endoscopic sphincterotomy in cases with a biliary etiology, together with intensive systemic support.

Since 1974, when John Ranson reported the first prognostic scoring system for acute pancreatitis, a large variety of multifactorial systems and single biochemical markers have been extensively evaluated with the aim of predicting the severity of the disease. Despite these research efforts, the need for early prognostic evaluation of acute pancreatitis has been strongly questioned for several reasons.

• The clinical relevance of the prognostic evaluation of acute pancreatitis was markedly limited by the lack of specific therapeutic consequences.

• A generally accepted definition of severe acute pancreatitis was not available before 1993, when the Atlanta classification was published. At that time, most

studies on prognostic evaluation of the disease had already been published. Because of this, different definitions of severe acute pancreatitis were applied in different studies and a direct comparison among studies was not possible.

• Most prognostic markers reported in the literature were evaluated under clinical research conditions. Thus, biological samples (serum, plasma, or urine) were obtained in optimal conditions, immediately frozen, and stored until analysis. Samples were then analyzed together by a highly motivated researcher. Therefore, it has been questioned whether the reported results for the sensitivity and specificity of these prognostic markers is reproducible under routine clinical conditions.

• Methods for determination of most markers, such as enzyme immunoassay or radioimmunoassay, are hardly applicable to the daily routine of an emergency laboratory.

• Finally, application of most prognostic scoring systems is cumbersome and needs up to 48 hours for quantification.

Why should severity of acute pancreatitis be predicted?

Despite the points mentioned above, severity prediction has received consistent attention over the last three decades. One of the most important reasons for this, from the very earliest studies to the most recent, was the possibility of providing stratification of disease severity and thus objective comparison of the response to any tested therapy in different patient populations. More-

47

over, comparisons among different series of patients and different centers would be possible.

The wide acceptance of the definitions provided by the Atlanta classification of acute pancreatitis has markedly improved the likelihood of both evaluating the accuracy of different prognostic markers and comparing the results obtained from different series of patients and centers. In addition, as a consequence of the international recognition of the Atlanta definitions of local and systemic complications of acute pancreatitis, our knowledge of the natural history of the severe disease and of the effect of several therapeutic measures on it has markedly improved.

Over the past few years, there has been important progress in our knowledge of the pathophysiology of severe acute pancreatitis. In this context, and independently of the cause of acute pancreatitis, the development of systemic inflammatory response syndrome (SIRS) is associated with a severe course of the disease. Since SIRS is an early event after the intrapancreatic activation of pancreatic enzymes, acute pancreatitis is characterized by a small therapeutic window, most probably limited to the first 72 hours from onset of the disease. Any therapeutic measure in acute pancreatitis should be applied early, within the time window of 72 hours from onset, so that it has a positive effect on morbidity and mortality.

Although no specific therapy is available for acute pancreatitis, several advances have occurred over the last few years. Randomized studies have shown that patients with acute necrotizing pancreatitis may benefit from early antibiotic prophylaxis of infected pancreatic necrosis. Furthermore, early enteral nutrition is able to reduce complications and even mortality in severe acute pancreatitis when compared with parenteral nutrition. It is also generally accepted that patients with severe gallstone-induced pancreatitis may benefit from early endoscopic sphincterotomy. Finally, several pharmacologic therapies, such as protease inhibitors and immune-modulator drugs (e.g., cytokine inhibitors and antiinflammatory drugs), may play an important therapeutic role in severe acute pancreatitis, provided they can be started early enough.

Taking all these aspects into consideration, it is nowadays absolutely necessary to identify in advance those patients at high risk of developing a severe course of acute pancreatitis. All presently used and future therapies for severe acute pancreatitis are expensive and not without complications and/or adverse events.

We should also not forget that the vast majority of patients with acute pancreatitis will have mild disease and thus will not benefit from any of the therapies mentioned above. Therefore, there is a real need for the use of a severity marker in clinical routine, which should be able to provide reliable prognostic information about acute pancreatitis within the first hours of evolution.

Simple and easily applicable laboratory methods for quantification of biochemical markers are being developed. In this way, simpler tests for the determination of markers such as polymorphonuclear (PMN) elastase or trypsinogen activation peptide (TAP), which were considered reliable for the prognostic evaluation of acute pancreatitis but not under clinically routine conditions, are now available or emerging. As other new biochemical methods are developed, the early prognostic evaluation of acute pancreatitis, even on admission, will be more widely accepted and applied to the clinical routine.

How can severity of acute pancreatitis be predicted?

Hundreds of papers have reported over the last three decades on a wide variety of clinical parameters, single biochemical markers, scoring systems, and imaging procedures for predicting severe pancreatitis. Most of these parameters have found no place in clinical practice, because of either low reliability or high complexity. The aim of this chapter is to focus on those parameters that have gained popularity among clinicians and on those with a high accuracy in the prognostic evaluation of acute pancreatitis.

Although it is well known that clinical examination on admission often fails to detect severe pancreatitis, even in experienced hands, it has been proposed that several clinical parameters influence the course of the disease. Despite some controversies, the etiology of acute pancreatitis should not be considered as associated with severity of the disease. Advancing age is associated with a higher mortality rate, whereas complications and even mortality are more frequent in obese patients. Fever, tetanus, palpable abdominal mass, paralytic ileus, and Cullen's sign and Grey Turner's sign have been related to severe pancreatitis. Finally, pleural effusion is also a sign of severe disease. However, none of these parameters *per se* are accurate enough to predict severe pancreatitis.

Imaging procedures, mainly contrast-enhanced computed tomography (CT), are able to detect and define the extent of pancreatic necrosis and retroperitoneal effusion and, as a whole, to define the degree of local severity of acute pancreatitis. Emil Balthazar discusses these procedures in detail in the next chapter of this book.

Multiple factor scoring systems, such as those reported by Ranson and the Glasgow group, or more recently the Acute Physiology and Chronic Health Evaluation (APACHE) II score have been widely used in clinical practice despite relative complexity and limited positive predictive value for severity. The usefulness of these systems is discussed below.

Among biochemical markers, necrosis markers such as methemalbumin or pancreatic ribonuclease, protease inhibitors such as α_1-protease inhibitor or α_2-macroglobulin, complement factors such as C3 or C4, and markers for leakage of pancreatic enzymes such as amylase, lipase, or trypsinogen-2 have been assayed without success. More recently, markers of inflammatory response and markers of pancreatic enzyme activation have demonstrated a high prognostic accuracy in the early stages of acute pancreatitis.

Scoring systems

Scoring systems consist of several clinical and laboratory parameters that correlate with the outcome of acute pancreatitis. Two general types of scoring system, depending on whether or not they were specifically developed for acute pancreatitis, have been evaluated. Specific scoring systems are those described by Ranson and the variants from the Glasgow and Hong Kong groups.

Ranson and Glasgow scores are applied worldwide. They consist of 8–11 variables that, in a multivariable model, are significantly associated with a severe outcome in acute pancreatitis (Tables 6.1 and 6.2). Whereas the Ranson score was defined for a population mainly comprising alcoholic pancreatitis, the Glasgow criteria were equally effective predictors of mortality regardless of etiology. Despite their wide use, extensive evaluation of these scoring systems has identified some important limitations that hinder their clinical usefulness.

1 They generally need 48 hours to be calculated. Taking into account the time from onset of the disease to admission, this additional 48-hour period for predic-

Table 6.1 Ranson's scoring system for the prognostic evaluation of acute pancreatitis. Severe pancreatitis is defined by the presence of three or more criteria.

At admission
Age > 55 years
White blood cells > 16 000/mm³
Lactate dehydrogenase > 350 U/L
Aspartate aminotransferase > 250 U/L
Glucose > 200 mg/dL

Within 48 hours
Hematocrit decrease > 10%
Blood urea nitrogen increase > 5 mg/dL
Serum calcium < 8 mg/dL
Pa_{O_2} < 60 mmHg
Base deficit > 4 mEq/L
Fluid sequestration > 6 L

Table 6.2 Glasgow scoring system for the prognostic evaluation of acute pancreatitis during initial 48 hours. Severe pancreatitis is defined by the presence of three or more criteria.

White blood cell > 15 000/mm³
Glucose > 10 mmol/L (no history of diabetes)
Serum urea > 16 mmol/L
Pa_{O_2} < 60 mmHg
Serum calcium < 2.0 mmol/L
Lactate dehydrogenase > 600 U/L
Aspartate aminotransferase/alanine aminotransferase > 250 U/L
Albumin < 3.2 g/dL

tion of severity limits the possibility of starting the appropriate treatment within the tight therapeutic window of acute pancreatitis.

2 These scoring systems have limited positive predictive value for severity. The accuracy of the Ranson and Glasgow criteria in the prognostic evaluation of acute pancreatitis has been extensively investigated, the sensitivity of these systems ranging from 40 to 88% and the specificity from 43 to 99%. It is accepted that the probability that a patient with zero to two Ranson or Glasgow criteria has a severe course of the disease is extremely low. In this sense, the negative predictive value for severity tends to be higher than 90% (starting from a probability of mild disease of 80%). Therefore, these

scoring systems could be useful for detecting those patients who do not require any intensive monitoring and therapy. However, the ability of these systems to predict severe disease is very low, with a positive predictive value consistently below 50% (starting from a probability of severe disease of 20%).

3 These scoring systems do not allow patients to be followed up and the course of the disease to be monitored. Because of all these limitations, Ranson and Glasgow scoring systems should no longer be applied in the prognostic evaluation of acute pancreatitis in clinical routine.

The APACHE II score was developed to predict the probability of death secondary to a variety of diseases. It consists of an acute physiology score and a preadmission health score (chronic health score) that is based on severe chronic preexistent diseases (Table 6.3). The main advantage of the APACHE II score is that it can be calculated on admission and daily thereafter, in comparison with the 48-hour wait required for the Ranson and Glasgow systems. In this way, the APACHE II score may be useful in the early prognostic evaluation of acute pancreatitis as well as for close monitoring of the disease.

Several studies have evaluated the accuracy of APACHE II system in the early prognostic evaluation of acute pancreatitis. Compared with Ranson and Glasgow criteria, APACHE II shows a similar sensitivity and specificity, with a negative predictive value for severity higher than 90% for scores equal to or less than 7. Similarly to Ranson and Glasgow criteria, APACHE II shows a positive predictive value for severity of around 50% for scores of more than 7. This accuracy is even lower if only the acute physiology score of the APACHE II classification is considered, the so-called simplified acute physiology score.

Nevertheless, APACHE II offers an opportunity to recalculate scores daily. This may be of clinical relevance, since severe attacks are associated with increasing scores over the first 48 hours, whereas mild attacks show decreasing scores. Therefore, the APACHE II system is widely used in clinical routine and should be preferred to Ranson or Glasgow criteria. In addition, APACHE II has been the prognostic classification system used for including patients in clinical trials on acute pancreatitis over the last few years. However, the low positive predictive value for severity and the complexity of evaluating and scoring so many variables (see Table 6.3) hinder the clinical usefulness of this scoring system.

The finding that obesity (O) is associated with a more severe course of acute pancreatitis has recently led several authors to add these clinical data to the APACHE II classification in the so-called APACHE-O score. Body mass index (BMI) is categorized as normal (score 0), overweight (BMI 26–30, score 1), or obese (BMI > 30, score 2). Addition of the score for obesity to the APACHE II score increases the predictive accuracy, and positive predictive values for severity higher than 70% have been reported.

Markers of protease activation

The role of protease activation markers in the early prognostic evaluation of acute pancreatitis is based on the positive correlation found between the degree of protease activation and the extent of pancreatic injury in the course of the disease. It is generally accepted that trypsinogen activation is one of the earliest events in the pathogenesis of acute pancreatitis. As a second step, the generated active trypsin is thought to be the key factor in the activation of other pancreatic proteases such as procarboxypeptidase B and prophospholipase A_2. Activation of proenzymes is produced by the cleavage of a peptide chain that masks the active site of the enzyme. During the process of enzyme activation, this peptide chain, usually called the activation peptide, is locally released; it enters the bloodstream and is finally excreted into the urine. Serum and urinary levels of activation peptides are therefore directly related to the amount of activated enzymes and are thus associated with the severity of local damage during acute pancreatitis. Among activation peptides, markers of trypsinogen, procarboxypeptidase, and prophospholipase A_2 activation are the most extensively studied.

TAP is the most studied activation peptide in acute pancreatitis. TAP concentrations in urine increase very early after the onset of the disease and reach maximal levels within the first 24 hours. This increase is significantly higher in patients with a severe course of acute pancreatitis than in those with mild disease. Urinary TAP levels decrease very quickly thereafter and this peptide is almost undetectable after 3–4 days. This rapid decrease limits the use of this prognostic marker to the time of admission. In addition, TAP is not useful in the daily monitoring of severity of the disease.

Together with several local studies, two large multicenter studies have investigated the predictive value of urinary TAP in detemination of severity in acute pan-

Table 6.3 APACHE II severity of disease classification system.

Physiologic variable	High abnormal range				0	Low abnormal range			
	+4	+3	+2	+1	0	+1	+2	+3	+4
Temperature, rectal (°C)	≥41	39–40.9		38.5–38.9	36–38.4	34–35.9	32–33.9	30–31.9	″29.9
MAP (mmHg)*	≥160	130–159	110–129		70–109		50–69		″49
Heart rate (bpm)	≥180	140–179	110–139		70–109		55–69	40–54	″39
Respiratory rate	≥50	35–49		25–34	12–24	10–11	6–9		″5
Oxygenation†									
A-aDo_2 (mmHg)	≥500	350–499	200–349		<200				
Pao_2 (mmHg)					>70	61–70		55–60	<55
Arterial pH	≥7.7	7.6–7.69		7.5–7.59	7.33–7.49		7.25–7.32	7.15–7.24	″7.15
Serum sodium (mmol/L)	≥180	160–179	155–159	150–154	130–149		120–129	111–119	″110
Serum potassium (mmol/L)	≥7	6–6.9		5.6–5.9	3.5–5.4	3–3.4	2.5–2.9		<2.5
Serum creatinine (mg/dL)‡	≥3.5	2–3.4	1.5–1.9		0.6–1.4		<0.6		
Hematocrit (%)	≥60		50–59.9	46–49.9	30–45.9		20–29.9		<20
White blood cells (×10³/mm³)	≥40		20–39.9	15–19.9	3–14.9		1–2.9		<1
Glasgow Coma Scale (GCS)					Score = 15 minus actual GCS				
Total acute physiology score (A) = sum of the 12 individual variable points									
Serum HCO₃⁻§	≥52	41–51.9		32–40.9	22–31.9		18–21.9	15–17.9	<15

B Age: < 44 years, 0 points; 45–54 years, 2 points; 55–64 years, 3 points; 65–74 years, 5 points; > 75 years, 6 points

C Chronic health points. If any of the following five categories is answered with yes, give +5 points for nonoperative or emergency postoperative patient
Liver: cirrhosis with portal hypertension or encephalopathy
Cardiovascular: class IV angina or at rest or with minimal self-care activities
Pulmonary: chronic hypoxemia or hypercapnia or polycythemia of pulmonary hypertension > 40 mmHg
Kidney: chronic peritoneal dialysis or hemodialysis
Immune: immune-compromised host

APACHE II score = **A + B + C**

* MAP, mean arterial pressure = (2 × diastolic + systolic)/3.
† Fio_2 > 0.5, record A-aDo_2; Fio_2 < 0.5, record only Pao_2.
‡ Double point for acute renal failure.
§ Venous mmol/L (not preferred, use instead of arterial pH if no arterial blood gas analysis is available).

creatitis. The results of these two studies are far from consistent, with sensitivities and specificities ranging from 58 to 100% and from 73 to 85% respectively. These findings, together with a rather low positive pre- dictive value for severity (as low as 35% at 48 hours in one of the studies), limit the clinical usefulness of uri- nary TAP measurement for prediction of severity in acute pancreatitis, which may be limited to the first 24 hours from onset of symptoms. In addition, TAP is quantified by an enzyme immunoassay that is still too complex and expensive to be applied for routine use in an emergency laboratory. New technologies based on rapid strips or "immunosticks" are being developed and could be an adequate tool for early prognostic evaluation of acute pancreatitis on admission.

The procarboxypeptidase activation peptide (CAPAP) is larger than TAP and thus more stable and easier to quantify. CAPAP levels in serum and urine correlate well with severity of the disease and show accuracy in the prognostic evaluation of acute pancreatitis that seems to be higher than that of TAP. As for TAP, the prognostic usefulness of CAPAP is limited to the first 24–48 hours from onset of symptoms and levels decrease quickly so that they are not useful for daily monitoring of the disease. Although a radioimmunoassay for CAPAP determination is commercially available, it is still too complex and expensive to be readily applied to clinical routine.

Recently, an enzyme immunoassay for quantification of phospholipase A_2 activation peptide (PLAP) has been developed. Although experience with PLAP determination is still limited, this may be a relevant marker in the future for evaluation of severity of acute pancreatitis. This is due to the fact that PLAP is released after activation of both pancreatic as well as granulocytic phospholipase A_2. In this way, a single parameter could reflect the intensity of the two central events in the pathogenesis of severe acute pancreatitis, i.e., pancreatic enzyme activation and the systemic inflammatory response.

Markers of inflammatory response

Independent of the etiology of acute pancreatitis, the initial cell damage in the gland induces the very early release of several inflammatory mediators such as interleukin (IL)-8 and oxygen-derived free radicals. These locally released inflammatory mediators attract granulocytes and monocytes/macrophages, which release large amounts of oxygen-derived free radicals, proteases, phospholipase, and cytokines. Excessive stimulation of the inflammatory and immune response leads to the development of SIRS, which is associated with the development of complications and a severe course of acute pancreatitis (Fig. 6.1). Therefore, quantification of circulating levels of inflammatory and immune markers allows evaluation of the intensity of the inflammatory and immune response, which correlates with the severity of acute pancreatitis.

Several inflammatory mediators have been evaluated in the context of acute pancreatitis. Among them, granulocyte (PMN) elastase, tumor necrosis factor (TNF), IL-6 and IL-8, and C-reactive protein (CRP) should be underlined. Although markers of inflammation are obviously not specific for acute pancreatitis, they can be used not only for early prognostic evaluation of the disease but also for monitoring its clinical course.

The correlation between plasma levels of PMN elastase and severity of acute pancreatitis is so close that it allows differentiation between mild and severe disease with high accuracy on admission, within the first 24 hours from onset of symptoms. Plasma PMN elastase reaches maximum levels between 24 and 48 hours after

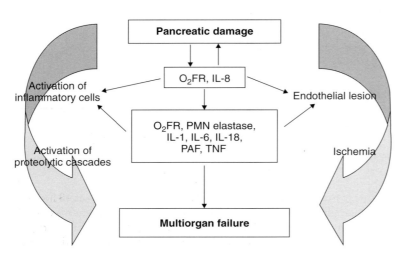

Figure 6.1 Pathophysiology of multiple organ failure in patients with acute pancreatitis. O_2FR, oxygen-derived free radicals; IL, interleukin; PMN, polymorphonuclear; PAF, platelet-activating factor; TNF, tumor necrosis factor.

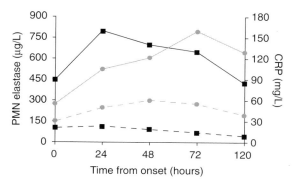

■—■ Serum PMN-elastase levels, severe attacks
■- -■ Serum PMN-elastase levels, mild attacks
●—● Serum CRP levels, severe attacks
●- -● Serum CRP levels, mild attacks

Figure 6.2 Circulating levels of polymorphonuclear (PMN) elastase and C-reactive protein (CRP) in patients with mild and severe attacks of acute pancreatitis. ■, Plasma PMN elastase; ●, serum CRP. Mild attacks of acute pancreatitis are shown as dashed lines, severe attacks as solid lines.

disease onset and then starts to decline over the following days (Fig. 6.2). Its sensitivity and specificity in the prognostic evaluation of acute pancreatitis are as high as 85–95%, with a negative predictive value for severity close to 100%. Most importantly, the positive predictive value for severity is even higher than 80% (starting from the known pretest probability of severe disease of 20%). The previous methodologic limitations related to quantification of PMN elastase by enzyme immunoassay have been overcome by the development of a method based on latex immunoagglutination. This method allows automated determination of PMN elastase that can be applied to the daily clinical routine.

Several interleukins have been evaluated in the early prognostic classification of acute pancreatitis. They are mainly released by activated monocytes/macrophages. Similarly to PMN elastase, circulating IL-1 and IL-6 levels increase within the first 24 hours of disease and allow differentiation between mild and severe acute pancreatitis with high accuracy. IL-8 is released even earlier, partly from damaged pancreatic cells, and circulating peak concentrations occur 12 hours from onset of acute pancreatitis. Results on TNF in acute pancreatitis are inconsistent because of the known intermittent release of this cytokine. As an alternative, circulating levels of soluble TNF receptor, which are

directly related to the amount of released TNF, have a longer half-life and can be more easily measured. Soluble TNF receptor levels are significantly increased in severe acute pancreatitis compared with mild disease, and are even more increased in severe patients who develop organ failure. Although cytokines could be reliable markers of severity in acute pancreatitis, their clinical applicability is hindered by methodologic complexity and costs.

The most widely used serum marker for the prognostic evaluation of acute pancreatitis is CRP. Liver synthesis of CRP is induced by released interleukins, mainly IL-1 and IL-6. Thus serum CRP levels in acute pancreatitis increase later than interleukins or PMN elastase, and peak about 72 hours from onset of symptoms (Fig. 6.2). The accuracy of serum CRP for the prognostic evaluation of acute pancreatitis has been extensively investigated. Serum CRP levels higher than 120–160 mg/L are likely associated with a severe course of the disease. The sensitivity and specificity of this marker for classification of severity in acute pancreatitis is to some extent lower than that reported for PMN elastase or interleukins, but higher than that of any scoring system. A strong correlation has been described between CRP and pancreatic and peripancreatic necrosis, which permits prediction of the presence of necrosis with a sensitivity and specificity greater than 80%. Based on this, serum CRP quantification may be an adequate marker for selecting those patients who require contrast-enhanced CT. Finally, since determination of CRP is technically simple, fast, and widely available, this marker can still be considered the reference for prognostic evaluation of acute pancreatitis. However, it should be remembered that the highest accuracy for CRP is reached at 72 hours from onset of symptoms, just at the end of the therapeutic window of acute pancreatitis, when most treatments should be already instituted. Therefore, CRP is far from being the optimal prognostic marker of acute pancreatitis and methodologic progress is awaited to help in the applicability of earlier and highly accurate markers for the prognostic evaluation of acute pancreatitis in clinical routine.

Early prognostic evaluation of acute pancreatitis in clinical practice

Prognostic evaluation of acute pancreatitis is a key step in the management of the disease immediately after diagnosis. This allows patients with mild disease to be treated conservatively, avoiding expensive therapies that are not without complications and adverse events. As important, intensive monitoring and therapies including enteral nutrition, antibiotic prophylaxis, and/or endoscopic sphincterotomy can be applied within the tight therapeutic window in patients classified as suffering from severe disease.

The relative complexity and principally the low positive predictive value for defining severity in acute pancreatitis limit the clinical usefulness of any scoring system. Ranson and Glasgow criteria are no longer recommended. Instead, APACHE II and mainly APACHE-O are more appropriate alternatives. Nevertheless, since the positive predictive value of these systems for detecting severity in acute pancreatitis is also low, they are basically recommended for monitoring the course of the disease and not for early prognostic evaluation.

The most accurate and earliest markers of severity in acute pancreatitis are those that reflect the intensity of the systemic inflammatory response and those related to the extent of pancreatic enzyme activation. With the exception of PMN elastase, the clinical applicability of these markers is hindered by methodologic limitations. Despite showing a delayed increase in serum, CRP is a valid alternative and useful in clinical practice because of technical simplicity and wide availability. Based on current consensus, severe acute pancreatitis is defined by a serum CRP concentration higher than 150 mg/L within the first 72 hours of disease.

New technologies are being developed for quantification of some of the early and accurate prognostic markers described above (TAP, cytokines, etc.). In addition, several new and promising markers are being evaluated and may change the concept of both early prognostic evaluation and disease monitoring in acute pancreatitis in the near future. Among these markers are serum amyloid A and especially procalcitonin, which are already used in many centers worldwide and could be easily applied to acute pancreatitis in clinical practice.

Recommended reading

Andrén-Sandberg A, Borgström A. Early prediction of severity in acute pancreatitis. Is this possible? *J Pancreatol* 2002;3:116–125.

Beechy-Newman N, Rae D, Sumar N, Hermon-Taylor J. Stratification of severity in acute pancreatitis by assay of trypsinogen and 1-prophospholipase A2 activation peptides. *Digestion* 1995;56:271–278.

Büchler M, Malfertheiner P, Schoetensack C et al. Sensitivity of antiproteases, complement factors and C-reactive protein in detecting pancreatic necrosis: results of a prospective study. *Int J Pancreatol* 1986;37:227–235.

DeBaux AC, Goldie AS, Ross JA et al. Serum concentrations of inflammatory mediators related to organ failure in patients with acute pancreatitis. *Br J Surg* 1996;83:349–353.

Dervenis C, Johnson CD, Bassi C et al. Diagnosis, objective assessment of severity and management of acute pancreatitis. *Int J Pancreatol* 1999;25:195–200.

Domínguez-Muñoz JE, Carballo F, García MJ et al. Clinical usefulness of polymorphonuclear elastase in predicting the severity of acute pancreatitis: results of a multicentre study. *Br J Surg* 1991;78:1230–1234.

Domínguez-Muñoz JE, Carballo F, García MJ et al. Evaluation of the clinical usefulness of APACHE-II and SAPS systems in the initial prognostic classification of acute pancreatitis: a multicenter study. *Pancreas* 1993;8:682–686.

Domínguez-Muñoz JE, Carballo F, García MJ et al. Monitoring of serum proteinase–antiproteinase balance and systemic inflammatory response in the prognostic evaluation of acute pancreatitis: results of a prospective multicenter study. *Dig Dis Sci* 1993;38:507–512.

Johnson CD, Toh SKC, Campbell MJ. Combination of APACHE-II score and an obesity score (APACHE-O) for the prediction of severe acute pancreatitis. *Pancreatology* 2004;4:1–6.

Kylänpää-Bäck ML, Takala A, Kemppainen EA et al. Procalcitonin strip test in the early detection of severe acute pancreatitis. *Br J Surg* 2001;88:222–227.

Lankisch PG, Blum T, Maisonneuve P, Lowenfels AB. Severe acute pancreatitis: when to be concerned? *Pancreatology* 2003;3:102–110.

Larvin M, McMahon MJ. APACHE-II score for assessment and monitoring of acute pancreatitis. *Lancet* 1989;ii:201–205.

Müller C, Appelros S, Uhl W et al. Serum levels of procarboxypeptidase B and its activation peptide in patients with acute pancreatitis and non-pancreatic diseases. *Gut* 2002;51:229–235.

Neoptolemos J, Kemppainen E, Mayer J et al. Early prediction of severity in acute pancreatitis by urinary trypsinogen activation peptide: a multicentre study. *Lancet* 2000;355:1955–1960.

Pezzilli R, Billi P, Miniero R et al. Serum interleukin 6, interleukin 8 and alpha-2 microglobulin in early assessment of severity in acute pancreatitis. *Dig Dis Sci* 1995;40:2341–2348.

Tenner S, Fernández del Castillo C, Warshaw AL *et al.* Urinary trypsinogen activation peptide (TAP) predicts severity in patients with acute pancreatitis. *Int J Pancreatol* 1997;21: 105–110.

Triester SL, Kowdley KV. Prognostic factors in acute pancreatitis. *J Clin Gastroenterol* 2002;34:167–176.

Viedma JA, Pérez-Mateo M, Domínguez-Muñoz JE, Carballo F. Role of interleukin-6 in acute pancreatitis: comparison with C-reactive protein and phospholipase A. *Gut* 1992;33: 1264–1267.

Werner J, Hartwig W, Uhl W, Müller C, Büchler M. Useful markers for predicting severity and monitoring progression of acute pancreatitis. *Pancreatology* 2003;3:115–127.

Role of imaging methods in acute pancreatitis: diagnosis, staging, and detection of complications

Emil J. Balthazar and Glenn Krinsky

Introduction

Even though a wide range of pathophysiologic alterations with different corresponding clinical manifestations characterize every case of acute pancreatitis, a simple and useful classification was proposed at the 1992 International Symposium on Acute Pancreatitis in Atlanta, Georgia. In order to define the severity of an acute attack, pancreatitis was divided on a practical clinically relevant basis into mild and severe acute pancreatitis. Mild pancreatitis, previously referred to as edematous or interstitial pancreatitis, occurs in 70–80% of individuals. It is a mild self-limiting disease that resolves rapidly, has practically no mortality or morbidity, and has absent or minimal systemic manifestations or organ failure. Severe acute pancreatitis, previously called hemorrhagic or necrotizing pancreatitis, occurs in the minority of patients and exhibits systemic physiologic alterations, distal organ failure, a protracted clinical course, local abdominal complications, and a significant mortality rate.

This classification is based on the early depiction of two pathophysiologic phenomena: (i) the presence and degree of systemic manifestations and distal organ dysfunction (clinical and laboratory parameters) and (ii) the presence and extent of pancreatic necrosis. The early detection of pancreatic necrosis, which mainly depends on computed tomography (CT) performed with intravenously administered contrast material, has greatly improved the initial evaluation of patients with acute pancreatitis. Mortality rates of less than 1% in patients with edematous pancreatitis undergo a striking increase to 10–23% in patients with pancreatic necrosis. Lethal incidence of up to 67% occurs in pa-tients with extensive infected necrosis of the pancreatic gland, and most complications occur in patients with necrotizing pancreatitis. Secondary contamination occurs in 40–70% of patients with pancreatic necrosis and represents a major risk of death. Additionally, there is a direct relationship between the development of gland necrosis and the degree of systemic functional alterations. Multiorgan failure is much more common and more severe in patients with necrotizing pancreatitis and the majority of patients with lethal outcome have pancreatic necrosis. The importance of early demonstration of pancreatic necrosis is obvious and is further underlined by the required therapeutic measures given to this group of individuals. Patients with necrosis are closely monitored in the intensive care unit, their metabolic and organ failures are corrected, and follow-up CT examinations are routinely performed in this setting.

Limitations in clinical diagnosis

The clinical diagnosis of acute pancreatitis hinges on the association of clinical findings, mainly abdominal pain, nausea, and vomiting, with elevation of serum amylase level. Physical signs and clinical symptoms, including more severe manifestations such as epigastric fullness, tenderness, tachycardia, tachypnea, hypotension, and leukocytosis, herald the development of an acute abdominal condition but have no specificity. Since 1929 when Elman first reported on the diagnostic utility of serum amylase elevation, the clinical diagnosis of acute pancreatitis could be confirmed in the majority of these patients. However, there remain two broad categories of limitations that affect the usefulness of hyperamylasemia in detecting acute pancreatitis.

First, since hyperamylasemia has become the gold standard diagnostic procedure, the real sensitivity of this test in patients with acute pancreatitis is difficult to establish. It varies in different clinical studies between about 80 and 95%. Several factors can substantially lower the diagnostic sensitivity of serum amylase in acute pancreatitis. Serum pancreatic amylase tends to increase at the beginning of an acute attack of pancreatitis but often will rapidly (24–72 hours) return to normal levels. Elevated serum lipase levels usually decrease more slowly, showing a superior sensitivity particularly when there is delay in the initial blood sampling. It has been noticed that in up to one-third of patients with alcoholic pancreatitis the serum amylase may be normal. In patients with hyperlipidemia and acute pancreatitis, the serum amylase concentration remains within the normal range. Moreover, slight elevations are not as useful in clinical practice, whereas twofold or threefold elevations of serum amylase levels show higher sensitivities in diagnosing acute pancreatitis.

Second, several metabolic and acute abdominal disorders may present with hyperamylasemia, decreasing the specificity of this test in diagnosing acute pancreatitis. Among these disorders, acute biliary disease, perforated peptic ulcer, small bowel obstruction, closed loop obstruction, mesenteric vascular occlusion, and infarcted bowel have similar, overlapping clinical features. In a large review of patients with acute abdominal disorders, 20% showed hyperamylasemia but only 75% of individuals with high serum amylase levels had acute pancreatitis. In the past, for these reasons, diagnostic laporatomies were often performed to confirm the suspected clinical diagnosis and exclude other life-threatening acute abdominal conditions.

It is fair to conclude that the clinical diagnosis of patients with acute pancreatitis is plagued by uncertainties in many instances. It has been reported that in 30–40% of patients with severe pancreatitis the correct diagnosis was not made until the time of autopsy.

Limitations in clinical staging

Conspicuous clinical manifestations such as hypotension, respiratory distress, oliguria, and fever may be seen in patients with severe pancreatitis; however these signs lack specificity, develop usually late, and individually are poor predictive indicators of severity. The development of flank ecchymosis (Grey Turner's sign) or periumbilical ecchymosis (Cullen's sign) are more specific but appear late and are rarely seen. Based on the clinical evaluation alone, a severe attack of pancreatitis can be detected in only 34–39% of patients at the beginning of clinical onset.

Abnormal values of some routine laboratory tests are often encountered in acute pancreatitis and they may be helpful in forecasting the occurrence of a severe attack. A low serum calcium level (< 7.5 mg/dL), an elevated serum glucose level (> 250 mg/dL), and/or a high serum creatinine level (> 2 mg/dL) correlate grossly with increased lethality. Furthermore, several biologically active substances (vasoactive peptides, inflammatory mediators, and cytokines) are found in the bloodstream, ascitic fluid, and urine of patients with acute pancreatitis. It has been postulated that measurements of some of these toxic compounds may reveal the development of an acute attack. Tumor necrosis factor, pancreatic ribonuclease, phospholipase A_2, polymorphonuclear elastase, and trypsinogen-activated peptide are only a few more commonly mentioned in the literature. The clinical usefulness of some of these solitary laboratory parameters is limited, whereas the utility of the others as reliable predictive indicators of severity remains to be proven.

Since individual clinical and laboratory parameters are unable to reliably identify patients with severe pancreatitis, numerical systems have been devised and used in clinical practice. These grading systems count the number of systemic and laboratory abnormalities (called prognostic indices, risk factors, or grave signs) and correlate them with mortality rates. The first numerical system, developed by Ranson and colleagues, is based on 11 objective signs, five calculated at the beginning of an acute attack and six within the first 48 hours. With an increasing number of grave signs there is a corresponding increase in morbidity and mortality. Patients with less than three grave signs are considered to have mild pancreatitis, whereas patients with more than six grave signs have severe pancreatitis and a very high mortality rate. Inaccuracies in staging and prediction of outcome are still seen in patients with three to six grave signs.

After 1974, several other grading systems, each using slightly different objective parameters, were proposed, with a prognostic ability similar to that of the Ranson system. Apparently a slightly more reliable numerical system is the Acute Physiology and Chronic Health Evaluation (APACHE II), which is being used not only at the onset of an acute attack but also to monitor patients' response to treatment in the intensive care unit.

Although useful in clinical practice, two serious shortcomings characterize numerical systems: overall accuracy is about 70–80% with a sensitivity of 57–85%. Additionally, it should be stressed that the depicted abnormalities reflect metabolic and distal organ dysfunction; they do not assess severity of intraabdominal disease and obviously they have no diagnostic specificity being seen in other acute abdominal conditions.

The use of imaging modalities and radiologic procedures are intended to complement the clinical diagnostic and staging systems in our quest to improve the evaluation and management of patients with acute pancreatitis.

Imaging modalities

Early attempts to use noninvasive radiologic procedures in the evaluation of patients suspected of having acute pancreatitis focused on conventional plain abdominal films, chest films, and barium gastrointestinal examinations. These studies were used mainly to confirm the clinical diagnosis and detect local complications following attacks of severe pancreatitis. Since the pancreatic gland could not be seen, only secondary abnormalities, mainly affecting adjacent segments of the gastrointestinal tract, could be detected. While sometimes useful, the drawbacks included lack of specificity and low sensitivity because only severe secondary findings presumed to be induced by acute pancreatitis could be perceived. In the past 25 years, with the development of more reliable noninvasive techniques, imaging evaluation of acute pancreatitis has shifted almost entirely toward CT imaging, with sonography and magnetic resonance imaging (MRI) as complementary modalities.

Ultrasonography

Despite technical improvements with the use of real-time high-resolution equipment, color and spectral Doppler analysis, and optimal scanning techniques, sonography plays only a secondary role in the evaluation of acute pancreatitis. Overlying bowel gas often hinders the visualization of the pancreatic gland, rendering the examination limited in scope and quality. Nevertheless, ultrasound examinations are performed in most patients with pancreatitis for at least two main reasons: detection of biliary stones and follow-up evaluation of fluid collections and pseudocysts.

The very high sensitivity (> 95%) of sonography in diagnosing gallstones, with a lower sensitivity (40–60%) in the detection of common duct stones, makes it an ideal method for diagnosing gallstone pancreatitis. This triage is beneficial since it is influencing the management of these patients. In some patients, endoscopic retrograde cholangiopancreatography (ERCP) and sphincterotomy procedures are performed; in others with cholecystolithiasis, cholecystectomy is advised on an elective basis to prevent the potential risk of a further attack of pancreatitis, which has been estimated to occur in as much as 60% of patients. When visualized, stones appear as echogenic foci within the fluid-filled gallbladder, with posterior acoustic shadow, a finding considered pathognomonic (Fig. 7.1). Abdominal sonography is the best imaging method for detecting gallstones; it is a rapid examination, noninvasive, mostly affordable, generally available, and extremely reliable. However, the examination is heavily operator dependent and somewhat limited in the detection of common duct stones.

When the pancreatic gland can be accurately seen by sonography, findings of acute pancreatitis can be detected. Interstitial edema will result in a diffusely enlarged and hypoechoic gland, with irregular contour. Focal intrapancreatic abnormalities are due to acute fluid collections, inflammation, and hemorrhage. Extrapancreatic fluid collections involving the anterior pararenal space and lesser sac may be detected. Pseudocysts are easily identified and appear as anechoic well-defined fluid collections with through transmission of sound. Abdominal ultrasound is an accepted modality for follow-up of patients with pancreatic pseudocysts. The essential limitations of abdominal ultrasound in evaluating acute pancreatitis rest on its inconstant results and dependence on the experience of a skillful operator. Reported data in the literature show that in patients with acute pancreatitis abnormal ultrasound findings are detected in 33–90% of patients.

Computed tomography

Abdominal CT, particularly after the introduction of

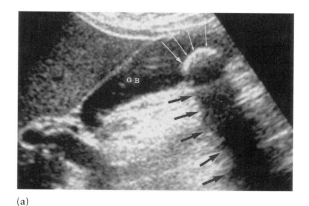

(a)

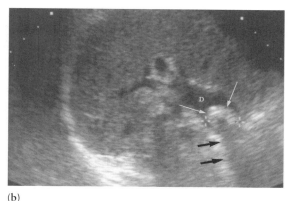

(b)

Figure 7.1 Sonographic demonstration of cholelithiasis. (a) Gallbladder (GB) stones detected as echogenic foci (small arrows) producing posterior acoustic shadowing (large arrows). (b) Large echogenic calculus (small arrows) is visualized in a distended common duct (D) with posterior acoustic shadowing (large arrows).

incremental dynamic bolus techniques and more recently helical and multidetector equipment, has become the most reliable and efficient method for evaluating patients with acute pancreatitis. Fast examinations, performed in only a few minutes using narrow collimation, have virtually eliminated most respiratory and streak artifacts. Remarkably, these procedures obtain high-resolution images that can be used to assess the gross morphology of the pancreas and detect pancreatic abnormalities in almost all individuals. Several important clinical objectives justify the use of CT in patients suspected of acute pancreatitis:

1 it can confirm the clinical diagnosis or depict pancreatitis when not suspected;

2 it is an essential component of early assessment of disease severity;

3 it can detect and follow up local life-threatening abdominal complications;

4 it can diagnose acute abdominal disorders clinically masquerading as acute pancreatitis.

Technique

Depending on the equipment used, technical parameters can vary, but our objective is to increase the conspicuity of the pancreatic gland by using narrow collimation and to acquire images during the administration of intravenous contrast material. Oral contrast agents are habitually given as well as one cup of water just before image acquisition begins. We administer a rapid 3–4 mL/s intravenous bolus injection of 150 mL of 60% nonionic contrast material after the digital scout film is taken.

With helical scanning, axial 5 mm collimation, pitch 1.5 over the upper abdomen, and 7 mm collimation, pitch 2 for the rest of the abdomen and pelvis is performed. Acquisition starts about 60 s after the beginning of intravenous contrast administration.

With multidetector row CT, a two-phase acquisition technique can be employed. The first, arterial-dominant phase starts at approximately 40–45 s and acquires images over the pancreatic gland, from the top of the vertebral body T12 to the superior edge of the vertebral body L4. Collimation of 2–2.5 mm, with a table speed of 3.75 mm is used. The second, portal-dominant phase starts at about 70 s and acquires images of 5 mm collimation with a table speed of 15 mm, from above the dome of the diaphragm to the pubic symphysis. Once data are generated, images can be viewed as planar two-dimensional axial images or can be reconstructed into coronal, oblique, or sagittal planes at a commercially available workstation. Images can be surveyed on printed films, workstation, or picture archiving and communication systems (PACS). For dual-phase multidetector examination with datasets containing hundreds of images, the use of films has become impractical.

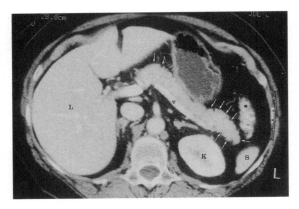

Figure 7.2 Normal pancreas in a 70-year-old woman with abdominal pain and hyperamylasemia (1400 IU/L) presumed to have gallstone pancreatitis. The visualized pancreas (arrows) shows normal size and homogeneous enhancement. K, kidney; L, liver; S, spleen; v, splenic vein.

Normal pancreas

The pancreatic gland is obliquely oriented in the upper abdomen with the head to the right, embraced by the duodenal sweep, body more superiorly crossing the spine, and tail located in the splenic hilum. On CT the gland appears as a sharply contoured, homogeneously enhancing structure, having a smooth contour or a slightly corrugated acinar configuration (Fig. 7.2). There are slight individual variations in the size of the gland, with smaller atrophic glands seen in older individuals. In most patients the head of the pancreas measures 3–4 cm in the anteroposterior diameter, body 2–3 cm, and tail about 1–2 cm, with a gradual transition between segments. The body of the pancreas is reliably located anterior to the splenic artery and vein, a relationship that helps identify the pancreas on more limited quality studies or in cachectic individuals who do not have retroperitoneal fat (Fig. 7.2). A more common variation to normal is a slightly enlarged tail, having a bulbous appearance but showing a similar texture and enhancing value as the rest of the gland. With high-resolution images, a normal pancreatic duct measuring no more than 1–2 mm in thickness is often seen together with a small (2–4 mm) common duct on the posterior aspect of the pancreatic head.

In the absence of intravenous contrast administration, baseline attenuation values of a normal pancreas are 40–50 Hounsfield units (HU), similar to the liver and spleen. Lower attenuation values should be ex-pected with fatty infiltration of the pancreas. During the administration of intravenous contrast, homogeneous enhancement of the entire normal pancreas occurs, with values as high as 150 HU in the arterial-dominant phase and about 100 HU in the portal-dominant phase of acquisition (Fig. 7.2). Individual density variations, usually no more than 10–20 HU, between different segments of pancreatic gland are sometimes seen in normal individuals. Congenital variations, such as lack of development of the dorsal gland (body and tail) or annular pancreas, can be detected by CT.

Diagnosis of acute pancreatitis

The severity and extent of the pancreatic and peripancreatic inflammatory reaction that occur in pancreatitis are reflected by the various CT findings. These findings are similar in appearance and are not dependent on the etiology of an acute attack. In the majority of cases the inflammatory process is diffuse, involving the entire pancreatic gland. Milder clinical forms show a slight to moderate enlargement of the gland and the development of subtle peripancreatic changes (Fig. 7.3). Interstitial heterogeneous densities appear and the degree of parenchymal enhancement is variable, depending on the extent of hyperemia and/or edema induced by the inflammatory process. There are subtle increased densities in the retroperitoneum, having a dirty, hazy, or lace-like appearance, induced by the extravasation of pancreatic exudate. Small, ill-defined, and heterogeneous fluid collections begin to develop, with attenuation values of 20–40 HU, which represent a combination of fat necrosis, extravasated pancreatic enzymes, inflammatory exudate, and hemorrhage (Fig. 7.4). In some cases, while the peripancreatic abnormalities are evident, the pancreatic gland retains its relatively normal size, configuration, and attenuation values (Fig. 7.4).

In more severe forms of acute pancreatitis, the extravasated retroperitoneal fluid collections are large and commonly located in the anterior pararenal space and lesser peritoneal sac (Fig. 7.5). Since most of the pancreas is located to the left of the spine, fluid collections tend to be more abundant and more common in the left anterior pararenal space (Fig. 7.4). When massive, fluid collections can dissect fascial planes and extend further down over the psoas muscles into the pelvis. Pancreatic exudates can thicken peritoneal surfaces, involve the mesocolon and small-bowel mesentery, enter the peritoneal cavity and present as ascites,

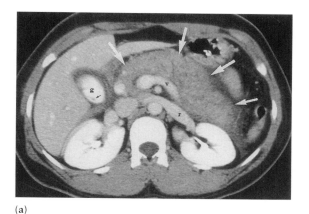

(a)

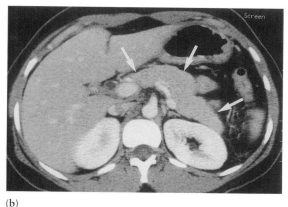

(b)

Figure 7.3 Endoscopic retrograde cholangiopancreato-graphy pancreatitis in a 27-year-old woman with cholelithiasis. (a) Pancreas is diffusely enlarged (arrows) with homogeneous but moderate enhancement because of interstitial edema. There is mild periglandular inflammatory reaction but no necrosis. CT severity index 2. Small stone is seen in the gallbladder (small arrow); g, gallbladder; r, renal vein; v, splenic vein. (b) Follow-up CT examination 7 days later shows resolution of the inflammatory changes. Pancreas has decreased in size with normal homogeneous enhancement (arrows).

and affect adjacent hollow segments of the gastrointestinal tract (Fig. 7.4). Small amounts of free intraperitoneal fluid are detected in about 7% of cases of acute pancreatitis, an incidence that depends on the severity of an acute attack (Fig. 7.5). Retroperitoneal fluid collections, which are demonstrated in about half the patients with acute pancreatitis, tend to slowly resolve in the majority of patients over a period of about 2 weeks. In some cases, however, fluid collections linger on, increase in volume, begin to form a capsule, and eventually develop into pseudocysts or become pancreatic abscesses. At the beginning of an acute attack of pancreatitis, the natural history of the fluid collections is difficult to predict, but in our experience their fate appears to be related to the association of conspicuous intrinsic parenchymal changes.

Failure of the diseased pancreas to enhance during the intravenous contrast administration is consistent with ischemia, and is the most distinguishing CT feature of severe pancreatitis. The process may affect only part of the gland or it may be diffuse and involve the entire gland (Figs 7.6 & 7.7). The demonstration of this phenomenon at the onset of an acute attack heralds the development of pancreatic necrosis, a protracted clinical course, and a severe outcome. Ischemic tissue initially present tends to liquefy within the first 2 or 3 days,

and when extensive it may disrupt the pancreatic ductal system, allowing larger amounts of pancreatic secretions to extravasate in the retroperitoneum for longer periods (Fig. 7.7). CT can also quantify the extent of pancreatic necrosis by grossly dividing necrosis into severe, involving more than 50% of the gland (Fig. 7.7); moderate, involving up to 50% of the gland; or mild, involving less than 30% of the gland (Fig. 7.6).

The CT abnormalities that occur in acute pancreatitis are characteristic and reliable with very few exceptions, and have a reported specificity approaching 100%. On the other hand, the diagnostic sensitivity of CT is reported to be lower (77–92%) and is heavily dependent on the severity of disease in the group of individuals tested. The decreased diagnostic sensitivity is attributed to the incidence of normal CT findings in some patients with acute pancreatitis. The frequency of this presentation is difficult to establish because surgical or pathologic proof is lacking and the diagnosis is based on nonspecific symptoms and on a rise in the serum amylase concentration (Fig. 7.2). Based on these criteria, a normal pancreas is visualized with CT in as many as 14–28% of patients with pancreatitis. However, there is extensive experience to attest that a normal CT examination is seen only with very mild forms of pancreatitis and that all patients with moderate or

61

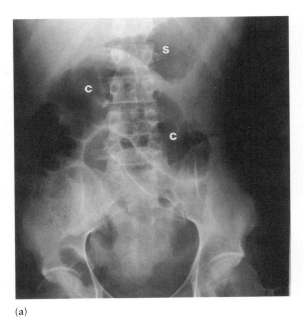

(a)

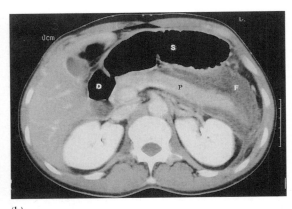

(b)

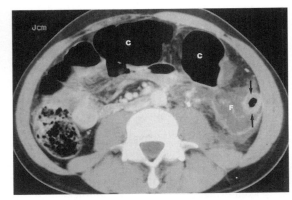

(c)

Figure 7.4 Acute pancreatitis with colon cutoff sign. (a) Conventional abdominal film reveals marked distension of the air-filled transverse colon (C) and air in the stomach (S) and small bowel. (b) Pancreas (P) has maintained its normal size with homogeneous attenuation values. Heterogeneous fluid collection (F) is present around body and tail of pancreas in the left pararenal space. CT severity index 3. (c) Fluid (F) is enveloping a narrowed and thickened splenic flexure (arrows), explaining the dilation of the proximal colon (C). D, duodenum; S, stomach.

severe pancreatitis will exhibit characteristic CT changes.

Segmental pancreatitis
A segmental form of acute pancreatitis has been reported in up to 18% of patients, often associated with a biliary etiology. This morphologic presentation occurs mainly after repeated episodes of pancreatitis; it affects predominantly the head of the pancreas and only rarely the tail of the gland. Discrete peripancreatic inflammatory changes, small fluid collections, and enlargement of the head or tail of the pancreas is noted on CT. The rest of the pancreatic gland appears normal or it may be only slightly enlarged. The focal distribution of the inflammatory process is associated with milder clinical forms of pancreatitis but on CT may be misinterpreted as a pancreatic neoplasm.

Groove pancreatitis
Groove pancreatitis can be described as a chronic and more severe form of segmental pancreatitis involving the head of the pancreas. The head of the pancreas is enlarged and heterogeneous in attenuation, and extravasated pancreatic exudate collects in the groove between the head of the pancreas and duodenal sweep (Fig. 7.8). The secondary extensive inflammatory reac-

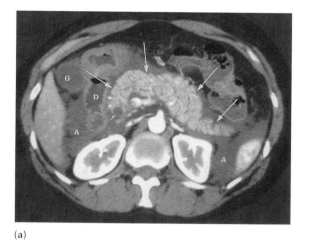

(a)

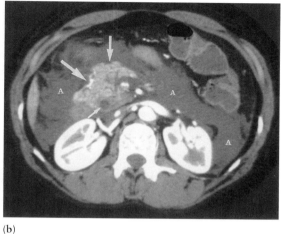

(b)

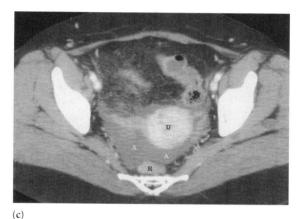

(c)

Figure 7.5 Gallstone pancreatitis in a 50-year-old woman. (a, b) Pancreas is enlarged (arrows) but reveals the normal expected attenuation values throughout. Large fluid collections are present in both anterior pararenal spaces and peritoneal cavity consistent with ascites (A). Distended common duct (small arrow) is visualized along the posterior aspect of the head of the pancreas. D, duodenum; G, gallbladder. (c) Ascites (A) is noted in the lower pelvis anterior to rectum (R) and posterior to uterus (U). CT severity index 4. Ascites resolved without abdominal complications.

tion that follows injures the duodenal wall as well as the distal common duct. Over time this development leads to several complications, such as duodenal stenosis, gastric outlet obstruction, and bile duct strictures. Duodenal stenosis and/or bile duct obstruction have been reported in about 50% of patients and they dominate the clinical aspects of this syndrome. Abdominal pain, vomiting, and obstructive jaundice are the common manifestations and the illness appears to be caused by excessive alcohol intake in most patients. The clinical presentation as well as the CT findings can be misleading, leading to an erroneous diagnosis of carcinoma of the head of the pancreas.

Acute exacerbation of chronic pancreatitis
Acute episodes of pancreatitis characterized by sudden

onset of abdominal pain and hyperamylasemia can occur in patients with chronic pancreatitis. This development is seen mainly in chronic alcoholics with stigmata of chronic pancreatitis on CT, and it is generally regarded as a mild self-limiting exacerbation of a chronic disease. CT examination detects parenchymal atrophy, dilatation of the main pancreatic duct, and/or intraductal calcifications, findings not seen in acute pancreatitis. When present, mild peripancreatic inflammatory reaction and/or small fluid collections betray the occurrence of an acute attack. Associated pseudocysts or pancreatic abscesses may be present. The intrinsic morphologic changes are permanent whereas the recent peripancreatic abnormalities and acute clinical symptoms usually resolve with conservative therapy.

63

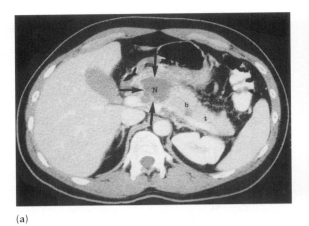

(a)

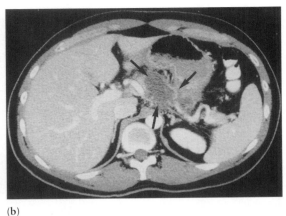

(b)

Figure 7.6 Necrosis of the neck of pancreas in a 33-year-old male with alcoholic pancreatitis. (a) Body (b) and tail (t) of the pancreas is enhancing while a small area of nonenhancement consistent with necrosis (N) is affecting the neck of the pancreas (arrows). (b) Associated fluid collection is seen in the lesser sac around the celiac axis (arrows). CT severity index 5.

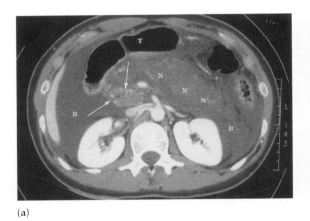

(a)

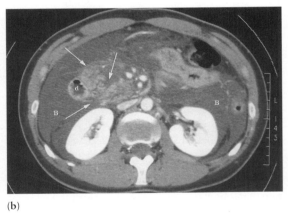

(b)

Figure 7.7 Massive sterile necrosis in a 27-year-old woman associated with intraperitoneal bleeding. (a, b) Head of the pancreas is enlarged, edematous but still enhancing. Rest of the gland shows no enhancement, consistent with massive necrosis (N) affecting more than 50% of pancreas. Large high-attenuated fluid collections consistent with blood (B) are detected in the abdomen. CT severity index 10. Findings proven at surgery. T, transverse colon.

Staging of acute pancreatitis

The management of patients with acute pancreatitis depends on the initial evaluation of severity of disease. To this end, objective clinical and laboratory parameters as well as CT are being used to better detect and quantify the severity of an acute attack. For a long time it has been known that the overall 2–10% mortality of acute pancreatitis is directly related to the development of pancreatic necrosis. More recently it has become evident that the necrotic pancreatic parenchyma, rather than representing the end result of a protracted form of severe pancreatitis, is a phenomenon that occurs at the beginning of an acute attack. Pancreatic necrosis therefore should not be considered a complication of pancreatitis but one end of a spectrum of manifestations of a severe attack, explaining the protracted clinical

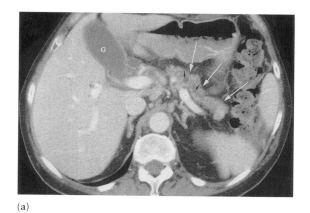

(a)

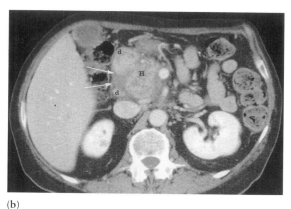

(b)

Figure 7.8 Groove pancreatitis in an alcoholic 37-year-old man with several previous episodes of pancreatitis. (a) Body and tail of the pancreas are normal in size (long white arrows) and pancreatic duct is dilated (short black arrows). G, gallbladder. (b) Head of pancreas (H) is enlarged and heterogeneous in attenuation secondary to inflammation and edema. Fluid is seen around the head of pancreas adjacent to duodenum (arrows). Endoscopic biopsies revealed severe inflammatory changes in duodenum (d).

course that follows. Thus the early detection of pancreatic necrosis by CT has acquired great clinical significance, being used as a grave prognostic indicator of the outcome in these patients (Figs 7.6 & 7.7). Consequently, CT has become a required and essential component of our new classification system.

Radiologic investigations have tried to assess the usefulness of CT in staging the severity of an acute attack of pancreatitis. In our initial 1985 report, we divided the CT features of acute pancreatitis into five separate grades (Table 7.1) and correlated the CT findings with the development of local complications and death. It became obvious that most morbidity and all lethal attacks occurred in individuals with grade D or E presenting with fluid collections (Figs 7.4–7.7). Combined mortality for patients with grades D and E was 14% and morbidity was 54%, compared with no mortality and a morbidity rate of only 4% in patients with grades A, B, and C (Fig. 7.9). Similar general observations were later published by other clinical researchers.

The advantages of our initial grading system are based on the ability to select a subgroup of patients with acute pancreatitis (grades D and E), at higher risk of morbidity and mortality. This CT grading is easy to perform, does not require intravenous contrast administration, or can be performed with slower injection rates, slower CT scanners, and 5–7 mm collimation.

Table 7.1 CT grading in acute pancreatitis.

A	Normal pancreas
B	Pancreatic enlargement
C	Inflammation of pancreas and/or peripancreatic fat
D	Single peripancreatic fluid collection
E	Two or more fluid collections and/or retroperitoneal air

The drawback is its inability to better predict morbidity in patients with fluid collections, since in the majority of these patients fluid resolves spontaneously. Furthermore, CT examinations performed on slower scanners, without intravenous contrast administration or with slower injection rates, are limited in their ability to detect pancreatic necrosis, decreasing the sensitivity of CT as a prognostic indicator of severity.

The causal relationship between lack of pancreatic enhancement and the development of pancreatic necrosis has been previously recognized. When the arterial flow is impeded or the capillary network is damaged, there is a striking decrease or a total lack of parenchymal enhancement consistent with ischemia, followed habitually by the development of necrosis. With few exceptions, necrosis appears at the beginning of an acute attack and remains stable in size and location. However, the necrotic tissue liquefies in the following few days

65

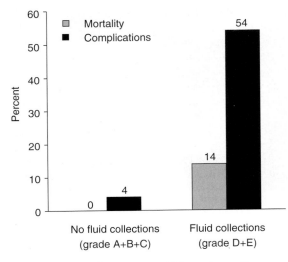

Figure 7.9 CT grading versus morbidity and mortality.

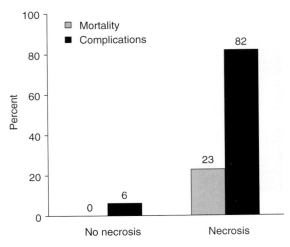

Figure 7.10 Pancreatic necrosis detected by CT versus morbidity and mortality.

and the normal glandular CT texture changes; the area of necrois becomes better defined and more easily appreciated when compared with the adjacent viable enhancing pancreatic tissue (Fig. 7.6).

The veracity of this concept and the clinical importance of CT detection of pancreatic necrosis was confirmed in our 1990 paper. Our data documented an excellent correlation between the early CT findings, the development of local complications, and mortality in patients with acute pancreatitis. Patients with normal pancreatic enhancement had no mortality and only a 6% morbidity rate, whereas patients with CT evidence of pancreatic necrosis (areas of lack of enhancement) exhibited a 23% mortality and 82% morbidity (Fig. 7.10). In addition, the extent of necrosis was found to have prognostic significance. Mortality and morbidity in individuals with extensive necrosis far exceeded those observed in patients with smaller patchy areas of necrosis. The combined morbidity in patients with over 30% necrosis was 94%, and the mortality was 29%. Surgical correlation studies have shown that CT has an overall sensitivity of 77–85% in detecting pancreatic necrosis, with higher percentages for extensive necrosis and lower percentages (50%) for smaller necrotic foci. These findings will probably improve following recent technical advances in abdominal CT imaging.

Although the early detection of necrosis by CT imaging is considered the most revealing prognostic indicator of disease severity, a smaller incidence of

complications (22% in our experience) should be expected in patients with fluid collections but with normally enhancing pancreatic glands. Therefore we have combined the previously described CT prognostic risk factors into a single CT grading system which we have called the "CT severity index."

CT severity index

The CT severity index is a scoring system that combines the initial grading system with the presence and extent of pancreatic necrosis as perceived by CT examination. Patients with grades A–E are assigned 0–4 points, to which are added 2 points for up to 30% necrosis, 4 points for up to 50% necrosis, and 6 points for greater than 50% necrosis (Table 7.2). The resulting severity score, divided into three broad categories (0–3, 4–6, 7–10), correlates well with the incidence of death and the developing local morbidity (Fig. 7.11). Patients with severity index of 0 or 1 are free of complications, whereas patients with a severity index of 7–10 have a 17% mortality and a 92% complication rate.

Limitations of CT evaluation

Most limitations of CT evaluation of the pancreas are related to poor-quality studies, motion artifacts, inadequate technique, and lack of intravenous contrast administration. When intravenous contrast administration is contraindicated (renal insufficiency, allergic reaction to contrast), some of the more subtle

Table 7.2 Acute pancreatitis CT staging.

CT Severity index (CTSI)				
CT Grade	Points	Necrosis	Points	CTSI Score
A	0			
B	1	None	0	1
C	2	<30%	2	4
D	3	30–50%	4	7
E	4	>50%	6	10

CTSI Score = CT grade + necrosis score (0–10).

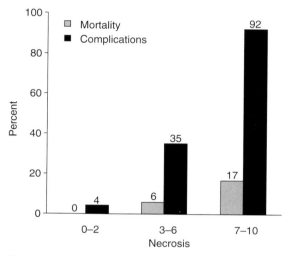

Figure 7.11 CT severity index versus morbidity and mortality. Stage A = 0, B = 1, C = 2, D = 3, E = 4. No necrosis = 0, one-third = 2, one-half = 4, more than one-half = 6.

parenchymal and peripancreatic abnormalities are harder to depict. Moreover, ischemic and necrotic changes become difficult to detect, particularly at the beginning of an acute attack, drastically reducing CT accuracy in staging acute pancreatitis.

CT imaging performed 2–3 days after the initial clinical onset has a higher accuracy in detecting and quantifying pancreatic gland necrosis. Although the presence of pancreatic ischemia is initially evident in most patients, the extent of necrotic involvement before liquefaction appears is more difficult to define at the beginning of an acute attack. Patients who exhibit early equivocal findings or who have large peripancre-

atic fluid collections should undergo a follow-up CT examination.

Extravasated pancreatic exudate severely affects retroperitoneal structures, with the development of inflammatory reaction, hemorrhage, saponification, and extensive fat necrosis. These pathologic changes can occur without recognizable intrinsic parenchymal changes and are difficult to reliably differentiate on CT. For this reason all residual, lingering, heterogeneous, retroperitoneal collections should be considered suspicious for fat necrosis. Secondary bacterial contamination in these collections cannot be ruled out unless diagnostic percutaneous needle aspiration is performed.

Complications of acute pancreatitis
Several complications may occur following an attack of acute pancreatitis that are responsible for the overall 2–10% mortality and a protracted clinical course. Most life-threatening complications should be expected in patients with necrotizing pancreatitis. Despite some overlap, these complications develop mostly in different time frames, following the clinical onset of an acute episode of pancreatitis. They can be divided into systemic toxic manifestations and local abdominal pathologic changes confined mainly to the pancreas and adjacent structures (Table 7.3).

Early complications Early complications, i.e., those occurring at the onset or within the first 2–3 days of an acute attack, are systemic in nature and account for the 20–50% mortality reported in acute pancreatitis. The underlying pathology is connected to the presence and extent of pancreatic necrosis, and its triggering mechanism to the production and release in the bloodstream of a variety of toxic compounds (inflammatory mediators, cytokines, vasoactive peptides). These toxic compounds induce metabolic, cardiovascular, pulmonary, and/or renal functional aberrations with various clinical expressions reflecting the severity of disease at the onset of an acute attack. Detection of these systemic complications is made by clinical means, is part of the numerical staging systems, and greatly influences management decisions and treatment options in these individuals.

Intermediate complications Several ominous abdominal complications can develop between the second and fifth week following an acute attack of pancreatitis,

Table 7.3 Complications of acute pancreatitis.

1 Early, 2–3 days: clinical manifestations of the cardiovascular, pulmonary, renal, and metabolic systems
2 Intermediate, 2–5 weeks: local, retroperitoneal infections, infected necrosis, abscess, pseudocysts, gastrointestinal and biliary complications, and solid organ involvement
3 Late, months–years: vascular and hemorrhagic complications and pancreatic ascites

after the violent systemic manifestations subside. These pathologic changes are frequently but not exclusively associated with gland necrosis and they are responsible for more than 50% of the mortality reported in acute pancreatitis. CT plays a crucial role in their detection and in the decision-making clinical management process.

Infected pancreatic necrosis One of the most foreboding consequences of pancreatic necrosis is secondary bacterial contamination of the liquefied parenchymal tissue, referred to as infected pancreatic necrosis. This complication occurs in about 40–70% of patients with devitalized pancreatic parenchyma, with a time-related incidence that increases to 60% after 3 weeks of hospitalization. Infected necrotic pancreatic tissue is a severe aggravating factor increasing the mortality rate in this cohort of patients. In the series of Beger and colleagues, patients with extensive infected necrosis had a 67% mortality rate as opposed to a 14% mortality rate in patients with a similar extent of sterile necrosis. If contamination does not occur, after the early systemic manifestations resolve, patients become clinically stable and the liquefied pancreatic tissue may resolve or organize into pancreatic pseudocysts (Fig. 7.12).

The source of contamination is the subject of intriguing and controversial theories but is probably multifactorial in origin. Translocation of bacteria (*Escherichia coli*, *Enterobacter*, *Klebsiella*, anaerobes, fungi) through the intestinal wall, via the blood or lymphatic system or due to microperforations, are some of the hypotheses offered.

Infected pancreatic necrosis should be suspected when sepsis (fever, chills, elevated white blood count) dominates the clinical syndrome in patients with known CT findings characteristic of gland necrosis (Fig. 7.13). The diagnosis can be confirmed by percuta- neous needle aspiration under sonography or CT guid- ance and bacteriologic examination. There are no spe- cific CT signs of infection unless bubbles of air are detected in the necrotic pancreatic gland (Fig. 7.13). An aggressive surgical approach consisting of necrosecto- my, débridement, sump drainage, and lavage is the treatment of choice. These invasive surgical procedures are able to substantially reduce the mortality rate to below 10% from the previously reported 40–80% death rate.

Pancreatic abscess A similar, often polymicrobial, contamination of residual retroperitoneal fluid collec- tions and fat necrosis that usually occurs in the vicinity of but outside the pancreas is referred to as pancreatic abscess. This complication can be defined as a partially encapsulated collection of pus that appears totally liquefied on CT (10–30 HU) and which develops in about 3% of patients with acute pancreatitis, mostly 3–4 weeks after the onset of an acute attack. Gas bub- bles are present in 12–18% of abscesses, confirming the clinical suspicion in septic patients. The diagnosis can be secured by percutaneous fine-needle aspiration under imaging guidance.

Recent literature emphasizes the importance of dif- ferentiating abscesses from infected necrosis since the mortality rate of infected necrosis is about twice that of pancreatic abscess. Infected necrotic gland tissue often has a thicker consistency and is thus more amenable to open surgical treatment. Abscesses, on the other hand, are composed mostly of infected, fluid, pancreatic exu- dates that can be effectively treated with less invasive percutaneous catheter drainage. Small abscesses may respond to conservative broad-spectrum antibiotic therapy. CT detection of solitary or multiple, poorly en- capsulated, low-attenuated peripancreatic collections that fail to resolve 3–4 weeks after onset of an acute episode of pancreatitis, in a symptomatic individual, should raise the suspicion of a developing abscess (Fig. 7.14).

Pancreatic pseudocysts Fluid collections that do not resolve, often communicate with the pancreatic ductal system, and slowly develop a circumferential capsule are called pancreatic pseudocysts. They should be dif- ferentiated from the early extravasated fluid collec- tions, having a dissimilar clinical significance and requiring a different therapeutic approach. Pseudo- cysts usually require more than 4 weeks to evolve, are

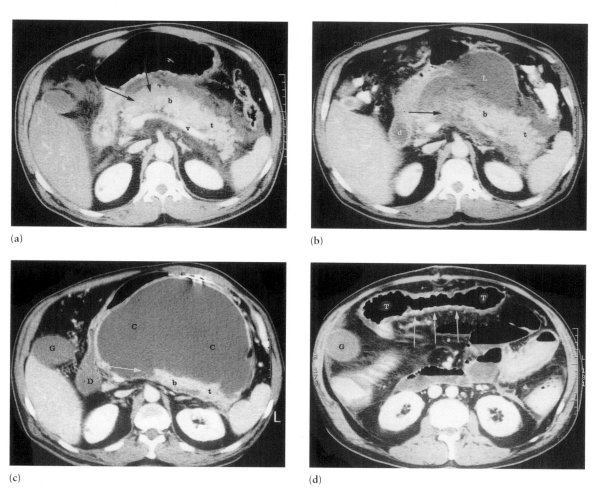

(a)

(b)

(c)

(d)

Figure 7.12 Acute pancreatitis in a 48-year-old man with CT demonstration of parenchymal ischemia followed by sterile liquefaction necrosis and pseudocyst formation. (a) Initial CT examination reveals a zone of decreased attenuation in the neck of pancreas (arrows) compared with attenuation of the body (b) and tail (t) of the gland. CT grading 4, necrosis less than 30% of gland, CT severity index 6. v, splenic vein. (b) Follow-up CT 10 days later reveals liquefaction of the neck of pancreas better defining the area of necrosis (arrow) and larger amount of partially encapsulated fluid collection in the lesser sac (L); b, body; d, duodenum; t, tail. (c) Follow-up CT 6 weeks from onset reveals development of a large pseudocyst (C). Body (b) and tail (t) of the pancreas are atrophic and necrotic liquefaction is seen in the neck of the gland (arrow). D, duodenum; G, gallbladder. (d) Transverse colon (T) has an inflamed thickened wall with a narrowed ahaustral appearance (arrows).

located either in the pancreas or more often in the proximity of the gland, are completely enveloped by a nonepithelialized granulation tissue or fibrotic capsule, and contain fluid with high amylase concentrations (Fig. 7.12). This complication occurs in about 3–10% of cases of acute pancreatitis, most likely secondary to foci of pancreatic necrosis that injure and disrupt the pancreatic ductal system. In my experience most developing acute pseudocysts evolve at the site, or close to the site, of an area of pancreatic necrosis (Figs 7.12 & 7.15).

On CT examination, pseudocysts are distinguished

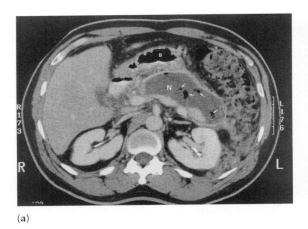

(a)

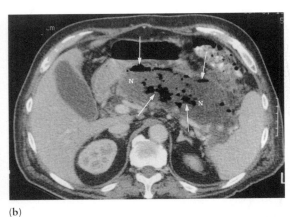

(b)

Figure 7.13 Two patients with massive infected pancreatic necrosis proven by surgical débridement and drainage. (a) CT image shows lack of enhancement of the entire pancreas with liquefaction necrosis (N). A few bubbles of air (arrows) are present in the encapsulated necrotic tissue; s, stomach. (b) Necrotic (N) liquefied pancreatic gland with larger collections of air and air–fluid levels (arrows).

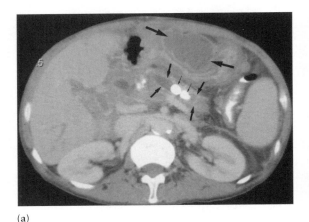

(a)

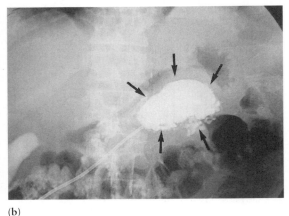

(b)

Figure 7.14 Pancreatic abscess in a 60-year-old alcoholic man with chronic pancreatitis. (a) CT reveals atrophy of the pancreas (medium-sized arrows) with dilation of the pancreatic duct and calcified calculi (small arrows). An encapsulated fluid collection is present anterior to the pancreas (large arrows) in the lesser peritoneal sac. (b) A large collection of pus was percutaneously drained (arrows).

by their obviously thin (1–2 mm) and symmetrical capsule, round or oval configuration, and low-attenuation (< 15 HU) fluid content (Figs 7.12 & 7.15). They may dissect fascial planes and travel away from the pancreas, from the lower mediastinum to the pelvis. In time, the capsule may become thicker and calcified and the luminal contents may be heterogeneous and higher in attenuation, consistent with necrotic tissue,

hemorrhage, or blood clots. Pseudocysts vary greatly in size (1–15 cm in diameter), have no septations and no nodular peripheral elements, and show no intraluminal enhancement (Figs 7.12 & 7.15). These morphologic traits enable pseudocysts to be distinguished from other pancreatic or retroperitoneal cystic tumors in most instances. Occasionally, however, if a relevant clinical history is not available, dif-

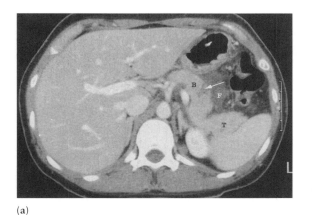

(a)

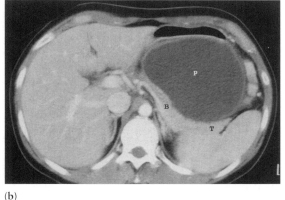

(b)

Figure 7.15 Focal pancreatic necrosis followed by the development of a large pseudocyst in a 34-year-old woman with gallstone pancreatitis. (a) Initial CT examination shows a small area of decreased attenuation in the body of the pancreas (arrow) with adjacent small fluid collection (F). CT severity index 5. B, body; T, tail. (b) Follow-up examination 6 weeks later reveals the development of a large fully encapsulated fluid collection in the lesser sac consistent with pseudocyst (p). B, body; T, tail.

ferentiation from a cystic neoplasm may be difficult (Fig. 7.16).

The fate of an acute pseudocyst evolving during an episode of pancreatitis is unpredictable. There appears to be an important relationship between the existence of a communication with the pancreatic ductal system and the natural development or resolution of a pancreatic pseudocyst. The maintenance of a patent fistulous tract of acute pseudocysts causes them to be unstable, amenable to fluctuations in size, and exposed to recurrences following drainage procedures. Conversely, chronic pseudocysts that lose the connection to the pancreatic ductal system become stable and persist a long time, but respond well to surgical or percutaneous invasive therapeutic measures. As expected young pseudocysts (< 6 weeks) have a high rate of resolution whereas older pseudocysts (> 12 weeks) tend not to resolve. These observations, and additional data documenting an 18–50% rate of complications (rupture, infection, bleeding), has led to an aggressive surgical approach of early operative drainage of most pseudocysts. More recently, CT observations have shown that complications are more common in large pseudocysts (> 6 cm) and that in asymptomatic individuals a more conservative approach, especially for smaller pseudocysts, may be justified since most of the cysts will eventually resolve.

Chronic pseudocysts incidentally detected during routine abdominal CT examinations do not resolve (Fig. 7.16). Spontaneous resolution occurs with acute pseudocysts, by drainage into the pancreatic ductal system, rupture into the peritoneal cavity, or spontaneous drainage into an adjacent hollow viscus such as stomach or transverse colon. Percutaneous or surgical internal drainage is reserved for large cysts (> 5 cm), cysts that are older or enlarging, and symptomatic cysts. Pain, nausea and vomiting, jaundice, infection with sepsis, and hemorrhage are all indications for a more aggressive therapeutic approach. When intervention is necessary, percutaneous catheter drainage with imaging guidance has proved to be successful in curing over 90% of patients. A retrospective study of 92 patients with pseudocysts found similar success rates with percutaneous compared with surgical drainage procedures.

Other complications A variety of other abdominal complications, all related to the extravasated pancreatic exudate, may occur in the first few weeks after the onset of pancreatitis. These complications affect mainly hollow and solid organs located in proximity to the pancreas, such as stomach, duodenum, transverse colon, biliary ducts, spleen, and liver. The extent and degree of enzymatic injuries depend on the severity of the acute episode and induce different clinical pictures.

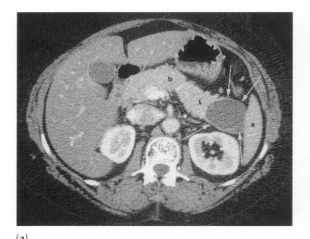

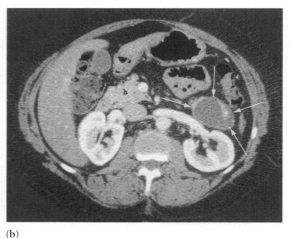

(a)

(b)

Figure 7.16 Pseudocyst in the tail of pancreas mimicking cystic pancreatic tumor, surgically proven. (a) Encapsulated low-attenuated cystic lesion (arrows) was incidentally detected in a 51-year-old woman presenting with left-sided abdominal pain. Body (b) and most of the tail (t) of the pancreas are normal; s, spleen. (b) A more caudal axial image reveals inferior extension of the cystic lesion (arrows) and suggestion of septation with a few flecks of calcium in the capsule; h, head of pancreas.

Functional spasm, bowel edema with thickened mucosal folds, and an ileus pattern appear early within the first few days and rapidly dissipate. A more lasting severe inflammatory spasm of the splenic flexure of the colon leads to massive dilation of the transverse colon, referred to as the colon cutoff sign (see Fig. 7.4). More severe enzymatic injuries may induce intestinal and biliary strictures, or sinus tracts and fistulas affecting duodenum, jejunal loops, and/or colon (Fig. 7.12). Inflammatory exudates can dissect into small bowel mesentery and mesocolon, and can invade solid organs such as spleen, liver, or kidneys. Subcapsular fluid collections, intraparenchymal collections that organize into pseudocysts, splenic infarcts, and splenic hemorrhage are complications that can develop a few weeks following the onset of severe acute pancreatitis.

Late complications Vascular and hemorrhagic complications. Vascular and severe hemorrhagic complications can appear at any time following an acute attack of pancreatitis but usually occur late and often after several acute episodes. Clinical presentation is mostly nonspecific and thus CT is essential for their detection and evaluation. Peripancreatic vessels are injured by the autodigestive action of the extravasated pancreatic exudate, explaining these complications.

Splenic vein thrombosis is the most common vascular complication, which develops in 1–3% of patients following pancreatitis. The developing syndrome, called left-sided portal hypertension, is defined by the obstruction of splenic vein with massive enlargement of the collateral short gastric and gastroepiploic veins, and the development of gastric varices on the posterior wall of the gastric fundus (Fig. 7.17). Since the main portal vein is patent, the collateral blood flow drains into the portal system via the coronary vein, avoiding the development of esophageal varices. Patients are commonly asymptomatic unless and until hematemesis intervenes. Contrast-enhanced CT is eminently suited for detecting this condition (Fig. 7.17).

Massive sudden occurrence of intraabdominal hemorrhage can be seen at the beginning of a severe attack of pancreatitis. However, this ominous complication often follows a long history of repeated acute attacks in patients with stigmata of chronic pancreatitis. In the series of Bretagne and colleagues it occurred 1–9 years (median 4 years) after the first episode, and in our experience as late as 8 years (mean 2.3 years) after the initial attack of pancreatitis. Most life-threatening episodes are attributed to ruptured pseudoaneurysm involving the splenic, gastroduodenal, or pancreaticoduodenal arteries (Fig. 7.18). Left gastric artery, middle colic

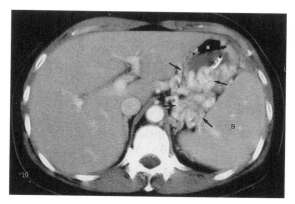

Figure 7.17 Gastric varices secondary to splenic vein thrombosis associated with previous episodes of acute pancreatitis in a 54-year-old woman. CT axial image reveals multiple, large, enhancing collateral veins (arrows) along the posterior aspect of the proximal stomach (s) and adjacent to an enlarged spleen (S).

artery, hepatic artery, or smaller arterial branches are less commonly affected.

Pseudoaneurysms are apparently common complications of pancreatitis, with an incidence as high as 10% reported in an angiographic survey. Clinical signs and symptoms attributable to hemorrhage manifest only when a slowly enlarging false aneurysm ruptures into the peritoneal cavity, or erodes into an adjacent hollow viscus (small bowel, colon) or into the pancreatic duct inducing hemosuccus pancreatitis. Other causes of abdominal hemorrhage attributed to pancreatitis are bleeding pseudocysts and diffuse venous or capillary bleeding, seen in patients with necrotizing pancreatitis (Figs 7.7 & 7.19). In individuals with chronic pancreatitis, an incidence of 3.2% for bleeding pseudoaneurysms and bleeding pseudocysts has been reported. In our experience, 60% of hemorrhagic complications were due to pseudoaneurysms (Fig. 7.18), 20% to hemorrhagic pseudocysts (Fig. 7.19), and 20% induced by massive capillary or small arterial bleeding related to extensive pancreatic necrosis (see Fig. 7.7).

Previous mortality rates of 25–60% have been reduced to about 11% with early detection by contrast-enhanced CT followed by angiographic embolization or, when required, an aggressive surgical approach. CT can detect pseudoaneurysms as sharply defined, round or oval, high-attenuated lesions located along or adja-

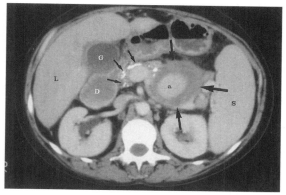

(a)

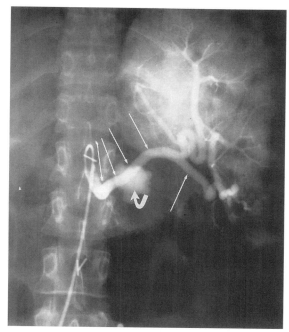

(b)

Figure 7.18 Splenic artery pseudoaneurysm in a 34-year-old woman with a long history of pancreatitis and stigmata of chronic pancreatitis. (a) Axial image in the upper abdomen reveals a round enhancing aneurysm (a) in a pancreatic pseudocyst (large arrows). Pancreas is atrophic with ductal calcifications (small arrows). D, duodenum; G, gallbladder; L, liver; S, spleen. (b) Selective angiogram of splenic artery (long arrows) reveals a saccular dilatation (small curved arrow) consistent with a false aneurysm or pseudoaneurysm. Surgical resection with ligation of the splenic artery was performed.

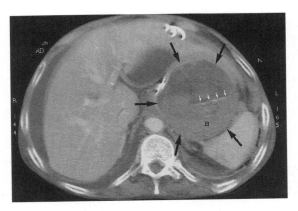

Figure 7.19 Bleeding pseudocyst in a 37-year-old alcoholic man with repeated episodes of acute pancreatitis. CT axial image reveals a large pseudocyst (arrows) in the left upper quadrant filled with high-attenuated fluid representing blood (B). Small active extravasation of intravenous contrast material is detected (small arrows). Findings proven at surgery.

cent to a peripancreatic artery (Fig. 7.18). Free spill of contrast material or high-attenuated (50–60 HU) collections of fresh blood implies rupture or, in the absence of a pseudoaneurysm, capillary bleeding (Figs 7.4 & 7.19). The sensitivity of CT for detecting false aneurysms depends on the size of the lesion, quality of examination, and skill of radiologic interpretation. Small nonbleeding false aneurysms can be easily overlooked during routine abdominal CT examinations.

Pancreatic ascites The overall incidence of free peritoneal fluid (ascites) detected by CT in patients with acute pancreatitis is about 7–12%. This range of occurrence as well as the amount of peritoneal fluid depends on the severity of the acute episode. Ascites is considered to be a sign of severity, yet the fluid usually resolves spontaneously. Conversely, the massive and chronic accumulation of intraperitoneal fluid, rich in amylase, caused by long-standing disruption of the pancreatic ductal system and formation of permanent fistulous communication defines a more specific syndrome called "pancreatic ascites."

Clinical diagnosis should be suspected in patients with long histories of pancreatitis who develop increasing abdominal girth and complain of pain and sometimes nausea and vomiting. CT can help in diagnosis,

revealing massive ascites often associated with retroperitoneal fluid and stigmata of chronic pancreatitis, such as pancreatic atrophy and dilated pancreatic ducts. Ascites tends to be massive because the normal pancreas produces in excess of 1 L of exocrine secretions a day, part of which is diverted into the peritoneal cavity. Definite confirmation, using percutaneous needle aspiration, can be obtained when the protein content in the ascitic fluid is greater than 3 g/dL and the amylase level is above 1000 IU/L.

Chronic pancreatic ascites is a serious debilitating complication difficult to properly manage and control. If spontaneous resolution does not occur, endoscopic retrograde pancreatography followed by dilation of strictures or stent placement is advocated. If not effective, surgical resections with pancreatico-jejunostomy can be attempted with various degrees of success. Operative mortality of about 20% and a recurrence rate of 15% have been reported.

Magnetic resonance imaging

Technique

The pancreas is best imaged at field strength of 1.5 T or higher using high-speed gradient coils and phased-array multicoils. This allows for faster imaging, higher signal to noise, and increased separation of water and fat frequencies. Several pulse sequences are useful in MRI of the pancreas, including T1-weighted, T2-weighted, fat-saturation and dynamic gadolinium-enhanced images, magnetic resonance cholangio-pancreatography (MRCP), and vascular imaging (Fig. 7.20). No single pulse sequence is adequate to evaluate the pancreas. However, a comprehensive examination can still be performed in as little as 15 min, essential when evaluating patients with severe acute pancreatitis.

T1-weighted images are essential for imaging the pancreas, especially valuable for depicting fat planes surrounding abdominal viscera and therefore essential for optimal delineation of the pancreas and demonstration of gross morphologic abnormalities. Fat suppression usually improves the conspicuity of pancreatic parenchyma. T1-weighted, fat-suppressed images are especially useful for detecting subtle focal or diffuse pancreatic abnormalities. These images are also exquisitely sensitive in the detection of blood products in necrotizing pancreatitis. Single-shot, fast spin-echo, T2-weighted images are most useful for depicting

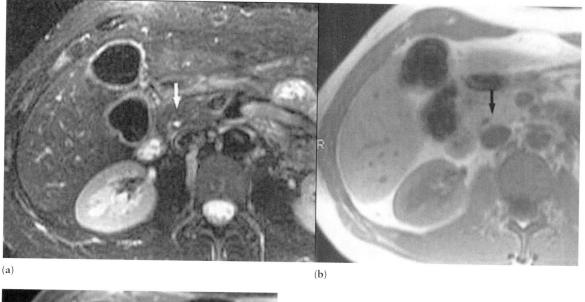

(a)

(b)

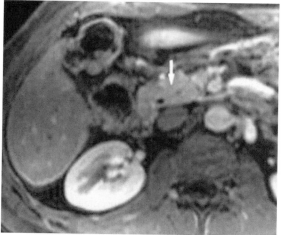

(c)

Figure 7.20 Normal pancreas on MRI. The normal pancreas is homogeneously hypointense on T2-weighted fat-suppressed imaging (a), hyperintense on T1-weighted gradient-echo imaging (b), and enhances homogeneously during the pancreatic phase on T1-weighted fat-suppressed imaging (c).

intrapancreatic or peripancreatic fluid collections and biliary/pancreatic duct calculi because they can be acquired without breath-holding and are free from motion artifacts; these images are invaluable when evaluating patients too ill to comply with simple commands.

The pancreas is a highly vascular organ that enhances intensely during the arterial phase of a dynamic bolus of intravenous gadolinium chelate. Contrast enhancement is typically performed with three-dimensional, fat-suppressed, breath-hold, T1-weighted gradient–echo (GRE) imaging. This technique maximizes the contrast between an enhancing normal pancreas and pancreatic necrosis. By using a three-dimensional volumetric technique with isotropic resolution, reconstructions can be performed in any plane without loss of spatial resolution. Maximum intensity projection (MIP) algorithms applied to the arterial phase acquisitions provide magnetic resonance angiograms capable of diagnosing vascular complications of acute pancreatitis, such as pseudoaneurysms.

MRCP is the generation of projectional or tomographic magnetic resonance images of the biliary tree and pancreatic duct using heavily two-dimensional or three-dimensional T2-weighted techniques. MRCP accurately depicts morphologic abnormalities of the biliary and pancreatic ducts in relation to parenchymal structures, and can replace diagnostic ERCP in most cases.

MRI versus CT for acute pancreatitis
CT is the gold standard for the diagnosis and staging of acute pancreatitis and its complications. It is widely available and can be performed quickly such that even the most critically ill patients can be studied. However, the limitations of CT include ionizing radiation and potentially nephrotoxic iodinated contrast agents. MRI of the pancreas can be performed without radiation and the contrast agents used have no nephrotoxicity. In addition, MRI is more sensitive than CT for the diagnosis of cholodocholithiasis and can better differentiate complex fluid collections from mature pseudocysts. However, MRI is more expensive, takes longer to perform, and is insensitive to small calcifications and small amounts of air. For these reasons, we recommend MRI instead of CT only in pregnant women, in patients with renal insufficiency or severe contrast allergy, and when evaluating common duct stones. The multiplanar capability of MRI may also be helpful prior to interventional or surgical therapy for complex fluid collections.

The morphologic changes of acute pancreatitis have been described based on CT findings. The MRI signal intensity of the pancreas in uncomplicated acute pancreatitis may be normal, but the pancreas may exhibit morphologic changes of either focal or diffuse enlargement, or peripancreatic fluid. Low-intensity peripancreatic stranding may be seen within the retroperitoneal fat on T1-weighted images. Peripancreatic fluid or stranding is best shown on T2-weighted, fat-suppressed images (Fig. 7.21) or post gadolinium chelate gradient-echo images.

Similar to CT, the presence and degree of pancreatic necrosis can only be assessed after the administration of gadolinium chelates. These extracellular agents behave in a similar fashion as iodinated CT agents, but without the nephrotoxicity or anaphylactoid reactions.

With gadolinium chelate enhancement, viable pancreas enhances normally during the arterial phase whereas necrotic pancreatic tissue does not enhance (Figs 7.22 & 7.23). The degree of pancreatic necrosis can be assessed in a similar manner as on CT. Hemorrhagic fluid collections/sterile necrosis often have debris with focal high signal on T1-weighted images and low signal on T2-weighted images (Fig. 7.24). It may be quite difficult to differentiate sterile necrosis from infected necrosis as MRI is insensitive to small bubbles of air. Recently, MRI has been used to identify pancreatic ductal disruption in patients with pancreatic ascites after trauma or severe acute pancreatitis. A poorly defined focal collection of fluid in the region of the pancreatic duct may be seen with ductal disruption.

Pseudocysts are depicted as homogeneous high-signal lesions on T2-weighted images without internal debris or blood products on T1-weighted images (Fig. 7.25). They typically communicate with the pancreatic duct, a finding seen much better on MRI than on CT. Other complications, including vascular thrombosis, pseudoaneurysm, and hepatic abscesses, are readily identified on MRI.

Summary

Newly developed radiologic imaging methods have achieved recognition and play a crucial role in the evaluation of patients with acute pancreatitis. Sonography, and to a large extent MRI, are secondary or complementary modalities while helical or mulitidetector contrast-enhanced CT has become the imaging examination of choice. In individuals suspected of acute pancreatitis, CT accomplishes several important aims.
1 Depending on the clinical presentation, CT can confirm the clinical suspicion, detect pancreatitis in clinically unsuspected patients, and depict other acute abdominal conditions that may be confused as pancreatitis.
2 Based on the detection of fluid collections and on its ability to diagnose pancreatic necrosis (CT severity index), CT is essential in the early assessment of severity of an acute attack of pancreatitis.
3 Local abdominal complications that develop during the natural history of severe pancreatitis can be detected by CT on follow-up examinations.

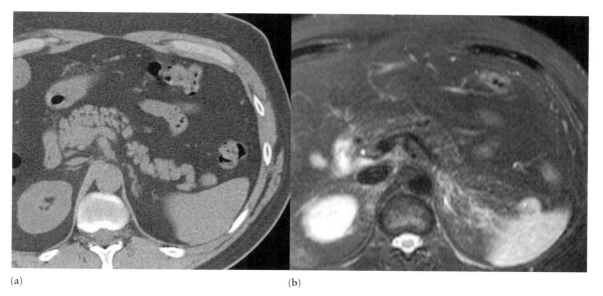

(a)

(b)

Figure 7.21 Mild acute pancreatitis better seen on T2-weighted MRI than unenhanced CT. (a) Unenhanced CT demonstrates a normal pancreas. (b) T2-weighted fat-suppressed image (performed 4 hours after CT) demonstrates normal pancreatic signal intensity but increased signal in the posterior peripancreatic fat consistent with mild acute pancreatitis.

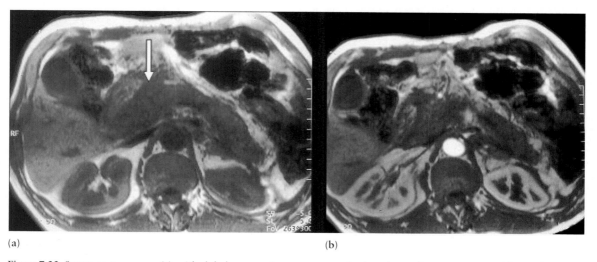

(a)

(b)

Figure 7.22 Severe acute pancreatitis with global pancreatic necrosis. (a) Unenhanced T1-weighted gradient-echo image demonstrates marked decreased signal throughout the pancreas (compare with Fig. 7.1a). (b) Gadolinium-enhanced pancreatic-phase image demonstrates no evidence of glandular enhancement consistent with diffuse pancreatic necrosis.

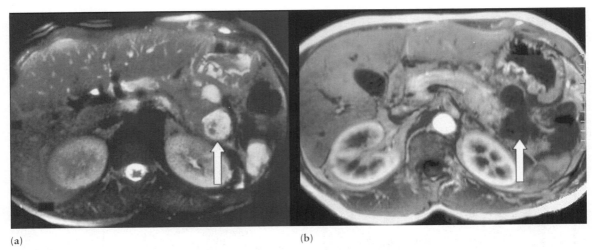

(a)

(b)

Figure 7.23 Focal pancreatic necrosis involving the tail. (a) T2-weighted fat-suppressed image shows a bilobed tail collection with extensive debris (arrow). (b) Gadolinium- enhanced pancreatic-phase image focal necrosis of the pancreatic tail with contiguous acute fluid collection (arrow).

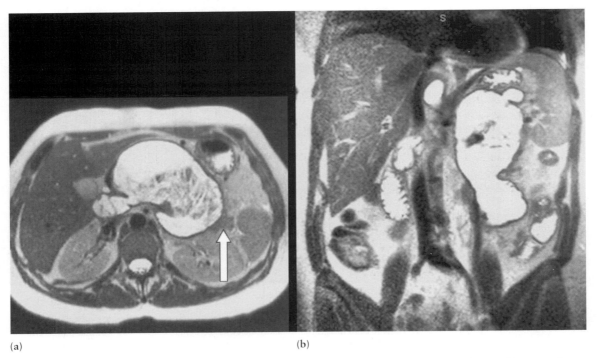

(a)

(b)

Figure 7.24 Sequelae of severe acute pancreatitis and necrosis. Coronal (a) and axial heavily T2-weighted MRI (b) shows replacement of the gland by a poorly defined fluid collection with extensive debris. Only a small amount of normal pancreatic tail is present (arrow).

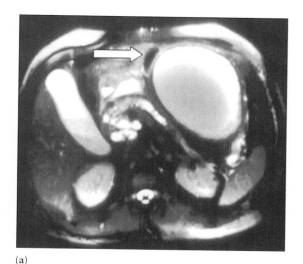

(a)

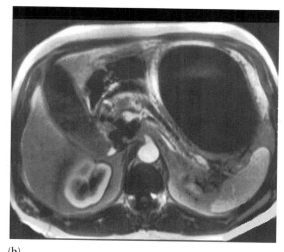

(b)

Figure 7.25 Mature pseudocyst from chronic pancreatitis with mass effect on the stomach. (a) T2-weighted fat-suppressed and (b) gadolinium-enhanced pancreatic-phase images show a well-circumscribed mature pseudocyst (no debris) displacing the antrum anteriorly (arrow). Diffuse pancreatic duct dilation with acinar atrophy is present.

Imaging modalities and particularly CT have become an indispensable diagnostic tool in the evaluation and management of patients with acute pancreatitis.

Recommended reading

Balthazar EJ. Acute pancreatitis: assessment of severity with clinical and CT evaluation. *Radiology* 2002;223:603–613.

Balthazar EJ. Complications of acute pancreatitis: clinical and CT evaluation. *Radiol Clin North Am* 2002;40:1211–1227.

Balthazar EJ, Fisher LA. Hemorrhagic complications of pancreatitis: radiologic evaluation with emphasis on CT imaging. *Pancreatology* 2001;1:306–313.

Balthazar EJ, Robinson DL, Megibow AJ *et al.* Acute pancreatitis: value of CT in establishing prognosis. *Radiology* 1990;174:331–336.

Balthazar EJ, Freeny PC, VanSonnenberg E. Imaging and intervention in acute pancreatitis. *Radiology* 1994;193: 297–306.

Belli AM, Jennings CM, Nakielny RA. Splenic and portal venous thrombosis: a vascular complication of pancreatic disease demonstrated on computed tomography. *Clin Radiol* 1990;41:13–16.

Bittner R, Block S, Buchler M *et al.* Pancreatic abscess and infected pancreatic necrosis: different local septic complications in acute pancreatitis. *Dig Dis Sci* 1987;32: 1082–1087.

Burke JW, Erickson SJ, Kellum CD *et al.* Pseudoaneurysms complicating pancreatitis: detection by CT. *Radiology* 1986;161:447–450.

Clavien PA, Hauser H, Meyer P *et al.* Value of contrast-enhanced computerized tomography in the early diagnosis of acute pancreatitis. A prospective study of 202 patients. *Am J Surg* 1988;155:457–466.

Freeny PC, Hauptmann E, Althaus SJ *et al.* Percutaneous CT guided catheter drainage of infected acute necrotizing pancreatitis: technique and results. *AJR* 1998;170:969–975.

Gerzof SG, Banks PA, Robbins AH *et al.* Early diagnosis of pancreatic infection by computed tomography-guided aspiration. *Gastroenterology* 1987;93:1315–1320.

Jeffrey RB. Sonography in acute pancreatitis. *Radiol Clin North Am* 1989;27:5–17.

London MJM, Neoptolemos JP, Lavelle J *et al.* Contrast-enhanced abdominal computed tomography scanning and prediction of severity of acute pancreatitis: a prospective study. *Br J Surg* 1989;76:268–272.

Lowham A, Lavelle J, Leese T. Mortality from acute pancreatitis. *Int J Pancreatol* 1999;25:103–106.

Megibow AJ, Lavelle MT, Rofsky NM. MR imaging of the pancreas. *Surg Clin North Am* 2001;81:307–320.

Merkle EM, Gorich J. Imaging of acute pancreatitis. *Eur Radiol* 2002;12:1979–1992.

Nordestgaard AG, Wilson SE, Williams RA. Early computerized tomography as a predictor of outcome in acute pancreatitis. *Am J Surg* 1986;152:127–132.

Piironen A, Kivisaari R, Kemppainen E *et al.* Detection of

severe acute pancreatitis by contrast-enhanced magnetic resonance imaging. *Eur Radiol* 2000;10:354–361.

Sugiyama M, Atomi Y. Endoscopic ultrasonography for diagnosis of choledocholithiasis: a prospective comparative study with ultrasonography and computed tomography. *Gastrointest Endosc* 1997;45:143–146.

VanSonnenberg E, Wittich GR, Casola G *et al.* Percutaneous drainage of infected and noninfected pancreatic pseudocysts: experience in 101 cases. *Radiology* 1989;170: 757–761.

Vujic I. Vascular complications of pancreatitis. *Radiol Clin North Am* 1989;27:81–91.

8 Basis of therapy in acute pancreatitis

Clement W. Imrie

Once the diagnosis of acute pancreatitis has been established on the basis of an appropriate clinical and biochemical presentation (usually sudden-onset upper abdominal pain with troublesome vomiting and significant elevations in blood and/or urine of amylase and/or lipase), there are several important therapeutic steps, outlined in Table 8.1 and Fig. 8.1. This is a dynamic disease process in which approximately 85–90% of patients will not develop signs of organ compromise. However, some patients will have organ failure at presentation to hospital and they constitute a high-risk group (Table 8.2). Of those who die from acute pancreatitis, approximately 50% succumb in the first 7–10 days of hospitalization. Patients in whom systemic inflammatory response syndrome (SIRS) is marked, and especially those in whom multiple organ dysfunction syndrome (MODS) is present, have a greater probability of death and major morbidity. Most patients with mild acute pancreatitis will settle with simple therapeutic measures to correct hypovolemia, hypoxemia, and pain. Especially in those with more severe disease and comorbidity, high dependency and/or intensive care will be necessary.

Hypovolemia

Correction of hypovolemia, even in mild acute pancreatitis, may necessitate provision of 3.5–4 L of simple electrolyte fluid in the initial 24 hours. In higher-risk patients, a central venous pressure line is essential. Urinary catheterization with careful aseptic technique is important as no patient should be producing less than 30 mL of urine per hour without the closest attention to fluid replacement requirements. In the severely ill patient those fluid requirements are akin to the patient with severe burns, such that 6–10 L of fluid may be necessary in the first 24 hours, with particularly high-volume input in the initial 6 hours of treatment. The major reasons for hypovolemia are the alteration of capillary permeability associated with the degree of insult from the acute pancreatitis, which causes loss of albumin from the intravascular space, and vomiting.

Hypoxemia

This is a hallmark of both moderate and severe acute pancreatitis. Initially it was thought that any single recording of arterial saturation of less than 60 mmHg (8 kPa) was an indication of severe acute pancreatitis, but in recent years it has been established that transient dips in arterial saturation are not associated with high morbidity and high mortality. It is the patient who has sustained nonresponsive hypoxemia to standardized humidified oxygen therapy who causes greatest concern. Respiratory insufficiency and failure is the single organ compromise most frequently encountered in this disease. The help of an intensive care expert and treatment in an intensive care unit with ventilator therapy is necessary for those with the most marked hypoxemia. Moderate hypoxemia is treated by protracted oxygen therapy, until the patient can manage without this support.

Treatment of pain and vomiting

This is very important. The first step is to pass a naso-

Table 8.1 Initial steps in therapy.

Analgesia
Aspirate stomach
Correct hypovolemia
Catheter in bladder
Central line
Oxygen (humidify)

Table 8.2 High-risk patients.

Elderly (> 70 years)
Obese (> 30 kg/m²)
Comorbidity (renal/respiratory/cardiac)
Organ failure at presentation

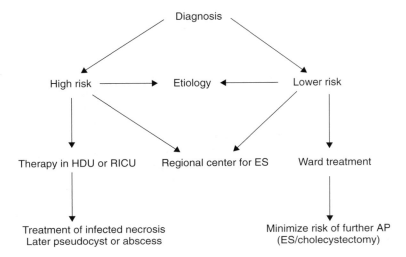

Figure 8.1 Algorithm of therapy of acute pancreatitis. ES, endoscopic sphincterotomy (papilla of Vater); HDU, high-dependency unit; RICU, respiratory intensive care unit.

gastric tube and aspirate all gastric contents. Occasionally, antiemetic drugs may be necessary to combat the vomiting problem. The volume of vomited fluid can contribute significantly to the degree of hypovolemia, which is primarily due to the loss of fluid from the intervascular space into the peritoneal cavity, retroperitoneal area, and pleural space.

Pain control is frequently achieved by intramuscular or intravenous opiate administration. Classically, meperidine (pethidine, Demerol) has been considered the drug of choice based on the incorrect belief that there was less of a problem with spasm of the sphincter of Oddi with this agent compared with morphine. Morphine is the better agent for pain relief, but both drugs at the dosage used to achieve analgesia cause sphincter spasm. For this reason some clinicians, particularly in continental Europe, favor the use of epidural analgesia. Patient-controlled analgesia can be useful but those with hypoxemia have to be monitored closely in case

opiates exacerbate the problem. Severe initial pain usually recedes by day 3 or 4 of the illness.

Cardiac failure

Cardiac failure is most commonly associated with comorbidity in older patients who have a history of hypertension, myocardial ischemia, atrial fibrillation, or combinations of these. Decisions regarding the place of inotropic support will usually be made in the early phase of management in the high-dependency or intensive-care setting. Expert cardiologic advice is very helpful in those patients taking cardiac support drugs prior to the episode of acute pancreatitis.

The initial management steps are therefore usually quite straightforward and in patients with mild acute pancreatitis improvement within 24–36 hours is usually quickly evident. The provision of adequate intravenous fluid replacement has greatly lowered the frequency of renal insufficiency and failure in this disease. Indeed it is most unusual to find a patient with renal failure who does not have a major degree of respiratory compromise or failure preceding the kidney problem. Hemofiltration or hemodialysis is necessary in some patients.

During the steps of early therapy an ultrasound scan will be performed and chest X-ray will monitor for early pleural effusions. Where diagnostic doubt is present, contrast-enhanced computed tomography is very helpful. This is also the gold standard for grading the morphologic ischemic damage to the pancreas and its location within the gland. Magnetic resonance imaging (MRI) may become more important as this technology improves.

Where a stone is judged to be stuck for an unusually long time in the ampulla on the basis of clinical, biochemical, and imaging evidence of obstructive jaundice with or without cholangitis, early endoscopic bile duct clearance may be necessary (see Chapter 13).

Antibiotics are essential where coincidental cholangitis is present but in the absence of this feature there is debate about the role of prophylactic imipenem, meropenem, tazobactam, or cephalosporins in severe acute pancreatitis as randomized controlled studies have been too small to show clear-cut benefit in lowering mortality. Metaanalysis tends to argue in favor of their use but concerns regarding the risks of fungal and rarer bacterial infections are real (see Chapter 11).

Biochemical abnormalities

A fall in blood albumin is a common early feature of severe acute pancreatitis due to the loss of albumin from the intravascular space. Replacement albumin is not usually administered nowadays partly because of its high cost and the increased infection risk associated with pooled human albumin. It is the fall in blood albumin levels that is mainly responsible for the hypocalcemia and is due to the loss of protein-bound calcium, which constitutes approximately 50% of circulating calcium.

Ionized calcium levels do tend to fall but rarely warrant replacement therapy. This is because the parathyroid hormone response is usually a very efficient homeostatic mechanism. When replacement calcium is administered, it is usually in the form of calcium gluconate and frequently the dosage given is almost insignificant against the background of the massive pool in bone usually being extracted by the homeostatic mechanisms of the body. If it is decided to give calcium gluconate, then a practical dose such as 50–60 mg/day should be tried.

Blood glucose levels tend to rise and may be poorly controlled in the initial phase of disease. Close control of blood sugar has been shown to be beneficial in the intensive-care setting in terms of improving both mortality and morbidity. The Belgian study that outlined this matter predominantly looked at patients immediately after cardiac surgery. It will be intriguing to determine whether maintaining a blood sugar in the range 4.0–6.1 mmol/L also proves beneficial in severe acute pancreatitis. This appears to be a new desirable therapeutic target.

Elevations of bilirubin, transferases, and alkaline phosphatase may all occur where a stone is impacted in the ampulla of Vater. This information, combined with imaging data from either ultrasound or MRI, may well prompt an early endoscopic inspection of the ampulla with a view to endoscopic sphincterotomy. Elevated levels of lactate dehydrogenase have been demonstrated to be associated with more severe disease and were utilized in both the Ranson and Glasgow prognostic scores. This observation also applies to elevated blood glucose and depressed calcium levels with regard to the Ranson criteria and the same factors plus blood albumin in the Glasgow prognostic score.

Elevations of triglycerides may be associated with primary hyperlipidemia as a cause of acute pancreatitis. However, our own group in Glasgow examined more than 300 consecutive patients with acute pancreatitis and found that most of the 4% of patients with elevated blood lipids had this entity observed as an epiphenomenon secondary to alcohol abuse. Appropriate investigation and therapy with regard to prophylaxis of further attacks is clearly important. In those with primary hyperlipidemia the treatment can be complex, including both dietary exclusions and drugs affecting lipid metabolism directly. Reliance on elevations in serum amylase during hyperlipidemia can be a technical problem for biochemists. Urinary amylase elevations still are measurable, and the diagnostic level is approximately 7.5 times the upper normal serum amylase value.

Elevated C-reactive protein is part of the acute-phase

response to injury and this has been a valuable marker of disease severity after the initial 48 hours of onset of disease. Levels of 150 mg/L are usually taken as an indicator of severe acute pancreatitis, although greater elevations in excess of 200 mg/L are a more useful indicator.

Hematologic abnormalities

In rare instances, hemoglobin levels fall due to bleeding in and around the pancreas. This is not common and it is most frequent to find hemoconcentration at the start of disease and thereafter the dilutional effect of providing intravenous fluids ensures a fall in hemoglobin. The necessity for blood as a replacement therapy is uncommon.

Blood platelet levels usually demonstrate a typical pattern, falling throughout the initial 3–5 days of illness and thereafter improving spontaneously. Only in patients with intravascular coagulation does the drop in platelet levels occasionally warrant therapy with normal or low-molecular-weight heparin. As part of the acute-phase response, factors V and VIII rise throughout the initial week of illness. Fibrinogen levels also show a very similar pattern.

Very uncommonly, disseminated intravascular coagulation can occur in which severe drops in hemoglobin as well as platelet count and fibrinogen occur. Heparin therapy may be helpful. Expert hematologic support is necessary.

Post-ERCP acute pancreatitis

This is often a mild condition but on occasions it can be particularly severe. Careful endoscopic retrograde cholangiopancreatography (ERCP) with nonionic contrast medium and the avoidance of high-pressure injection are important prophylactic steps. In patients with a history of sphincter of Oddi dyskinesia, there is a much higher risk of inducing pancreatitis at the time of manometry. More modern manometric methods have lowered the risk of acute pancreatitis being induced.

In therapeutic terms, interleukin (IL)-10 and the much cheaper analgesic diclofenac have been shown to be beneficial in the management of this problem. IL-10 is very expensive and its efficacy is contested in different studies. Only one study has examined the potential use of diclofenac and this readily available analgesic can be given as a suppository prior to ERCP in the high-risk patient or immediately after should the operator have concern in a particular patient.

The problem of early mortality

In severe acute pancreatitis, especially the most severe types of disease characterized by a Marshall score of 2 or more persisting for greater than 36 hours, the mortality rate is in the region of 50%. Approximately 45% of patients who achieve a Marshall score of 2 or more (Table 8.3) have this feature present on admission to hospital. The remainder develop such features more than 24 hours after admission to hospital. It is mandatory that these patients be treated in an intensive-care

Table 8.3 Modified Marshall organ failure score (hepatic index excluded).

	0	1	2	3	4
Cardiovascular system (systolic blood pressure, mmHg)	>90	<90 and fluid responsive	<90 and fluid unresponsive	<90 and pH<7.3	<90 and pH 7.2
Respiratory system (F_{IO_2}/P_{O_2})	>400	301–400	201–300	101–200	<101
Glasgow Coma Score	15	13–14	10–12	6–9	<6
Coagulation (platelets, 10^9/L)	>120	81–120	51–80	21–50	<21
Renal system (creatinine, μmol/L)	<134	134–169	170–310	311–439	>439

setting and the efficacy of this approach will only be able to be measured in the years ahead. Such patients constitute less than 20% of those who have met previous criteria of severe disease based on an APACHE II score of 6 or more, a CRP of greater than 150 mg/L, or a Ranson or Glasgow score of 3 or more.

In the last decade it has been appreciated that many prospective randomized studies of acute pancreatitis reveal that within the group who have fatal acute pancreatitis almost 50% succumb within the first week of illness. Nearly all these patients die from multiorgan failure and the majority are over 70 years of age. Indeed, in the retrospective national study from Scotland of almost 14 000 patients over an 11-year period, close examination of the deaths in the first week identified that most of these patients died within 96 hours. Only rapid access to an intensive-care bed with full back-up has the potential to reduce the mortality rate in such patients at this time.

A host of potential specific therapies for severe acute pancreatitis, including aprotinin and gabexate mesylate (both antiproteases), octreotide (synthetic somatostatin analog), peritoneal lavage, and lexipafant (platelet-activating factor antagonist), have all failed when subjected to randomized controlled study.

Recurrent pancreatitis

Finally, it is very important that the risk of further attacks of acute pancreatitis be minimized. Numerically, gallstone-induced disease is the most common etiology, and all guidelines on management of acute pancreatitis rightly emphasize optimum therapy to include cholecystectomy with clearance of common duct stones within the same admission. In older or very unfit patients endoscopic sphincterotomy is a reasonable alternative therapy for gallstone acute pancreatitis. It is usually a small stone of 5 mm diameter (or less) that causes this disease.

Recommended reading

Allam BF, Imrie CW. Serum ionised calcium in acute pancreatitis. *Br J Surg* 1977;64:665–668.

Blamey SL, Imrie CW, O'Neill J, Gilmour WH, Carter DC. Prognostic factors in acute pancreatitis. *Gut* 1984;25:1340–1346.

Buter A, Imrie CW, Carter CR, Evans S, McKay CJ. Dynamic nature of early organ dysfunction determines outcome in acute pancreatitis. *Br J Surg* 2002;89:298–302.

Dervenis C, Johnson CD, Bassi C *et al*. Diagnosis, objective assessment of severity and management of acute pancreatitis. Santorini consensus conference. *Int J Pancreatol* 1999;25:195–210.

Dickson AP, O'Neill J, Imrie CW. Hyperlipidaemia, alcohol abuse and acute pancreatitis. *Br J Surg* 1984;71:685–688.

Glazer G, Mann DV. United Kingdom Guidelines in the management of acute pancreatitis. *Gut* 1998;42(Suppl 2):S1–S13.

Imrie CW, Allam BF, Ferguson JC. Hypocalcaemia of acute pancreatitis: the effect of hypoalbuminaemia. *Curr Med Res Opin* 1976;4:101–116.

Imrie CW, Murphy D, Ferguson JC, Blumgart LH. Arterial hypoxia in acute pancreatitis. *Br J Surg* 1977;64:185–188.

Imrie CW, Beastall GH, Allam BF, O'Neill J, Benjamin IS, McKay AJ. Parathyroid hormone and calcium homeostasis in acute pancreatitis. *Br J Surg* 1978;65:717–720.

Isenmann R, Rau B, Beger HG. Early severe acute pancreatitis: characteristics of a new subgroup. *Pancreas* 2001;22:274–278.

Johnson CD, Kingsnorth AN, Imrie CW *et al*. Double blind, randomised, placebo controlled study of a platelet activating factor antagonist, lexipafant, in the treatment and prevention of organ failure in predicted severe acute pancreatitis. *Gut* 2002;48:62–69.

Knaus WA, Wagner DP, Draper EA, Zimmerman JE. APACHE II final form and national validation results of a severity of disease classification system. *Crit Care Med* 1984;12:213–223.

McKay CJ, Curran F, Sharples C, Baxter JN, Imrie CW. Prospective placebo-controlled randomised trial of Lexipafant in predicted severe acute pancreatitis. *Br J Surg* 1997;84:1239–1243.

McKay CJ, Evans S, Sinclair M, Carter CR, Imrie CW. High early mortality rate from acute pancreatitis in Scotland, 1984–1995. *Br J Surg* 1999;86:1302–1305.

Marshall JC, Cook DJ, Christou NU. Multiple organ dysfunction score, a reliable descriptor of a complex clinical outcome. *Crit Care Med* 1995;23:83–92.

Mayer AD, McMahon MG, Bowen M, Cooper EH. C-reactive protein: an aid to assessment and monitoring of acute pancreatitis. *J Clin Pathol* 1984;37:207–211.

Murray B, Carter R, Imrie C, Evans S, O'Suilleabhain C. Diclofenac reduces the incidence of acute pancreatitis after endoscopic retrograde cholangiopancreatography. *Gastroenterology* 2003;124:1786–1791.

Puolakkainen P, Valtonen V, Paananen A, Schroder T. C-reactive protein (CRP) and serum phospholipase A2 in the assessment of the severity of acute pancreatitis. *Gut* 1987;28:764–771.

Ranson HJC, Rifkind KM, Roses DF, Fink SD, Eng K, Spencer FC. Prognostic signs and the role of operative management in acute pancreatitis. *Surg Gynecol Obstet* 1974;139: 69–81.

Thune A, Baker RA, Saccone GTP, Owen H, Toouli J. Differing effects of pethidine and morphine on human sphincter of Oddi motility. *Br J Surg* 1990;77:992–995.

Uhl W, Warshaw A, Imrie C *et al*. IAP guidelines for the surgical management of acute pancreatitis. *Pancreatology* 2003;2:565–573.

van den Berghe G, Wouters P, Weekers F *et al*. Intensive insulin therapy in critically ill patients. *N Engl J Med* 2001;345: 1359–1367.

Wilson C, Heads A, Shenkin A, Imrie CW. C-reactive protein, antiproteases and complement factors as objective markers of severity in acute pancreatitis. *Br J Surg* 1989;76: 177–181.

Guidelines for the treatment of pain in acute pancreatitis

Juan Martínez and Miguel Pérez-Mateo

Pain is the main symptom in acute pancreatitis. Abdominal pain occurs during almost all episodes of acute pancreatitis. Usually there is epigastric or upper abdominal pain, which rapidly becomes more severe, accompanied by nausea and vomiting, leading the patient to ask for attention at the emergency department. It is thought that the pain is caused by the action of activated pancreatic enzymes and the release of cytokines by inflammatory cells, which stimulate visceral pain receptors in the pancreas and peritoneal somatic receptors. Abdominal distension and ileus also play a role in causing abdominal discomfort.

The sensation of pain in acute pancreatitis is transmitted along the different sensory fibers found throughout the pancreas to the celiac plexus and then, via the splanchnic nerves, to the sympathetic chain between T5 and T9. The nerve bodies of these fibers are found in the dorsal root ganglia.

No study has shown any correlation between the degree of pain and the severity of the pancreatitis. However, it tends to last longer in patients with severe pancreatitis and contributes to their hemodynamic instability. Similarly, the presence or absence of pain is an important factor in resuming normal eating. A relationship has been shown between prolonged pain and its recurrence when oral feeding is started.

Usually, the initial pain in acute pancreatitis lasts only a few days and disappears spontaneously when the local inflammatory reaction improves. Sometimes it may recur during the course of the illness if complications such as pseudocysts, pancreatic infections, peptic ulcer, or biliary obstruction develop. In this chapter we refer to the initial pain, although obviously the recommendations for treatment given below may

be applicable at any stage of the pancreatitis, whenever the recurrence of abdominal pain is due to this condition.

Treatment of pain in acute pancreatitis

General aspects

There are several measures available to relieve pain. It is advisable for the patient to fast, at least initially. This limits pancreatic stimulation and improves the abdominal distension secondary to acute pancreatitis. When ileus is present, passing a nasogastric tube may improve symptoms. Obviously, these measures alone are not sufficient to control the pain as this requires suitable medication. The management of abdominal pain associated with acute pancreatitis follows the same general rules as the treatment of other acute pain, namely the staged use of analgesics, but the oral route is ruled out. The pharmacologic treatment of pancreatitis therefore requires parenteral or other alternative routes of administration. Basically, since the pain is continuous, analgesics should be prescribed at regular intervals or even as a continuous perfusion following an initial loading dose to control the pain rapidly. Once the pain is under control, analgesics may be prescribed as needed by the patient.

Patient-controlled analgesia

In recent years patient-controlled analgesia (PCA) pumps have been used for intravenous administration. This technique provides small doses of analgesic drugs as required by the patient by means of a perfusion pump controlled by a microcomputer. Theoretically, greater efficacy should be achieved with lower dosage. PCA pumps may also be used for subcutaneous or epidural medication. Some authors recommend continuous perfusion of analgesic drugs administered via PCA. Because of the stability of the serum levels of these drugs, this modality provides higher pain relief during sleep intervals and decreases the number of loading doses self-administered by the patient. However, the possibility of overdosage is present. On the other hand, PCA without continuous perfusion allows the dosage of drug to be matched to the patient's requirements with low risk of overdosage, but patients need to be trained in this technique and decreased effectiveness during sleep intervals might occur.

Some concepts must be taken into account when programming a PCA.

• Loading dose: generally a high dose of the analgesic drug is programmed by the physician. This allows an analgesic effect to be achieved quickly.

• Incremental dose: dose self-administered by the patient when pain is present.

• Lockout interval: interval between two incremental doses. It represents a security measure to avoid overdose.

We recommend a program with high incremental doses and long lockout intervals. Some examples of PCA are shown in Table 9.1.

Parenteral drug treatment

Nonsteroidal antiinflammatory drugs

Nonsteroidal antiinflammatory drugs (NSAIDs) are generally used as the initial treatment of pain of any origin. They are therefore the analgesics most often used in acute pancreatitis. They provide limited analgesia but are associated with antiinflammatory and antipyretic effects. NSAIDs are usually well tolerated. Unlike other analgesics, they have an upper limit of therapeutic effectiveness, above which no further benefit is expected. Their analgesic effect is due to the inhibition of prostaglandin synthesis by inhibition of peripheral cyclooxygenase, thus reducing the peripheral inflammatory effects, although it is thought that they probably also affect central neurotransmission. Adverse effects may occur, the most dangerous of which is upper gastrointestinal bleeding. This complication is important in acute pancreatitis since it is one of the criteria of severity in this disease. Hypersensitivity reactions, bone marrow impairment, renal involvement (especially when there is intravascular volume depletion as is common in acute pancreatitis), and hepatotoxicity may also be seen. It has been shown experimentally that they improve the outcome of acute pancreatitis, although it has not been confirmed in humans. Recently, they have been recommended in the prevention of pancreatitis after endoscopic retrograde cholangiopancreatogra-

Table 9.1 Administration of analgesics and local anesthetics using patient-controlled analgesia (PCA).

	Drug	Loading dose (mg/kg)	Loading dose duration (hours)	Infusion (mg/hour)	Bolus (mg)	Lockout interval (min)
Opioids (i.v.)	Morphine	0.05	3–4	1–2	0.5–2	60
	Meperidine	0.5	3–4	10–20	5–30	60
	Tramadol		6–8	15–25	15–30	60
Opioids (epidural)	Morphine	0.015	6–24	0.2–0.4	0.1–0.2	60
	Meperidine		4–8	10–15	20–25	60
	Fentanyl	0.001	2–4	0.05–0.075	25–30	30
	Tramadol			8	4	30
	Bupivacaine + fentanyl			7.5	2.5	10
				0.015–0.03	10	
NSAID (i.v.)	Metamizol			320	320	30

i.v., intravenous; NSAID, nonsteroidal antiinflammatory drug.

phy. In acute pancreatitis one of the most widely used NSAIDs is metamizol. It is a pyrazolone and seems to be less gastroerosive than other NSAIDs since it does not affect the synthesis of prostacyclin. However, it has the disadvantage of causing agranulocytosis in a small proportion of cases. The usual dose is 2000 mg intravenously every 6–8 hours.

Local anesthetics

These drugs reversibly prevent the genesis and transmission of nervous stimuli in any excitable membrane (membrane-stabilizing effect). This property favors a decrease in pain sensitivity in a determined region of the organism. Parenteral procaine has been shown to be useful in the management of pain associated with acute pancreatitis. It is the analgesic of choice for the treatment of acute bouts of chronic pancreatitis as recommended by the German consensus conference on the treatment of chronic pancreatitis. It should be used carefully in patients with renal failure, and adverse effects such as weakness, dizziness, hypertension, and skin rash may occur when patients are sensitive to the drug. It is therefore advisable to check whether there is hypersensitivity to the drug before using it. The recommended dose is 2000 mg given as an intravenous perfusion over 24 hours.

Pancreatic enzymes

These are used to treat pain associated with chronic pancreatitis on the assumption that they inhibit pancreatic secretion by negative feedback due to the intraduodenal release of proteases. However, these enzymes have not been shown to be useful for analgesia in acute pancreatitis.

Opioids

These drugs represent the next stage in the treatment of pain. Their analgesic effect is due to the stimulation of specialized opiate receptors found in the central nervous system, where they interfere with nociceptive transmission by reducing the release of excitatory neurotransmitters. Although they may be given by the oral, sublingual, rectal, or transdermal route, parenteral use is recommended in acute pancreatitis. The disadvantage of this route is the short drug half-life (usually < 4 hours), so continuous perfusion would be advisable if a continuous analgesic effect is required. In general, the recommended dose of opioids is only a guide since pain is subjective and the specific dose required by each particular patient should be used. The development of adverse effects would be the only limiting factor.

Although opioids are more powerful analgesics than NSAIDs, they have major adverse effects. In the case of seriously ill patients, respiratory depression is the most important; almost all opiates cause it in a dose-dependent fashion. This adverse effect is especially important in acute pancreatitis where opioids may contribute to the occurrence of respiratory failure or aggravate it when it is already present. They may also cause euphoria, drowsiness, nausea and vomiting, reduced peristalsis, urinary retention, cardiac dysrhythmias, pruritus, mental clouding, physical dependency, and tolerance. Another adverse effect relevant to acute pancreatitis is the supposed effect that some opioids produce on the sphincter of Oddi (see below). The opioids most widely used are described below.

1 *Morphine*: the paradigm of this group of drugs and the reference for comparison of the potency of the other opioids. It is therefore the best known and most widely studied. Since it does not cross the blood–brain barrier readily, it causes less central nervous system excitation. Although plasma levels of its metabolite morphine 3-glucuronide are raised in renal failure, this metabolite is not associated with central nervous system alterations. The dose is 5–15 mg intramuscularly or subcutaneously every 4–5 hours or 0.01–0.04 mg/kg per hour as an intravenous perfusion.

2 *Meperidine* has weaker analgesic effect than morphine. As with most opioids it has a short half-life (3–4 hours), although its metabolite (normoperidine) stays in the bloodstream for much longer. This metabolite is potentially neurotoxic and may cause hyperexcitation of the central nervous system with the development of seizures, particularly in cases of renal failure, reduced seizure threshold, simultaneous use of monoamine oxidase inhibitors, some antiretroviral agents, alcoholism, or drug addiction. It also has an anticholinergic effect and becomes cardiotoxic when high doses are administered. For these reasons, continuous infusion is not recommended. Parenteral dosage is 1–1.5 mg/kg every 4 hours.

3 *Buprenorphine* has a beneficial effect on the course of acute pancreatitis in experimental animals, although this condition has not been demonstrated in humans. It is approximately 30 times more potent than morphine. Intoxication with buprenorphine is difficult to overcome with antagonists (such as naloxone) because of the strength with which it binds to opiate receptors. It is almost completely metabolized by the liver to inactive

or only weakly active metabolites. Thus it may be used safely in cases of renal failure. It does not cause seizures. Nevertheless, it has an important emetic effect that is sometimes difficult to manage. When used sublingually the dose is 0.2–0.4 mg every 6–8 hours. The usual parenteral dose is 0.3–0.6 mg intramuscularly or intravenously every 6 hours or 0.002 mg/kg per hour as an intravenous perfusion.

4 *Tramadol*: although it has agonist effects on opioid receptors, it also shows analgesic activity due to other mechanisms. It is a weaker analgesic than morphine (about eight times). Since its half-life is slightly longer, it is used parenterally at a dose of 100–150 mg every 6–8 hours (0.17 mg/kg per hour in perfusion). In cases of renal failure the drug accumulates in the bloodstream and it is advisable to increase the interval between doses. It favors the development of seizures in the conditions described for meperidine. Unlike most opiates it does not cause addiction.

5 *Hydromorphone* is eight times more potent as an analgesic than morphine. The recommended dose is 0.5 mg every 3 hours intravenously or 1–2 mg intramuscularly or subcutaneously. A dose of 0.2–1 mg/hour may be given as a perfusion.

6 *Fentanyl* is 80 times more potent than morphine. It is hardly used parenterally in pancreatitis but the transdermal route, which allows slow drug release, is used especially to treat chronic pain. Recently, this treatment has also been used successfully in acute pancreatitis (see below).

Effect on the sphincter of Oddi Traditionally, several opioids, including morphine, have been rejected as treatments for pain in acute pancreatitis on the assumption that they increase biliary pressure. This was based on the findings of preliminary studies that indirectly measured biliary pressure after the use of these drugs. However, opioids such as meperidine did not cause pressure changes and consequently it has become the narcotic of choice in acute pancreatitis. However, as commented before, morphine has several advantages over meperidine in the management of this disorder: it is more potent, its management is more widely known, and it is safer in cases of renal failure with less risk of seizures.

Direct manometric studies of the sphincter of Oddi have not fully confirmed the initial hypothesis (Table 9.2). In these studies both morphine and meperidine significantly increased the frequency of the phasic waves of the sphincter, whereas buprenorphine and tramadol did not seem to have any effect. The increase in frequency of the phasic waves causes a reduction in passive filling of the sphincter segment and results in an increase in biliary pressure (confirming the result of the preliminary studies). However, only high cumulative doses of morphine cause a significant increase in the basal pressure of the sphincter of Oddi. Furthermore, no study has yet shown that the increased basal pressure of the sphincter caused by this dose of morphine has a deleterious effect on patients with acute pancreatitis. Therefore it is possible to use morphine (or any

Table 9.2 Effect of opioids on sphincter of Oddi dynamics (direct measurement).

Drug	Study	Dose	Results
Morphine	Helm *et al.* (1988)	Successive dose: 2.5, 2.5, 5, 10 µg/kg every 5 min i.v.	2.5–5 µg/kg: increased frequency 10–20 µg/kg: increased basal pressure, frequency and amplitude
	Thune *et al.* (1990)	Cumulative dose: 2.5, 5, 10 µg/kg every 2 min i.v.	Increased frequency of phasic waves
Meperidine	Elta & Barnett (1994)	1 mg/kg i.v.	Increased frequency of phasic waves
	Thune *et al.* (1990)	Cumulative dose: 25, 25, 50 µg/kg every 2 min i.v.	Decreased frequency of phasic waves
	Sherman & Lehman (1996)	1 mg/kg to 75 mg i.v.	Increased frequency of phasic waves
Buprenorphine	Staritz *et al.* (1986)	0.3 mg i.v.	No changes
	Cuer *et al.* (1989)	0.3 mg i.v.	No changes
Tramadol	Staritz *et al.* (1986)	50 mg i.v.	No changes

i.v., intravenous.

other opioid) in the management of pain in acute pancreatitis, although more studies are still necessary to confirm this hypothesis.

Controlled studies Despite the number of therapeutic drugs used to treat pain in acute pancreatitis, there are few published controlled studies that compare these drugs with each other or with a placebo (Table 9.3).

In 1984, Blamey and colleagues compared the use of intramuscular buprenorphine with intramuscular meperidine in 32 patients with acute pancreatitis. These authors found similar analgesic responses to these drugs in both the intensity and duration of pain relief. Adverse effects were minimal (nausea and vomiting) and occurred in the same proportion in both types of treatment. A year later, Ebbehoj *et al.* studied the analgesic effect of rectal indomethacin (indometacin) compared with a placebo in 30 patients with acute pancreatitis. In this study, treatment with indomethacin significantly reduced the number of days with pain and the amount of other analgesics (opiates) given. In 1995 Patankar *et al.* reported another controlled study comparing the use of pancreatic enzymes with a placebo in 23 patients with acute pancreatitis. No difference was found in the analgesia obtained by these patients. The main adverse effect seen was nausea, which occurred in approximately half the patients in both groups. Recently, Jakobs and colleagues compared the analgesic effects of intravenous buprenorphine and procaine. In 40 patients with acute pancreatitis or acute bouts of chronic pancreatitis, buprenorphine produced higher pain relief and reduced the need for additional analgesics. Apart from slight sedation of the buprenorphine-treated group, the secondary effects were few and comparable. Another recent German controlled trial confirmed the lower analgesic effects

Table 9.3 Controlled studies with analgesics in acute pancreatitis.

Study	No. of patients	Drugs	Pain assessment	Outcome	Adverse effects
Blamey *et al.* (1984)	32	Buprenorphine 0.3 mg i.m. Meperidine 100 mg i.m.	Standard lineal scale Categories scale	Similar relief Similar duration of pain relief	Similar (nausea, vomiting)
Ebbehoj *et al.* (1985)	30	Indomethacin 50 mg twice (rectal) Placebo	Visual analog scale	Indomethacin group: less number of days with pain and opiate administration	None
Patankar *et al.* (1995)	23	Oral pancreatic enzymes (7800 U protease daily) Placebo	Visual analog scale	Similar pain relief and analgesic requirements	Similar (nausea)
Jakobs *et al.* (2000)	40	Buprenorphine 0.3 mg (bolus i.v.) + 2.4 mg (infusion i.v.) per 24 hours Procaine 2 g (infusion i.v.) per 24 hours	Visual analog scale	Buprenorphine group: higher pain relief and less additional analgesic requirements	Buprenorphine group: higher sedation rate
Stevens *et al.* (2002)	32	TTS fentanyl + meperidine Placebo + meperidine	Self-reported pain intensity	Fentanyl group: less pain intensity at 36, 45, and 60 hours from admission	None reported
Kahl *et al.* (2004)	107	Pentazocine 30 mg (bolus i.v.) per 6 hours Procaine 2 g (infusion i.v.) per 24 hours	Visual analog scale	Pentazocine group: lower pain scores over 72 hours	None

i.m., intramuscular; i.v., intravenous; TTS, transdermal therapeutic system.

of procaine. Finally, Stevens *et al.* reported that transdermal fentanyl (plus meperidine for further relief) failed as compared with placebo (plus meperidine) in obtaining significant pain relief during the first 24 hours in hospital in 32 patients with acute pancreatitis. However, fentanyl was more effective for pain relief after the first 36 hours in hospital.

Thus although there is scanty evidence, we must conclude that the use of certain opioids such as meperidine and buprenorphine is safe and effective for pain control in patients with acute pancreatitis. Further controlled studies are needed to confirm whether opioids in general are more effective than theoretically less potent but more widely used drugs such as NSAIDs and to clarify the role of morphine (more potent and safer than meperidine) in pain management in this condition.

Epidural analgesia

Epidural analgesia is becoming widely used in delivery and in the immediate postoperative period after abdominal or gynecologic surgery. When this route of administration is used, the drug is concentrated where the painful impulses enter the spinal cord (i.e., on the spinal nerve roots). This permits the use of doses substantially lower than those required for oral or parenteral administration. Systemic adverse effects are thus decreased. The procedure involves the insertion of a catheter 3 cm into the epidural space between T5 and T9 (usually T8) and analgesia is instituted by injection of an analgesic drug through the catheter. Because dural puncture is not intended, the site of entry may be at any vertebral level that permits a segmental blockade approximately limited to the chosen region. Usually local anesthetics such as bupivacaine or opioids such as fentanyl or morphine, or a combination of both types of drugs, are used. The association of both agents permits the use of lower doses, minimizing local anesthetic-induced complications of motor blockade and opioid-induced complications. The dose of local anesthetic used can produce high concentrations in blood following absorption from the epidural space, which is rich in venous plexuses. On the other hand, since conduction in autonomic, sensory, and motor nerves is not affected by opioids, blood pressure, motor function, and nociceptive sensory perception typically are not influenced by epidural opioids. Pruritus, nausea, vomiting, and urinary retention may appear. Delayed respiratory depression and sedation, presumably from cephalad spread of opioid within the cerebrospinal fluid, occurs infrequently with the doses of opioids currently used.

The technique may involve a single dose but to achieve analgesia over a prolonged period a catheter should be placed for either intermittent dosage or continuous perfusion. As previously mentioned, PCA pumps can be applied. If continuous perfusion is administered, stable analgesic levels are obtained. Therefore, early patient mobilization, improvement in muscular tone, and fewer episodes of hypotension are expected. After correct placing of the epidural catheter, it is necessary to administer a single dose; if adverse effects do not develop, a continuous perfusion should be programmed with variable rate according to the analgesic level obtained. Table 9.4 shows some examples of epidural administration of analgesic drugs.

This type of analgesia has reduced postoperative morbidity and mortality. Recently, a systematic review reported that in patients undergoing laparotomy epidural administration of local anesthetics and opioids provided higher postoperative analgesia than the use of local anesthetics alone. However, local anesthetics were found to be associated with less gastrointestinal

Table 9.4 Epidural administration of opioids and local anesthesics.

	Loading dose	Infusion (per hour)	Bolus
Morphine	1–2 mg	0.2–0.4 mg	0.1–0.2 mg/hour
Meperidine	25–50 mg	10–15 mg	20–25 mg/hour
Fentanyl	100 μg	50–75 μg	25–50 μg/hour
Fentanyl + bupivacaine (0.0625%)	75 μg + 3.75 mg (6 mL)	50 μg + 2.5 mg (4 mL/hour)	12.5 μg + 0.0625 mg/30 min (1 mL)
Morphine + bupivacaine (0.0625%)	1 mg + 5 mg	0.15 mg + 1.8 mg (3 mL)	0.15 mg + 1.8 mg/30 min (3 mL)

paralysis than when systemic or epidural opioids were used.

In patients with acute pancreatitis, this type of analgesia has many theoretical advantages. Firstly, it permits a reduction in high doses of opioids when these are excessive and/or associated with adverse effects (as previously mentioned, opioids facilitate the occurrence or aggravation of respiratory failure and some show increased neurotoxicity in the presence of renal failure). Also, it allows severely ill patients to achieve a sitting or semi-sitting position readily and therefore improves gas exchange and reduces the incidence of respiratory infections. Intestinal blood flow and motility is also said to improve. Finally, in postoperative patients, epidural analgesia reduces the metabolic response and improves catabolism. All these beneficial effects favor mobilization, reduce the incidence of complications, and permit early resumption of oral feeding. Unfortunately, there are still no controlled studies of patients

with acute pancreatitis which confirm the theoretical benefits of this type of analgesia.

Nevertheless, this type of analgesia may have adverse effects, such as hypotension (due to involvement of the sympathetic nervous system when the catheter is inserted or medication administered), headache, urinary retention, radicular damage, or catheter migration. The most serious, though infrequent, complication is the development of epidural hematoma or abscess. Epidural analgesia is contraindicated in hypovolemic shock, severe coagulopathy, infection, or radiculopathy at the level of catheter insertion. As previously mentioned, since variable amounts of the drugs reach the peripheral blood, systemic adverse effects of local anesthetics or opioids might develop.

Large series of patients with acute pancreatitis treated by epidural anesthesia have been reported to have had excellent pain control, with no neurologic or septic complications. Finally, there have been sporadic

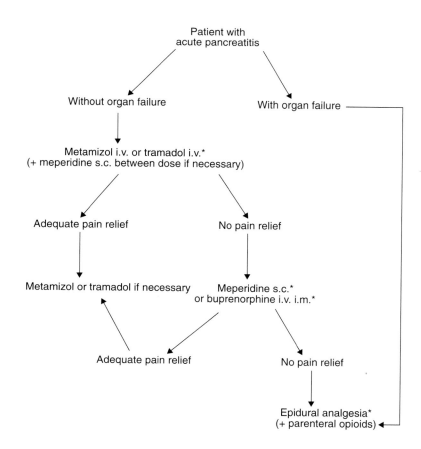

Figure 9.1 Guidelines for the treatment of pain in acute pancreatitis. *, Patient-controlled analgesia, if possible; i.m., intramuscular; i.v., intravenous; s.c., subcutaneous.

reports of good pain relief following percutaneous pharmacologic blockade of the celiac plexus.

Guidelines for the management of pain in acute pancreatitis

Pain due to acute pancreatitis should be treated from the very onset of the disease by regular analgesic administration. In general terms, PCA pumps are recommended (see Table 9.1). Staged treatment should be given (Fig. 9.1). Thus we may use metamizol (2000 mg every 6–8 hours intravenously) or tramadol (100 mg every 8 hours intravenously), with meperidine (50–100 mg subcutaneously as a single dose) for rescue between doses. When pain control is satisfactory or the pain disappears, the same dosage may be used on demand by the patient. However, if the pain is not controlled, opioids become necessary. Until studies confirm the safety of morphine and its derivatives, the use of meperidine (50–100 mg every 4 hours subcutaneously) or buprenorphine (0.3–0.6 mg every 6 hours parenterally; 0.2–0.4 mg every 6 hours sublingually; 0.002 mg/kg per hour as intravenous continuous perfusion) is recommended.

Patients who require high doses of opioids for adequate pain control, and especially those with organ failure (mainly renal and/or respiratory failure), should be treated with epidural anesthesia using either local anesthesics alone or, better, local anesthesics plus opioids (see Table 9.4). This kind of analgesia may be administered in addition to systemic opioids, the dose of which can then be reduced, or can be used as the sole treatment.

Recommended reading

Blamey SL, Finlay IG, Carter DC, Imrie CW. Analgesia in acute pancreatitis: comparison of buprenorphine and pethidine. *BMJ* 1984;288:1494–1495.

Cuer JC, Dapoigny M, Ajmi S *et al.* Effects of buprenorphine on motor activity of the sphincter of Oddi in man. *Eur J Clin Pharmacol* 1989;36:203–204.

Ebbehoj N, Friis J, Svendsen B, Bülow S, Madsen P. In-domethacin treatment of acute pancreatitis. A controlled double-blind trial. *Scand J Gastroenterol* 1985;20:788–800.

Elta GH, Barnett JL. Meperidine need not be proscribed during sphincter of Oddi manometry. *Gastrointest Endosc* 1994;40:7–9.

Helm JF, Venu RP, Geenen JE *et al.* Effects of morphine on the human sphincter of Oddi. *Gut* 1988;29:1402–1407.

Holte K, Kehlet H. Epidural anaesthesia and analgesia: effects on surgical stress responses and implications for postoperative nutrition. *Clin Nutr* 2002;21:199–206.

Isenhower HI, Mueller BA. Selection of narcotic analgesics for pain associated with pancreatitis. *Am J Health Syst Pharm* 1998;55:480–486.

Jakobs R, Adamek MU, von Bubnoff AC, Riemann JF. Buprenorphine or procaine for pain relief in acute pancreatitis. A prospective randomized study. *Scand J Gastroenterol* 2000;35:1319–1323.

Jorgesen H, Wetterslev J, Moiniche S, Dahl JB. Epidural local anaesthesics versus opioid-based analgesic regimens for postoperative gastrointestinal paralysis, PONV and pain after abdominal surgery. *Cochrane Database Syst Rev* 2003;4:CD001893.

Kahl S, Zimmerman S, Pross M *et al.* Procaine hydrochloride fails to relieve pain in patients with acute pancreatitis. *Digestion* 2004;69:5–9.

Patankar BV, Chand R, Johnson CD. Pancreatic enzyme supplementation in acute pancreatitis. *HPB Surg* 1995;8:159–162.

Rodgers A, Walker N, Schung S *et al.* Reduction of postoperative mortality and morbidity with epidural or spinal anaesthesia: results from overview of randomised trials. *BMJ* 2000;321:1–12.

Sherman S, Lehman G. Opioids and the sphincter of Oddi. *Gastrointest Endosc* 1996;44:239–242.

Staritz M, Poralla T, Manns M *et al.* Effect of modern analgesic drugs (tramadol, pentazocine and buprenorphine) on the bile duct sphincter in man. *Gut* 1986;27:567–569.

Stevens M, Esler R, Asher G. Transdermal fentanyl for the management of acute pancreatitis pain. *Appl Nurs Res* 2002;15:102–110.

Thompson DR. Narcotic analgesic effects on the sphincter of Oddi: a review of the data and therapeutic implications in treating pancreatitis. *Am J Gastroenterol* 2001;96:1266–1272.

Thune A, Baker RA, Saccone GT *et al.* Differing effects of pethidine and morphine on human sphincter of Oddi motility. *Br J Surg* 1990;77:992–995.

10 Nutrition in the acute phase of pancreatitis: why, when, how, and how long?

Konstantina Paraskeva, Costas Avgerinos, and Christos Dervenis

Acute pancreatitis is a disease with a wide spectrum of clinical courses, ranging from the mild form with minimum morbidity and almost zero mortality, to the severe form with a high percentage of complications and high risk for a lethal outcome.

In about 80% of patients, the inflammatory process is self-limited, involving only the pancreas and immediate pancreatic tissues, and resolves spontaneously within less than a week. These mild cases require only a short period of fasting, intravenous hydration, electrolytes, and analgesia. Patients can usually start an oral low-fat diet within 3–7 days of the onset of their pain, resulting in minor and usually easily reversible nutritional defects.

This is not the case in severe acute pancreatitis, which is characterized by various degrees of necrosis of pancreatic parenchyma as well as local and systemic complications such as systemic inflammatory response syndrome (SIRS) and multiple organ failure (MOF). This form of the disease represents a typical hypermetabolic septic model, with increased resting energy requirements and considerable protein catabolism that leads to severe malnutrition.

As a result nutritional support in acute pancreatitis should be one of the main therapeutic aims and nutritional management should depend on the underlying pancreatic disease.

Malnutrition and metabolic changes in acute pancreatitis: why?

Regardless of the etiology, all cases of acute pancreatitis share a common pathogenetic pathway that involves the premature activation of trypsinogen to trypsin, after which a cascade of pancreatic enzyme activation begins that leads to autodigestion of the pancreas and peripancreatic tissues. At the same time, a number of powerful inflammatory mediators are produced locally and systemically, with cytokines being the most important because they initiate or amplify an inflammatory cascade and induce the development of SIRS and remote organ failure. Later in the course of the disease, infective complications may occur, particularly infected pancreatic necrosis, consequent sepsis, and sepsis-related MOF, that further increase energy requirements. The release of inflammatory mediators, particularly tumor necrosis factor (TNF)-α and interleukin (IL)-6, and in cases of sepsis the release of catabolic hormones (catecholamines, cortisol, glucagon), change protein and energy metabolism in ways that increase both energy demands and urinary nitrogen excretion, which, in parallel with the reduction of food intake, result in the development of protein–energy malnutrition.

Clinical studies have shown that patients with acute pancreatitis have a resting energy expenditure (REE) that is 1.2–1.5 times that predicted by the Harris–Benedict equation, depending on the severity of the disease. Septic patients are the ones with the greater protein–energy needs, since they are in marked metabolic stress. These patients exhibit accelerated catabolism and protein breakdown and have a decreased blood supply to vital organs due to hypovolemia or decreased cardiac performance during the inflammatory process.

As already mentioned, nitrogen loss during severe disease is increased. While a healthy adult loses approximately 12 g of nitrogen daily in the urine in the fasting state, patients with acute pancreatitis complicated by sepsis commonly lose up to 40 g of nitrogen daily, with most of this loss coming from the skeletal muscle. Negative nitrogen adversely affects host defenses and immune competence balance and is associated with increased morbidity and mortality.

Another metabolic response to severe inflammation and energy deprivation is endogenous gluconeogenesis from protein degradation, which can only partially be inhibited by exogenous glucose. Intravenous administration of high doses of glucose carries the risk of hyperglycemia as the insulin response is often impaired. Furthermore, insulin release is also frequently impaired as a result of the inflamed pancreas, rendering the patient susceptible to hyperglycemia in 40–90% of cases. It has been suggested that transient hyperglycemia may impair complement fixation, evoking an immunosuppressive state. Parenteral nutrition is associated with an additional risk for hyperglycemia and careful monitoring of blood glucose levels is necessary in these patients.

Finally, lipid metabolism is also altered in acute pancreatitis via a mechanism that is not entirely clear. Increased serum triglycerides may either be the cause or the result of acute pancreatitis. Increase in cholesterol and free fatty acids in serum have also been reported. After the acute phase subsides, serum lipids tend to return to normal. Infusion of exogenous fat does not seem to interfere with the development or the course of acute pancreatitis and is therefore not contraindicated, provided that patients are monitored for hypertriglyceridemia.

Energy supply in acute pancreatitis

Patients with severe acute pancreatitis manifest increased basal energy requirements, accentuated protein catabolism, and endogenous gluconeogenesis. The goals of nutritional support in this setting are (i) to lessen nitrogen wasting, (ii) to support organ structure and function, and (iii) to positively affect the clinical course of the disease if possible.

Individual protein–calorie needs vary widely depending mostly on the severity of the disease, as well as the age, body size (height and weight), and sex of the patient. The most accurate method of measuring caloric requirement is indirect calorimetry, which is also useful for determining the fuel mix being oxidized and for assessing the metabolic stress level. Unfortunately, it is not often available, and therefore the most

commonly used method for estimation of REE is the equation devised by Harris and Benedict. The formulas for calculating REE (in kcal/day), using the four variables age, height, weight, and sex, are as follows:

$$BMR_{women} = 655 + 9.5W + 1.8H - 4.7A$$
$$BMR_{men} = 66 + 13.7W + 5H - 6.8A$$

where W is the actual or usual weight (kg), H is height (cm), and A is age (years). In patients with acute pancreatitis, REE as determined by indirect calorimetry varies from 77 to 158% of the energy expenditure predicted by the Harris–Benedict equation, being higher in patients with pancreatitis complicated by sepsis or MOF. These results make the Harris–Benedict equation a very rough method for estimating the energy demands of these patients.

Even simpler REE equations are often used in clinical practice and it should be remembered that these may overestimate or underestimate the measured values by 20 or even 30% for any individual. In severely ill patients, REE is usually about 25–35 kcal/kg daily and 1.2–1.5 g of protein per kilogram dry body weight, adjusting for obesity. With increasing metabolic stress, calories and protein should be increased, except in critically ill patients. During the early catabolic stage, 15–25 kcal/kg and 1.5 g/kg of protein are more suitable in nonsurgical patients with MOF.

During artificial nutrition, energy should be provided in the form of mixed fuel, with 60–70% given as glucose and 30–40% as lipid emulsion. Patients with severe disease and MOF often have high serum glucose and triglyceride levels. Intravenous infusion of glucose and fat does not suppress endogenous production and may therefore result in further elevations of blood glucose and triglycerides. Hyperglycemia predisposes to fluid retention (due to increased insulin requirements) and immunosuppression. High-dose lipid emulsion is also immunosuppressive and hypertriglyceridemia may exacerbate pancreatitis; therefore blood glucose levels should be monitored and should not exceed 10 mmol/L, while serum triglyceride concentrations should not exceed 1.5–2 times normal. Requirements for protein can be adjusted by performance of a nitrogen balance study.

Hypocalcemia is the most frequent mineral aberration seen in patients with acute pancreatitis, and a marked reduction of serum calcium is associated with a poor prognosis. Systemic endotoxin exposure appears to play a significant role in the development of hypocalcemia in severe attacks. In cases where ionized calcium is low and this is not a false reduction due to hypoalbuminemia, an attempt to correct this reduction should be made. Excessive calcium infusion may induce pancreatitis.

Patients with pancreatitis may also benefit from glutamine supplementation, as it is an important fuel for the gastrointestinal tract (pancreatic islets, acinar cells, and enterocytes). The oxidation of one molecule of glutamine produces 30 mmol of ATP, which makes this amino acid a very rich energy source. It appears that although enterocytes are rich in glutamine and may even synthesize it endogenously, this amino acid is an essential nutrient in stressed patients.

Attempts to favorably modulate the immune and inflammatory responses of severely ill patients led to efforts to enrich nutrition with various immune-enhancing nutrients. This has become known as immunonutrition. Of the various nutrients that have been suggested as beneficial, glutamine, arginine, ω-3 fatty acids, and nucleotides have been introduced into clinical use in the form of several standard formulas, often in combination preparations. There are a number of reports, mainly in severely injured patients, dealing with the role of immune-enhanced enteral diets in these cases. A metaanalysis of 1009 patients from 11 trials showed that immune-modulated regimens resulted in a significant reduction of infective complications and length of hospital stay, but with no effect on survival. Only one study dealt with the use of glutamine in acute pancreatitis, as a supplement in standard total parenteral nutrition (TPN). This investigation found that glutamine improved leukocyte activity and reduced proinflammatory cytokine release in acute pancreatitis. No conclusions can be drawn from these studies and although it seems possible that immune-enriched diets could play a role, further studies are needed to clarify this issue.

In the light of the emerging evidence regarding the primary role of the intestine in the pathophysiology of acute pancreatitis, enteral feeding is now considered the preferred mode of nutritional support in these patients. Enteral feeding has proved to be safe and in the majority of patients may cover caloric needs. Due to its beneficial effect on gut integrity, it should be started very early in the course of the disease (during the first 24 hours) and should be continued until the patient tolerates oral feeding. In cases where the caloric goal cannot be achieved by enteral nutrition, combined parenteral nutrition should be used. Even a low volume of low-residue enteral diet given in cases where TPN is used is sufficient to protect the intestinal mucosa. Recently, it was suggested that gastric feeding may be feasible in patients with severe pancreatitis. The optimal feeding formula has yet to be determined, but an elemental or immune-enhancing diet (10–30 mL/hour) continuously perfused to the jejunum is suggested.

Total parenteral nutrition in acute pancreatitis

Traditionally, TPN has been the only nutrient-providing treatment in patients with acute pancreatitis and prolonged starvation. TPN achieves energy and protein provision without stimulating pancreatic exocrine secretion. Although Feller et al. in 1974, in an uncontrolled retrospective study, showed a decrease in the mortality rate of patients with acute pancreatitis who received intravenous hyperalimentation, several other similar retrospective uncontrolled clinical trials have failed to reproduce these results. On the contrary, other authors observed a higher incidence of catheter-related sepsis among TPN groups but no difference in total mortality.

Two prospective nonrandomized trials have been published on this subject. In 1989, Sitzmann et al. divided 73 patients with acute pancreatitis into three groups depending on their ability to tolerate glucose-free, lipid-based, and lipid-free nutrition. Within 15 days most patients in all groups achieved improvement in nutritional status. A higher mortality was observed in the fat-free group as well as among patients with persistent negative nitrogen balance. A high incidence of catheter sepsis was also documented. In 1991, Kalfaretzos et al. divided 67 patients with severe acute pancreatitis (more than three Ranson criteria) into two groups of early (within 72 hours after admission) and late (after 72 hours) onset of TPN. They noted a significantly lower incidence of complications and mortality in the early group but a high incidence of catheter-related sepsis as well.

The only prospective randomized controlled trial on the effects of early parenteral nutrition versus no nutritional support in patients with acute pancreatitis was published by Sax et al. in 1987. During this study, 54 patients were randomized to receive either supporting treatment alone or supportive treatment with early

TPN (within 24 hours of admission). TPN had no significant effect on clinical outcome, duration, and pancreatitis-related complications, but patients in the TPN group had a ninefold increase in the incidence of catheter sepsis. A significant drawback of this study is the fact that all patients studied had mild pancreatitis (mean Ranson score 1) and hence had low complication and mortality rates with conventional treatment.

In conclusion, it can be stated that there is no strong information regarding the role of TPN in acute pancreatitis and more trials are needed in order to establish any benefit. The use of TPN does not seem to interfere with the progress of the disease but indicates a trend in improvement of morbidity and mortality in patients with severe pancreatitis who achieve a state of positive nitrogen balance and in those who require prolonged starvation (i.e., persistent pancreatic inflammation, abscess, and pancreatic fistula). TPN is associated with certain disadvantages, such as an increased rate of catheter-related infections, metabolic disturbances such as hyperglycemia, effects on gut permeability, and increased cost.

Role of the gut in acute pancreatitis

Contamination of pancreatic necrosis and consequent sepsis is the main cause of death in severe pancreatitis, although in the early period of the disease SIRS remains the main fatal cause. The organisms responsible for secondary pancreatic infection are usually Gram-negative bacteria of the same type that colonize the gastrointestinal tract. This suggests gut barrier dysfunction, increased intestinal permeability, and subsequent bacterial translocation through the gut wall.

Indeed, changes in intestinal permeability have been proven to occur in acute pancreatitis and are directly related to the severity of the disease. Patients with severe acute pancreatitis have increased intestinal permeability compared with healthy controls or those with mild attacks, and patients who develop MOF have even greater changes compared with those with severe disease and more favorable outcome. Intestinal permeability changes occur within 72 hours of the onset of pancreatitis and normalize during recovery.

It has been proposed that intestinal permeability may allow bacteria and bacterial components to migrate from the intestinal lumen to extraintestinal sites. In fact, bacterial translocation from the lumen to the pancreas and mesenteric lymph nodes is well documented in animal models but has not been convincingly demonstrated in humans. Nevertheless there are some data that support the hypothesis. Firstly, it has been demonstrated that 50% of patients with pancreatic necrosis have gut-origin bacteria colonizing the pancreas, and that colonization is maximal during the second to third week after the onset of the disease. Secondly, intestinal colonization with Gram-negative organisms precedes pancreatic infection and represents an early risk factor for developing a pancreatic infection. Thirdly, clinical studies indicate an association between gut dysfunction and infection, acute respiratory distress syndrome, and MOF. However, studies in patients with acute pancreatitis have demonstrated that the changes in gut permeability occur early, whereas pancreatic infection usually occurs during the second to third week after the onset of the disease, and patients with increased permeability do not necessarily have more septic complications.

The early changes in intestinal permeability have been also correlated with corresponding levels of endotoxemia. Endotoxins derive from Gram-negative bacteria and have systemic toxic effects, such as tachycardia, hypotension, and pyrexia, and also derange the immune system. Endotoxemia appears to correlate with the severity, incidence of systemic complications, and mortality of patients with acute pancreatitis. Patients with severe attacks have higher serum concentrations of endotoxin compared with those with mild disease, and the same was found in nonsurvivors compared with survivors and in patients with MOF as opposed to those without it. Nevertheless, in a study conducted by Moore et al. on severely injured trauma patients, it was not possible to document bacteria or endotoxin in the portal blood, even in patients with MOF. Selective gut decontamination seems to reduce infection complications, but it does not increase patients' survival.

Overall, the maintenance of intestinal structure and function is a complicated and multifactorial process that requires the adequate delivery of energy and oxygen. Enterocytes use glutamine and short-chain fatty acids as primary fuel. The presence of these nutrients in the lumen stimulates the proliferation of mucosal cells and enhances gut integrity. Fasting leads to mucosal atrophy, increased rate of enterocyte apoptosis, decreased glutamine and arginine transport, and altered mucin composition of goblet cells. These changes may develop as early as the first week and intestinal permeability changes occur within 48–72 hours of the disease onset. Furthermore, the impairment of gut motility that occurs within 12 hours of the onset of acute pancreatitis favors bacterial overgrowth and contributes to endotoxemia and bacterial translocation. Enteral feeding repairs the mucosal damage caused by fasting and, if given very early, preserves epithelial integrity and bacterial ecology, therefore helping to maintain gut barrier function.

The intestinal barrier is particularly susceptible to ischemia and therefore an adequate blood supply is of great importance for its function. Severe acute pancreatitis produces hypovolemia and third-space fluid losses that induce splanchnic vasoconstriction and subsequent intestinal ischemia. The hypoxia that occurs early in patients with acute pancreatitis may further contribute to mucosal ischemia. The ischemic effect is also enhanced by the local production of various inflammatory mediators. Intestinal reperfusion causes further damage through the production of oxygen free radicals and inflammatory mediators. Severe acute pancreatitis is associated with priming and subsequent overactivation of leukocytes, which may be the main cause of intestinal injury, by inducing gut ischemia, amplifying inflammation, and releasing oxygen free radicals. Fluid replacement and resuscitation is essential in order to maintain microcirculation and prevent ischemia and reperfusion injury.

Recently, the role of the gut in acute pancreatitis has expanded beyond the bacterial translocation and endotoxin phenomenon, as emerging evidence has indicated that the gut may be a source of cytokines and a site of neutrophil priming. It appears that intestinal ischemia and reperfusion injury results in the overactivation of gut macrophages and gut-associated lymphoid tissue, which in turn release excessive cytokines and other mediators. The release of cytokines contributes to SIRS and MOF.

Enteral nutrition

Based on the above, efforts have been made to find a more natural way of delivering nutrients in patients with pancreatitis. Despite concerns for the possible stimulatory effect of oral feeding on pancreatic secretion and for disease exacerbation, several experimental and clinical trials have shown that delivery of nutrients

to the jejunum does not increase pancreatic secretion and is well tolerated with no increase in complications. More specifically, although administration of lipid into the duodenum is a strong stimulatory factor for pancreatic exocrine secretion, jejunal delivery of the same amount of lipid causes minimal pancreatic reaction. Similar minor effects of intravenous lipid infusion have been shown in human studies. Gastric or duodenal protein or carbohydrate administration is also a strong stimulus for pancreatic secretion, whereas jejunal delivery of the same nutrients is harmless to the pancreas.

Additionally, it has been confirmed that enteral feeding is technically feasible and clinically safe even in critically ill patients with severe disease, and provides efficient nutrition support. Severe paralytic ileus is not a contraindication to nasojejunal feeding, but in rare cases it may prevent adequate calorie intake. From the practical point of view, enteral feeding is achieved by the insertion of a nasojejunal feeding tube, usually placed endoscopically or under radiologic screening, distal to the ligament of Treitz. Occasionally, correct feeding tube location and maintenance of its patency may be troublesome.

Five randomized controlled studies have been published that compare enteral nutrition (EN) with TPN. Kalfaretzos et al. randomized 38 patients, all with severe acute pancreatitis, in two groups (EN vs. TPN). They found a significant reduction in total, including septic, complications in the EN group. The cost was three times lower in the EN than the TPN group, and the authors suggested that the use of EN is preferable in all patients with severe disease. In another other study, by Windsor et al., 34 patients were randomized in EN and TPN groups. In this study patients with moderate and severe disease were included. Patients who received EN fared better after 7 days with respect to APACHE II score and C-reactive protein (CRP) levels compared with the TPN group. The authors also reported an increase in serum IgM anti-endotoxin antibodies in the TPN group, levels of which remained unchanged in the EN group. The total antioxidant capacity was less in the former group. They concluded that patients on EN were exposed to less endotoxin levels. This was probably related to preserved host defense.

More recently, Abou-Assi and O'Keefe demonstrated earlier recovery, shorter hospital stay and shorter duration of nutritional support, better tolerance to restarting oral feeding, and much cheaper cost for nutrition in a group of 17 enterally fed patients with acute pancreatitis compared with 16 patients who received TPN. Catheter-related sepsis and hyperglycemia necessitating insulin were significantly more common in the TPN group but overall mortality was no different. Olah *et al.* compared conventional parenteral nutrition with early jejunal nutrition in 89 patients admitted with acute pancreatitis. The rate of septic complications, need for surgery, MOF, and death was higher in the TPN group but differences were not statistically significant. Conversely, Powell *et al.* have published the only randomized controlled study that compared EN with no nutritional support and which studied the effect of early EN on markers of the inflammatory response in predicted severe pancreatitis. Serum IL-6, TNF receptor 1, and CRP were used as inflammatory markers. Despite previous findings the authors documented that early EN did not ameliorate the inflammatory response in patients with severe acute pancreatitis compared with no nutritional intervention. An ongoing randomized study by our group is trying to identify the role of early EN, compared with standard TPN, in reducing the need for surgery in patients with predicted severe acute pancreatitis. We have reported preliminary results in which we showed that early EN seemed to reduce surgical interventions in the EN group by reducing the incidence of sepsis (9% vs. 33%).

The above studies provide compelling evidence that enteral feeding is safe and most probably beneficial in patients with severe acute pancreatitis. Enteral jejunal feeding can be started during the first 24 hours after admission and be continued until the patient is able to feed orally. At present there is no definite evidence that artificial nutrition support, either TPN or EN, alters the outcome in patients with mild or moderate acute pancreatitis, unless malnutrition is also a problem. Diagnosis of acute pancreatitis is not itself an indication for instituting artificial nutrition, unless severity of the disease is the case. EN is safe, well tolerated, and does not stimulate the pancreas, and therefore should be used preferably in the treatment or prevention of malnutrition and probably immunosupression and infection in patients with severe acute pancreatitis.

Finally, larger, well-conducted trials are needed before any conclusive statement about the benefits of nutritional support on outcome can be made. These trials should recruit only patients with severe pancreatitis and should stratify them for disease severity, nutritional status, and etiology of pancreatitis before randomization.

Recommended reading

Abou-Assi S, O'Keefe SJD. Nutrition support during acute pancreatitis. *Nutrition* 2002;18:938–943.

Ammori BJ. Role of the gut in the course of severe acute pancreatitis. *Pancreas* 2003;26:122–129.

Ammori BJ, Leeder PC, King PF *et al.* Early increase in intestinal permeability in patients with severe acute pancreatitis: correlation with endotoxemia, organ failure and mortality. *J Gastrointest Surg* 1999;3:252–262.

Beaux AC, O'Riordain MG, Ross JA *et al.* Glutamine-supplemented total parenteral nutrition reduces blood mononuclear cell interleukin-8 release in severe acute pancreatitis. *Nutrition* 1998;14:261–265.

Dervenis C, Johnson CD, Bassi C *et al.* Diagnosis, objective assessment of severity and management of acute pancreatitis: Santorini consensus conference. *Int J Pancreatol* 1999; 25:195–210.

Dickerson RN, Vehe KL, Mullen JL *et al.* Resting energy expenditure in patients with pancreatitis. *Crit Care Med* 1991;19:484–490.

Eatock FC, Brombacher GD, Steven A *et al.* Nasogastric feeding in severe acute pancreatitis may be practical and safe. *Int J Pancreatol* 2000;28:23–29.

Edelmann K, Valenzuela JE. Effect of intravenous feeding on human pancreatic secretion. *Gastroenterology* 1983;85: 1063–1068.

Flint RS, Windsor JA. The role of the intestine in the pathophysiology and management of severe acute pancreatitis *HPB Surg* 2003;5:69–85.

Hernandez G, Velasco N, Wainstein C *et al.* Gut mucosal atrophy after a short enteral fasting period in critically ill patients. *J Crit Care* 1999;14:73–77.

Heys SD, Walker LG, Smith I *et al.* Enteral nutrition supplementation with key nutrients in patients with critical illness and cancer: a metaanalysis of randomized controlled trials. *Ann Surg* 1999;229:467–477.

Imrie CW, Carter CR, McKay CJ. Enteral and parenteral nutrition in acute pancreatitis. *Best Pract Res Clin Gastroenterol* 2002;16:391–397.

Kalfarentzos FE, Karavias DD, Karatzas TM, Alevizatos BA, Androulakis LA. Total parenteral nutrition in severe acute pancreatitis. *J Am Coll Nutr* 1991;10:156–164.

Kalfarentzos F, Kehagias J, Mead N *et al.* Enteral nutrition is superior to parenteral nutrition in severe acute pancreatitis: results of a randomised prospective trial. *Br J Surg* 1997; 83:349–353.

Luiten EJ, Hop WC, Endtz HP *et al.* Prognostic importance of Gram negative intestinal colonization preceding pancreatic infection in severe acute pancreatitis. Results of a controlled clinical trial of selective decontamination. *Intensive Care Med* 1998;24:438–445.

Meier R, Beglinger C, Layer P *et al.* ESPEN guidelines on

nutrition in acute pancreatitis. *Clin Nutr* 2002;21:173–183.

Olah A, Pardavi G, Belagyi T, Nagy A, Issekutz A, Mohamed GE. Early nasojejunal feeding in acute pancreatitis is associated with a lower complication rate. *Nutrition* 2002;18:259–262.

Powell JJ, Murchison JT, Feavon KCH *et al.* Randomized controlled trial of the effect of early enteral nutrition on markers of the inflammatory response in predicted severe acute pancreatitis. *Br J Surg* 2000;87:1357–1381.

Pupelis G, Austrums E, Jansone A *et al.* Randomized trial of safety and efficacy of postoperative enteral feeding in patients with severe pancreatitis. Preliminary report. *Eur J Surg* 2000;166:383–387.

Sax AC, Warner BW, Talamini MA, Hamilton FN, Bell RH Jr, Fischer JE. Early total parenteral nutrition in acute pancreatitis: lack of beneficial effects. *Am J Surg* 1987;153:117–124.

Sitzmann JV, Steinborn PA, Zinner MJ, Cameron JN. Total parenteral nutrition and alternate energy substrates in treatment of severe acute pancreatitis. *Surg Gynecol Obstet* 1989;168:311–317.

Vu MK, Van Der Veek P, Frolich M *et al.* Does jejunal feeding activate exocrine pancreatic secretion? *Eur J Clin Invest* 1999;29:1053–1056.

Windsor AC, Kanwar S, Li AG *et al.* Compared with parenteral nutrition, enteral feeding attenuates the acute phase response and improves disease severity in acute pancreatitis. *Gut* 1998;42:431–435.

11 Antibiotic prophylaxis for acute pancreatitis in clinical practice: rationale, indications, and protocols for clinical practice

Giovanni Butturini, Roberto Salvia, Nora Sartori, and Claudio Bassi

Introduction

Acute pancreatitis is characterized by a wide range of clinical manifestations, ranging from mild self-limiting to severe life-treatening. The gold standard for treatment of acute pancreatitis is conservative management with fluid balance correction and administration of opiates. Patients with the more severe forms may also be kept in intensive care. In severe pancreatitis, prognosis is strictly related to the extension of glandular necrosis as the risk of infection depends on the extent of pancreatic necrosis. The aim of antibiotic prophylaxis is to prevent superinfection of necrotic tissues. The indication for the prophylactic schedule includes the presence of glandular necrosis as demonstrated by computed tomography (CT) or a serum value of C-reactive protein (CRP) that surpasses 150 mg/dL in a sample obtained at least 48 hours after onset of disease. The accepted antibiotic protocols advocate the use of broad-spectrum antibacterial agents such as imipenem, which are particularly active against Gram-negative bacteria of intestinal origin.

Rationale

The presence of infected necrosis is the single most important negative prognostic index during the course of severe acute pancreatitis and is the major factor responsible for mortality and morbidity. The infection rate is related to the amount of necrosis, and infection is present in about 30–40% of patients with more than 30% necrosis. The infectious organisms able to reach the necrotic parenchyma are mostly Gram-negative bacteria of intestinal origin (Table 11.1). They access the pancreatic necrosis through the intestinal mucosal barrier, which may have been previously damaged during acute pancreatitis by several factors, including cytokine activation and ischemia. Data from experimental models and early microbiologic cultures of necrotic tissue have demonstrated that infection is an initial consequence of severe pancreatitis. Therefore, the efficacy of antibiotic prophylaxis (or, as we prefer, early antibiotic treatment) is strictly dependent on the pharmacologic therapy used, as well as its appropriate timing. Initial efforts to demonstrate the efficacy of prophylactic therapy in the 1970s failed due to the use of ampicillin, an antibiotic not able to penetrate into pancreatic tissue. The different pattern of tissue penetration demonstrated in clinical/microbiologic studies by other antibiotics (Table 11.2) led to a new series of prospective randomized trials in the 1990s. From those studies, it was concluded that early antibiotic treatment reduces morbidity, and in one instance mortality was also decreased (Table 11.3). The metaanalyses by Golub *et al.* and Sharma and Howden revealed that antibiotic prophylaxis also reduces the rate of mortality.

In our experience, imipenem–cilastatin reduced the incidence of bacterially infected necrosis compared with a homogeneous control group of patients without treatment (12.2% vs. 30.3%; $P < 0.01$, Mann–Whitney U-test). No significant reduction in overall mortality was observed in the treated group with respect to controls, possibly due to the relatively small number of patients ($n = 74$) and to the number of deaths in the treated patients who had early surgery for multiorgan failure without pancreatic sepsis. Moreover, the number of patients who either died or underwent surgical interven-

Table 11.1 Infectious organisms found in over 1100 cases of infected necrotizing pancreatitis.

Escherichia coli	35%
Klebsiella pneumoniae	24%
Enterococcus spp.	24%
Staphylococcus spp.	14%
Pseudomonas spp.	11%

Table 11.2 Antibacterial agents and penetrative capacity in pancreatic tissue.

Good penetrators
Clindamycin
Fluoroquinolone
Imipenem
Metronidazole
Mezlocillin

Poor penetrators
Aminoglycosides
Ampicillin
Cephalosporins
Moxalactam
Tetracyclines

tion for infected necrosis or abscess was twice that in the group not receiving antibiotic therapy with respect to the group of patients treated with prophylactic imipenem. In 35.7% of cases with severe necrosis (>50% of glandular volume), imipenem did not prevent superinfection.

We have also compared the efficacy of imipenem (500 mg three times daily) with pefloxacin (400 mg twice daily) in patients suffering from severe necrosis (>50% of glandular volume) using a multicenter, prospective, randomized study involving 60 patients. Patients treated with pefloxacin had a significantly higher infection rate compared with the imipenem-treated group (37% vs. 10%), despite its theoretic potential. Thus, the latter antibiotic is still the therapy of choice for prophylactic treatment. Again, no significant differences in mortality rates between the different treatment groups were observed, most likely due to the relatively low number of patients.

Indications

Early antibiotic treatment is indicated in all patients suffering from necrotizing pancreatitis, although there is still wide debate about the criteria that should be used to identify this subgroup of patients with acute pancreatitis. The need to select only patients with necrosis for early therapy is related to the broad-spectrum antibiotic nature of the administered drugs and their potential capacity to select for multiresistant strains. Our current

Table 11.3 Pancreatic infection and mortality rate in six randomized controlled trials of antibiotic prophylaxis.

Study	No. of patients	Antimicrobial agents	Pancreatic infection rate (%)		Mortality (%)	
			Control	Case	Control	Case
Pederzoli *et al.* (1993)	74	Imipenem	30	12*	12	7
Luiten *et al.* (1995)	102	SDD and i.v. cefotaxime	38	18**	35	22
Sainio *et al.* (1995)	60	Cefuroxime	40	30	23	3***
Delcenserie *et al.* (1996)	23	Ceftazidime, amikacin, metronidazole	58	0**	25	9
Schwarz *et al.* (1997)	26	Ofloxacin, metronidazole	53	61	15	0
Bassi *et al.* (1998)	60	Pefloxacin vs. imipenem	34	0**	24	10

i.v., intravenous; SDD, selective digestive decontamination (see text).
* $P < 0.01$; ** $P = 0.03$; *** $P = 0.028$.

policy is to determine CRP after 48 hours from the onset of acute pancreatitis, and a serum level greater than 150 mg/dL is considered a reliable cutoff for necrosis. CT is also performed after 48–72 hours to detect and quantify the amount of necrosis. Furthermore, in our experience, other measurements taken during the first 24 hours of hospital admission, such as serum creatinine (values > 2 mg/dL) and pulmonary involvement (pleural effusions or parenchymal densifications), may be of prognostic significance and have been successfully tested in combination to predict severity in a multicenter study. Although all patients with pancreatic necrosis might benefit from early antibiotic treatment on the basis of available clinical data, some experienced pancreatic surgeons believe that this therapy should be abandoned or at least limited to highly selected cases. In a recent editorial, Beger and Imrie underlined the increasing problem of antibiotic resistance and fungal infection. This was also revealed by a survey conducted in the UK and Ireland in 1999.

In our experience the microbiologic findings in patients with infected necrosis in the latest trial were rather different from those of the first clinical trial; in particular, higher rates of infection with *Staphylococcus aureus* (methicillin-resistant), *Candida glabrata*, and *Pseudomonas aeruginosa* were observed. As previously reported, this observation is in agreement with several recent reports and represents a grave problem, since methicillin-resistant species and fungal infection, even when appropriately treated, leads to a high mortality rate.

Protocols

The antibiotic of choice for early prophylactic treatment in necrotizing pancreatitis is imipenem, as demonstrated in our two randomized trials. This finding was recently confirmed by Mitchell and colleagues in an article published in *Lancet*. Imipenem must be started early at a dose of 500 mg intravenously every 8 hours and administered for 2 weeks. In order to avoid the development of multiresistant infective agents, patients with acute pancreatitis requiring prophylactic therapy should be carefully selected. As soon as possible, the administration of total enteral nutrition through a nasoenteric feeding tube placed beyond the ligament of Treitz (rather than total parenteral nutrition) should also be combined with antibiotics. As it is

well demonstrated that enteral nutrition is able to prevent gut mucosal damage and bacterial translocation, this is the most rational therapeutic strategy proposed to date. The decision to implement antifungal therapy with fluconazole in addition to the antibiotic prophylaxis appears to give rise to other problems, such as the development of multiresistant *Candida* species, although definitive data are not yet available. Patients should be selected for antibiotic therapy based on the extent of necrosis. When the necrosis is over 50%, the infection rate is significantly higher, while in the subgroup with less than 30% necrosis, the rate of infection is only about 20%. Careful clinical monitoring may avoid antibiotic therapy or at least limit its use to 5–7 days as opposed to the conventional 2 weeks. As soon as possible, fine-needle aspiration of pancreatic necrosis has to be done in the subgroup with worsening clinical conditions in order to obtain early data about the infectious organisms present. The choice between surgical débridement or antibiotic therapy in infected necrosis is a matter of debate, even if surgery still remains the preferred standard.

Summary

The rationale for early antibiotic treatment in necrotizing pancreatitis is based upon the evidence that mortality in this pathology is strictly correlated with superinfection. The most common infectious agents are Gram-negative bacteria of intestinal origin, whose transmission is facilitated by the damage to the gut barrier and subsequent translocation. Several prospective randomized trials have demonstrated that prophylaxis reduces the rate of infection of the necrotic areas and leads to additional advantages in terms of morbidity and, in metaanalysis, of mortality.

The indications for antibiotic prophylaxis are all forms of severe necrotizing pancreatitis; the assessment and classification of early pancreatitis is imperative in order for prophylaxis to be undertaken as soon as possible.

The protocols are mainly based on antibiotics able to penetrate both the necrotic and viable tissues of the pancreas (imipenem 500 mg three times daily for 2 weeks or 1 g three times daily for 10 days). It is reasonable to assume that in necrotizing pancreatitis limited to less than 30% of the glandular parenchyma, patients able to start early enteral nutrition with a good response (decrease in CRP) may benefit by antibiotic prophylaxis lasting only 5–7 days, thereby avoiding fungal infection.

Acknowledgments

We are grateful to Dr Patrick Moore, senior researcher at our university, for his review of the English version of this chapter.

Recommended reading

Ammori BJ. Role of the gut in the course of severe acute pancreatitis. *Pancreas* 2003;26:122–129.

Bassi C, Falconi M, Talamini G *et al*. Controlled clinical trial of pefloxacin versus imipenem in severe acute pancreatitis. *Gastroenterology* 1998;115:1513–1517.

Beger HG, Rau B, Mayer J, Pralle U. Natural course of acute pancreatitis. *World J Surg* 1997;21:130–135.

Beger HG, Isenmann R, Imrie CW. Diagnosis, objective assessment of severity, and management of acute pancreatitis. Santorini Consensus Conference by C. Dervenis *et al*. *Int J Pancreatol* 1999;26:1–3.

Buchler M, Malfertheiner P, Friess H *et al*. Human pancreatic tissue concentration of bactericidal antibiotics. *Gastroenterology* 1992;103:1902–1908.

Buchler MW, Gloor B, Muller CA, Friess H, Seiler CA, Uhl W. Acute necrotizing pancreatitis: treatment strategy according to the status of infection. *Ann Surg* 2000;232:619–626.

Butturini G, Salvia R, Bettini R, Falconi M, Pederzoli P, Bassi C. Infection prevention in necrotizing pancreatitis: an old challenge with new perspectives. *J Hosp Infect* 2001;49: 4–8.

Delcenserie R, Yzet T, Ducroix JP. Prophylactic antibiotics in treatment of severe acute alcoholic pancreatitis. *Pancreas* 1996;13:198–201.

Golub R, Siddiqi F, Pohl D. Role of antibiotics in acute pancreatitis: a meta-analysis. *J Gastrointest Surg* 1998;2:496–503.

Grewe M, Tsiotos GG, Luque de-Leon E, Sarr MG. Fungal infection in acute necrotizing pancreatitis. *J Am Coll Surg* 1999;188:408–414.

Howard TJ, Temple MB. Prophylactic antibiotics alter the bacteriology of infected necrosis in severe acute pancreatitis. *J Am Coll Surg* 2002;195:759–767.

Isenmann R, Rau B, Beger HG. Bacterial infection and extent of necrosis are determinants of organ failure in patients with acute necrotizing pancreatitis. *Br J Surg* 1999;86: 1020–1024.

Kalfarentzos F, Kehagias J, Mead N, Kokkinis K, Gogos CA. Enteral feeding is superior to parenteral nutrition in severe acute pancreatitis: results of a randomized prospective trial. *Br J Surg* 1997;84:1665–1669.

Luiten EJ, Hop WC, Lange JF, Bruining HA. Controlled clinical trial of selective decontamination for the treatment of severe acute pancreatitis. *Ann Surg* 1995;222:57–65.

Lumsden A, Bradley EL III. Secondary pancreatic infections. *Surg Gynecol Obstet* 1990;170:459–467.

Mitchell RMS, Byrne MF, Baillie J. Pancreatitis. *Lancet* 2003;361:1447–1455.

Nordback I, Sand J, Saaristo R, Paajanen H. Early treatment with antibiotics reduces the need of surgery in acute necrotizing pancreatitis. A single centre randomized study. *J Gastrointest Surg* 2001;5:113–118.

Pederzoli P, Bassi C, Vesentini S, Campedelli A. A randomized multicenter clinical trial of antibiotic prophylaxis of septic complications in acute necrotizing pancreatitis with imipenem. *Surg Gynecol Obstet* 1993;176:480–483.

Powell JJ, Campbell E, Johnson CD, Siriwardena AK. Survey of antibiotic prophylaxis in acute pancreatitis in the UK and Ireland. *Br J Surg* 1999;86:320–322.

Robbins EG, Stollman NH, Bierman P *et al*. Pancreatic fungal infections: a case report and review of the literature. *Pancreas* 1996;12:308–312.

Sainio V, Kemppainen E, Puolakkainen P *et al*. Early antibiotic treatment in acute necrotising pancreatitis. *Lancet* 1995;346:663–667.

Schwarz M, Isenmann R, Meyer H, Beger HG. Antibiotic use in necrotizing pancreatitis. Results of a controlled study. *Dtsch Med Wochenschr* 1997;122:356–361.

Sharma VK, Howden CW. Prophylactic antibiotic administration reduces sepsis and mortality in acute necrotizing pancreatitis: a meta-analysis. *Pancreas* 2001;22:28–31.

Talamini G, Bassi C, Falconi M *et al*. Risk of death from acute pancreatitis. Role of early, simple "routine" data. *Int J Pancreatol* 1996;19:15–24.

Talamini G, Uomo G, Pezzilli R *et al*. Serum creatinine and chest radiographs in the early assessment of acute pancreatitis. *Am J Surg* 1999;177:7–14.

Windsor AJC, Kanwar S, Li AJK *et al*. Compared with parenteral nutrition, enteral feeding attenuates the acute phase response and improves disease severity in acute pancreatitis. *Gut* 1998;42:431–435.

12 Modulation of the inflammatory response in acute pancreatitis: what can be expected?

Colin J. McKay

Background

In the past decade, increased understanding of the pathophysiology of acute pancreatitis has led to an interest in the potential of cytokines or cytokine antagonists to prevent or treat the systemic complications of the disease. In this chapter, the importance of the innate inflammatory response to the outcome from acute pancreatitis will be explored and potential therapeutic targets discussed.

Natural history of acute pancreatitis

Before examining the possible benefit of any treatment in acute pancreatitis, we need first to consider the natural history of the disease. Regardless of etiology, the majority of cases of acute pancreatitis are self-limiting and require no treatment other than intravenous fluid and appropriate analgesia. Severe attacks occur in 10–20% of cases and are characterized by varying degrees of systemic organ dysfunction. The most common clinical manifestation of this is respiratory insufficiency, which is seen to some extent in almost all patients with severe acute pancreatitis. Some, although by no means all, of these patients will have evidence of pancreatic necrosis on contrast-enhanced computed tomography and are therefore at risk of developing late septic complications. Two phases of mortality are recognized: (i) early deaths occur within the first week and are usually caused by overwhelming multiple organ failure; (ii) later deaths are more commonly associated with infected pancreatic necrosis, although this is also complicated by multiple organ failure in fatal cases.

While there is continuing debate about the relative importance of early and late mortality to overall outcome from acute pancreatitis, there can be no doubt that the key event in patients at risk of death from acute pancreatitis is the development of multiple organ dysfunction syndrome (MODS).

Recent prospective studies in patients with severe acute pancreatitis have demonstrated that in those patients who go on to develop systemic complications some evidence of systemic organ dysfunction is present at the time of hospital admission in 70% of cases, and develops within 48 hours of admission in the remainder. Worsening organ dysfunction during the first week of illness is associated with mortality approaching 50%. A clinically useful system for prediction of those patients who will develop MODS, or for the identification of those patients with MODS in whom early resolution is unlikely, has yet to be developed. Multifactorial predictive systems, such as the widely used Ranson and Glasgow criteria, have proved insufficiently accurate to influence decision-making in acute pancreatitis, and use of the Acute Physiology and Chronic Health Evaluation (APACHE) II scoring system is limited to selection of patients for clinical trials and monitoring of patient progress. Careful observation of patients for the development of systemic complications and appropriate supportive care remain the basis of management.

Despite advances in supportive care and improved understanding of the natural history of the disease, there is little evidence that mortality from acute pancreatitis has reduced. In a population study over a 12-year period in Scotland, we found no evidence of a reduction in case mortality from acute pancreatitis. Some specialist units have recently reported that early deaths from MODS can be largely prevented by appropriate supportive care, but outside specialist units such deaths continue to account for up to 50% of total mortality from acute pancreatitis.

It is clear from these data that if we are to improve overall mortality in acute pancreatitis, the patients to whom specific treatment should be targeted are those with MODS. It is here that modulation of the inflammatory response is most likely to be of value.

Role of the inflammatory response in the development of MODS in acute pancreatitis

The inflammatory response is mediated by a complex system of cytokines and cytokine inhibitors and has been widely studied in many acute and chronic illnesses. In the early stages of acute pancreatitis, proinflammatory cytokines such as tumor necrosis factor (TNF), interleukin (IL)-8, IL-6, and IL-1 are released by mononuclear phagocytes. These cytokines induce margination and infiltration of neutrophil polymorphs, neutrophil priming and degranulation, and induction of the hepatic acute-phase response. Clinically, this is manifested as the systemic inflammatory response syndrome (SIRS), characterized by fever, tachycardia, and leukocytosis. Under most circumstances, this process is tightly regulated and self-limiting but in a small number of patients there is an overwhelming inflammatory response that results in MODS. Although this process is far better understood than was the case a decade ago, the precise mechanisms leading to this overwhelming, dysregulated inflammatory response remain unclear.

Cytokine response in acute pancreatitis

Tumor necrosis factor and interleukin-1

TNF and IL-1 are both produced predominantly by monocytes and macrophages and not only have direct effects on endothelial cells but can also induce production of most other cytokines, resulting in amplification and prolongation of the inflammatory response. Studies in experimental acute pancreatitis have identified IL-1 and TNF as the earliest mediators of the inflammatory response. These are detectable within the pancreatic parenchyma within 30 min of the onset of acute pancreatitis and are produced by infiltrating leukocytes, and possibly also pancreatic acinar cells. It has proven difficult to assess the role of these cytokines in clinical acute pancreatitis as their action is mainly at a paracrine level and the quantity in tissue is therefore of considerably more importance than serum levels. TNF can be detected in the serum of one-third of patients with severe acute pancreatitis, but IL-1 is rarely found in the systemic circulation. Increased production of TNF, and to a lesser extent IL-1, has been demonstrated in circulating mononuclear cells taken from patients with severe acute pancreatitis. This finding demonstrates that mononuclear cells are primed *in vivo* and may be induced to release proinflammatory cytokines in response to a systemic trigger. Systemic production of these cytokines is associated with the development of pulmonary injury in experimental models but the factors responsible for the induction of TNF and IL-1 release in the lungs and other systemic organs are unknown.

The release of TNF and IL-1 is normally tightly controlled, although the mechanisms are at present only partly understood. Soluble TNF receptors are released and may serve to regulate the local and systemic effects of TNF. Similarly, soluble IL-1 receptor antagonist (IL-1ra) is released in tandem with IL-1. In addition, TNF and IL-1 induce the release of antiinflammatory cytokines, of which IL-10 is perhaps the most important. There are therefore mechanisms in place that serve to "mop-up" cytokines released by inflammatory cells and also to rapidly downregulate the inflammatory response. The failure of these mechanisms is presumed to be central to the pathophysiology of MODS in acute pancreatitis and other acute illnesses such as sepsis.

Certain pancreatic enzymes (elastase, carboxypeptidase A, and lipase) have been demonstrated to induce TNF production by monocytes *in vitro*, although other mechanisms may well be involved.

In the absence of TNF and IL-1, it appears that the subsequent inflammatory response is greatly attenuated. Inhibition of TNF and IL-1 translation reduces the severity of pancreatic damage in experimental acute pancreatitis and prevents the induction of later cytokines such as IL-6. In fact, because of the synergistic action of TNF and IL-1, inhibition of either cytokine greatly decreases the magnitude of the subsequent inflammatory response and ameliorates the effect of experimental pancreatitis. However, by the time patients with acute pancreatitis present to hospital, the inflammatory response is well established. This is clearly seen in those studies that have examined systemic serum cytokine levels, mainly with a view to their use as prognostic indices. Secondary cytokines, such as IL-6, IL-8, and IL-10, are frequently elevated at the time of hospital admission and, as will be discussed later in this chapter, most patients who develop systemic complications have evidence of organ dysfunction at this early stage.

Interleukin-6

IL-6 is produced by monocytes, macrophages, endothelial cells, T cells, and neutrophil polymorphs in response to various stimuli including TNF and IL-1. It is responsible for induction of the hepatic acute-phase response, resulting in the induction of C-reactive protein (CRP), fibrinogen, and α_1-antitrypsin. Many of these acute-phase proteins have important roles in controlling hemostasis (as with fibrinogen) or modulating the potentially toxic effects of enzymes derived from inflammatory cells (as with α_1-antitrypsin). IL-6 levels correlate with levels of CRP in peripheral blood but peak levels precede those of CRP by 24 hours, leading to the investigation of IL-6 as a possible early predictor of severe acute pancreatitis. Most patients with severe attacks have elevated IL-6 levels at admission to hospital. IL-6 levels correlate with objective measurements of systemic illness and are also linked to mortality. One study has demonstrated a fivefold increased risk of death with early IL-6 levels greater than 1000 pg/mL and others have reported significant differences in admission IL-6 levels when patients with mild and severe pancreatitis are compared. However, although high levels of IL-6 correlate with disease severity and mortality, it is entirely possible that this represents an adaptive process designed to control the inflammatory response and initiate the regenerative process.

Interleukin-8

IL-8 was originally discovered as a chemokine responsible for activating neutrophils after stimulation of monocytes by lipopolysaccharide. Its main role in acute pancreatitis is the induction of neutrophil priming, aggregation, and activation. Neutrophils are key effector cells of the inflammatory response, responsible for the release of free oxygen radicals at tissue level that induce endothelial damage and the widespread capillary leak typical of MODS. Although less widely studied than IL-

6, raised levels of IL-8 are seen in patients with severe acute pancreatitis. IL-8 levels peak within 24 hours of symptom onset and remain raised in those patients with systemic complications.

Platelet-activating factor

Platelet-activating factor (PAF) is a phospholipid released from cell membranes in response to a variety of physiologic stimuli. It is released from many of the key cells involved in MODS, including monocytes, macrophages, neutrophils, platelets, and endothelial cells. PAF is capable of inducing the release of many proinflammatory cytokines and acts on other inflammatory cells to induce its own production, thereby amplifying the inflammatory response. PAF itself also increases endothelial permeability and primes and activates neutrophils. Experimental pancreatitis is associated with increased levels of PAF in peritoneal exudates and blood. When injected into the gastroduodenal artery or intraperitoneally, PAF can induce the changes of acute pancreatitis and PAF inhibitors ameliorate the effects of experimental acute pancreatitis. For these reasons, PAF was seen as an ideal target for therapeutic intervention and the PAF antagonist lexipafant has been studied in several large clinical trials.

Interleukin-10

IL-10 is a potent antiinflammatory cytokine produced by monocytes and macrophages and inhibits the transcription of proinflammatory cytokines such as TNF and IL-1. Higher levels of IL-10 are seen in patients with severe acute pancreatitis and sustained high levels are associated with the most severe episodes. This demonstrates that, in parallel with the proinflammatory cytokine response, there is a compensatory antiinflammatory response (CARS). It is unclear why there is continuing proinflammatory activity despite an apparently adequate CARS in severe acute pancreatitis. One suggestion is that in severe acute pancreatitis, although the antiinflammatory response is activated, there may be a relative deficiency of such cytokines as IL-10. Evidence supporting this comes from a study from New Zealand in which a reduced IL-10/IL-8 ratio was observed in severe attacks compared with mild acute pancreatitis. Similar findings have been reported in patients with severe sepsis. Another explanation may be a failure of the antiinflammatory response at a key stage early in the development of MODS. There is evidence that the capacity of an individual to produce IL-10 may, like other cytokines, be genetically determined, leading to the recent suggestion that low IL-10 productive capacity may be associated with more severe attacks of acute pancreatitis.

Chemokines

Chemokines are inflammatory mediators involved in recruitment and activation of inflammatory cells and an increasing number have been studied in acute pancreatitis. Monocyte chemoattractant protein (MCP)-1 levels are increased in the serum of patients with acute pancreatitis and correlate with the severity of systemic complications. Similar finding have been reported with other chemokines, including macrophage inhibitory factor, growth-related oncogene, and epithelial neutrophil-activating protein-78.

Potential therapeutic targets

Tumor necrosis factor and interleukin-1

Given the pivotal role of TNF and IL-1 in the pathophysiology of acute pancreatitis, these cytokines would seem the most obvious candidates for appropriate therapeutic targeting. Although there have been no clinical studies to date, a number of experimental studies have been reported. Pretreatment of rats with a polyclonal anti-TNF antibody reduced the biochemical severity of acute pancreatitis. In a separate study in a similar model, anti-TNF antibody reduced pancreatic histologic damage and significantly improved survival. Antagonism of TNF using recombinant TNF receptor also improved survival in a murine model of acute pancreatitis. Interestingly, this effect was most marked when administration of TNF receptor was delayed until pancreatitis was established, but before the maximal peak in serum cytokine levels. Similarly, pretreatment with recombinant IL-1ra reduced amylase release and the extent of pancreatic necrosis in a rat model of acute pancreatitis. Both pretreatment and delayed treatment with IL-1ra were associated with reduced mortality in a murine model. This effect was associated with a marked reduction in cytokine levels.

Another approach to IL-1 inhibition has been the use of inhibitors of IL-1 converting enzyme. This enzyme is responsible for the cleavage of IL-1 into its biologically active form and its inhibition has been reported to improve outcome if given before or after induction of experimental acute pancreatitis.

Although none has been tested in the clinical setting of acute pancreatitis, large-scale trials of anti-TNF antibody, TNF receptor, and IL-1ra have been carried out in patients with sepsis. Unfortunately, none of these agents has improved outcome in severe sepsis, perhaps because any therapeutic window that may exist in these patients has long passed by the time the clinical manifestations of MODS are apparent.

Interleukin-10

IL-10 is a potent antiinflammatory cytokine and evidence from experimental models suggests that augmenting IL-10 production may improve outcome in acute pancreatitis. Prophylactic and therapeutic IL-10 gene therapy have been demonstrated to reduce severity of experimental acute pancreatitis. IL-10 itself reduces the severity of experimental acute pancreatitis, even if given 2 hours after onset. Of considerable interest is the randomized placebo-controlled trial from Belgium demonstrating that a single dose of recombinant human IL-10 can reduce the incidence of acute pancreatitis following endoscopic retrograde cholangiopancreatography. Unfortunately, a study from Ohio failed to confirm this finding and there have been no therapeutic studies carried out in the treatment of acute pancreatitis. There is little evidence to suggest that the IL-10 response in acute pancreatitis is anything other than an adaptive homeostatic response and the potential effects of augmentation of this response are unclear. It has been suggested that increased susceptibility to secondary septic complications may result from the balance of the inflammatory response swinging toward CARS.

Other cytokine targets

Antibodies against intracellular adhesion molecule (ICAM)-1 have been assessed in two experimental studies. ICAM-1 is upregulated by proinflammatory cytokines and mediates leukocyte adhesion and infiltration. In both studies, monoclonal anti-ICAM-1 antibody was associated with beneficial effects. In the second study, reduced capillary leakage was also demonstrated using antibodies to the receptor of another vasoactive mediator, endothelin-A. Met-

RANTES, a chemokine antagonist, reduced the extent of lung injury in a murine model of acute pancreatitis. Similar effects have been reported with antibodies to another cytokine, macrophage inhibitory factor.

PAF antagonism

In the 1990s, it was hoped that lexipafant, a potent PAF antagonist, would lead to reduced mortality from MODS in severe acute pancreatitis. Pretreatment with PAF antagonists reduced the local and systemic manifestations of acute pancreatitis in experimental models. Lexipafant is a potent PAF receptor antagonist and was shown to reduce the effects of experimental pancreatitis when given before or shortly after induction. These findings led to four randomized trials of this agent in patients with acute pancreatitis.

Phase II studies
In a phase II randomized study from Liverpool, Kingsnorth and colleagues reported the effect of lexipafant on biochemical markers of severity in 83 patients with acute pancreatitis of all severity grades. Patients admitted to five UK hospitals were recruited if they had pain of less than 48 hours' duration. Patients were given 15 mg of lexipafant by intravenous bolus for a maximum of 12 doses. Biochemical markers, serum cytokines, and organ failure scores were monitored. Lexipafant treatment was associated with a reduction in IL-8 levels at day 1 and nonsignificant reductions in IL-6 and E-selectin. There was also a reduction in organ failure scores and no patient receiving lexipafant developed new organ dysfunction after admission. These encouraging results were reinforced by a study from our unit in Glasgow. In this study, 100 mg lexipafant was given by continuous intravenous infusion over 24 hours and continued for up to 7 days. Of 188 patients admitted to 11 participating hospitals, 50 were recruited to the study on the basis of an admission APACHE II score of more than 5 (although 43/50 had an APACHE II score > 8). The primary end point of this study was reduction in organ failure scores. Overall mortality was 18%, and 62% had evidence of organ failure. There was a significant reduction in organ failure scores at the completion of the 7-day treatment period. Five patients in the placebo group developed new organ failure after entering the study compared with two in the lexipafant group. In both of the lexipafant-treated patients the organ failure was transient. On the basis of these en-

couraging data, a large multicenter study was conducted within the UK.

UK multicenter study
Between 1994 and 1996, a multicenter trial was conducted in 78 UK hospitals. The aim of this study was to examine the effect of lexipafant on the development of organ failure in severe acute pancreatitis. The phase II studies had demonstrated an effect on organ failure scores, but for this study a firm clinically relevant end point was required. The study was powered on the basis of demonstrating a 40% reduction in the incidence of systemic complications. As with the Glasgow study, 100 mg lexipafant was administered over 24 hours for up to 7 days. From a total of more than 2000 patients screened, 290 were eventually recruited; 44% of patients had evidence of organ failure at the time of admission to hospital, with only 14% developing new organ failure after admission. Therefore, in 75% of patients who had systemic complications, evidence of this was present at study onset, thereby invalidating the primary end point. Of further concern was the fact that, unlike the two previous studies, there was no reduction in the incidence of new organ failure in patients receiving lexipafant. In addition, unlike the Glasgow study, there was no significant effect of lexipafant on organ failure scores at 7 days (although a significant reduction at 3 days was observed). However, in a *post-hoc* analysis, the lexipafant-treated group had a reduction in mortality if treated within 48 hours of symptom onset. The potential reduction in mortality was given further reinforcement by a metaanalysis of the Glasgow and UK studies, which came close to demonstrating a significant reduction in mortality with lexipafant treatment. When patients in the two studies were combined, mortality in the lexipafant-treated patients was 9.8% compared with 16.8% in the placebo groups ($P = 0.06$). In addition, the results from the combined patient group demonstrated a marked effect on organ failure scores (Fig. 12.1 & Table 12.1).

International study
The suggestion of a reduction in mortality in those treated within 48 hours led to a large-scale international study that aimed to recruit 1500 patients with predicted severe acute pancreatitis. In this study, only those with symptoms of less than 48 hours' duration were eligible for recruitment, compared with 72 hours in the previous studies. Patients were randomized to

one of two doses of lexipafant (10 or 100 mg daily) or to placebo, with the primary end point being all-cause 28-day mortality. Secondary end points were 7-day and 90-day mortality, the development of MODS, local complications, and various physiologic and biochemical markers of severity. A total of 1518 patients were randomized, of whom 1501 were included in the final analysis. There were 121 deaths within 28 days, resulting in a surprisingly low mortality rate of only 8%. This figure is similar to the mortality rate for acute pancreatitis overall, and is the lowest reported in any series of patients with predicted severe attacks. The mortality rates in the placebo, lexipafant 10 mg, and lexipafant 100 mg groups were 8.1%, 8.3%, and 7.7% respectively. Not only was there no difference in mortality between groups, but the incidence of local complications, length of intensive care stay, hospital stay, and change in organ failure scores were similar in all three study groups. Following these disappointing results, further development of lexipafant in acute pancreatitis was abandoned.

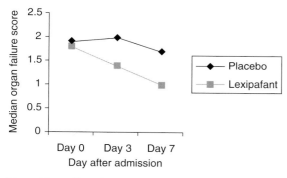

Figure 12.1 Effect of lexipafant on organ failure scores, Glasgow and UK multicenter studies combined. $P = 0.01$ (day 3) and $P = 0.03$ (day 7).

Enteral nutrition

Recent years have seen a change in the nutritional management strategy for patients with acute pancreatitis. Previous algorithms involving total gut rest and total parenteral nutrition (TPN) have been largely replaced by an enthusiasm for enteral routes of feeding. This follows several randomized trials demonstrating a reduction in septic complications when compared with TPN. In parallel, there has been interest in the role of the intestine in the pathophysiology of multiple organ failure in critical illness, with loss of gut barrier function potentially leading to endotoxemia and SIRS. Enteral nutrition is associated with improved gut barrier function but there is evidence that supplementing the enteral formula with key nutrients may have additional effects on the immune system. There have been many trials comparing so-called "immunonutrition" with standard enteral feed in critically ill patients, and the majority demonstrate significant reductions in septic complications with the supplemented feeds. In acute pancreatitis, nasojejunal feeding has been shown to reduce the incidence of septic complications when compared with TPN, although these findings relate mainly to chest and urinary tract infections and there is no evidence that the incidence of infected pancreatic necrosis is reduced. In the Leeds study, enteral feeding was associated with a reduction in SIRS scores and attenuation of the rise in IgM antibodies to endotoxin. One small study has assessed the effect of early jejunal feeding compared with no feeding in a group of patients with acute pancreatitis. This study was designed to assess the effect of feeding on the inflammatory response and measured serum cytokines sequentially during the first week of illness. No difference in the inflammatory response was observed in the enterally fed patients. The effects of immunonutrition on early organ failure

Table 12.1 Phase II and III UK studies of lexipafant in acute pancreatitis.

Study	No. of patients	Selection	Effect on organ failure scores	Effect on MODS
Kingsnorth *et al.* (1995)	83	None	Less at 3 days	No new MODS
McKay *et al.* (1997)	50	APACHE II > 5	Less at 7 days	No new MODS
Johnson *et al.* (2001)	290	APACHE II > 6	Less at 3 days	No effect

APACHE, Acute Physiology and Chronic Health Evaluation; MODS, multiple organ dysfunction syndrome.

and the inflammatory response have not been assessed in acute pancreatitis but such a study seems justified given the results from studies in other acute illnesses.

Future studies

It is now clear that some patients with early organ failure have progressive deterioration whereas others have rapid resolution. The reasons behind this remain obscure but for a therapeutic agent to be clinically useful it must be capable of both preventing organ failure and limiting its progression. In the lexipafant studies, more than 70% of patients who developed organ failure had evidence of this at admission to hospital or shortly thereafter. It is therefore likely that the "therapeutic window" for intervention is short or even nonexistent. Evidence from studies in established organ failure due to sepsis effectively rules out therapy with anti-TNF, anti-endotoxin antibody, or IL-1ra as being of likely benefit in acute pancreatitis.

It is also clear that any future study will need to be on a very large scale and focused on those with the most severe attacks. Smaller studies have proven misleading and the use of surrogate markers of outcome, such as organ failure scores, has led to inappropriate optimism. Clear, clinically relevant end points are necessary and, of these, the only one likely to lead to a change in practice is mortality. Unfortunately, as demonstrated in the largest lexipafant study, very large numbers of patients need to be recruited. In this study, despite restriction to patients with predicted severe acute pancreatitis, overall mortality was less than 10%. In the absence of an accurate early predictive tool it continues to be difficult to identify those patients to whom future trials should be targeted, but it is clear from this study that currently available predictive systems are insufficiently accurate.

Conclusion

Despite a decade of enthusiastic research and huge financial investment in clinical trials, there is no immediate prospect of cytokine or anticytokine therapy in the clinical management of patients with acute pancreatitis. In the immediate future, the only likely development is the use of early enteral nutrition but this approach has not yet been clearly shown to reduce the incidence or severity of systemic complications. Improved supportive care, avoidance of unnecessary or ill-timed surgical intervention, and the involvement of a dedicated multidisciplinary team are the best hopes for improving outcome at the present time. It seems likely that unless modulation of the inflammatory response is demonstrated to improve outcome in the more common setting of sepsis, it is unlikely to become a clinical reality in patients with acute pancreatitis.

Recommended reading

Brivet F, Emilie D, Galanaud P et al. Pro- and anti-inflammatory cytokines during acute severe pancreatitis: an early and sustained response, although unpredictable of death. Crit Care Med 1999;27:749–755.

Buter A, Imrie CW, Carter CR, Evans S, McKay CJ. Dynamic nature of early organ dysfunction determines outcome in acute pancreatitis. Br J Surg 2002;89:298–302.

Johnson CD, Kingsnorth AN, Imrie CW et al. Double blind, randomised, placebo controlled study of a platelet activating factor antagonist, lexipafant, in the treatment and prevention of organ failure in predicted severe acute pancreatitis. Gut 2001;48:62–69.

Kingsnorth AN, Galloway SW, Formela LJ. Randomized, double-blind phase II trial of Lexipafant, a platelet-activating factor antagonist, in human acute pancreatitis. Br J Surg 1995;82:1414–1420.

McKay CJ, Curran F, Sharples C et al. Prospective placebo-controlled randomized trial of lexipafant in predicted severe acute pancreatitis. Br J Surg 1997;84:1239–1243.

Norman J. The role of cytokines in the pathogenesis of acute pancreatitis. Am J Surg 1998;175:76–83.

13

Early endoscopic sphincterotomy in acute pancreatitis: is it indicated, advisable, not indicated, or contraindicated? A proposal for clinical practice

Jennifer Barro, Roy M. Soetikno, and David L. Carr-Locke

Background

Gallstones are the leading etiology of acute pancreatitis in Western and Asian countries. Although most patients will recover from an attack of acute pancreatitis, 15–25% of patients will have significant morbidity. Severe acute pancreatitis can carry up to a 13% risk of mortality. Investigators have hypothesized that gallstones, through mechanical means, initiate pancreatitis as they pass through the distal common bile duct (CBD). It is also believed that persistent obstruction due to a CBD stone causes more severe pancreatic injury.

Early surgical doctrine recommended aggressive removal of gallstones in all patients with suspected acute biliary pancreatitis (ABP), while endoscopic retrograde cholangiopancreatography (ERCP) was avoided due to concern for procedure-related complications. However, a few case reports suggested a benefit from immediate endoscopic removal of CBD stones in ABP. These early studies led to the performance of a number of randomized clinical trials.

Four randomized controlled trials have evaluated the impact of early ERCP with or without endoscopic sphincterotomy (ES) in patients with ABP. These studies involved over 800 patients in Western and Asian countries. Overall, the data suggested a benefit from early ERCP in patients with biliary obstruction or indices predicting severe pancreatitis, although the results from one study were contradictory. Due to the conflicting findings, two metaanalyses have been performed in an attempt to clarify the controversy. Important conclusions can be drawn from the available data and are useful for guiding clinical practice. In order to devise and employ a treatment algorithm in ABP, it is important to discuss the potential mechanism of pancreatic injury and how to distinguish biliary pancreatitis from other etiologies of pancreatitis.

Gallstones and pancreatitis

A relationship between gallstones and pancreatitis was first described over 100 years ago by Opie. He detailed a patient who died from severe pancreatitis and who, on autopsy, was found to have a stone impacted at the ampulla of Vater. Opie proposed that ampullary obstruction led to bile reflux into the pancreatic duct, which precipitated pancreatic injury. More recent animal studies suggest that reflux of bile into the pancreatic duct may not be sufficient to initiate pancreatic injury, but obstruction of the pancreatic and bile ducts may be required to cause pancreatic injury.

Although the exact mechanism is not yet understood, there is extensive evidence in the literature for a link between gallstones and acute pancreatitis. Gallstones can be recovered from the stool in 85–95% of patients with ABP. Conversely, only 10% of patients with symptomatic cholelithiasis without pancreatitis have gallstones in their stool. Approximately 60–70% of patients with ABP have CBD stones found on ERCP or at surgery performed within 48 hours of admission. A few published studies suggest that even very small stones or biliary sludge are associated with pancreatitis.

Diagnosis of acute gallstone pancreatitis

It is important to distinguish between biliary (gall-

113

stone) pancreatitis and other etiologies of pancreatitis. A diagnosis of ABP is established by combining the patient history and clinical presentation with laboratory and radiographic findings.

There are a number of biochemical parameters and radiographic studies that are useful in predicting a biliary etiology for pancreatitis. Amylase levels tend to be higher in patients with biliary pancreatitis compared to those with alcoholic pancreatitis; in particular, an amylase level greater than 1000 U/L suggests a biliary etiology. Abnormal liver biochemistries, specifically an alanine aminotransferase (ALT) level greater than three times normal, are predictive of a biliary etiology. Elevated bilirubin and alkaline phosphatase are not necessarily specific for ABP.

Documenting gallstones can help suggest a biliary etiology. Although abdominal imaging may be useful in detecting gallbladder stones, ultrasound and computed tomography (CT) can often fail to detect stones, especially CBD stones or microlithiasis. Also, an absence of biliary dilation on ultrasound or CT may not be a predictive finding early in the course of ABP. Neoptolemos *et al.* reported that ultrasound within 72 hours of admission did not detect gallstones in 18.5% of patients later diagnosed with a biliary etiology for acute pancreatitis. Recent studies have suggested that endoscopic ultrasound has a sensitivity and specificity of 84–98% and 95–100% for detecting choledocholithiasis. This is much more sensitive than transabdominal ultrasound, estimated at 25–63%. Performance characteristics for magnetic resonance cholangiopancreatography (MRCP) are similar to endoscopic ultrasound with slightly lower specificity. However, it is not clear how the newer imaging modalities of endoscopic ultrasound and MRCP play into the algorithm of ABP management.

Grading the severity of pancreatitis

Approximately 75–80% of patients with ABP will have a mild attack and recover. Criteria have been developed to identify patients who are likely to develop severe pancreatitis. Ranson developed an 11-factor system to predict severity on admission based on age over 55 years, white blood cell count greater than $16\,000/mm^3$, blood glucose greater than 200 mg/dL, serum lactate dehydrogenase (LDH) greater than 350 U/L, and aspartate aminotransferase (AST) greater than 250 U/L.

Additional factors were evaluated at 48 hours: decrease in hematocrit greater than 10%, increase in blood urea nitrogen greater than 5 mg/dL, serum calcium less than 8 mg/dL, arterial oxygen tension less than 60 mmHg, base deficit greater than 4 mEq/L, and fluid sequestration greater than 6 L. If a patient has three or more criteria within the first 48 hours, they are predicted to have a 28% risk of mortality compared with a 0.9% risk for patients with less than three criteria. A modified and simplified form of Ranson's criteria (Glasgow or Imrie) uses patient age, white blood cell count, glucose, blood urea nitrogen, LDH, albumin, calcium, serum transaminases, and arterial oxygen tension within 48 hours of admission to predict outcome. Hemoconcentration (admission hematocrit > 44%) may be an important risk factor by itself for predicting poor outcome. Some investigators have employed the Acute Physiology and Chronic Health Evaluation (APACHE) system for grading pancreatitis severity. This system includes variables from seven major organ systems and can be used to grade other disease processes as well as pancreatitis. CT findings can be used to predict severity of pancreatitis. The Balthazar CT grading system uses signs of pancreatic edema, the presence of retroperitoneal fluid collections, and/or pancreatic necrosis early in the hospital course to predict prognosis, with the highest score predicting 92% morbidity and 17% mortality rate compared with 2% and 0% respectively for patients with a low severity score.

The use of standardized scoring systems for grading pancreatitis assists in comparing studies performed at different institutions. Unfortunately, prior published studies examining ERCP outcomes in ABP have not all employed the same method of predicting pancreatitis severity and one study used criteria that have not been validated. This potentially confounds the interpretation of the studies discussed below.

Early surgical studies

Most of the early studies were retrospective and did not standardize the type of surgical procedure performed. Most surgical procedures involved a cholecystectomy with bile duct exploration as indicated and occasional transduodenal sphincterotomy. Some investigators report better outcomes with early surgical intervention and others found a significant increase in mortality when operating on patients with early acute pancreatitis. Another investigator reported no difference in morbidity and mortality between early and late surgical groups. Some of the studies were biased by the fact that patients with more severe illness had earlier surgical intervention. Thus, a more definitive study was needed. A prospective randomized trial of 165 subjects found that patients undergoing surgery within 48 hours of admission had a 30.1% morbidity and 15.1% mortality rate compared with 5.1% and 2.4% ($P < 0.005$) in patients undergoing delayed surgery. Such reports of high morbidity and mortality shifted surgical opinion toward avoiding early intervention in ABP.

Studies evaluating ERCP in ABP

Early case reports of ERCP and ES performed in patients with ABP suggested some benefit while not showing an increase in procedure-related complications. These reports led to further investigation and publication of four randomized controlled trials. While reviewing the clinical trials of early ERCP with or without ES in ABP, it is important to note that the studies differ somewhat in the grading of pancreatitis, randomization to ES, timing of ERCP, etiology of pancreatitis, and/or exclusion of patients with jaundice. Three of the available randomized controlled trials are published as full reports and the fourth in abstract form. These studies were designed to establish the safety and efficacy of early ERCP in ABP. Table 13.1 summarizes the designs and findings of the four randomized controlled trials.

UK study

Neoptolemos *et al.* in 1988 published the first randomized controlled trial evaluating the role of urgent ERCP in ABP. These authors randomized 121 of 146 consecutive patients with presumed ABP to ERCP within 72 hours of admission or to conventional management. The investigators established a diagnosis of biliary pancreatitis with ultrasound and biochemical criteria. Patients with a history of alcohol or other etiology for pancreatitis were excluded. Pancreatitis severity was predicted within 48 hours of admission by the modified Glasgow criteria; 44% of patients in this study were predicted to have severe pancreatitis. A single, highly skilled endoscopist performed all ERCP examinations. Patients were randomized to ERCP but not to performance of sphincterotomy. ES was performed only if stones were found on ERCP. After day 5, patients in the conventional treatment arm were permitted to have an ERCP if clinically indicated and no patients crossed over before this time; 23% of the conventional group did have an ERCP after day 5. Patients were followed by serial ultrasound or CT for the development of local complications such as ascites or pseudocyst. Outcomes were assessed based on development of local complications (pseudocyst, ascites, duodenal obstruction) or systemic complications (renal failure, disseminated intravascular coagulation, stroke, respiratory failure, cardiovascular failure, or death).

ERCP was successful in 94% of patients with predicted mild disease and 80% with predicted severe pancreatitis. The authors found that overall complications were less common in those patients undergoing early ERCP [10/59 (17%) vs. 21/62 (34%); $P = 0.03$] irrespective of predicted pancreatitis severity. However, on closer inspection, the complication rate was only significantly lower in the group predicted to have severe pancreatitis undergoing early ERCP compared with those predicted to have severe pancreatitis who were managed conventionally. The overall complication rate was 12% in both treatment groups for patients predicted to have mild pancreatitis. One case of lumbar osteitis was reported as an ERCP complication, but no cases of bleeding, cholangitis, or hemorrhage due to ERCP were noted.

Notably, mortality rates were not significantly different between the treatment groups [intervention vs. conventional: 1/59 (1.7%) vs. 5/62 (8%); $P = 0.23$]. All patients who died had been predicted to have severe pancreatitis. In patients predicted to have severe pancreatitis, mortality and morbidity were lower in the early ERCP group (4% and 24% respectively) compared with the conventional group (18% and 61% respectively). The length of stay was also shorter for patients with severe pancreatitis who underwent early ERCP compared with conventional management (median 9.5 vs. 17 days respectively; $P < 0.035$), whereas it was not significantly different for those predicted to have a mild case (9 vs. 11 days respectively). In each treatment group, gallstones could not be confirmed by ERCP, ultrasound, or necropsy in nine patients. This may call into question the true etiology of the pancreatitis, but the authors hypothesize that stones may have been passed or microlithiasis may have been the cause. The groups are too small to establish

Table 13.1 Results of four randomized controlled trials of early endoscopic retrograde cholangiopancreatography (ERCP) with or without endoscopic sphincterotomy (ES) compared with conservative therapy in acute biliary pancreatitis (ABP). (Modified from Soetikno *et al.* 1998.)

Study	Study period	No. of patients	Study design	Study findings
UK	1983–87	121	Single center. Consecutive patients suspected of having ABP were included	ERCP could be safely performed in ABP. Morbidity of severe ABP significantly reduced with ERCP (24% vs. 61%). Hospital stay for severe ABP reduced by about 50% with early ERCP
Hong Kong	1988–91	195	Single center. Consecutive patients who had acute pancreatitis including some patients with nonbiliary etiology	Incidence of biliary sepsis in acute pancreatitis was significantly reduced (0% vs. 12%). Patients with "ABP" had significantly reduced morbidity with early ERCP (16% vs. 33%)
Germany	1989–94	238	Multicenter (22). Patients suspected of having ABP were enrolled. Patients who had bilirubin > 5 mg/dL were excluded	Morbidity rates between the two groups similar, but patients who had early ERCP developed more severe complications (respiratory failure). Mortality was nonsignificantly increased in patients with early ERCP (12% vs. 6%)
Poland	1984–95	280	Single center. Consecutive patients suspected of having ABP were studied. Immediate ERCP was performed in all patients; those who had stone impaction underwent ES. Others were randomized	Early ERCP significantly reduced both morbidity (17% vs. 36%) and mortality (2% vs. 13%)

whether patients without proven gallstones benefited from ERCP.

Other authors have argued that most of the benefit from ERCP in ABP comes from early treatment of acute cholangitis. In this study 10% (6/59) of early ERCP patients had cholangitis compared with 8% (5/62) in the conventional group. The authors examined their data excluding patients with acute cholangitis. In patients without cholangitis, complications occurred in 6/53 (11%) patients undergoing early ERCP versus 19/57 (33%) patients treated conventionally ($P = 0.02$). The difference was also significant when the analysis was limited to patients predicted to have severe pancreatitis [3/20 (15%) vs. 15/25 (60%); $P = 0.003$].

This study was the first to evaluate early ERCP in ABP in a prospective, randomized, controlled manner.

The results suggest that ERCP with or without ES is safe in acute pancreatitis when performed by a skilled endoscopist. Early ERCP with or without ES was associated with fewer complications and reduced hospital stay for patients predicted to have severe pancreatitis compared with those undergoing conventional management. The data for impact on mortality, as well as on a mild pancreatitis course, were not conclusive.

Hong Kong study

The next study on the subject came from Hong Kong in 1993. Fan *et al.* randomly assigned 195 patients with acute pancreatitis to ERCP within 24 hours or to conservative management. Patients underwent ES during ERCP only if CBD or ampullary stones were detected.

Nearly one-third of patients in the conservative management group with a deteriorating course were also allowed to have an early ERCP within 72 hours of admission. The remaining patients underwent ERCP after resolution of the acute course. Urgent ERCP was successful in 90% of cases. In this study, 127 patients had confirmed biliary stones (65%) and half of the remaining patients had an alternative etiology for their pancreatitis. The authors used a scoring system based on blood urea nitrogen and glucose at admission to grade pancreatitis severity after randomization. They report similar severity stratification when comparing their scoring system to Ranson's criteria.

Complications of acute pancreatitis, both local and systemic, were not statistically different between the intervention and conventional groups (18% vs. 29%; $P = 0.07$). The overall mortality rate was 5% in the intervention group and 9% in the conservative group ($P = 0.4$). If only patients with gallstones in any part of the biliary tract were analyzed, the morbidity was 16% in the intervention group and 33% in the conservative management group ($P = 0.03$). The mortality rate was also lower in the intervention group, but not significantly different. Biliary sepsis occurred less often in patients undergoing early ERCP (0/97, 0%) compared with conservative management (12/98, 12%; $P = 0.001$). The authors report a decreased rate of total complications and biliary sepsis in patients predicted to have severe pancreatitis of biliary etiology who underwent early ERCP.

Since all the patients ultimately underwent ERCP, either early or late, the authors commented on timing of ERCP in relation to complication rate. Early procedures were not different from late procedures in terms of procedure-related complications. Four patients in each treatment group had bleeding after sphincterotomy. Although patients with early ERCP had higher amylase levels after the procedure than those who underwent late ERCP, there was no difference in exacerbation of abdominal pain after the procedure.

These investigators argue that ERCP did not have an adverse effect on patients with nonbiliary pancreatitis and therefore in regions where the incidence of biliary pancreatitis is high, early ERCP should be employed even in the absence of a definitive diagnosis of biliary pancreatitis. This study demonstrated reduced morbidity with early ERCP for patients with CBD or ampullary stones, i.e., those with a clear biliary etiology for pancreatitis. There was also a decreased frequency of biliary sepsis in patients predicted to have severe pancreatitis who underwent early ERCP. The authors advocate early (within 24 hours) intervention because the course in pancreatitis is unpredictable and can deteriorate rapidly after admission. Notably, there were no differences in overall survival or ERCP complications between the study groups. The primary benefit of early ERCP was to decrease the incidence of biliary sepsis and this benefit was stronger for patients predicted to have severe pancreatitis.

Polish study

Nowak *et al.* published the largest randomized trial in abstract form in 1995. They evaluated 280 consecutive patients presenting with ABP suspected on the basis of imaging (CT, ultrasound, or ERCP), microlithiasis in a bile sample, and biochemical criteria. All patients underwent duodenoscopy within 24 hours of admission. Patients with evidence of an impacted stone at the papilla ($n = 75$) had an immediate sphincterotomy. The remaining patients were randomized to immediate ES ($n = 103$) or to conventional management ($n = 102$). Disease severity was predicted with Ranson's criteria.

In the randomly assigned groups, those undergoing ES had a significantly lower morbidity rate compared with the conventional group (17% vs. 36%; $P < 0.001$). The early, randomized, sphincterotomy group also had a significantly lower mortality rate compared with the conventional group (2% vs. 13%; $P < 0.001$). The results did not change when the nonrandomized group with obvious ampullary stones was added to the analysis. The authors report that their results held for patients predicted to have severe and mild pancreatitis, and regardless of presence or absence of CBD stones, jaundice, and biliary sepsis (data not shown). This study has been the strongest support for early ERCP with or without ES, but has been criticized for lack of full publication years after the initial abstract was released.

German study

Fölsch *et al.* conducted a prospective multicenter trial of 238 patients with ABP randomized to ERCP within 72 hours of symptom onset versus conservative treatment. Patients underwent sphincterotomy if CBD stones were found during ERCP. Patients who were randomized to conservative management had an ERCP for persistent biliary pain, fever greater than 39°C, or an increase in bilirubin of more than 3 mg/dL in 5 days. Notably, these authors excluded patients with jaundice (bilirubin > 5 mg/dL) in an attempt to discover whether patients without obvious biliary complications would benefit from early ERCP. They selected patients with biliary etiology for pancreatitis, defined as radiographic evidence of gallstones (ultrasound/CT) or the presence of two of the following: alkaline phosphatase greater than 125 U/L, ALT greater than 75 U/L, or bilirubin greater than 2.3 mg/dL. A modified Glasgow system was used to determine pancreatitis severity; 12–14% of patients in each treatment group were labeled as undefined severity.

The authors report a 96% procedure success rate for patients randomized to early ERCP. Of the conservative management group, 20% had ERCP performed during the first 3 weeks for jaundice, fever, or biliary pain and 86% of these patients had bile duct stones. Two patients in the intervention group had bleeding after sphincterotomy (2.8%); one required transfusion and later died from sepsis. Less than 20% of patients in the study were predicted to have severe pancreatitis. Only 46% of the ERCP group had bile duct stones and underwent ES. The study was terminated at the second planned interim unblinded analysis (238/380 patients recruited) when a higher percentage of deaths was found in the treatment group and the authors felt they were unlikely to prove their hypothesis that the invasive treatment was superior.

Although the mortality rate was higher in the treatment group, there was no statistical difference between the early ERCP and conventional groups (11% vs. 6%; $P = 0.10$). The authors also reported no difference between the treatment groups with regard to frequency of local and systemic complications when patients were stratified according to pancreatitis severity. Since the study was terminated early, it is possible that it may have been underpowered to detect real differences between the groups. Although the rate of complications was also not different between the groups, those patients who underwent early ERCP had more severe complications, primarily respiratory failure [15/126 (12%) vs. 5/112 (4%); $P = 0.03$]. Approximately half the patients with respiratory failure died. Jaundice occurred significantly more often in the conservative management group [12/112 (11%) vs. 1/126 (0.8%); $P = 0.02$]. There were no deaths attributed to biliary complications in the conservative group

despite more frequent jaundice. The authors concluded that patients with ABP without biliary obstruction or biliary sepsis do not benefit from early ERCP and in fact there may be a higher rate of respiratory complications.

Other authors have criticized the Fölsch study for the unusually high incidence of respiratory complications and have suggested that the multicenter nature of the study may have included endoscopists with a low ERCP case load and hospitals with a very low patient accrual rate.

Summary of the randomized controlled trials

These four randomized controlled trials certainly differ in their designs, for example in the grading of pancreatitis, randomization to ES, timing of ERCP, etiology of pancreatitis, and/or exclusion of patients with jaundice. These differences make summary of the aggregate data somewhat difficult. The data obtained, limited to patients with a biliary etiology of pancreatitis, are summarized in Tables 13.2 and 13.3 and the corresponding calculated absolute risk reductions are shown in Figs 13.1 and 13.2. Three of the four trials demonstrated the safety of early ERCP in ABP. These studies also suggest a reduction in morbidity and possibly mortality in patients with severe pancreatitis who undergo early ERCP. One of these studies, the Polish study, reports benefit of ERCP in all patients with ABP, regardless of predicted disease severity. The German study calls into question the impact of intervention in ABP by reporting that patients without evidence of jaundice do not benefit from early ERCP.

Metaanalyses

Given the somewhat mixed conclusions of the four randomized controlled trials, other authors have attempted to pool the data. There have been two metaanalyses that examined the role of ERCP with or without ES in ABP. One was published as a full report and the second in abstract form.

Sharma and Howden published a metaanalysis using published data from the four trials, including the patients with nonbiliary pancreatitis in the Hong Kong study. Although the procedures in this metaanalysis are described as ERCP plus sphincterotomy, it is important to note that roughly 60% of patients had a sphincterotomy only if CBD stones were found on

Table 13.2 Outcomes of patients with predicted mild acute biliary pancreatitis in four randomized controlled trials. (Modified from Soetikno *et al.* 1998.)

Study	Morbidity, *n* (%)		Mortality, *n* (%)		Total number of cases	
	ERCP ± ES	Conventional	ERCP ± ES	Conventional	ERCP ± ES	Conventional
UK	4 (12)	4 (12)	0 (0)	0 (0)	34	34
Hong Kong	6 (18)	6 (17)	0 (0)	0 (0)	34	35
Germany	35 (42)	36 (47)	2 (2)	0 (0)	84	76
Poland	8 (10)	19 (25)	0 (0)	4 (5)	53	65
All	53 (23)	65 (30)	2 (0)	4 (2)	232	220

Note: 32 patients from the German study were excluded from analysis due to inability to stratify pancreatitis severity; 75 patients from the Polish study were excluded because they underwent immediate nonrandomized endoscopic sphincterotomy (ES) for an ampullary stone. ERCP, endoscopic retrograde cholangiopancreatography.

Table 13.3 Outcomes of patients with predicted severe acute biliary pancreatitis in four randomized controlled trials. (Modified from Soetikno *et al.* 1998.)

Study	Morbidity, *n* (%)		Mortality, *n* (%)		Total number of cases	
	ERCP ± ES	Conventional	ERCP ± ES	Conventional	ERCP ± ES	Conventional
UK	6 (24)	17 (61)	1 (4)	5 (18)	25	28
Hong Kong	4 (13)	15 (54)	1 (3)	5 (18)	30	28
Germany	17 (65)	14 (70)	6 (23)	2 (10)	26	20
Poland	9 (39)	20 (74)	1 (4)	9 (33)	23	27
All	36 (35)	66 (64)	9 (9)	21 (20)	104	103

Note: 32 patients from the German study were excluded from the analysis due to inability to stratify pancreatitis severity; 75 patients from the Polish study were excluded because they underwent immediate nonrandomized endoscopic sphincterotomy (ES) for an ampullary stone. ERCP, endoscopic retrograde cholangiopancreatography.

cholangiogram. The authors report a statistically significant difference in complication rate between early ERCP plus ES versus control (25% vs. 38.2%; $P < 0.001$). Although the data for mortality reached statistical significance only in the Polish study, the pooled data did show a significant decrease in mortality for the early ERCP group compared with control (5.2% vs. 9.1%; $P < 0.05$). The authors report relative and absolute risk reduction of 34.6 and 13.2 in complications and 42.9 and 3.9 in death with early ERCP plus ES. The authors did not perform a subgroup analysis based on the predicted severity, citing lack of relevant data from two of the four trials. They concluded that ERCP plus ES is safe in early ABP and is effective in reducing the morbidity and mortality, with a possible stronger benefit for patients with severe pancreatitis.

Soetikno *et al.* reviewed the same four trials, but included only the 695 patients with a diagnosis of acute gallstone pancreatitis in their analysis by collecting unpublished data from the senior authors of the studies. This eliminated 143 patients with an alternative etiology for pancreatitis. Their summary statistics showed that early ERCP with or without ES reduced the odds of morbidity and mortality compared with conservative treatment, but were statistically significant only for patients with severe pancreatitis. Figures 13.1 and 13.2 show that there is an overall absolute risk reduction in morbidity and mortality for patients with severe ABP

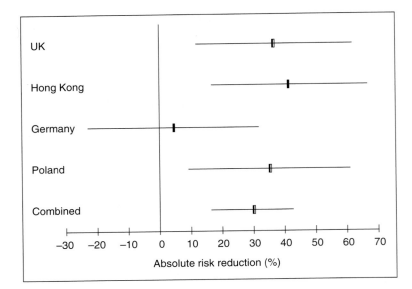

Figure 13.1 Absolute risk reduction (± 95% confidence interval) for morbidity in severe acute biliary pancreatitis (ABP) in four randomized controlled trials. These calculations exclude patients without biliary etiology for pancreatitis. The pooled data show a significant reduction in the morbidity rate with early endoscopic retrograde cholangiopancreatography with or without endoscopic sphincterotomy compared with conventional management (P < 0.0001) in severe ABP. Results were calculated from data presented by Soetikno et al. (1998).

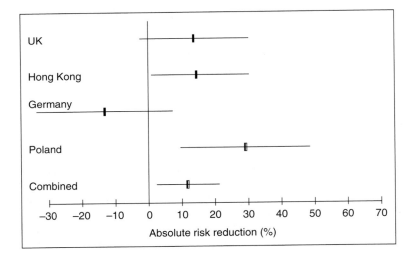

Figure 13.2 Absolute risk reduction (± 95% confidence interval) for mortality in severe acute biliary pancreatitis (ABP) in four randomized controlled trials. These calculations exclude patients without biliary etiology for pancreatitis. The pooled data show a significant reduction in the mortality rate with early endoscopic retrograde cholangiopancreatography with or without endoscopic sphincterotomy compared with conventional management (P = 0.028) in severe ABP. Results were calculated from data presented by Soetikno et al. (1998).

who undergo early ERCP. The results for mild pancreatitis did not show a consistent reduction in absolute risk reduction with early ERCP.

Although prior randomized controlled trials report some conflicting data, the weight of the evidence suggests that patients with predicted severe pancreatitis are not harmed by, and will actually avoid morbidity with, early ERCP. The data for impact on mortality and for patients predicted to have mild pancreatitis are inconclusive. There is a suggestion that patients with CBD stones may benefit from early intervention, possibly by avoiding obstructive complications. Investigators have tried to establish noninvasive methods to predict the likelihood of CBD stones and identify patients who may benefit from intervention.

Predicting CBD stones

Predicting which patients have bile duct stones is self-evidently important. Chang *et al.* evaluated 122 consecutive patients with gallstone pancreatitis in order to identify predictors of CBD stones. They made a diagnosis of ABP by detection of stones with ultrasound and by excluding other potential etiologies. Their previous work suggested that patients with elevated total bilirubin (≥ 1.7 mg/dL) or elevated amylase (≥ 150 U/L) beyond hospital day 4 had an increased likelihood of a retained CBD stone. High-risk patients without cholangitis were randomized to either precholecystectomy ERCP or intraoperative cholangiography (IOC) with a postoperative ERCP if stones were found. Patients deemed low risk for CBD stones based on ultrasound, bilirubin, and amylase had an IOC. Procedures were performed on hospital day 6–7 (mean). A total of 21 patients (21%) had CBD stones on IOC or ERCP. The authors found that an elevated bilirubin (> 1.35 mg/dL) on day 2 had 90.5% sensitivity and 63% specificity for predicting CBD stones at ERCP or IOC. Patients with bile duct stones were more likely to have an increase in bilirubin from day 1–2 than those without stones.

Cohen *et al.* retrospectively evaluated 154 patients with gallstone pancreatitis who had ERCP or IOC during their hospitalization. Of these patients, 18% were identified as having a persistent bile duct stone on cholangiography at a median of 4 days into hospitalization. The authors reported that a rise in *any* biochemical parameter (amylase, lipase, total bilirubin, alkaline phosphatase, AST, or ALT) between admission and 24–48 hours was seen more often in patients with CBD stones than in those without (positive predictive value 31%, negative predictive value 92%, sensitivity 76%, specificity 60%; $P < 0.05$). There was also a significant increase in complication rate when a patient had an increase in any of the above indices over the same time course compared with patients who had no rise in laboratory values (21% vs. 8%; $P < 0.05$). Notably, transabdominal ultrasound was only 29% sensitive (performed at a median of 7 hours after presentation) for the detection of CBD stones. Standard criteria for predicting severe pancreatitis also failed to predict a CBD stone. Patients with persistent CBD stones had a higher morbidity (29% vs. 12%) and mortality (11% vs. 1%) than those without retained stones ($P < 0.05$). Neoptolemos *et al.* also reported that retained CBD stones were found more often in patients predicted to have severe pancreatitis compared with patients predicted to have a mild course (25% vs. 63%; $P = 0.03$).

Newer techniques to image the biliary tract include MRCP and endoscopic ultrasound. Studies suggest that endoscopic ultrasound and MRCP have high sensitivity and negative predictive value for the detection of choledocholithiasis. These modalities are attractive because they may help identify patients at risk for complications of ABP without the risk of ERCP. It must be recognized that these studies would often need to be performed in the setting of critical illness. They also do not offer a therapeutic option and therefore may be somewhat limited in their utility.

Acute cholangitis with ABP

In the literature the incidence of cholangitis in the setting of ABP varies from 3 to 14%. Since emergent ERCP to remove CBD stones and reestablish bile drainage has been shown to be efficacious in cholangitis, it can also be expected that ABP patients with concurrent cholangitis will benefit from early biliary decompression. Neoptolemos *et al.* recommend ERCP/ES in ABP patients with acute cholangitis given the high percentage of CBD stones found in such patients (47%). In addition, investigators have shown a reduced incidence of biliary complications (jaundice and cholangitis) in ABP patients undergoing early ERCP.

Bile duct crystals and biliary pancreatitis

Biliary sludge or microlithiasis can cause acute pancreatitis. Biliary sludge is defined as a suspension of crystals, either cholesterol monohydrate or calcium bilirubinate, in bile. These clusters of small stones have been postulated to incite acute pancreatitis by transiently obstructing the papilla. Lee *et al.* evaluated 31 patients with idiopathic acute pancreatitis; 74% had evidence of biliary sludge on ultrasound or microscopic evaluation of the bile. Most importantly, the authors showed that patients with biliary sludge who underwent cholecystectomy or sphincterotomy had a decreased risk of recurrent pancreatitis [1/10 (10%) vs. 8/11 (72%); $P = 0.01$]. Ros *et al.* examined bile from 51 patients after recovery from idiopathic acute pancreatitis and found that 67% contained sediment. They showed that patients who were not treated with cholecystectomy or ursodeoxycholic acid had a higher frequency of pancreatitis relapse than the treated group

(67% vs. 16%). Kohut *et al.* evaluated 15 patients with suspected acute pancreatitis without clear evidence of gallstones or an alternative etiology. They analyzed bile collected from the CBD within 24 hours of admission; 80% of patients had cholesterol monohydrate or calcium bilirubinate crystals present. Although biliary sludge appears to be a risk factor for recurrent pancreatitis, the role of sphincterotomy in the setting of acute pancreatitis in this subset of patients without overt CBD stones has not been established.

Optimal timing of ERCP

The majority of patients with ABP will recover from their attack without significant morbidity or mortality. If one intervenes at the onset of symptoms, procedures might be done in patients who would have recovered spontaneously. If one delays intervention, it is possible that a window of opportunity to alter the severity and duration of disease may be missed. The aforementioned randomized controlled trials did not specifically address the issue of ERCP timing. In those studies interventions were performed 24–72 hours into admission.

Nowak *et al.* published a prospective, nonrandomized, observational trial suggesting that the best outcomes were achieved if ERCP was performed within 24 hours of symptom onset and that morbidity and mortality were higher after a 72-hour delay. The authors followed 307 patients who had urgent ERCP for ABP. For those treated within 24 hours of symptom onset there were no deaths and a 7% complication rate. For patients treated between 24 and 72 hours, there was 2% mortality and a 16% complication rate. Patients treated with ERCP after 72 hours did worst, with 13% mortality and a 32% complication rate. Although statistically significant for both mild and severe pancreatitis groups, the authors noted that the trend for ERCP timing was more dramatic in the severe group. In our practice we perform ERCP in patients fitting criteria for severe pancreatitis as soon as the diagnosis and severity stratification is confirmed.

Outcomes of ERCP with ES in patients who are not candidates for cholecystectomy

Cholecystectomy is the recommended definitive treat-

ment for preventing relapse of gallstone pancreatitis. For the group of patients who are not good surgical candidates due to comorbid medical conditions, there are data to support the use of ES to prevent recurrence of pancreatitis. Wellbourn *et al.* reported on 51 patients who had ES for gallstone pancreatitis without subsequent cholecystectomy. After a mean follow-up of approximately 27 months, none of 47 patients with successful sphincterotomy had recurrent acute pancreatitis. Two of three patients with incomplete ES had recurrent pancreatitis over the same time course. Targarona *et al.* randomized 98 patients with a history of biliary pain, jaundice, or ABP to open cholecystectomy or ES. Although the authors showed that there was a higher recurrence of biliary symptoms in the ES group, there was no recurrence of pancreatitis in either group over the 17 months of follow-up. Kaw *et al.* reported in a prospective observational study that patients undergoing ES versus cholecystectomy had the same recurrence rate of ABP (2.4–2.9%) over a 33-month follow-up period. For patients with a history of CBD stones, other authors have reported a 5–10% recurrence of biliary symptoms (colic or jaundice) after ES alone, but no recurrence of ABP. Evidence suggests that ABP will recur in more than 50% of patients who do not undergo cholecystectomy or ES. Many authors therefore recommend ES in ABP patients who cannot undergo cholecystectomy and who have evidence for CBD or gallbladder stones.

Proposed algorithm for use of ERCP with or without ES in ABP

The available literature summarized above provides guidance for managing patients with ABP (Fig. 13.3). We recommend performing ERCP on patients with predicted severe pancreatitis as soon as this classification is applied to an individual. Patients with mild pancreatitis and evidence of cholangitis, jaundice, or a dilated CBD should undergo ERCP due to risk for CBD stone and complications of cholangitis. Also, for patients with a deteriorating course of ABP, ERCP should be considered. We perform sphincterotomy in patients with choledocholithiasis confirmed on cholangiography. We have a lower threshold for performing ES in patients who are not candidates for cholecystectomy and who have stones in the gallbladder or a dilated CBD. It should be noted that ERCP in acute and

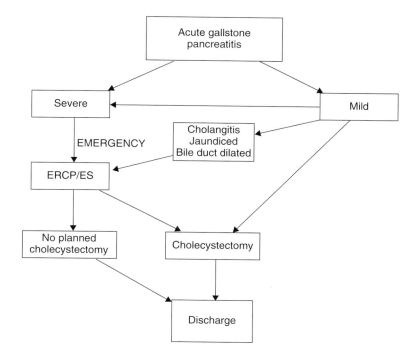

Figure 13.3 Proposed algorithm for treatment of patients with acute biliary pancreatitis. ERCP, endoscopic retrograde cholangiopancreatography; ES, endoscopic sphincterotomy.

severely ill patients can be complex and it has been shown that patients benefit from having an ERCP performed at a high-volume center by an experienced endoscopist.

Recommended reading

Acosta JM, Ledesma CL. Gallstone migration as a cause of acute pancreatitis. *N Engl J Med* 1974;290:484–487.

Acosta JM, Pellegrini CA, Skinner DB. Etiology and pathogenesis of acute biliary pancreatitis. *Surgery* 1980;88: 118–125.

Balthazar EJ, Robinson DL, Megibow AJ *et al*. Acute pancreatitis: value of CT in establishing prognosis. *Radiology* 1990;174:331–336.

Chak A, Hawes RH, Cooper GS *et al*. Prospective assessment of the utility of EUS in the evaluation of gallstone pancreatitis. *Gastrointest Endosc* 1999;49:599–604.

Chang L, Lo SK, Stabile BE *et al*. Gallstone pancreatitis: a prospective study on the incidence of cholangitis and clinical predictors of retained common bile duct stones. *Am J Gastroenterol* 1998;93:527–531.

Fan ST, Lai ECS, Mok FPT *et al*. Early treatment of acute biliary pancreatitis by endoscopic papillotomy. *N Engl J Med* 1993;328:228–232.

Fölsch U, Nitsche R, Ludtke R *et al*. Early ERCP and papillotomy compared with conservative management for acute biliary pancreatitis. *N Engl J Med* 1997;336:237–242.

Hill J, Martin DF, Tweedle DEF. Risks of leaving the gallbladder in situ after endoscopic sphincterotomy for bile duct stones. *Br J Surg* 1991;78:554–557.

Kelly TR. Gallstone pancreatitis: the timing of surgery. *Surgery* 1980;88:345–350.

Lee SP, Nicholls JF, Park HZ. Biliary sludge as a cause of acute pancreatitis. *N Engl J Med* 1992;326:589–593.

Neoptolemos JP, Carr-Locke DL, Leese T *et al*. Acute cholangitis in association with acute pancreatitis: incidence, clinical features and outcome in relation to ERCP and endoscopic sphincterotomy. *Br J Surg* 1987;74:1103–1106.

Neoptolemos JP, London NJ, James D *et al*. Controlled trial of urgent endoscopic retrograde cholangiopancreatography and endoscopic sphincterotomy versus conservative treatment for acute pancreatitis due to gallstones. *Lancet* 1988; ii:979–983.

Nowak A, Nowakowska-Dulawa E, Marek TA *et al*. Final results of the prospective, randomized controlled study on endoscopic sphincterotomy versus conventional management in acute biliary pancreatitis (abstract). *Gastroenterology* 1995;108:A380.

Nowak A, Nowakowska-Dulawa E, Marek TA *et al*. Timing of endoscopic sphincterotomy for acute biliary pancreatitis. *Gastrointest Endosc* 1996;43:391.

Ranson JHC. Etiological and prognostic factors in human acute pancreatitis: a review. *Am J Gastroenterol* 1982;77: 633–638.

Sharma VK, Howden CW. Meta-analysis of randomized controlled trials of endoscopic retrograde cholangiography and endoscopic sphincterotomy for the treatment of acute biliary pancreatitis. *Am J Gastroenterol* 1999;94:3211–3214.

Soetikno RM, Carr-Locke DL, Neoptolemos JP *et al.* Does early ERCP ± ES reduce the morbidity and mortality of acute gallstone pancreatitis? A meta-analysis. *Gastrointest Endosc* 1998;47:AB130.

Stone HH, Fabian TC, Dunlop WE. Gallstone pancreatitis. *Ann Surg* 1981;194:305–312.

Targarona EM, Perez Ayuso RM, Bordas JM *et al.* Randomised trial of endoscopic sphincterotomy with gallbladder left in situ versus open surgery for common bile duct calculi in high-risk patients. *Lancet* 1996;347: 926–929.

Tenner S, Dubner H, Steinberg W. Predicting gallstone pancreatitis with laboratory parameters: a meta-analysis. *Am J Gastroenterol* 1994;89:1863–1866.

14 Indications for surgery in acute pancreatitis

Oscar Joe Hines and Howard A. Reber

Acute pancreatitis is usually a self-limited disease that resolves in a few days, and surgery is rarely needed. However, 10% of cases may be complicated by pancreatic necrosis, infection, or multisystem organ failure, and operative management may be life-saving. The indications for surgery in the face of active pancreatitis following the resolution of the acute phase of this disease are listed in Table 14.1. In the following discussion, we review these indications and explain the logic for these surgical approaches to management.

Uncertain diagnosis

With the wide availability of sophisticated imaging techniques such as computed tomography (CT) and magnetic resonance imaging, the diagnosis of acute pancreatitis is rarely overlooked today. Nevertheless, an occasional patient with severe abdominal pain may undergo diagnostic laparoscopy or laparotomy only to find acute pancreatitis is the underlying problem. The severity of the pancreatitis should be assessed with a minimum of manipulation of the pancreas. With acute edematous pancreatitis and no evidence of pancreatic or peripancreatic necrosis, neither drainage nor débridement is indicated, but the gallbladder should be removed if it is inflamed or if gallstones are present. Irrigation, drainage, and débridement may be appropriate for severe pancreatitis with infected necrosis (see later).

Abdominal compartment syndrome

In patients with severe pancreatitis, intraabdominal pressures may rise due to bowel edema and sequestration of fluid in the abdominal cavity. This may compromise blood flow to vital intraabdominal organs and result in abdominal compartment syndrome, defined as combination of the following.

1 Urinary bladder pressure greater than 25 mmHg.
2 Progressive organ dysfunction: urinary output <0.5 mL/kg per hour, or Pao_2/Fio_2 <150, or peak airway pressure >45 cmH$_2$O, or cardiac index <3 L/min per m^2 despite resuscitation.
3 Improved organ function after decompression.

Abdominal decompression will result in improved cerebral blood flow, cardiac dynamics, respiratory compliance, and intestinal and renal perfusion. The midline abdominal fascia should be opened and an interposition material, such as an opened intravenous fluid bag or "Bogotá bag," is attached to the fascial or skin edges to prevent bowel evisceration. Although this procedure can be performed at the bedside in the intensive care unit, the operating room is preferred. As the patient improves and bowel edema resolves, plans can be made to remove the bag and close the abdomen in a more conventional way.

Gallstones

Gallstones are a very common cause of pancreatitis. If the pancreatitis is mild to moderate in severity, a laparoscopic cholecystectomy can be performed safely, often within the first 48–72 hours of admission. By this time, the abdominal pain has largely resolved and the serum amylase level is returning to normal. The former practice whereby the pancreatitis was allowed to

Table 14.1 Indications for intervention in acute pancreatitis.

Indication	Procedure
Unknown diagnosis	Exploratory laparotomy
	Diagnostic laparoscopy
Abdominal compartment syndrome	Decompressive laparotomy
Gallstones	Cholecystectomy (open or laparoscopic)
	Common duct exploration (open or laparoscopic)
	Endoscopic retrograde cholangiopancreatography
Infected pancreatic necrosis	Pancreatic débridement
Sterile pancreatic necrosis	Pancreatic débridement (rarely)
Hemorrhage	Angiographic embolization
	Operative suture ligation/packing
Pancreatic abscess	Percutaneous drainage (primary)
	Operative drainage (secondary)
Pseudocyst	Cystgastrostomy/cystjejunostomy
	Endoscopic drainage
	Radiologic drainage
Pancreatic fistula	Roux-en-Y pancreaticojejunostomy

resolve, the patient discharged from hospital, and then readmitted for elective cholecystectomy 6 weeks later is unnecessary, more expensive, and can be associated with recurrence of pancreatitis during the wait. As many as 60% will experience recurrent gallstone pancreatitis within 6 months. Of course, some patients with prohibitive coexisting medical conditions may never be surgical candidates. In this case, endoscopic sphincterotomy should be performed, which will decrease the incidence of recurrent pancreatitis to between 2 and 5% over 2 years.

About 1 in 12–15 patients with gallstone pancreatitis has choledocholithiasis. The common duct stones should be removed, but the pancreas should not be disturbed. Rarely, a stone impacted at the ampulla may require duodenotomy for stone removal under direct vision and T-tube decompression of the bile duct.

In patients with severe pancreatitis (fluid collections, necrosis), cholecystectomy should be delayed until the pancreatitis has resolved, some weeks or even months later. If acute cholecystitis is present, an interval cholecystostomy may be required. If the common duct is obstructed, an endoscopic sphincterotomy and/or stent may be indicated.

Emergency endoscopic sphincterotomy with stone extraction may be life-saving in some patients with severe biliary pancreatitis. It should be used when a patient with pancreatitis is known to have gallstones, the serum bilirubin concentration is elevated (> 4 mg/dL), the alkaline phosphatase concentration is elevated, and the clinical course does not improve within 24–36 hours with normal resuscitative efforts. At least four randomized studies have evaluated the utility of this approach (Table 14.2) and they have all demonstrated lower complication rates in those patients who received endoscopic retrograde cholangiopancreatography and stone extraction. Three of the studies also demonstrated lower mortality rates in this group. However, only a small minority of patients will need this intervention.

Pancreatic necrosis

In cases of severe pancreatitis, patients should undergo abdominal CT to confirm the diagnosis, determine the presence of local complications, and determine whether any of the pancreatic tissue has died as a result of the inflammatory process. This is especially important because the likelihood of pancreatic infection is greater with greater degrees of pancreatic necrosis, and infection is an indication for surgery. The role of pancreatic surgery in severe pancreatitis has evolved since the early part of the twentieth century. For a time, a total pancreatectomy was recommended, which

Table 14.2 Early endoscopic retrograde cholangiopancreatography (ERCP) and endoscopic sphincterotomy (ES) in acute and severe gallstone pancreatitis.

Study	Treatment	Complications (%)	Deaths (%)
Neoptolemos *et al.* (1988)	ERCP/ES	19	0
	Conservative	63	13
Nowak *et al.* (1995)	ERCP/ES	14	1
	Conservative	34	11
Fan *et al.* (1993)	ERCP/ES	20	3
	Conservative	76	18
Folsch *et al.* (1997)	ERCP/ES	17	5
	Conservative	14	3

included resection of living pancreas as well as that portion which had undergone necrosis. The reasoning was that removal of the entire gland would abort the inflammatory process, and recovery would then begin. Although some of those patients also had pancreatic and/or peripancreatic infection, infection itself was not a critical determinant in the decision for operation. This approach was eventually abandoned because of unacceptably high mortality rates in these critically ill patients. As the twenty-first century begins, most surgeons believe that surgery is indicated only when the necrotic pancreas has become infected, and that the procedure should consist primarily of débridement and drainage of the infected material. Viable pancreas is not removed. The systemic organ failure ultimately responsible for the demise of such patients is partly caused by this infected tissue.

There remains a group of critically ill patients with severe acute pancreatitis, usually with significant pancreatic and/or peripancreatic necrosis, in whom infection is not present. The role of surgery in these patients with so-called sterile necrosis continues to be controversial. In general, evidence is accumulating that this group is managed effectively by nonsurgical means in the majority of cases. If surgery is performed, it is done in an attempt to drain and débride the necrotic tissue that is the putative source of various noxious substances believed to be responsible for the ongoing illness. Or it may even be that infection was present but its diagnosis was overlooked. The validity of this approach is as yet unproven.

Risk factors for pancreatic infections

Secondary infection of necrotic pancreatic and peripancreatic tissue is a common source of morbidity in acute pancreatitis. The origin of the bacteria is usually the gastrointestinal tract, although hematogenous seeding from infected intravenous lines or other sources is possible. Infections are more likely to occur in patients with extensive pancreatic necrosis and severe pancreatic inflammation. Pancreatic necrosis develops in about 10% of all patients with acute pancreatitis, and of these about 30% become infected.

The use of prophylactic antibiotics in the face of severe necrotizing pancreatitis has been somewhat controversial since it is not clear that the patients benefit and there is the risk of selecting for more virulent bacterial strains or fungi. However, there does appear to be an advantage for prophylaxis with antibiotics that can reach concentrations in the pancreas that effectively inhibit infection. A recent metaanalysis that examined all the trials using antibiotic prophylaxis found six randomized studies of which only three were adequate for analysis (Table 14.3). Overall, antibiotic prophylaxis reduced sepsis by 21% and mortality by 12.3% compared with no prophylaxis. There were also fewer pancreatic infections but this was not statistically significant.

When does the necrotic tissue become infected? Beger found that in patients who underwent surgical exploration within the first week after the onset of pancreatitis, 24% had infected pancreatic necrosis. From

Table 14.3 Studies of randomized prophylactic antibiotics in acute pancreatitis

Study	Antibiotic prophylaxis	No. of patients		Pancreatic infection		Sepsis		Mortality	
		Drug	Control	Drug	Control	Drug	Control	Drug	Control
Pederzoli *et al.* (1993)	Imipenem (500 mg t.i.d.)	41	33	5	10	6	16	3	4
Sainio *et al.* (1995)	Cefuroxime (1.5 g t.i.d.)	30	30	9	12	11	13	1	7
Schwarz *et al.* (1997)	Ofloxacin (200 mg b.i.d.), metronidazole (500 mg b.i.d.)	13	13	8	7	4	6	0	2

the second to the third week there was an increase of 36–71%, and then a decline to an infection rate of 32.5% when operation was done after the fourth week. Similar results were reported for CT-guided fine-needle aspiration (FNA) of pancreatic necrosis.

Diagnosis of infected pancreatic necrosis

The diagnosis of pancreatic infection is made most reliably by CT or ultrasound-guided FNA with Gram staining and culture of the aspirate. The material should be sent for bacterial and fungal culture. The technique is safe, accurate, and can be performed rapidly. Although it is tempting to only perform FNA in patients who exhibit a septic clinical picture (e.g., high fever, white cell count), some patients with infection have a low-grade fever and a white cell count of less than 15 000/mm^3. Thus, in most patients FNA should be performed in those who have evidence of necrosis and fluid collection on CT. In a minority of patients, gas bubbles in the area of the pancreas are evident on CT. If this case, FNA is unnecessary since the gas should be assumed to be the product of bacterial fermentation from infection, and surgery is indicated.

Most pancreatic surgeons treat patients with necrotizing pancreatitis with prophylactic broad-spectrum antibiotics, in the hope that this will decrease the chance of infection of the necrotic material. However, in patients with proved infection, antibiotic therapy is adjunctive treatment only. Proof of infection is an indication for laparotomy and surgical drainage and débridement of the infected and necrotic material.

Definitive management requires surgery

Except in the unusual situation of fulminating acute pancreatitis with organ failure and a rapidly progressive downhill course soon after admission to hospital, most patients should not undergo operation during the first week of their illness. When clinical deterioration is rapid and surgery is undertaken during the first week, most of these patients die. The outcome is better when surgery is postponed at least until the second week or later, when the margins of the pancreatic necrosis have become better defined and the acute inflammation has subsided somewhat. Fortunately, in most cases the disease has been ongoing for a week or more by the time the diagnosis of infected pancreatic necrosis has been established and the need for surgery is evident. The patient's condition should be optimized, and surgery should be undertaken within 24–48 hours.

The goals of surgery are to remove infected and devitalized pancreatic and peripancreatic tissue, drain pus and other fluid collections, and leave drains behind that can be used for continuous postoperative lavage of the affected areas. CT provides a map to those areas which require drainage, so that uninvolved tissue planes do not need to be opened and unnecessarily contaminated. During operation viable pancreatic parenchyma should be preserved. Hemostasis may require suture ligation of bleeding vessels, but significant bleeding usually indicates that the surgeon should limit further dissection in that area. Once most of the necrotic material has been removed and all the fluid collections drained, several large sump drains are placed in the most involved areas for postoperative lavage. The fascia of the abdominal wound is closed but the skin left open. Patients with extended areas of infected necrotic tissue or large multiloculated or multiple abscesses may be treated better by open drainage and packing. The operative procedure is the same, but the débrided areas are packed and both the fascia and skin are left open. Normal saline at a rate of 1 L/hour is perfused through the drains for at least the first 24 hours, and then the rate is decreased over a number of days according to the patient's clinical course and the character of the drainage.

Patients who are treated by the open packing technique are committed to at least several reoperations before they recover completely. However, about 20% of patients treated with the closed technique also require at least one reoperation to drain recurrent or persistent areas of infection. An abdominal CT scan obtained at weekly intervals helps guide further therapy and documents improvement during the postoperative course.

Internationally, there has been some experience with laparoscopic and percutaneous approaches to infected pancreatic necrosis. The pancreatic bed can be approached through the stomach, the mesocolon, or the retroperitoneum. However, since the experience has been limited to date, these cases should be highly selected.

The most common local postoperative complications are hemorrhage and intestinal fistulas. Enterocutaneous fistulas (pancreatic, duodenal, small bowel, or colon) occur in up to 30% of patients. They can be caused directly by the necrotizing infection, or by iatrogenic trauma at the time of débridement or erosion into the bowel of an adjacent surgical drain. Most of the bowel fistulas eventually close spontaneously without operative intervention.

The mortality rate for all patients with acute pancreatitis is about 10%. Necrotizing pancreatitis associated with infection has a mortality rate of about 20%, although there is some evidence that earlier diagnosis of infection and aggressive surgical intervention may lower this figure.

Sterile pancreatic necrosis

Almost all patients with sterile pancreatic necrosis should be treated with conservative nonsurgical management in the intensive care unit. Most will eventually recover. Nevertheless, some patients fail to improve after weeks of treatment or may even begin to deterio-

rate. In these patients consideration for surgery still seems reasonable for the reasons presented earlier. The timing of operation in this small group of patients cannot be given precisely. In general, it seems best to continue to treat them conservatively for at least 3–4 weeks before concluding that surgery should be performed.

Hemorrhage

Hemorrhage is associated with a high mortality rate, as bleeding often occurs from major peripancreatic blood vessels (e.g., splenic, superior mesenteric or portal veins, gastroduodenal or pancreatic arteries). Arteriography with embolization of bleeding vessels can be effective and should be the first choice as long as the patient is able to be resuscitated and demonstrates reasonable hemodynamic stabilization before the procedure. Otherwise some patients will require urgent operation to stop the bleeding. Operative control of hemorrhage in the face of severe pancreatitis is difficult given the significant distortion of the anatomy in these cases. Ultimately, suture ligation and packing should suffice.

Pancreatic abscess

A pancreatic abscess is a collection of purulent material within a defined cavity, and with little if any associated necrosis. It is different from infected pancreatic necrosis and an infected pancreatic pseudocyst. Pancreatic abscesses usually require 3–4 weeks to become apparent. Diagnosis should be suspected when the patient begins to run a septic course, and it can be confirmed with CT and percutaneous FNA of the pus. An external drain should be left in place. Unlike infected pancreatic necrosis, radiologically placed tube drainage may be effective treatment and surgery may be unnecessary. However, unless the patient improves rapidly within 24–48 hours of external drainage, surgical drainage of the abscess is required. Antibiotics are adjunctive management only.

Pseudocyst

A pancreatic pseudocyst is a collection of fluid usually in the vicinity of the pancreas that develops in association with a leak of pancreatic juices from the inflamed parenchyma or from a disrupted duct. The wall of the pseudocyst is composed of fibrous nonepithelialized tissue. Occasionally a pseudocyst may present at great distance from the pancreas (e.g., thorax, groin) when the fluid dissects through tissue planes. As many as 30% of patients with acute pancreatitis form acute fluid collections around the time of the acute attack, but these must be distinguished from chronic pseudocysts. The majority of these acute "pseudocysts" resolve without intervention. Only about 5% of these patients develop chronic pseudocysts, which are characterized by their ovoid or spherical shape and well-formed wall. Because of this natural history, acute "pseudocysts" (fluid collections) should be managed expectantly. If they develop into chronic pseudocysts, they may require treatment.

The management of pseudocysts varies according to their size and the presence of associated symptoms. Asymptomatic pseudocysts up to 5–6 cm in diameter may be safely observed, and are usually followed with either serial ultrasound or CT examinations. Larger cysts or pseudocysts of any size that are symptomatic require treatment.

Symptoms are most often due to gastrointestinal obstruction, when the cyst distorts the stomach or duodenum, or to abdominal pain. Serious complications can also occur, although they are uncommon (< 5% of cases). These include hemorrhage into the cyst, perforation of the cyst, and infection of the cyst. Hemorrhage is usually caused by erosion of the splenic or gastroduodenal artery or other major vessel within the wall of the cyst, and the bleeding is usually confined to the cyst lumen. The diagnosis should be suspected if there are clinical signs of hypovolemia and a falling hematocrit. There may be abdominal pain, and a mass may be palpable. Abdominal CT shows the cyst with the contained blood clot. Angiography confirms the diagnosis, and the radiologist should attempt to embolize the bleeding vessel. If this is not successful, emergency surgery with ligation of the vessel or excision of the cyst is required. Perforation of a pseudocyst is a surgical emergency characterized by the sudden onset of intense abdominal pain with peritonitis. Patients require urgent surgery with irrigation of the peritoneal cavity and usually external cyst drainage. Infection of a pseudocyst should be suspected if signs of sepsis develop. Diagnosis by CT and treatment by percutaneous cyst aspiration and drainage are usually effective.

In the absence of a life-threatening complication, elective surgery of pseudocysts is usually delayed until the cyst has developed a mature wall that will hold sutures at the time of repair. For those cysts that develop following an episode of acute pancreatitis, this requires 4–6 weeks. In most cases the patient can eat and be discharged from hospital during the interval. Pseudocysts that resolve spontaneously usually will do so during this time.

Pseudocysts may be treated surgically or by endoscopic or radiologic drainage. Endoscopic methods require the placement of a plastic stent through the stomach or duodenal wall into the adjacent cyst. The stent is eventually removed, and in about 80% of cases the cyst is permanently eradicated. These endoscopic techniques require expertise, which is becoming more widely available. Radiologic approaches usually consist of percutaneous external drainage of the cyst with eventual removal of the drainage catheter many weeks later. Many of these pseudocysts recur. Surgical treatment usually consists of drainage of the cyst internally to either the stomach (cystgastrostomy) or to a Roux-en-Y limb of jejunum (cystjejunostomy). Both are safe and effective, with recurrence rates of less than 10%. If the pseudocyst is in the tail of the pancreas, a distal pancreatectomy with excision of the cyst may be best. The recurrence rate is less than 1% in this case.

Finally, many authors have reported excellent results with laparoscopic techniques for the drainage of pancreatic pseudocysts. These cysts can be drained through transgastric or intragastric approaches or a Roux limb can be used for definitive treatment.

Pancreatic fistula

In the setting of acute pancreatitis, a pancreatic fistula is usually the result of a ductal disruption associated with pancreatic necrosis and usually becomes apparent as the patient recovers from operative débridement. In a large series of 556 patients, pancreatic fistulas occurred in 9% of patients with necrotizing pancreatitis. The diagnosis is made by finding a high amylase level (usually many thousands of units per liter) in the drain effluent, and it is treated by leaving the drain in place. Many such fistulas will close spontaneously, provided that ductal continuity can be reestablished as healing occurs, infection is eradicated, and nutrition is adequate. Parenteral nutrition is usually not required and most patients are able to eat a regular diet. There is no evidence that oral intake delays resolution of the fistula. The use of somatostatin does not appear to hasten fistula closure, although if it is a high-output fistula (i.e., > 200 mL/day) the secretory inhibitor may simplify management of the patient. Fistulas that persist for as long as 1 year or those whose anatomic characteristics preclude spontaneous closure (e.g., duct obstruction between fistula and duodenal lumen, duct discontinuity) will require operative repair. This is best done by creating an anastomosis between the pancreatic duct at the point of the leak and a Roux-en-Y limb of jejunum. The success rate of operative repair is greater than 90%.

International guidelines for the surgical management of acute pancreatitis

In 2002, an international group of physicians interested in the treatment of acute pancreatitis published a consensus statement on the surgical management of acute pancreatitis. These recommendations reinforce much that has been described in this chapter and include the following. Mild acute pancreatitis is not an indication for pancreatic surgery. The use of prophylactic broad-spectrum antibiotics reduces infection rates in CT-proven necrotizing pancreatitis but may not improve survival. FNA for bacteriology should be performed in order to differentiate between sterile and infected pancreatic necrosis in patients with sepsis syndrome. Infected pancreatic necrosis in patients with clinical signs and symptoms of sepsis is an indication for intervention including surgery and radiologic drainage. Patients with sterile pancreatic necrosis (with negative FNA for bacteriology) should be managed conservatively and only undergo intervention in selected cases. Early surgery within 14 days after onset of the disease is not recommended in patients with necrotizing pancreatitis unless there are specific indications. Surgical and other forms of interventional management should favor an organ-preserving approach, which involves débridement or necrosectomy combined with a postoperative management concept that maximizes postoperative evacuation of retroperitoneal debris and exudate. Cholecystectomy should be performed to avoid recurrence of gallstone-associated acute pancreatitis. In mild gallstone-associated acute pancreatitis, cholecystectomy should be performed as soon as the patient has recovered and ideally during the same hospital admission. In severe gallstone-associated acute pancreatitis, cholecystectomy should be delayed until there is sufficient resolution of the inflammatory response and clinical recovery. Endoscopic sphincterotomy is an alternative to cholecystectomy in those who are not fit to undergo surgery in order to lower the risk of recurrence of gallstone-associated acute pancreatitis. However, there is a theoretical risk of introducing infection into sterile pancreatic necrosis.

Recommended reading

Ammori BJ. Laparoscopic transgastric pancreatic necrosectomy for infected pancreatic necrosis. *Surg Endosc* 2002; 16:1362.

Beger HG, Bittner R, Block S, Buchler M. Bacterial contamination of pancreatic necrosis: a prospective clinical study. *Gastroenterology* 1986;91:433–438.

Carter CR, McKay CJ, Imrie CW. Percutaneous necrosectomy and sinus tract endoscopy in the management of infected pancreatic necrosis: an initial experience. *Ann Surg* 2000; 232:175–180.

Fan ST, Lai EC, Mok FP, Lo CM, Zheng SS, Wong J. Early treatment of acute biliary pancreatitis by endoscopic papillotomy. *N Engl J Med* 1993;328:228–232.

Folsch UR, Nitsche R, Ludtke R, Hilgers RA, Creutzfeldt W. Early ERCP and papillotomy compared with conservative treatment for acute biliary pancreatitis. The German Study Group on Acute Biliary Pancreatitis. *N Engl J Med* 1997; 336:237–242.

Gagner M. Laparoscopic treatment of acute necrotizing pancreatitis. *Semin Laparosc Surg* 1996;3:21–28.

Gerzof SG, Banks PA, Robbins AH *et al*. Early diagnosis of pancreatic infection by computed tomography-guided aspiration. *Gastroenterology* 1987;93:1315–1320.

Hammarstrom LE, Stridbeck H, Ihse I. Effect of endoscopic sphincterotomy and interval cholecystectomy on late outcome after gallstone pancreatitis. *Br J Surg* 1998;85:333–336.

Mori T, Abe N, Sugiyama M, Atomi Y, Way LW. Laparoscopic pancreatic cystgastrostomy. *J Hepatobiliary Pancreat Surg* 2000;7:28–34.

Neoptolemos JP, Carr-Locke DL, London NJ, Bailey IA, James D, Fossard DP. Controlled trial of urgent endoscopic retrograde cholangiopancreatography and endoscopic sphincterotomy versus conservative treatment for acute pancreatitis due to gallstones. *Lancet* 1988;ii:979–983.

Nowak A, Nowakowska-Dulawa E, Marek TA, Rybicka J. Final results of the prospective, randomized, controlled study on endoscopic sphincterotomy versus conventional management in acute biliary pancreatitis. *Gastroenterology* 1995;108:A380.

Patti MG, Pellegrini CA. Gallstone pancreatitis. *Surg Clin North Am* 1990;70:1277–1295.

Pederzoli P, Bassi C, Vesentini S *et al.* A randomized multi-center clinical trial of antibiotic prophylaxis of septic complications in acute necrotizing pancreatitis with imipenem. *Surg Gynecol Obstet* 1993;176:480–483.

Roth JS, Park AE. Laparoscopic pancreatic cystgastrostomy: the lesser sac technique. *Surg Laparosc Endosc Percutan Tech* 2001;11:201–203.

Sainio V, Kemppainen E, Puolakkainen P *et al.* Early antibiotic treatment in acute necrotizing pancreatitis. *Lancet* 1995; 346:663–667.

Schwarz M, Isenmann R, Meyer H *et al.* Antibiotic use in necrotizing pancreatitis. Results of a controlled study. *Dtsch Med Wochenschr* 1997;122:356–361.

Sharma VK, Howden CW. Prophylactic antibiotic administration reduces sepsis and mortality in acute necrotizing pancreatitis: a meta-analysis. *Pancreas* 2001;22:28–31.

Thompson MH, Tranter SE. All-comers policy for laparoscopic exploration of the common bile duct. *Br J Surg* 2002;89:1608–1612.

Uhl W, Warshaw A, Imrie C *et al.* International Association of Pancreatology. IAP Guidelines for the Surgical Management of Acute Pancreatitis. *Pancreatology* 2002;2:565–573.

Widdison AL, Karanjia ND, Alvarez C, Reber HA. Sources of pancreatic pathogens in acute necrotizing pancreatitis. *Gastroenterology* 1991;100:A304.

15 Surgical approaches to acute necrotizing pancreatitis

Laureano Fernández-Cruz and Hans G. Beger

Surgical approach to necrotizing pancreatitis

The development of extensive pancreatic necrosis is a major cause of death in patients with severe pancreatitis. However, the question remains, which is the best method to identify individuals developing severe necrosis who require surgical intervention? There are patients in whom surgery should rarely or never be contemplated. Multisystem failure is an important marker of fulminant disease, and a rising pulse rate, serum creatinine, fever, and white cell count, in conjunction with difficulty in maintaining arterial blood pressure and Pao_2, are ominous signs. These are the patients who, after 10–14 days of disease onset, are characterized by a systemic inflammatory response syndrome (SIRS) maintained by the release of various inflammatory mediators. In other patients it is apparent from the onset that multisystem failure is present and worsening, whereas others fail to thrive or improve temporally before beginning to deteriorate. In these cases, it is evident that spontaneous resolution is unlikely and surgery should be performed as soon as pancreatic infection is proved by positive fine-needle aspiration (FNA).

At present there are no biochemical markers that indicate the need for surgery in patients with severe acute pancreatitis. The most useful, the acute-phase protein C-reactive protein (CRP), is a nonspecific index of injury, inflammation, sepsis, and ischemia. This serum marker is the one most commonly used in clinical practice to monitor the progress of the individual patient, and an elevated CRP level is an early indicator of the need for computed tomography (CT) to define the presence and extent of pancreatic and peripancreatic necrosis. Elevation of CRP above 120 mg/L is an indication of the presence of pancreatic necrosis, although no correlation has been found between serum CRP levels and the presence of infected necrosis.

The mortality rate for patients with infected pancreatic necrosis is more than 30%, and up to 80% of fatal outcomes in acute pancreatitis are due to septic complications. Several randomized controlled trials have provided evidence that prophylactic antibiotics may prevent the development of septic complications. However, about one-third of patients given prophylactic antibiotics that penetrate the pancreas will develop infected necrosis. The conservative management of infected pancreatic necrosis with multiple organ failure has a mortality rate of up to 100%. Based on this, there is no doubt that extensive necrosis and in particular the presence of infected necrosis are strong indications for surgery.

The gold standard in the diagnosis of infected pancreatic necrosis is FNA guided by either CT or ultrasound, with Gram staining and culture of the aspirate. In published series, the sensitivity for prediction of infected necrosis ranges from 90 to 100%, with specificity ranging from 96 to 100%. However, important questions remain on the appropriate indications, timing, and frequency for FNA. In a recent paper by Büchler *et al.* the indications for FNA included the following: newly developed signs of metabolic disorders and deterioration of organ failure of lung, kidney or cardiovascular system, or newly developed increase in blood leukocytes or fever (> 38°C) after initial response to conservative treatment. The timing is usually at a mean of 17 days. Interestingly, in 20% to more than 40% of patients the initial FNA was sterile and subsequent aspirate was positive for infection only after two, three, or more FNAs. These findings suggest that sterile necrosis does not necessarily remain sterile and that continued vigilance and surveillance by repeated FNA is mandatory until the patient is certifiably recovered. Also, the finding of an initially negative FNA that eventually becomes positive should be regarded as of benefit to the patient because it extends the interval to operation, permitting more organization of the necrosis (Fig. 15.1).

The management of patients with sterile pancreatic necrosis remains a matter of controversy. A number of prospective studies have supported the value of nonoperative therapy in sterile pancreatic necrosis. Recently, Büchler *et al.* have reported a death rate of 1.8% in patients with sterile pancreatic necrosisis managed without surgery compared with 24% in patients with infected pancreatic necrosis. On the other hand, the group from the Massachusetts General Hospital has reported that débridement and drainage in patients with SIRS can be carried out with a mortality of 6.2%, with no difference between infected and sterile necrosis. Outcomes were best if the operation was not delayed past 4 weeks. The authors suggest that patients who have unresolving or significant new signs of SIRS, even with negative FNA, should be considered for débridement by the fourth week after onset of pancreatitis. The latter report emphasizes that a nonoperative approach to sterile pancreatic necrosis should not be a rigid policy but should take into account the clinical condition of the patient as the most important factor in the decision to operate (Fig. 15.1).

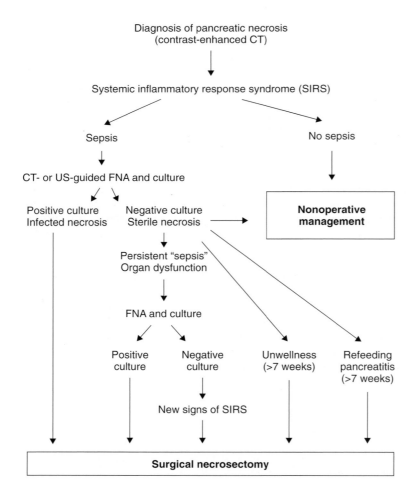

Figure 15.1 Management of patients with pancreatic necrosis. CT, computed tomography; FNA, fine-needle aspiration; SIRS, systemic inflammatory response syndrome.

Other indications for surgery in patients with necrotizing pancreatitis include residual pain, difficulty in eating, malaise, and general lack of well-being that prevents them from returning to work and other normal activities for many months. These patients may benefit symptomatically from clearance of the burden of necrotic tissue. In the series of Fernández del Castillo, 39% of patients were operated on for such persistent ill health, most of them at more than 7 weeks and one at 300 days, after several hospitalizations (Fig. 15.1).

Another group of patients can benefit from surgical débridement. These patients develop "refeeding" pancreatitis, characterized by abdominal pain and hyperamylasemia 6–8 weeks following recovery from a bout of severe sterile necrotizing pancreatitis. These patients can be restored by débridement of the necrotic tissue. Bradley has suggested that the pathophysiologic mechanism appears to be one of obstruction of the pancreatic duct secondary to the necrotic process (Fig. 15.1).

Finally, Adler *et al.* from the Mayo Clinic have suggested that patients with infected pancreatic necrosis but clinically stable would best avoid the operative risks of débridement and the possible postoperative complications and can be managed conservatively with prolonged targeted antibiotics. In addition, in patients ultimately requiring débridement, a delay in operation might provide the surgeon with a well-demarcated organized collection leading to a simplified procedure.

According to Beger and Isenmann, the rationales for a surgical approach in necrotizing pancreatitis include the following.

1 Removal of the necrotic pancreatic and peripancreatic parenchyma will stop the progression of necrosis and allow resolution of the disease process.

2 Bacteria and their toxic components are released into the circulation and are responsible for remote organ failure. As organ failure is a main determinant of outcome in patients with severe acute pancreatitis, the removal of infected pancreatic material is a therapeutic necessity in patients with infected pancreatic necrosis.

3 Formation of late complications, such as pancreatic abscess, can be prevented by removing the infected debris.

4 Preservation of viable pancreatic tissue will achieve good long-term results with respect to pancreatic exocrine and endocrine function.

The principles of the operation, independent of the technique chosen, are widely accepted. Dead and liquefied pancreas is removed and dead retroperitoneal tissue is débrided thoroughly. Blunt (finger dissection) necrosectomy is used and care should be taken in removing viable pancreas unnecessarily and incurring a high risk of insulin-dependent diabetes. Inspection of the transverse colon may detect areas of necrosis, and colon resection should be performed with creation of a temporary colostomy. The operation is completed with an intraoperative peritoneal lavage and the area of pancreatic bed must be adequately drained.

Surgical treatment

A number of surgical techniques are currently in use: conventional drainage, open or semiopen procedures, and closed procedures (Table 15.1).

Conventional drainage

Conventional drainage involves necrosectomy with placement of standard surgical drains. It is associated with persistent intraabdominal infections and a high rate of reoperations (by the presence of fever, leukocytosis, or lack of improvement on imaging studies). The success rate has been shown to depend on the extent and completeness of débridement.

Open or semiopen management

Open or semiopen management involves necrosectomy and either repeated laparotomies or open packing, which leaves the abdominal wound exposed for frequent changes of dressing. Fernández del Castillo

Table 15.1 Surgical treatment modalities in necrotizing pancreatitis.

Conventional treatment
Resection or necrosectomy with drainage
Reoperations on demand
Open procedures
Resection or necrosectomy and scheduled relaparotomies
Open abdominal management (open procedure)
Temporary abdominal closure (semiopen procedure)
Closed procedures
Necrosectomy and continuous closed local lavage
Reoperations on demand
Minimally invasive necrosectomy and lavage

et al. evaluated the results in 64 consecutive patients treated with necrosectomy followed by closed packing with gauze-stuffed Penrose drains, in addition to placement of a soft silicone-rubber closed suction drain in each major extension of the cavity. Between 6 and 10 days after surgery the stuffed Penrose drains were removed, one at a time, on sequential days to allow the cavity to collapse. The closed suction drains were the last to be removed and were not withdrawn until their output was minimal. Of the patients evaluated, 56% had infected pancreatic necrosis. The approach was successful in 44 patients (69%) and these had no further need for surgical or other interventions. The overall mortality rate was 6.2%, much lower than the 25% seen by these authors in 1992. The authors found a correlation between duration of pancreatitis and outcome and favored the practice of delaying surgery beyond the fourth week with good surgical conditions (well-demarcated necrosis with easier safer necrosectomy).

The experience of the Mayo Clinic was reviewed by Tsiotos *et al.* In 72 patients they employed blunt débridement, gauze packing, zipper closure, and planned reoperation. Infected pancreatic necrosis was found in 57 patients (79%) and was the main indication for surgery. These results were challenged by Bradley, whose own series employed a similar technique. The incidence of procedure-induced gastrointestinal fistulas in the Mayo Clinic's experience was comparatively high at 20.8% compared with 5.8% in Bradley's series; the number of deaths attributable to infection was also higher in the Mayo Clinic series compared with Bradley's series [11/18 (61%) vs. 4/15 (27%)]. Bradley has suggested that since the principal value of planned reoperation is to prevent reaccumulation of infected necrotic tissue, it is possible that the high rate of fatal infections may have resulted from a reduction in the average number of planned reoperations (2.2 in the Mayo series vs. 5.6 in Bradley's series). The overall hospital mortality rate achieved by the Mayo group was 25%, much less than the 39% observed by the Utrecht group using similar techniques. The Atlanta group has reported a remarkably low mortality rate (12%) with necrosectomy and staged reoperation. Tsiotos *et al.* have found that Acute Physiology and Chronic Health Evaluation (APACHE) II score greater than 13 at admission, extensive parenchymal necrosis, and postoperative hemorrhage were indicative of a worse outcome. An alternative such as laparostomy

(upper and lower edges of the opening in the gastrocolic omentum are sutured to the upper and lower edges of the wound) offers the theoretic advantage of open and continuous drainage of an infected or necrotic focus, avoiding the need to move the patient to the operating room. Using this technique the mortality rate observed by Függer *et al.* was 32%.

Necrosectomy and continuous closed lavage

Necrosectomy and continuous closed lavage and reoperations on demand best address the pathophysiologic background of the disease. Necrosectomy of necrotic infected material implies careful removal of necroses and infected fluids and preservation of vital pancreatic tissue. This simple change in intraoperative management decreases mortality from 30–80% to about 15–30%. The course of recurrent sepsis is mulifactorial, but is most commonly due to either inadequate peripancreatic drainage or incomplete necrosectomy as a result of the necrotizing process. In an attempt to provide further evaluation of infected peripancreatic exudates as well as to promote further débridement, the employment of postoperative closed local lavage of the lesser sac and necrotic cavities provides atraumatic and continuous evacuation of necrotic and infected material as well as biologically active compounds. The use of this mechanical "flow-through" technique in the later postoperative period means there is no need for routine reoperations (Fig. 15.2).

After surgical débridement, an extensive intraoperative lavage is performed, using in the first few postoperative days 24 L (1 L/hour) of isotonic saline or continuous ambulatory peritoneal dialysis (CAPD) solution. For postoperative continuous local lavage, large-bore single (Charrière 24–34) and double-lumen (Charrière 18) catheters are placed in the lesser sac and brought out through the right and left upper-lateral wall of the abdomen; two to five drainage tubes are used. If the peritoneal cavity is also affected, local lavage is combined with short-term peritoneal lavage. Lavage therapy is stopped when the effluent has no signs of active pancreatic enzymes and shows negative bacteriology. During the lavage treatment, monitoring in the intensive care unit (ICU) is necessary.

The overall mortality of closed management in necrotizing pancreatitis is 15–25% in reviewed series. Short-term closed lavage lasting 6–10 days is more beneficial than long-term closed lavage of up to 3 weeks.

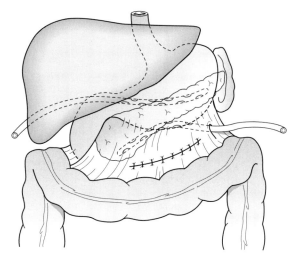

Figure 15.2 Continuous postoperative closed lavage of the lesser sac. Lavage is carried out using several double- and single-lumen catheters.

Minimally invasive necrosectomy and lavage

A critical analysis of the three different surgical techniques in necrotizing pancreatitis shows that these approaches are associated with a postoperative mortality of around 25–35% in experienced hands. Unfortunately, prospective studies comparing these surgical techniques are still lacking.

In an attempt to reduce the high mortality and morbidity with the classical open approach, Fagniez *et al.* first reported a retroperitoneal approach for pancreatic necrosectomy through the left flank just anterior to the twelfth rib in 40 patients with necrotizing pancreatitis. The retroperitoneal approach allows direct and complete removal of necrotic tissue and adequate drainage of the cavities with infected necrosis through the retroperitoneum without involving other organs in the abdominal cavity. The overall mortality rate was 33%, but only 18% in the 22 patients in whom the retroperitoneal approach was the only abdominal procedure performed. However, the technique was associated with a high rate of complications (50%), especially colonic fistula. This technique was used recently by Nakasaki *et al.* in eight patients, with two deaths, five reoperations, and a mean hospital stay of 48 days. We believe this approach has certain advantages over laparotomy in selected patients with localized infected necrosis.

The retroperitoneum can be approached by using an endoscopic technique. An endoscopic retroperitoneal approach was performed by Gambiez *et al.* in 20 patients via a 6-cm lumbotomy centered on the twelfth rib. A 23-cm mediastinoscope was used to perform débridement of the necrotic material with a suction device under direct visualization. A tube drain was left for postoperative irrigation. The wound was left open and a planned repeat lumboscopy (mean 5 ± 4) was performed as a second-look procedure every 5 days until definitive elimination of all the debris. The authors reported a 10% mortality rate. This technique mimics the open necrosectomy technique with planned relaparotomies. Castellanos *et al.* have used a translumbar retroperitoneal approach (incision 15 cm long) combined, in some patients 10 days after surgery, with repeated retroperitoneoscopy (8–10 sessions) in the ICU with no requirement to return to the operating room.

In recent years laparoscopic surgery has been used for pancreatic necrosectomy. Three alternatives have been described by Gagner: retrogastric–retrocolic débridement, retroperitoneal débridement, and transgastric pancreatic débridement. The choice of which laparoscopic technique to use depends upon the location of retroperitoneal collections in the abdomen. This approach has been reported as anecdotal cases and results from large series of patients are awaited.

The technique of laparoscopy in conjunction with percutaneous drainage has already been proposed as an alternative by Alves *et al.* and more recently by Horvath *et al.* The concept underlying the technique is that percutaneous drainage is the primary therapeutic modality whereas laparoscopic-assisted drainage of the particular debris is secondary. Location of the percutaneous catheters and information from the post-drain CT scan are used for port placement. A postoperative lavage system and the placement of drains allow for continued drainage of the debris. This approach may have a role in selected patients with localized disease (Fig. 15.3).

A combination of percutaneous radiologically controlled procedures and minimally invasive techniques was developed by Carter *et al.* from Glasgow. In this experience, the first four patients were treated by repeated sinus tract endoscopy following establishment of the tract at open laparotomy with percutaneous necrosectomy; there were two deaths. This approach was recently investigated by Connor *et al.* from Liverpool in

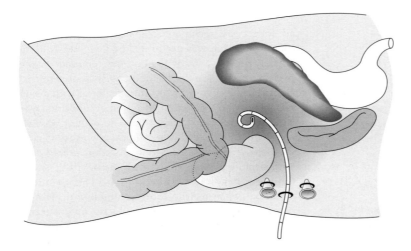

Figure 15.3 Computed tomography-guided percutaneous drainage followed by endoscopy hecrosectomy.

24 patients, although it was not possible to complete the technique in three patients for technical reasons. A total of 88 procedures were performed, with a median of four (range 0–8) per patient; 88% of patients developed 36 complications during the course of their illness. Five patients required an additional open procedure, while six (25%) patients died. The median postoperative hospital stay was 51 (range 5–200) days. The authors believe that this minimally invasive retroperitoneal approach is not suitable for all patients with pancreatic necrosis, especially in those with disease involving the head and uncinate process, as percutaneous access is not always possible. Removing the debris from the necrotic cavity can be time-consuming as only small amounts can be removed at a time. The hospital stay may also be longer and, combined with the increased number of procedures, the cost compared with open necrosectomy is likely to be higher. We hope that these promising preliminary results will encourage the development of better instruments to apply this technique in patients severely ill with varying degrees of organ dysfunction awaiting an open laparotomy. The minimally invasive retroperitoneal approach might get the patient through the initial high-risk period of the illness until they are well enough to tolerate the further insult of a definitive laparotomy.

Complications in the postoperative course

Complications of pancreatic necrosis may result from spread of the inflammatory process to adjacent organs (transverse colon or mesocolon, duodenum, portal vein, and splenic vessels) or adverse effects at the time of surgical treatment.

Most complications involve colon necrosis, intestinal fistulas, bleeding, and pancreatic fistulas. Colon necrosis develops early in the course of the disease as a result of spread of intrapancreatic and peripancreatic necrosis, the dangers being the increase in translocation of the bacteria causing infection of the necrotic material and, eventually, bowel perforation and peritonitis. Colonic perforation may result as a consequence of aggressive local treatment. Sarr *et al.* have reported an incidence of 22% for colonic fistula in a series of 23 consecutive patients with necrotizing pancreatitis treated by planned staged relaparotomies with repeated lavage. Gastrointestinal fistulas occurred in 13–27% of patients with pancreatic necrosis but over half were iatrogenic, mostly after open packing. In a study by Nordback *et al.*, gastrointestinal fistulas were major problems of laparostomy and developed in 55% of their patients. Besides the influence of the surgical approach on the occurrence of enteric fistulas, a poorly positioned drain causing pressure necrosis on adjacent hollow viscera is an additional iatrogenic cause of fistulization. According to Tsiotos *et al.*, most upper-gut fistulas close spontaneously and only one-third require operative closure. However, colonic fistulas appear to require operative intervention, usually colon resection and proximal colostomy.

In about 30% of the patients undergoing necrosectomy and continuous closed lavage a reoperation is necessary because of formation of an abscess, with reappearance of the clinical consequences of sepsis syndrome. The development of postoperative sepsis syndrome is caused by the separation of infected material that is not drained or by the formation of a retroperitoneal abscess in areas of necrosis not primarily included in the necrosectomy protocol. Contrast-enhanced CT demonstrates the location of the abscess. The first-choice treatment for an abscess appearing after necrosectomy is interventional CT-guided puncture and drainage. In cases where interventional drainage fails to interrupt the septic clinical course, an open reoperation with surgical evacuation is mandatory.

Intraabdominal bleeding has been reported in 20% of cases of necrotizing pancreatitis, and was more frequently venous than arterial probably due to erosive vasculitis secondary to activated pancreatic fluid and bacteria. The splenic or mesocolonic vessels and the portal vein are the most common sites of bleeding. Correct positioning of suction drains is important to avoid hemorrhage. Also, when using open packing it is recommended that a nonadherent interphase between viscera or exposed blood vessels and the intraabdominal gauze packing is used in order to reduce the risk of both fistulization and hemorrhage. Prompt surgical intervention is the preferred treatment, although angiography may be helpful for localization and, potentially, definitive therapy.

Pancreatic fistulas are invariably associated with pancreatic parenchymal necrosis and develop secondary to disruption of ductal continuity within the necrotic pancreas. Uomo et al. reported that 30% of patients with pancreatic necrosis had main pancreatic duct disruption and were therefore prone to pseudocyst formation and, if externally drained, to fistula formation. This complication occurred in 19–55% of patients after débridment for necrotizing pancreatitis. Surgical trauma may play an important role in the frequency of this complication. The great majority of patients are managed conservatively with gradual drain advancement. However, in those in whom it persists, either an endoscopic sphincterotomy or placement of a pancreatic stent usually results in resolution.

There have been a number of studies evaluating the functional or morphologic changes (or both) that occur after acute pancreatitis. Most showed that pancreatic exocrine function is seriously impaired during the first few days after pancreatitis. According to Fernández-Cruz et al., at a later stage the pancreas gradually recovers its normal function, although the recovery is not complete in all patients. Certain of these studies should be mentioned here. Angelini et al. observed, after a 4-year follow-up study of 27 patients, that pancreatic exocrine function, which was impaired immediately after the acute pancreatitis, gradually returned to normal. Changes in the pancreatic duct persisted. Büchler et al. examined pancreas morphology using CT and endoscopic retrograde cholangiopancreatography. They found morphologic alterations after 12 months in 95% of patients with alcohol-induced necrotic pancreatitis and in 81% of those with biliary-induced pancreatitis. These abnormalities persisted after 40 months in 91% of alcoholic patients and in 47% of the biliary patients. Exocrine pancreatic insufficiency was present after 12 months in 95% of the alcohol-induced cases; after 40 months, exocrine pancreatic insufficiency persisted in 68% of alcoholic patients and 30% of the biliary patients. After edematous pancreatitis, alcoholics again had significantly more frequent exocrine pancreatic insufficiency than patients with biliary lithiasis once the episode was over.

All these studies indicate that the factors that appear to have an effect on morphologic and functional changes occurring after acute pancreatitis include the severity of the episode and the etiology of the pancreatitis. Thus most patients who suffer necrotic pancreatitis exhibit functional exocrine pancreatic insufficiency during the first year after the attack. Some patients subsequently regain normal function, but this alteration persists in a high proportion.

Etiology is another of the determining factors in the changes that take place after an attack of acute pancreatitis. Whereas with biliary-induced pancreatitis the pancreatic functional alterations rarely persist beyond a year, chronic alcoholism leads to exocrine pancreatic dysfunction that can persist for months and may even fail to return to normal. Morphologic changes too are seen to be more related to the alcoholic etiology than to biliary etiology.

Recommended reading

Adler DG, Chari ST, Dahl TJ, Farnell MB, Pearson RK. Conservative management of infected necrosis complicating severe acute pancreatitis. *Am J Gastroenterol* 2003;98: 98–1003.

Angelini G, Pederzoli P, Caliari S *et al.* Long-term outcome of acute necrohemorrhagic pancreatitis: a 4-year follow-up. *Digestion* 1984;30:131–137.

Beger HG, Isenmann R. Surgical management of necrotizing pancreatitis. *Surg Clin North Am* 1999;79:783–800.

Bradley EL. Necrotizing pancreatitis. *Br J Surg* 1999;86:147–148.

Büchler MW, Gloor B, Müller CA, Friess H, Seüer ChA, Uhl W. Acute necrotizing pancreatitis: treatment strategy according to the status of infection. *Ann Surg* 2000;232:619–626.

Carter RC, Mackay CJ, Imrie CW. Percutaneous necrosectomy and sinus tract endoscopy in management of infected pancreatic necrosis: an initial experience. *Ann Surg* 2001;232:175–180.

Castellanos G, Piñero A, Serrano A, Parrilla P. Infected pancreatitis necrosis. Translumbar approach and management with retroperitoneoscopy. *Arch Surg* 2002;137:1060–1063.

Connor S, Ghaneh P, Raraty M *et al.* Minimally invasive retroperitoneal pancreatic necrosectomy. *Dig Surg* 2003;20:270–277.

Fagniez PL, Rotman N, Dracht M. Direct retroperitoneal approach to necrosis in severe acute pancreatitis. *Br J Surg* 1989;76:264–267.

Fernández-Cruz L, Navarro S, Castells A, Sáenz A. Late outcome after acute pancreatitis: functional impairment and gastrointestinal tract complications. *World J Surg* 1997;21:169–172.

Fernandez Del-Castillo C, Rattner DW, Makary MA, Mostafavi A, McGrath D, Warshaw A. Debridement and closed packing for the treatment of necrotizing pancreatitis. *Ann Surg* 1998;228:676–684.

Függer R, Schulz F, Rogy M, Herbst F, Mirza D, Fritsch A. Open approach in pancreatic and infected pancreatic necrosis: laparostomies and preplanned revisions. *World J Surg* 1991;15:516–520.

Gambiez LP, Denimal FA, Porte HL, Saudemont A, Chambon JPM, Quandalle PA. Retroperitoneal approach and endoscopic management of peripancreatic necrosis collections. *Arch Surg* 1998;133:66–72.

Horvath KD, Kao LS, Ali A, Wherry KL, Pellegrini CA, Sinanan MN. Laparoscopic assisted percutaneous drainage of infected pancreatic necrosis. *Surg Endosc* 2001;15:677–682.

Nakasaki H, Tajima T, Fujii K, Makuuchi H. A surgical treatment of infected pancreatic necrosis: retroperitoneal laparotomy. *Dig Surg* 1999;16:506–511.

Pamoukian VN, Gagner M. Laparoscopic necrosectomy for acute necrotizing pancreatitis. *J Hepatobiliary Pancreat Surg* 2001;8:221–223.

Rau B, Uhl W, Büchler MW, Beger HG. Surgical treatment of infected necrosis. *World J Surg* 1997;21:155–161.

Sarr MG, Nagorney DM, Mucha PJ, Farnell MB, Johnson CD. Acute necrotizing pancreatitis: management by planned, staged pancreatic necrosectomy/debridement and delayed primary wound clousure over drains. *Br J Surg* 1991;78:576–581.

Tsiotos GG, Luque de León E, Soreide JA *et al.* Management of necrotizing pancreatitis by repeated operative necrosectomy using a zipper technique. *Am J Surg* 1998;175:91–98.

Uomo G, Molino D, Visconti M, Ragozzino A, Manes G, Rabitti G. The incidence of main pancreatic duct disruption in severe biliary pancreatitis. *Am J Surg* 1988;176:49–52.

16 Management of acute pancreatic pseudocyst: when to observe, when and how to drain

René Laugier

Introduction

Fortunately, most patients presenting with acute pancreatitis develop only an edematous nonsevere form without pancreatic necrosis and thus have no risk of developing a necrotic collection. In contrast, patients with severe acute pancreatitis almost always develop, because of necrosis, acute fluid collections (often still called, erroneously, "phlegmon"). Necrosis can develop from interstitial and interlobular fat tissue or from periductular areas but severity is mainly related to necrosis of acinar pancreatic parenchyma.

In about 30–50% of patients presenting with severe forms of acute pancreatitis, these collections turn into pseudocysts over a period of several weeks (from 1 to 6, usually more than 3). Pseudocysts can become infected by intestinal bacteria and can thus transform into genuine abscesses. Translocation of bacteria from the gut is greatly enhanced by the increased permeability of the intestinal epithelium. In severe acute pancreatitis, only a minority of these pancreatic pseudocysts resolve spontaneously.

Initially, pseudocysts are limited in size by the neighboring organs or structures. They contain a mixture of necrosis, blood, and fragments of pancreatic tissue. Later, the necrotic contents can simply liquefy, whereas in other cases necrosis induces ductal rupture and pancreatic juice effusion into or outside the initial cavity. After the fourth week of evolution, the peripheral zone of the cyst becomes fibrous but without an individual wall. Analysis of the physical state of the cystic contents is crucial in order to administer the most appropriate treatment.

Clinical evolution: when to observe

It is generally accepted that pancreatic pseudocysts do not resolve spontaneously after a period of 6 weeks: this is completely wrong! Indeed, when lack of complications prompts no treatment, it is preferable to wait as long as possible without any invasive treatment (as long as the general condition of the patient does not deteriorate). Delcenserie *et al.* reported that 83% of patients with severe acute pancreatitis (score E of Balthazar on computed tomography (CT)) resolved completely in 20–280 days, with a complication rate of only 7.8%. Maringhini *et al.* reported a 56% healing rate of cysts in 1 year, and Yeo *et al.* have reported that, among 75 such patients, only 50% of them required surgical treatment. Thus, whenever possible, it is always better to manage patients without special treatment, for example following them up medically in the intensive care unit (ICU) and performing CT every 3 weeks. In our institution, contrary to what happens in North America, we use ultrasonography as the main method for observing the constituents and level of organization of fluid collections in these patients—it is easier to bring the ultrasonography equipment to the patient than the patient to the CT suite. Moreover, ultrasound appears to be more reliable than CT for determining the presence of liquid in a cyst and the level of liquefaction: the reinforcement of ultrasonic transmission behind a cavity is a more precise sign than either the pattern or the density measured on CT. Finally, it is quicker and easier to perform an ultrasound-guided transcutaneous puncture than a CT-guided puncture. Such transcutaneous punctures (which sometimes have to be regularly repeated) allow the maturation of the cystic contents and any infection that may follow to be monitored. Such investigations contribute to the decision about the necessity for, and type of, antibiotics required.

In most cases, the patient becomes symptomatic because of the evolution of these cavities. Pain is by far the most frequent symptom, and in about 85% of cases it represents the first sign. Typically, pancreatic pain is associated with nausea or vomiting. The persistence of such symptoms for more than 7–10 days should alert the physician to such a clinical eventuality. Fever is also often present, sometimes with a very elevated temperature. An increase in white blood cells is always present with signs of severe inflammation, such as enhanced C-reactive protein (CRP), the level of which is considered a good predictor of outcome for the patient. Such severely ill patients should undergo an imaging examination in order to precisely delineate and analyze the development, size, content, and evolution of necrosis of possible liquid collections.

More worrying complications, such as signs of severe infection leading to septic shock, may develop; in such cases, the clinical condition of the patient deteriorates very rapidly, prompting specific treatment. A palpable mass or epigastric tenderness may develop, while in other cases signs of peritonitis appear. All treatments include antibiotic administration according to the bacteriologic data provided by puncture and drainage of the cavities. It is not necessary to define the pathogenicity of the bacteria or fungi found in these collections (Gram-negative, aerobic, anaerobic), since several infectious factors are usually associated. Drainage can be performed surgically, percutaneously, or endoscopically: it must be discussed regularly with all the different specialists involved in order to choose the most appropriate method at the most appropriate time.

In other cases, the pseudocyst complicates locally: it may induce compression of neighboring organs and thus be responsible for specific symptoms. A collection may induce jaundice by compression of the main bile duct within the pancreas. The patient may either develop a silent isolated jaundice, identical to that produced by carcinoma of the head of the pancreas, or more frequently an angiocholitis, which is not always easy to diagnose in patients who already have sepsis. Increased fever and chills are associated with a progressive increase in biological cholestasis and progressive jaundice, sometimes of variable intensity. Once again, imaging techniques such as ultrasonography or CT

are essential for proving that distension of the main bile duct is due to compression and for showing the precise localization of the obstacle as well as its nature. In some cases, the collection may be relatively distant from the bile duct but nonetheless is able to block the bile duct by one of its extensions. Gastric compression, especially of the antral part of the stomach, may be responsible for exacerbation of vomiting. Besides imaging techniques, a gastroscopy will demonstrate the gastric or duodenal compression and its precise anatomic localization.

Fistulization of the cyst may lead to a sudden clinical improvement if this occurs directly within the digestive tract itself (duodenum, stomach, or even jejunum). After a short symptomatic exacerbation, the collection will decrease in size, as can be demonstrated clinically or by imaging techniques. In contrast, if the opening develops in a noncommunicating space, specific complications will occur: infected ascites (which will not be rich in pancreatic enzymes), responsible for peritoneal infection with a high risk of peritonitis; or an infected pleural effusion, responsible for respiratory failure. The perforation of a cystic cavity within the colon is particularly dramatic: acute liquid diarrhea and sudden enhancement of preexisting infection, together with peritoneal infection, make the situation very difficult to manage, whatever the treatment initiated, and associated with a very high mortality.

Finally, the presence of variable amounts of pancreatic enzymes inside a pseudocyst may induce some erosion of vessels neighboring the limits of the cyst (well-organized walls are unusual) and thus bleeding ensues, the severity of which will depend on the type of vessel (artery or vein) disrupted and its anatomic location (in the cyst or in the digestive tract or an anatomic cavity). The vessel involved is also important. Unfortunately, in most cases, this is one of the three branches of the celiac axis. In this case, acute or subacute pain will be associated with hematemesis and sudden loss of red blood cells leading to acute anemia; at the same time, imaging techniques will demonstrate a parallel increase in the diameter of the collection. In this situation, one must be very careful before performing a puncture (either endoscopic or transcutaneous) because this could induce sudden but nonlimited decompression of the cystic contents and thus a noncontrolled relapse of hemorrhage, with a very poor prognosis.

In the latter case, unfortunately the most usually encountered, the hemorrhagic syndrome will be unmistakable, associated with hematemesis and melena of extreme severity and thus of very high mortality, whatever the treatment initiated. In these conditions, the most effective treatment is radiologic embolization of the bleeding artery and not surgery. The final clinical picture is represented by sudden ascites or pleural effusion that develops with the blood loss. Here again, a puncture of significant volume could be very deleterious.

Treatment: when and how to drain

It has already been mentioned that as long as the clinical condition of the patient does not deteriorate, it is always best to wait. If symptomatic treatments initiated in the ICU are sufficient to manage the clinical problems presented by the patient, nothing particular has to be performed, except total parenteral nutrition and gastric aspiration, which are mandatory. Improvement in care in general, and especially in the ICU, is probably the most important factor for the decreased mortality observed in patients with severe acute pancreatitis. Enteral nutrition, directly administered into the jejunum, has proved to be as effective as the parenteral route with less specific complications. Of course, the search for a cystic infection must be continued, including results of repeated punctures of the cyst in order to follow the level of liquefaction. As soon as an area of pancreatic necrosis or a pseudocyst has been demonstrated to be infected, specific antibiotic therapy, guided by bacteriologic data, should be initiated intravenously.

Schematically, therefore, two scenarios are possible in this kind of situation: either the patient does not require any special drainage and no specific treatment has to be initiated for a number of weeks (see above) or a complication, whatever it is, develops and drainage becomes essential. In the case of a rapid clinical recovery without local pancreatic complications, even though important collections may be detected on CT, it is not necessary to attempt drainage. These collections may produce no clinical symptoms for some patients for a number of months: as long as any secondary spontaneous infection or portal segmental hypertension does not develop, it is best to resist the temptation to treat these silent cavities. Only in the second scenario does treatment need to be envisaged: the type of therapeutic approach will depend on the size of the collection and its localization within the pancreas. In this case, as in the much more frequent one of a complicated evolution, the question of cyst drainage will emerge. Several techniques are available and are discussed below.

Percutaneous puncture or drainage

The simplest approach consists of percutaneous puncture with aspiration of the cystic contents. The puncture can be guided using either ultrasonography or CT, depending on availability and custom (including skillfulness of radiologists or gastroenterologists in charge of the patient). This simple technique is usually performed under local anesthesia. A relatively large needle should always be preferred to one of smaller diameter (ranging from 19 to 12 French gauge). Part of the aspirated liquid should be sent for biological and bacteriologic analysis. This direct approach is only effective in pseudocysts with relatively well-organized walls, without any communication with the ductal system, and with nonsevere infection; the content has also to be homogeneous and relatively fluid in order to allow aspiration through the fine needle. All these restrictions readily explain why only a few percent of patients heal with a single puncture. It can, of course, be repeated with no special risks, if the cyst contents are fluid enough to allow reasonable hope of treating the patient adequately.

If the cyst relapses soon after an initial percutaneous puncture, one can complete this therapeutic approach by using permanent drainage. The drain is usually introduced using the Seldinger technique, over a guidewire, under ultrasonographic control. The diameter of the drain is chosen to suit the viscosity of the cyst contents: 7–10 French gauge if the liquid is very fluid; up to 20 or even 30 French gauge in the more frequent case of infected contents (pus, necrotic debris, or pancreatic juice). The most direct route should be followed in order to avoid any risk of perforating the colon, liver, or spleen. The healing rate of infected collections treated using this technique has been reported very differently in the literature, between 21 and 75% according to different series. All the reported results mention the importance of recurrence rate, which ranges from 16 to 32%. The weak point of this technique is its duration, from 20 days to more than 3 months, with important risks for secondary infections due to the catheter itself. Morbidity and mortality are also associated with hemorrhage and fistulas, which can partly explain the long duration of treatment.

143

Surgical treatment

The oldest and probably the most used treatments are surgical. External drainage is no longer used: it was only chosen in cases of infected collections with immature walls that were unable to accept any surgical suture. Since echo-guided punctures now allow the level of maturity of cysts to be followed, this technique has become redundant. Pseudocyst excision is usually only performed in cases of chronic pancreatitis, which is not the subject of this chapter.

The most widely used surgical technique is classical cystogastrostomy, described as the Juracz intervention (Fig. 16.1). In most cases, large collections are located just behind the posterior wall of the stomach, a situation favorable for the surgeon. At the beginning of the

operation, the cyst contents are aspirated into a syringe; then both the anterior and posterior gastric walls are opened as is the anterior wall of the cyst. A large suture (6–9 cm or even more) is introduced between the cyst and stomach. If a hemorrhage is detected at aspiration, the origin of the bleeding has to be meticulously searched for and eliminated. Symptoms disappear rapidly in most cases, although complications and recurrences are not unusual (10–30% and 5–31%, respectively). Mortality is around 5%.

When the anatomic location of the collection is favorable, i.e., a smaller cyst in the right part of the head of the pancreas, a cystoduodenostomy using the same technique could be performed (Fig. 16.2). This has the same rate of complications as the Juracz intervention. In France, a cystojejunostomy on a Roux-en-Y is often

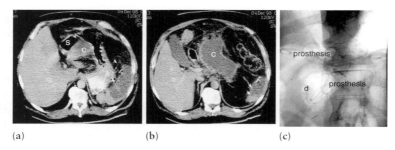

(a) (b) (c)

Figure 16.1 Cystogastrostomy. (a, b) Computed tomography scans demonstrate the close relationship between the stomach (s) and cyst (c). (c) The cystogastrostomy was equipped with two double-pigtail

endoprostheses, one being within the duodenum while the other is in the cyst and also in a nasocystic drain for some days (d).

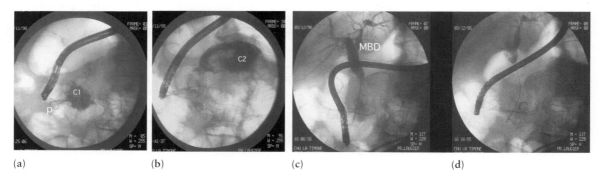

(a) (b) (c) (d)

Figure 16.2 Double cystoduodenostomy using the same orifice performed with a needle knife (Boston Scientific). (a) After opacification of the first cyst (c1), the first double-pigtail prosthesis is inserted (p). (b) Opacification of the second cyst (c2) and insertion of a simple pigtail prosthesis.

(c) Injection of the strictured main bile duct (MBD) drained by a temporary biliary endoprosthesis. (d) Due to infection of the cavities, an external temporary nasocystic drain was also inserted, allowing lavages of the cyst.

preferred but is far less easy to perform than in cases of chronic pancreatitis.

Finally, pancreatectomy is sometimes performed when the collection is tightly associated to the pancreatic tail, although mortality and morbidity are significantly higher than with the other surgical techniques and thus it should be avoided as often as possible, especially if the pancreas is still pathologic.

Endoscopic treatment

Over the last 13 years, endoscopic approaches to pancreatic cysts and infected collections have improved tremendously. All these techniques depend on the anatomic location of the cyst to be treated. Thus every endoscopic approach begins with a careful examination of the upper digestive tract using a side-viewing duodenoscope equipped with a large working channel (4.2 mm). The first attempt was reported by Liguory and coworkers in 1990. A large cyst located in the body or tail of the pancreas frequently bulges into the posterior wall of the stomach; this bulging, which represents a proximity (< 10 mm) between the cystic and gastric walls, must be investigated first. At the point of maximum bulging, under both visual and X-ray guidance, a diathermic needle is introduced into the cyst cavity. Immediately after this, the communication between the cyst and the stomach is secured by the deep introduction of a guidewire into the cyst; several loops are usually preferable in order to delineate cyst size without having to inject contrast medium. A catheter is introduced over the guidewire in order to aspirate cyst contents for laboratory analysis. Usually, the best description of the anatomy is obtained by injection of contrast medium.

The cystogastrostomy can now be performed, either by cutting the gastric wall up to 10 mm with a papillotome or, preferably, by dilating the communication up to 8 or 10 mm using an inflatable hydraulic balloon; this technique almost eliminates the risk of hemorrhage. In order to maintain the patency of the communication, the cystogastrostomy is equipped with one, preferably two, double-pigtail plastic stents, the diameter of which range from 7 to 10 French gauge (Fig 16.1, p. 144). Their length is adapted to the distance between the two cavities (Fig 16.3). Often, when the cyst contents are too viscous and heterogeneous, it is preferble

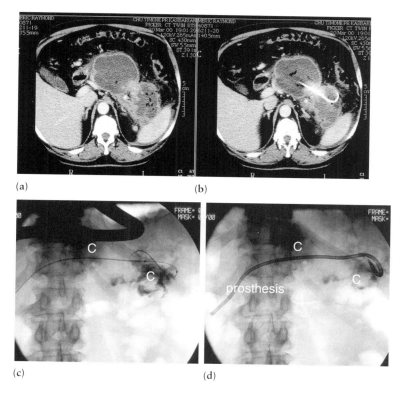

Figure 16.3 (a, b) Computed tomography scans delineate the two cysts in the body and tail of the pancreas. (c) Opacification demonstrates communication between the pancreatic duct and the bilocular cavity (C). (d) A transpapilllary simple pigtail prosthesis was inserted deep up to the left part of the cyst.

to also insert nasocystic external temporary drainage: this allows the inside of the cavity to be flushed regularly and the washing liquid to be aspirated thereafter. The same kind of internal drainage can also be performed after endosonography for determining a zone of puncture devoid of vessels or directly through an echoendoscope as described by Giovannini *et al*. The same principle has also been described using a combination of percutaneous and endoscopic methods, the stent between stomach and cyst being delivered over an echo-guided percutaneous catheter and correctly positioned using the gastroscope.

Such internal endoscopic drainage has a morbidity evaluated at around 10%, mainly due to perforation or hemorrhage. Recurrence is often observed, which should prompt another endoscopic intervention consisting of an exchange of stents with careful washing of the inside of the cyst. Sometimes, enlargement of the communication has to be performed. Eventually, cystoscopies (endoscopic examination of the inside of a cystic cavity) can be performed.

Of the last 16 patients we have treated using this kind of endoscopic approach, direct cystogastrostomy has been performed five times. One case was complicated by a hemorrhage that was treated endoscopically by injection of local vasoactive agent. The mean size of the cavities was over 18 cm. Another patient had to be operated on because of recurrence and massive infection after the first endoscopic procedure. The other three patients healed completely after four endoscopic procedures, as described earlier.

The second endoscopic approach is cystoduodenostomy, which is very similar to but easier and safer than cystogastrostomy; it necessitates a well-defined bulging of the cyst into the second or third part of the duodenum (Fig 16.2, p. 144). The surgeon can also perform this kind of communication in the third part of the duodenum with the help of an echoendoscope. The technique is absolutely identical to that used through the stomach. Mortality and morbidity rates are lower than those for cystogastrostomy because of the much closer relationship between duodenum and pancreas than between stomach and pancreas. However, fewer patients with large necrotic collections after acute pancreatitis are suitable for this approach: in our series, only 3 of 16 patients could be treated by this safe method. Those patients with a long distance and, therefore, communication between the cyst and the duodenum require a larger number of endoscopic interventions (mean of seven).

The third endoscopic technique is indirect access to the collection through the main pancreatic duct itself (Fig 16.3, p. 145). When the cyst does not bulge obviously within the digestive tract, communication between the cyst and the ductal system has to be investigated. After injection of contrast material into the duct through the papilla (the main one or, in some cases, the minor one), some leak is often demonstrated, leading to the possibility that this route can be used for treatment. A hydrophilic guidewire is introduced into the origin of the leak via the papilla, thus accessing the collection. Once the guidewire has been deeply introduced into the collection, an inflatable hydraulic balloon, introduced over the guidewire, dilates the communication and thereafter a simple pigtail endoprosthesis is pushed up inside the cyst in order to perform cystoduodenostomy. This technique has the tremendous advantage of being completely bloodless and thus there is no risk of bleeding or perforation. In contrast, its disadvantage is the limitation in the size and number of drainage catheters that can be placed through the papilla because of the generally small diameter of the main pancreatic duct in patients without previous pancreatic pathology. This method of treatment has been used in 11 of our patients, including two cases where access was through the minor papilla; in other words, some patients have had more than one approach to optimize the drainage. Four interventions were performed in each of these patients. The anatomic localization of the collection is not a limitation for this transpapillary approach: in five cases, the pseudocyst was located in the tail of the pancreas. The observed complications included an increase in septic syndrome in five cases, all treated medically and endoscopically, these patients requiring an exchange of the drainage material as an emergency. In two patients with a caudal pancreatic lesion, a 10 F endoprosthesis was introduced up to the left part of the abdomen and a colonic fistula was observed; this was treated medically with total parenteral nutrition for 10 days, antibiotics, and endoprosthesis exchange.

In this series of 15 very severely ill patients following severe acute pancreatitis, only one of them died because of an antibiotic-resistant infection that was impossible to drain either endoscopically or surgically, the patient having been operated twice, before and after the endoscopic attempt. Four patients did require delayed surgery, which appeared of less gravity due to the much better general condition of the patients and the better maturation of the cyst wall.

In conclusion, consideration should be given to treating these very large, complicated, and infected postnecrotic pseudocysts endoscopically, i.e., without initial surgery but with more interventional procedures that yield healing times ranging from 1 to 11 months.

Conclusions

The treatment of complicated severe acute pancreatitis is changing, the most important decrease in mortality having been achieved by improvements in medical care. The decrease in early surgery has also participated in the improved rate of survival. Pseudocysts and necrotic collections are no longer the main problem presented by these patients: so many different techniques of treatment have been described and progressively improved recently. The place of each of them in treatment is still a matter of debate but, with time, one can adapt more precisely the best approach to each individual case.

When cysts are not symptomatic and as long as the general condition of the patient is not deteriorating, there is no indication for drainage, which is always difficult and adventurous, whatever the technique.

In contrast, if a complication prompts drainage, in our opinion surgery should not be the first option. Depending mainly on the time elapsed between the acute phase and maturation of the collection, a simple puncture (with or without associated percutaneous drainage) should be preferred if the cystic contents are particularly fluid and not severely infected, i.e., when the cyst is relatively "organized." When the pseudocyst is immature, it is best to wait as long as necessary, while following the level of organization and liquefaction of the cystic content. As soon as the cyst is considered suitable for treatment, different techniques are available, although there has been no demonstration of clear-cut advantages of one over another.

In our experience, we feel that an initial approach with endoscopy may avoid surgery completely or postpone it up to the time where surgical drainage becomes easy and thus safe and effective in one single procedure. For us, the only contraindication lies in surgical drainage in patients presenting with an immature cyst; in these circumstances, there is a risk that surgery could worsen the clinical picture.

Finally, one has always to keep in mind that these modalities are not incompatible but complementary in most of the situations presented by the most difficult patients.

Recommended reading

Balthazar AJ, Freeny PC, Van Sonnenberg E. Imaging and intervention in acute pancreatitis. *Radiology* 1994;93: 97–306.

Barthet M, Bugallo M, Moreira L, Bastid C, Sastre B, Sahel J. Traitement des pseudokystes de pancréatites aigües. Etude rétrospective de 45 patients. *Gastrontérol Clin Biol* 1992; 16:853–859.

Beger H, Bittner R, Block S, Buchler M. Bacterial contamination of pancreatic necrosis. A prospective clinical study. *Gastroenterology* 1986;91:433–438.

Delcenserie R, Koller J, Delamarre J, Dupas JL. Score clinicobiologique et tomodensitométrique précoce et évolution des pancréatites aigües traitées médicalement: la nécrose est peu fréquente ou régresse. *Gastroentérol Clin Biol* 1988; 12:A14.

Feller J, Brown R, MacLaren-Toussant G *et al.* Changing method of treatment of severe pancreatitis. *Am J Surg* 1974;127:196–201.

Freeny PC, Lewis G, Traverso M, Ryan J. Infected pancreatic fluid collections: percutaneous catheter drainage. *Radiology* 1988;167:435–441.

Gerolami R, Giovannini M, Laugier R. Endoscopic drainage of pancreatic pseudocysts guided by endosonography. *Endoscopy* 1997;29:106–108.

Giovannini M, Bernardini D, Seitz JF. Cystogastrostomy entirely performed under endosonographic guidance for pancreatic pseudocyst: results in 6 patients. *Endoscopy* 1998;48:200–203.

Hancke S, Henriksen FW. Percutaneous pancreatic cystogastrostomy guided by ultrasound scanning and gastroscopy. *Br J Surg* 1985;72:916–917.

Laugier R, Ries P, Grandval P. Endoscopic drainage of large necrotic pseudocysts and abscess after acute pancreatitis is feasible and efficient. *Endoscopy* (in press).

Liguory C, Lefebvre JF, Vitale G. Endoscopic drainage of pancreatic pseudocysts. *Can J Gastroenterol* 1990;4:568–571.

Maringhini A, Uomo G, Patti R *et al.* Pseudocysts in acute non alcoholic pancreatitis. Incidence and natural history. *Dig Dis Sci* 1999;44:1669–1673.

Maule W, Rebert H. Diagnosis and management of pancreatic pseudocysts, pancreatic ascites and pancreatic fistulas. In: *The Pancreas: Biology, Pathobiology and Diseases*. New York: Raven Press, 1993.

Reynolds J. Enteral nutrition in acute pancreatitis. In: CD Johnson, CW Imrie (eds) *Pancreatic Disease Towards the Year 2000*. London: Springer-Verlag, 1999: 115–122.

Van Sonnenberg E, Wittich G, Gasola G *et al*. Percutaneous drainage of infected and non infected pancreatic pseudocysts. *Radiology* 1989;170:751–756.

Waade JW. Twenty-five year experience with pancreatic pseudocysts. Are we making progress? *Am J Surg* 1985; 149:705–708.

Yeo C, Bastidas J, Lynch-Nyhan A, Fishman E, Zinner M, Cameron J. The natural history of pancreatic pseudocysts documented by computed tomography. *Surg Gynecol Obstet* 1990;170:411–417.

17 Therapeutic approach to pancreatic abscess

Luis Sabater-Ortí, Julio Calvete-Chornet, and Salvador Lledó-Matoses

Definition, clarification of concepts, and frequency

Pancreatic abscess is currently defined as a circumscribed intraabdominal collection of pus, usually in proximity to the pancreas, containing little or no pancreatic necrosis that arises as a consequence of acute pancreatitis or pancreatic trauma. This definition contains two key concepts: the presence of pus (i.e., infection) and the fact that the result of the infection is bounded by adjacent tissues and organs (i.e., is encapsulated).

It is extremely important to discriminate pancreatic abscess from infected pancreatic necrosis, the other local septic complication in acute pancreatitis, and from other nonseptic local complications (sterile necrosis, pseudocysts, and fluid collections). Thus, it is worthwhile reviewing concepts and pointing out the differences among these entities.

Pancreatic necrosis is a diffuse or focal area of nonviable pancreatic parenchyma demonstrated by imaging techniques, specifically contrast-enhanced computed tomography (CT). Characteristically it is associated with peripancreatic fat necrosis that spreads diffusely through the retroperitoneum without signs of encapsulation. When the presence of bacteria or fungi is demonstrated within these areas of nonviable parenchyma or peripancreatic fat necrosis, the diagnosis of infected pancreatic necrosis is established. A pseudocyst is a collection of pancreatic juice enclosed by a wall of fibrous or granulation tissue, and thus the content of the collection differentiates a pancreatic abscess from a pseudocyst. Finally, the differences between pancreatic abscess and acute fluid collection are

the nature of the material (pus versus exudative or serosanguineous fluid), timing of occurrence (late versus early), and especially encapsulation (present in the case of pancreatic abscess versus absent in acute fluid collection).

A precise estimation of the real frequency of pancreatic abscess was not possible until clear definitions of acute pancreatitis complications were established. Since then, the main series of secondary pancreatic infections have referred to an incidence of pancreatic abscess in 3–9% of all patients with acute pancreatitis. This represents approximately one-third to half of the cases reported as infected pancreatic necrosis. Therefore, it must be clearly stated that the most frequent local septic complication in severe acute pancreatitis is infected necrosis, pancreatic abscess being less common.

Pathogenesis

The origin of a pancreatic abscess is probably the necrotic pancreatic tissue contaminated with bacteria. The ability of the human organism to maintain the infection within certain limits by forming a rim of granulation tissue leads to localized progressive liquefaction of the necrotic tissues and pus formation. On the other hand, when the infection spreads in an unlimited way within the devitalized surrounding tissues, the consequence is infected pancreatic necrosis. In this sense, the immunologic capacity of the patient may play an important role, since in pancreatic abscess host defenses seem better able to confine the infection than in infected pancreatic necrosis.

Microbiology

The species of pathogens isolated from the infected pancreas suggest an enteric origin in both pancreatic abscess and infected pancreatic necrosis. Nevertheless, the origin and route of the bacteria leading to infection of the pancreatic gland in acute pancreatitis are still unclear. Several mechanisms have been proposed to explain how these enteric bacteria reach the pancreas: translocation of bacteria from the gut, infection from the biliary tree or duodenum, as well as hematogenous or lymphatic spread from other sites.

Pancreatic abscesses are more frequently polymicrobial (57%) than monomicrobial (43%). This fact contrasts with infected pancreatic necrosis, where monomicrobial infection is usually found. The most commonly isolated microorganisms in pancreatic abscesses are *Escherichia coli*, *Enterococcus* spp., *Klebsiella pneumoniae*, and *Enterobacter* spp.; less frequent are *Staphylococcus* spp., *Pseudomonas aeruginosa*, *Streptococcus* spp., and *Bacteroides*. Up to now anaerobes and fungi have rarely been reported; however, the bacterial spectrum may change in the near future due to the use of specific antibiotics leading to an increase in different microorganisms, especially fungi.

Pathology

As previously defined, a pancreatic abscess is a collection of pus, usually with little or no necrotic tissue and surrounded by a more-or-less distinct inflammatory capsule or pseudocapsule. Abscesses are usually multiple and can be unilocular or multilocular. The extension may involve the entire gland (20%), or may be predominantly right-sided (35%) and related to the head of the gland, or predominantly left-sided (45%) in the proximity of the body or pancreatic tail. Abscesses commonly extend to one or more of the following areas: the transverse mesocolon, the root of the mesentery, the paracolic or subdiaphragmatic spaces.

Clinical and laboratory features

The general unpredictable and variable course of acute pancreatitis can also be applied to its complications. In this regard, the clinical presentation of pancreatic abscess may vary from an indolent, almost asymptomatic course to a severe septic status.

In most patients the clinical expression of acute pancreatitis complicated with pancreatic abscess exhibits a *biphasic evolution*: after completion of the toxic phase during the first and second weeks of the disease, the patient enters into a variable period of well-being for several (2–4) weeks that usually ends with the onset of clinical signs of sepsis. Thus, and this is a very important characteristic of this complication, the diagnosis of pancreatic abscess will usually be late, no earlier than the fourth or fifth week from the onset of pancreatitis. Differing from this clinical pattern, infected pancreatic necrosis is characterized by an *overlapping biphasic* trend. After an initial "toxic" phase, clinical elements of concomitant sepsis appear, without the period of recovery and improvement outlined above. Therefore, the diagnosis of infected pancreatic necrosis is usually earlier, within the second or third week of the onset of the disease. This different clinical pattern may be helpful from a clinical point of view for distinguishing between infected pancreatic necrosis and pancreatic abscess, since signs and symptoms are usually the same and nonspecific.

Secondary pancreatic infections are usually associated with fever and pyrexia greater than 38°C: in the case of pancreatic abscess the fever adopts an undulating pattern, arising from transient bacteremia, different from the more constant pattern of the fever in infected pancreatic necrosis. Also, most patients complain of epigastric pain, frequently radiating to the back or flank and associated with nausea and vomiting. A great variety of other abdominal features can be observed, among them distension, guarding, rebound, and palpable mass. This latter sign is identified in approximately 40% of cases.

Patients with pancreatic abscess usually have a lower Ranson score and Acute Physiology and Chronic Health Evaluation (APACHE) II score than those with infected pancreatic necrosis. The lesser morbidity, especially systemic complications, associated with pancreatic abscess is the reason why these scores are lower in pancreatic abscess than in infected pancreatic necrosis.

Although pancreatic abscess is generally less severe than infected pancreatic necrosis, a series of life-threatening complications may appear secondary to the evolution of the abscess that the medical team should be aware of. Especially relevant are bleeding in the gastrointestinal tract, perforation into the free peritoneal cavity or neighboring hollow viscera, hemorrhage into the abscess cavity, pancreatopleural fistula with empyema, endocarditis, and finally diabetes due to progressive destruction of pancreatic tissue.

There are no specific and useful laboratory parameters for the diagnosis of pancreatic abscess. In fact the most frequent laboratory finding is leukocytosis and, if any other, the absence of specific signs of acute pancreatitis such as hyperamylasemia and elevated C-reactive protein. An additional consideration must be made regarding blood cultures: they are rarely positive due to the fact that bacteremia from an abscess tends to be intermittent and transient.

Diagnosis

The diagnosis of pancreatic abscess is based on clinical suspicion, imaging techniques, and demonstration of infection. Since clinical presentation may be very variable, pancreatic infection should be suspected in any patient with fever or suggestive signs or symptoms of sepsis within the context of acute pancreatitis. Pancreatic abscess should be highly suspected when fever appears during the fourth or fifth week of evolution.

During the first 2 weeks of the disease, fever and signs of sepsis will probably reflect the inflammatory process and the presence of necrosis, but not necessarily infection. After the second week of disease, clinical features suggesting sepsis will probably reflect infection. Between the second and third weeks of the disease, infection of the necrosis should be suspected. When such signs appear later, and specifically if they appear after a period of well-being, the first suspected diagnosis should be pancreatic abscess.

A differential diagnosis can be established by contrast-enhanced CT. This imaging technique is considered at present the gold standard and should always be available when treating patients with acute pancreatitis. The information obtained from this exploration is very concrete:
• Whether or not there is necrosis of the pancreas, its extent and location.
• The presence of fluid collections, their number, location, characteristics, and whether they are surrounded by a wall (Fig. 17.1): for this purpose good bowel opacification with oral contrast is important for discriminating abdominal fluid collections from loops of bowel during CT examination.

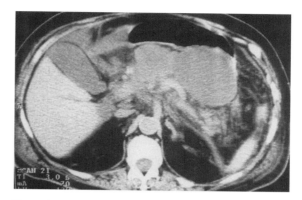

Figure 17.1 Computed tomography scan reveals a large unilocular pancreatic abscess. Aspiration yielded purulent fluid.

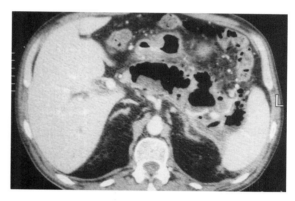

Figure 17.2 Computed tomography scan shows irregular and multilocular gas-filled abscesses.

• The presence of gas bubbles within the fluid collections, a pathognomonic feature of pancreatic infection (Fig. 17.2).
However, the limits of this exploration must be taken into account: firstly, in the absence of gas bubbles, CT cannot recognize the presence of infection; secondly, CT cannot discriminate between an abscess and a pseudocyst.

The final step for definitive diagnosis is demonstration of infection by needle aspiration. This can be achieved by several methods: via the percutaneous route guided by ultrasonography or CT, or via the gastrointestinal tract guided by endoscopic ultrasonography. The aspirated sample is immediately Gram-stained and cultured under aerobic and

Table 17.1 Local septic complications in acute pancreatitis: differential diagnosis between pancreatic abscess and infected pancreatic necrosis.

	Pancreatic abscess	Infected pancreatic necrosis
Definition	Collection of pus encapsulated	Nonviable pancreatic parenchyma
Timing	Fourth to fifth week	Second to third week
Clinical course	Biphasic (with an interphase of recovery)	Overlapping biphasic
Microbiology	Polymicrobial	Monomicrobial
Systemic complications	Rare	Frequent
Imaging (computed tomography)	Encapsulated material high density (> 15 HU)	Lack of enhancement in ≥ 30% of pancreas (< 50 HU)

anaerobic conditions. Depending on the characteristics of the fluid, the aspiration should also be examined for its content of pancreatic enzymes. The combination of imaging techniques and aspiration permits a precise diagnosis in 90–95% of cases.

A summary of the differences between pancreatic abscess and infected pancreatic necrosis is shown in Table 17.1.

Treatment

Once a pancreatic abscess has been diagnosed the treatment is complete drainage. Pancreatic abscesses do not resolve spontaneously and, if untreated, the prognosis of a patient is almost invariably death. Nowadays, two different approaches can be considered for primary drainage of a pancreatic abscess: surgical and percutaneous.

Classically, drainage of a pancreatic abscess was always surgical. As a result of the mortality and complications associated with operative therapy and with the advances in methodology of percutaneous drainage of abdominal abscesses, during the last decade there was great enthusiasm for the transcutaneous route as primary treatment of pancreatic abscesses. Nevertheless, subsequent studies have shown the limitations of this approach, resulting in a lower rate of success than was initially believed. Although by definition a pancreatic abscess contains little or no necrotic tissue, clinical practice shows that there is always a proportion of necrotic tissue and solid debris within the abscess cavity that cannot pass through the catheters; hence the limitations of percutaneous treatment. This is why the first

therapeutic approach to pancreatic abscess in patients fit for surgery should still be surgical and not radiologic, as occurs with intraabdominal abscesses of nonpancreatic origin.

Surgical techniques

The aims of the primary surgical intervention are to perform a thorough extraction and cleansing of the purulent material, unroofing of the abscess cavities, débridement, removal of necrotic tissue, and placement of drains. Surgery starts with a midline or bilateral subcostal incision, reaching the pancreas through the gastrocolic omentum. These maneuvers allow entry to the abscess cavity, thus enabling the surgeon to drain and aspirate its content of pus. A large window is made in the abscess capsule, and the necrotic tissue contained within the abscess is removed. Débridement must be performed very carefully by blunt dissection, using one's fingers or sponge forceps. Extensive irrigation with a certain degree of pressure on the cavity helps to release fragments of necrotic debris.

Management of the abscess cavity includes several options. The first approach is closed continuous local lavage. In this technique, two or more large double silicone rubber tubes are inserted within the lesser sac and infected areas (Fig. 17.3). Gastrocolic and duodenocolic ligaments are then sutured to create a closed retroperitoneal lesser sac compartment for the postoperative continuous lavage. The lavage provides atraumatic and continuous evacuation of devitalized tissues and detritus that mechanically cleans the inflamed area. During the postoperative course the amount of lavage fluid is 1 L/hour; as outflow fluid becomes cleaner dur-

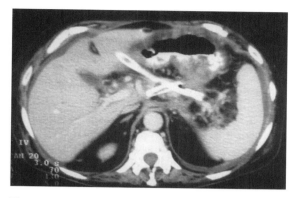

Figure 17.3 Position of drainage tubes for local lavage of the abscess cavity.

ing the following days, lavage can be stopped and the drainage tubes removed stepwise. This is, in our opinion, the recommended technique for the majority of cases of pancreatic abscess. The results of this approach are excellent, with a mortality rate of 8–29%. However, with this technique lavage is limited to the lesser sac and therefore if the process extends beyond this anatomic compartment or there is a great proportion of necrotic tissue, this technique may not be the most advisable.

The second approach for management of the residual cavity is the open-packing technique. With this method the entire lesser sac and all extensions of the pancreatic abscess are packed with moist pads, the abdomen is left open, and the patient undergoes re-explorations every 48 hours for further drainage and débridement until the cavity has begun granulation. This technique shows its major benefits in patients with an extensive component of necrosis accompanying the abscess, especially those with necrosis beyond the colonic flexures. The mortality rate with this technique ranges from 9 to 22%, its main drawbacks being a high incidence of intestinal fistulas due to the repeated reex-plorations and of incisional hernias due to secondary healing of the wound.

Finally, there is a third option, which involves inserting a series of soft silicone rubber closed-suction drains (Jackson–Pratt) and Penrose drains stuffed with gauze into all extensions of the abscesses. Once the drains have been inserted the abdomen is closed. As the patient improves the drains are slowly advanced out to allow the cavity to collapse as healing occurs. The

mortality rate with this approach has been described as low as 5% for pancreatic abscess, the main complication being a high incidence of pancreatic fistula.

The present tendency is to consider each approach as equally valid, the choice depending on the case. These techniques could also complement each other: for example, in a case of a very extensive pancreatic abscess with a high proportion of necrotic tissue, it would be advisable to start with an open-packing technique and, as the cavity heals, to insert the drains for lavage and close the abdomen.

Percutaneous drainage

Transcutaneous drainage has been proposed as an alternative to surgery for the primary treatment of pancreatic abscess. Exceptional series aside, results have been disappointing and this treatment is generally no longer considered to be the most adequate. Nonetheless, the two situations in which percutaneous drainage is considered the first option for treatment of pancreatic abscess are, firstly, residual or recurrent pancreatic abscesses after a primary surgical approach in which most of the necrotic or solid material has been removed; and, secondly, as a temporary measure in exceedingly high-risk patients. In the first situation the percutaneous approach is usually successful, avoids a difficult reoperation with the associated risk of intestinal fistula, and therefore has become a well-established indication. The rationale for using this therapy in patients presenting an extremely high surgical risk is to give them time to recover in readiness for the operation. However, this latter indication has a much lower rate of success than the drainage of postoperative pancreatic abscesses.

Image-guided percutaneous catheter drainage is carried out under local anesthesia. Localization of the abscess or abscesses is performed by imaging techniques, basically CT, and once identified, a catheter or multiple catheters of different sizes are inserted into the cavities. These catheters remain in place until drainage ceases, the clinical situation improves, and follow-up CT reveals resolution of the abscess. Nevertheless, the high rate of success when treating residual or recurrent pancreatic abscesses does not imply it is an easy therapy, since patients will require the insertion of several catheters, frequent catheter manipulations and changes, and a long duration of catheter drainage.

153

Role of antibiotics

Sepsis is the main cause of death in secondary pancreatic infections. Therefore the use of antibiotics associated with drainage in pancreatic abscesses is almost universal. Appropriate antibiotic therapy depends on the identification of the causative microorganisms and sensitivity testing. Meanwhile several options have been recommended: a combination of ceftazidime and clindamycin; a combination of ciprofloxacin and metronidazole; or carbapenems as a single agent due to its extremely broad spectrum of activity. The recommended duration of antibiotic therapy is unknown, but common sense suggests maintaining the treatment as long as the septic state persists.

Prognosis

Infected pancreatic necrosis and pancreatic abscess are at present the main causes of mortality in acute pancreatitis. The single most important factor leading to a poor outcome in patients with pancreatic abscess is late diagnosis. The prognosis improves greatly with a prompt diagnosis and adequate treatment, resulting in mortality rates of 5–10%, whereas infected pancreatic necrosis shows higher mortality rates (20–50%).

An important factor that needs special attention is the possible changes in endocrine and exocrine function after treating pancreatic abscesses. Thus, monitoring both pancreatic functions becomes essential for the care of these patients.

Looking at the future: therapeutic perspectives

Advances in medical technology may open a door to new approaches that would minimize the aggressiveness of current techniques when draining pancreatic abscesses, while achieving a high rate of success. Thus, the armamentarium for treatment of pancreatic abscess is already increasing with the new procedures currently under investigation.

Let us consider firstly laparoscopic-assisted percutaneous drainage: this approach, which combines the advantages of the percutaneous route for draining fluids of the abscess cavity with the laparoscopic route that allows removal of the debris in the cavity, overcomes the limitations of percutaneous catheter drainage. A second idea currently under investigation is to drain the abscess cavity through the gastrointestinal tract by endoscopic means. The endoscopic transmural technique aims to drain the abscess cavity into the gastrointestinal lumen by endoscopic fistulization and subsequently place stents in the cavity. To determine the site for fistulization and also to rule out the presence of vascular structures, endoscopic ultrasound is proving to be a remarkable aid. Additionally, this technique allows insertion of nasopancreatic abscess drains for irrigation of the cavity. Thirdly, although related to the previous method, the endoscopic transpapillary drainage technique drains the abscess by inserting stents through the papilla of Vater.

These techniques, albeit attractive, remain at present within the context of investigation and cannot as yet be recommended for routine use.

Acknowledgments

The authors thank Ms. Landy Menzies for reviewing the manuscript and technical assistance.

Recommended reading

Bittner R, Block S, Büchler M, Beger HG. Pancreatic abscess and infected pancreatic necrosis. Different local septic complications in acute pancreatitis. *Dig Dis Sci* 1987;32:1082–1087.

Bradley EL III. A clinically based classification system for acute pancreatitis. *Arch Surg* 1993;128:586–590.

Bradley EL III. Pancreatic abscess. In: JL Cameron (ed.) *Current Surgical Therapy*, 6th edn. St Louis: Mosby, 1998: 502–506.

Cinat ME, Wilson SE, Din AM. Determinants for successful percutaneous image-guided drainage of intra-abdominal abscess. *Arch Surg* 2002;137:845–849.

Giovannini M, Pesenti C, Rolland A-L, Moutardier V, Delpero J-R. Endoscopic ultrasound-guided drainage of pancreatic pseudocysts or pancreatic abscesses using a therapeutic echo-endoscope. *Endoscopy* 2001;33:473–477.

Isenman R, Schoenberg MH, Rau B, Beger HG. Natural course of acute pancreatitis: pancreatic abscess. In: HG Beger, AL Warshaw, MW Büchler *et al.* (eds) *The Pancreas*. Oxford: Blackwell Science, 1998: 461–465.

Lumsden A, Bradley EL III. Secondary pancreatic infections. *Surg Gynecol Obstet* 1990;170:459–467.

Mithöfer K, Mueller PR, Warshaw AL. Interventional and surgical treatment of pancreatic abscess. *World J Surg* 1997;21:162–168.

Rotman N, Mathieu D, Anglade M-Ch, Fagniez P-L. Failure of percutaneous drainage of pancreatic abscesses compli-cating severe acute pancreatitis. *Surg Gynecol Obstet* 1992;174:141–144.

van Sonnenberg E, Wittich GR, Chon KS *et al.* Percutaneous radiologic drainage of pancreatic abscesses. *Am J Roentgenol* 1997;168:979–984.

18 Is there a place for laparoscopic surgery in the management of acute pancreatitis?

Gregorio Castellanos, Antonio Piñero, and Pascual Parrilla

Introduction

Following the consensus reports of Atlanta and Santorini, acute pancreatitis is defined as an acute inflammatory process of the pancreatic gland with involvement of the peripancreatic tissues and remote organ systems.

Mild acute pancreatitis is associated with minimal organ dysfunction, without local or systemic complications, and recovery is complete after initial conservative medical treatment together with supportive measures and clinical surveillance. Once pancreatic enzymes return to normal, and when the etiology is biliary, surgery is limited to laparoscopic cholecystectomy prior to hospital discharge to avoid further attacks.

Severe acute pancreatitis (SAP) is the clinical expression of the presence of pancreatic necrosis. It can evolve into multiple organ failure and local and/or systemic complications and requires early medical treatment in an intensive care unit to prevent and adequately treat the complications. It also requires close collaboration with the surgeon in order to prevent and diagnose infection of the necrotic tissue as early as possible, and to decide when to operate and what technique to use.

Pancreatic necrosis is regarded as a focal or diffuse area of nonviable pancreatic tissue that is principally sterile and associated with necrosis of the peripancreatic fat. It is diagnosed by dynamic computed tomography (CT) and initially given conservative treatment. If there is clinical suspicion of infection, CT with needle aspiration and culture of the material is necessary, and confirmation requires emergency surgical drainage due to its high mortality rate. The aims of surgical treatment are to eliminate the toxic pancreatic exudate, débride the devitalized pancreatic tissue and peripancreatic fat while conserving the healthy pancreatic tissue, and regularly check the retroperitoneum to evacuate newly formed necrosis.

Optimum surgical drainage in infected pancreatic necrosis (IPN) is still controversial, and the unacceptably high postoperative morbidity and mortality rates following conventional closed débridement has led surgeons in search of new technical alternatives.

The aim of this chapter is to analyze the role currently played by laparoscopic surgery as a minimally invasive technique in the treatment and management of SAP with IPN. The various modalities of laparoscopy-related treatment are detailed here together with the results obtained, conclusions, and future prospects.

Laparoscopy-related therapeutic modalities in SAP

Several techniques have been described for the approach, débridement, and management of IPN. We have divided these into (i) direct laparoscopies, (ii) percutaneous punctures assisted by laparoscopic instruments, and (iii) techniques for necrosectomy assisted by endoscopic instruments.

Direct laparoscopic techniques

These techniques consist of laparoscopic access to the retroperitoneal space via the transgastric or retrogastric and retrocolic or paracolic approaches. This provides sufficient guarantee of ample drainage and débridement of the pancreatic area, and the possibility of tube placement for continuous lavage and drainage in the postoperative period, as occurs in open surgery but with less operative trauma and lower rates of morbidity and mortality. These techniques may be indicated in early or late stages of IPN, when there is a predominance of fluid collections of pancreatic exudate or pus and a scarce solid component of debris and necrosis.

Various types of laparoscopic approach have been designed for accessing the retroperitoneum depending on the images obtained by three-dimensional CT.

Transperitoneal approach to the retroperitoneum
Transgastric necrosectomy is performed through a window opened lengthways by laparoscopic instruments in the posterior gastric wall along the axis of the pancreas, which under direct vision allows drainage, débridement, and lavage of the retroperitoneal space leaving communication open to the stomach, without placement of tubes for lavage or drainage. It is indicated in late-appearing IPN located in the pancreatic body, when adhesions and fibrosis between the posterior gastric wall and the retroperitoneal space are solidly formed.

Retrogastric necrosectomy (Fig. 18.1) is performed through two windows opened by laparoscopic instru-

ments in the gastrocolic and gastrohepatic omentum. It allows drainage, débridement, and placement of tubes for continuous lavage and drainage of the retroperitoneal space and contaminated peritoneal cavity. It is indicated in early stages of IPN when there is still only edema and liquid exudate with scarce necrosis and no inflammatory adhesions or fibrosis between the posterior wall of the stomach and the peripancreatic space.

If IPN extends to the flanks, down along the lumbar quadrate and psoas major muscles, the retroperitoneum must be accessed via the retrocolic, infracolic, or paracolic approach, with the two gutters detached by laparoscopic instruments to mobilize the right and/or left colon (Fig. 18.2).

Extraperitoneal approach to the retroperitoneum
Laparoscopic access to the retroperitoneum is direct and totally extraperitoneal, via the translumbar route through the anterior pararenal space. For this a balloon trocar is used, through which carbon dioxide is insufflated to create a virtual cavity for placement of the scope and trocars.

This approach is recommended in initial pancreatic necrosis that requires drainage for any reason, because the edema and the moderate inflammatory response facilitate dissection of the tract.

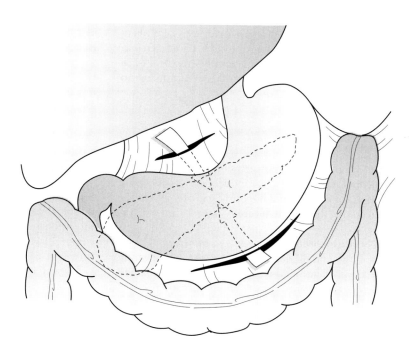

Figure 18.1 Retrogastric access route to the retroperitoneum using the transperitoneal approach.

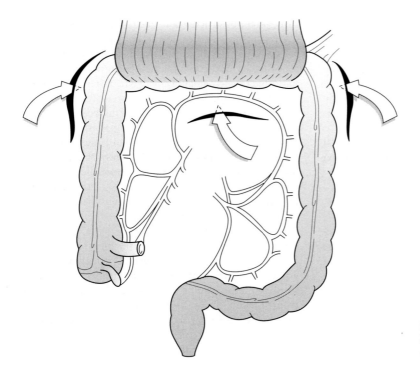

Figure 18.2 Infracolic–paracolic access route to the retroperitoneum using the transperitoneal approach.

Results

Experience and results with transperitoneal laparoscopic approaches in IPN are very limited, and only short series and isolated cases have been published, with discordant data as regards results. Using different laparoscopic approaches some authors report a 62% rate of morbidity and 25% rate of reoperation, but no technique-related mortality.

Techniques for percutaneous puncture assisted by laparoscopic instruments

These dynamic CT-guided percutaneous puncture techniques allow drainage, the possibility of obtaining material for culture, and use of the catheter as a guide for accessing the pancreatic area.

Direct transperitoneal percutaneous puncture

This is the standard technique for managing septic collections of intraabdominal fluid. The value of the technique in the presence of solid pancreatic necrosis is limited, because if débridement is not performed well solid foci will be left to act as nests of continuous infection.

The procedure is safe and effective as initial treatment for IPN in which the fluid component (pancreatic exudate/pus) predominates over the solid component (debris/necrosis). A one-way catheter is placed for lavage and discontinuous drainage and then exchanged for others of a larger caliber until a suitable diameter is reached for performing débridement, continuous lavage, and aspiration. For greater efficiency, one or several large-caliber two-way catheters must be used to facilitate continuous lavage and drainage of the cavity and avoid obstruction. Occasionally, when it is difficult to remove compact viscous necrosis, the aid of laparoscopic instruments is required. Multiple sessions and radiologic follow-up with contrast are required to assess the residual cavity or reveal any intestinal or pancreatic fistulous tract. Follow-up by three-dimensional CT gives information on volume, composition, topography, and communications between collections.

These drains may be indicated early or late:

1 in initial pancreatic necrosis in hemodynamically stable patients, in an attempt to avoid the high morbidity and mortality rates of surgical débridements;

2 in pancreatic necrosis in seriously ill patients with a

high anesthetic or surgical risk, as the sole therapeutic alternative;

3 in pancreatic necrosis with clinical suspicion of infection, in order for culture samples to be taken, leaving the drain as a guide in the translumbar approach;

4 in pancreatic necrosis with a predominance of fluid, when decompression of the pneumoperitoneum is required;

5 in single or multiple collections, other than IPN, that require drainage, but should not be used in the context of an IPN where solid or semisolid collections of necrosed tissue are present.

The main problems with these single or multiple punctures include discontinuous lavage, drain obstructions, and the need to use several drains for greater efficiency in multiple sessions, all of which carry a high rate of morbidity, particularly enterocutaneous and/or pancreatic fistulas, bleeding phenomena, and residual abscesses, which require new percutaneous drains or open surgery. Likewise, to work efficiently and give good results the drains require special care and maintenance by skilled personnel in order to avoid obstruction or loosening.

Transperitoneal percutaneous puncture as a guide for laparoscopic assistance

This laparoscopic technique allows pancreatic necrosis to be removed and débrided under vision until seen to be completely clean. A direct CT-guided puncture is made to the IPN in order to drain the cavity and obtain material for culture, with the catheter left as a guide if access to the retroperitoneum is necessary. The laparoscopic instruments consist of a trocar for the scope and another two to be used as working channels. Once the cavity has been entered, the material is aspirated, the cavity washed thoroughly, and the trocars removed and replaced by thick tubes for continuous lavage and drainage. Generally, several laparoscopic accesses are required for the cavity to be cleaned properly. This procedure may be indicated in any type of IPN irrespective of the composition of the cavity contents.

Among the drawbacks of the technique is a greater possibility of intestinal fistula formation, contamination of the abdominal cavity, the difficulty posed by the rigidity of the laparoscope, and the need to use a minimum of three entry ports.

Lumbotomy-associated extraperitoneal percutaneous puncture with laparoscopic assistance

This technique consists of direct percutaneous puncture of the retroperitoneal space via the lumbar approach. Placement of a drain will guide the lumbotomy, through which the colon will be freed to facilitate posterior laparoscopic access to the prerenal fascia. As the peritoneal cavity remains intact at all times, morbidity is reduced considerably.

Results

The results are rather inconsistent, depending on the diameter and number of drains used, the time they have been left, and the routes for lavage and drainage. The main complication is digestive and/or pancreatic fistulas.

In the few series published, direct percutaneous puncture with simple or multiple drainage has a mortality rate of 0–20%, a morbidity of 26–66% (basically intestinal and pancreatic fistulas and local bleeding), and a reoperation rate for surgical necrosectomy of 10–24%. The chances of this percutaneous treatment being insufficient in IPN are very high, and in various series the technique is reported to have avoided surgery in 9–14% of cases (Table 18.1).

Techniques for necrosectomy assisted by endoscopic instruments

The first necrosectomy with the aid of a direct-vision endoscope was performed by Chmelizek in 1985, who, following an initial laparoscopy reconverted to laparotomy, carried out complementary necrosectomies via the anterior transperitoneal approach with the aid of a mediastinoscope. Three different techniques are currently described.

Transgastric retroperitoneal endoscopic necrosectomy

This is performed via direct gastric transmural access under the vision of a flexible endoscope. A lengthways opening is made along the axis of the pancreas in the posterior wall of the stomach and dilated with the aid of a balloon to create a gastric window, through which débridement, lavage, and endoscopic aspiration of the cavity are performed and which is left open without drainage tubes to act as an internal drain to the stomach. If solid material persists in the pancreatic area, endoscopic débridement of the cavity is repeated until it is seen to be clean and granulation begins. It is recommended in late IPN in which the posterior gastric wall is closely attached to the retroperitoneal cavity by fibrosis.

Table 18.1 Direct transperitoneal percutaneous punctures.

Study	No. of patients	Approach, drainage, lavage	Morbidity (%)	Mortality (%)	Reoperation (%)
Freeny *et al.* (1998)	34	CT + TPP Early simple drainage Discontinuous lavage	26	0	24
Echenique *et al.* (1998)	20	CT + TPP Multiple drains Continuous lavage	50	0	10
Gouzi *et al.* (1999)	32	CT + TPP Late multiple drains Continuous lavage/drainage	66	15	19
Carter *et al.* (2000)	10	CT + TPP Simple drainage Continuous lavage	40	20	10

CT, computed tomography; TPP, transperitoneal percutaneous puncture.

Among the drawbacks of the technique is the difficulty in leaving thick tubes for continuous lavage and drainage, the need to perform multiple sessions of endoscopy over the first 2 weeks, and the risk of closure of the gastric window, which allows internal drainage of the cavity to the stomach.

Transperitoneal percutaneous puncture and necrosectomy with endoscopic management
First, a transperitoneal percutaneous puncture is performed, and then the initial tract is dilated to a suitable diameter. After removal of the drains, a flexible endoscope is inserted through the tunnel created by these drains, and lavage and aspiration of the cavity is performed under vision for as often as necessary, with the drains reinserted on completion of the exploration.

This technical modality allows regular supervision of the patient depending on clinical evolution, follow-up of the process, and status of the pancreatic area using transperitoneal retroperitoneal endoscopy.

Transperitoneal or translumbar surgical approach and necrosectomy with endoscopic management
First, the extraperitoneal, transperitoneal, or translumbar open surgical approach is used, followed by drainage and ample débridement with lavage and aspiration, and several thick tubes are left for continuous lavage and drainage in the postoperative period. A week later the drainage tubes are temporarily removed and a flexible endoscope is inserted through the tracts created for postoperative follow-up and management of the infected pancreatic area under direct vision (Fig. 18.3).

After performing dynamic CT with direct retroperitoneal puncture of the pancreatic necrosis and verifying from culture that it is infected, we leave the drain to act as a guide in the surgical approach. Drainage is done under general anesthesia (with the patient placed in the lateral decubitus position) through an 8-cm-long posterior translumbar incision situated on the midline between the last rib and the iliac crest. The muscles of the abdominal wall are dissected, and the posterior parietal peritoneum and colon are pushed aside toward the midline in order to give access to the pancreatic area via the extraperitoneal route through the anterior pararenal space. In the same operation, and under direct vision, a flexible endoscope is inserted, the pancreatic area drained, and a superficial necrosectomy performed by flushing and endoscopic aspiration; the necrosed tissue is left adhering to the pancreas. Any small hemorrhage can be resolved with endoscopic coagulation or packing with hemostatic material. The translumbar incision is closed in layers, with placement of an 18 CH tube for continuous lavage and a 32 CH tube in the more sloping area for drainage of any infected necrosed material that falls away.

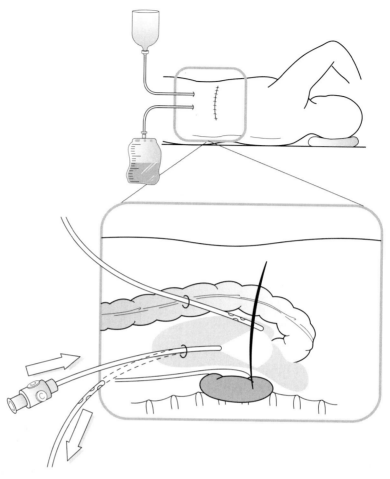

Figure 18.3 Extraperitoneal translumbar endoscopy route to the retroperitoneum.

Follow-up and lavage/aspiration of the pancreatic area are performed by translumbar retroperitoneal endoscopy (TRE) without insufflation, which can be done at the bedside with the patient intubated or awake under mild sedation. The patient is positioned on his or her side, and the flexible endoscope is inserted into the drainage tube orifice once the drain has been removed. These sessions are begun at least a week into the immediate postoperative period. They can be repeated as often as necessary depending on the patient's clinical evolution and on the three-dimensional imaging of helical CT until the retroperitoneum is seen to be completely clean.

This imaging technique is a very useful exploratory procedure in the monitoring and follow-up of IPN, as the detailed information it provides on volume, composition, and contents of the collection, the correct anatomic situation, the relationship of this situation in the retroperitoneal space, and communications with other collections is very useful in making a therapeutic decision. To radiologically assess the evolution of the retroperitoneal space and rule out the possibility of there being any intestinal or pancreatic fistulous tract, we perform retroperitoneography to contrast the cavity through the drainage catheter.

In our opinion the extraperitoneal lumbar approach is a good alternative for drainage of IPN. The anatomic communication of the pancreatic region with the pararenal spaces, the root of the mesentery and the transverse mesocolon, together with the proximity of the transcavity of the omenta, explain the certainty of draining these different territories via a right and/or left lumbar approach, guided by a direct-vision flexible endoscope, which enables us to move through all

161

these areas performing lavage and aspiration. The advantages of the procedure include the following.

• It is a direct approach to the areas of necrosis and can access the whole of the pancreatic gland and retroperitoneal layers.

• Good-quality necrosectomy by flushing.

• Protection, against infection and fistulas, of the peritoneal cavity and its contents, especially the inframesocolic space of the abdomen, thus facilitating the use of enteral nutrition.

• It limits trauma and complications of the abdominal wall.

• Low postoperative morbidity and mortality rates.

• Good patient tolerance of management and follow-up of the pancreatic area with repeated TRE.

The main drawback of the technique is that it cannot be used on the gallbladder when the etiology is biliary, but if there are no complications in the papilla that require endoscopic retrograde cholangiopancreatography, laparoscopic cholecystectomy can be performed in the short or long term after the acute episode.

Results

Transgastric endoscopic drainage has been performed in carefully selected patients (apart from initial pancreatic necrosis in the course of SAP) with organized sterile collections of necrotic fluid, using a pigtail stent with nasocavitary lavage; there was a 36% rate of cavity infection and 64% rate of morbidity. The different series using direct retroperitoneal surgical approaches yield results for mortality of 0–33%, morbidity of 0–57% for local complications (15–50% colonic and intestinal

fistulas, retroperitoneal hemorrhages, and gastric and pancreatic fistulas), and a mean of two reoperations per patient.

Our experience embraces a total of 24 patients with SAP and IPN documented by puncture. The first 13 cases received only the translumbar approach for drainage of the pancreatic area and blind superficial necrosectomy by flushing; thick tubes were left for continuous lavage and drainage in the postoperative period, and the incision was closed in layers. We observed a mortality rate of 23% due to multiple organ failure, a morbidity rate of 30.7% (due to spontaneously closing low-debit pancreatic, duodenal, and colonic fistula and pancreatic insufficiency requiring temporary monitoring of glycemia and oral antidiabetics), and no surgical reinterventions.

The remaining 11 cases, on completion of their initial translumbar drainage and during the same surgical intervention, had superficial necrosectomy with flushing and aspiration under the vision of a flexible endoscope; two thick tubes were fitted for lavage and drainage, and the incision was closed in layers. Management of the retroperitoneum was done periodically with TRE, averaging five procedures per patient depending on their clinical evolution and three-dimensional CT data. The mortality rate was 27% due to nontechnique-related multiple organ failure, and there was no morbidity or reoperations.

Other authors have recently corroborated our results in IPN using drainage and necrosectomy via an extraperitoneal posterior approach to the pancreatic area, reporting no morbidity, mortality, or reoperations (Table 18.2).

Table 18.2 Direct retroperitoneal approaches.

Study	No. of patients	Mortality (%)	Local morbidity (%)	Second-look operation (mean/patient)
Fagniez *et al.* (1989)	40	33	50	3.6
Villazón *et al.* (1991)	18	22	33	2.6
Von Vyve *et al.* (1992)	20	20	20	1.4
Chambon *et al.* (1995)	14	0	57	5
Nakasaki *et al.* (1999)	8	25	50	5 cases (62%)
Carter *et al.* (2000)	4*	0	25	2 cases (50%)
Castellanos *et al.* (2001)	24†	25	17	0 (5 TRE/patient)
Halkic *et al.* (2003)	3	0	0	0

TRE, translumbar retroperitoneal endoscopy.
* All four cases with management via transperitoneal retroperitoneal endoscopy.
† Eleven cases with management via translumbar retroperitoneal endoscopy.

Conclusions and recommendations regarding the different laparoscopy-related therapeutic modalities in SAP with IPN

Direct laparoscopic techniques and techniques for percutaneous puncture assisted by laparoscopic instruments

1 Laparoscopic surgery is indicated in the treatment and management of SAP with IPN in order to perform necrosectomy via the direct approach, lavage with aspiration, and placement of drains.

2 Laparoscopic pancreatic necrosectomy is feasible, although at times does not offer much guarantee of success, as the viscosity of the necrosis makes evacuation of the material difficult. When there is a predominance of debris and necrosis and the necrosectomy is incomplete, open surgery and regular monitoring of the pancreatic area under direct vision must be employed.

3 Laparoscopic pancreatic necrosectomy may have major advantages over open necrosectomy techniques because it fulfills the same objectives but with lower rates of morbidity and mortality. Despite attempts with this technique to avoid the morbidity and mortality rates of surgical débridement, it is not yet a reality.

4 The laparoscopic approach is less aggressive, involves less pain and tissue trauma, and causes fewer laparotomy hernias. The main drawbacks of the approach are rigidity of the instruments and limitation of the operating field, difficulty in evacuation and aspiration of necrotic material due to its consistency and viscosity, formation of enterocutaneous or pancreatic fistulas, and infection of the abdominal cavity.

5 Despite laparoscopic pancreatic necrosectomy being theoretically useful, it is currently not possible to draw more accurate or evidence-based conclusions. Comparative prospective studies are necessary to outline the specific indications of the technique.

6 Direct transperitoneal percutaneous puncture is a safe efficient technique that is minimally aggressive and has a future as a valid alternative. It is useful in hemodynamically stable patients for draining pancreatic and/or peripancreatic collections in which the fluid component predominates over debris and necrosis. It can likewise be used as a guide for laparoscopic assistance.

Techniques for necrosectomy assisted by endoscopic instruments

1 IPN requires early vigorous drainage and, in our opinion, the initial extraperitoneal translumbar approach for evacuating, débriding, and washing the pancreatic area is a suitably efficient surgical intervention.

2 The subsequent management of the pancreatic area can be carried out by regular programmed TRE. It is a minimally invasive technique that explores under visual control, offers a wider field of action due to the flexibility of the endoscope (with a single tube for vision and operation), and can be performed at the bedside. With the results obtained, we consider TRE to be a useful and efficient therapeutic alternative to open surgery of the abdomen in the follow-up and management of the retroperitoneum in IPN.

3 The open extraperitoneal translumbar access has advantages in that it avoids infection of the abdominal cavity, performs an ample necrosectomy with endoscopic flushing and aspiration, avoids reoperations, respects the integrity of the abdominal wall, and considerably reduces the rates of morbidity and mortality and both exocrine and endocrine pancreatic insufficiency.

Future prospects for laparoscopy in SAP with IPN

Despite progress in the knowledge and management of SAP, the mortality figures are still high, which means that diagnosis and treatment must be considered consensually by a multidisciplinary team of intensivists, radiologists, gastroenterologists, and surgeons.

As a result of its complex management, patients with SAP must be treated initially in the intensive care unit so that they can be monitored and given proper systemic support. A correct medical approach from the outset allows early detection of complications and improved patient survival. No disease responds better to work well done than SAP; its mortality rate must be less than 30%, with 80% related to IPN.

Reducing the role for surgery in patients suffering from SAP with IPN is a future challenge that can be met thanks to the new treatments for reducing systemic inflammatory response syndrome and preventing necrosis infection. There is still debate over the role of the surgeon, the time of operation, and the most suitable technique. The surgical indication, the technique of choice, and the appropriate time to perform it must be considered in each patient. The decision about when to perform the operation must take into account the reduction in surgical risk with time and the risk–benefit ratio of the wait. Surgical delay in SAP must not be regarded as a failure, but rather as the success of properly administered conservative treatment. Techniques with different degrees of aggression are performed, but the rationale for these techniques is similar, i.e., excision of devitalized tissue and lavage and drainage of the pancreatic area.

For some years laparoscopy, a minimally invasive surgical procedure, has been gaining ground and now represents an alternative to conventional surgical treatment in patients with SAP. It is less aggressive than surgery, allowing determination of the extent of the disease, irrigation and drainage of the cavity, and decompression of the pancreatic area.

Future challenges must be aimed at:

1 perfection of the technique to make laparoscopic pancreatic necrosectomy competitive with open techniques;

2 evaluation with controlled comparative studies to confirm its advantages over open transperitoneal approaches;

3 availability of large series to validate the technique (to counteract the present lack of experience and lack of prospective studies and protocols);

4 clear and accurate patient selection, criteria, indications, approaches, limitations, and advantages and disadvantages, in order to contrast the results of these different laparoscopic techniques.

Only in this way can we meet the challenge still posed in our hospitals by SAP.

Recommended reading

Direct laparoscopic techniques

Ammori BJ. Laparoscopic transgastric pancreatic necrosectomy for infected pancreatic necrosis. *Surg Endosc* 2002; 16:1362.

Cuschieri A. Pancreatic necrosis: pathogenesis and endoscopic management. *Semin Laparosc Surg* 2002;9:54–63.

Gagner M. Laparoscopic treatment of acute necrotizing pancreatitis. *Semin Laparosc Surg* 1996;3:21–28.

Hamad GG, Broderick TJ. Laparoscopic pancreatic necrosectomy. *J Laparoendosc Adv Surg Tech A* 2000;10:115–118.

Pomoukian VN, Gagner M. Laparoscopic necrosectomy for acute necrotizing pancreatitis. *J Hepatobiliary Pancreat Surg* 2001;8:221–223.

Zhu JF, Fan XH, Zhang XH. Laparoscopic treatment of severe acute pancreatitis. *Surg Endosc* 2001;15:1239–1241.

Techniques for percutaneous puncture assisted by laparoscopic instruments

Alverdy J, Vargish T, Desai T, Frawley B, Rosen B. Laparoscopic intracavitary débridement of peripancreatic necrosis: preliminary report and description of the technique. *Surgery* 2000;127:112–114.

Carter CR, McKay CJ, Imrie CW. Percutaneus necrosectomy and sinus tract endoscopy in the management of infected pancreatic necrosis: an initial experience. *Ann Surg* 2000; 232:175–180.

Connor S, Ghaneh P, Raraty M et al. Minimally invasive retroperitoneal pancreatic necrosectomy. *Dig Surg* 2003; 20:270–277.

Echenique AM, Sleeman D, Yrizarry J et al. Percutaneous catheter-directed debridement of infected pancreatic necrosis: results in 20 patients. *J Vasc Interv Radiol* 1998;9:565–571.

Freeny PC, Hauptmann E, Althaus SJ, Traverso LW, Sinanan M. Percutaneous CT-guided catheter drainage of infected acute necrotizing pancreatitis: techniques and results. *Am J Roentgenol* 1998;170:969–975.

Gouzi JL, Bloom E, Julio C et al. Drainage percutané des necroses pancréatiques infectées: alternative à la chirurgie. *Chirurgie* 1999;124:31–37.

Horvath KD, Kao LS, Wherry KL, Pellegrini CA, Sinanan MN. A technique for laparoscopic-assisted percutaneous drainage of infected pancreatic necrosis and pancreatic abscess. *Surg Endosc* 2001;15:1221–1225.

Techniques for necrosectomy assisted by endoscopic instruments

Baron TH, Thaggard WC, Morgan DE, Stanley RJ. Endoscopic therapy for organised pancreatic necrosis. *Gastroenterology* 1996;111:755–764.

Castellanos G, Serrano A, Piñero A et al. Retroperitoneoscopy in the management of drained infected pancreatic necrosis. *Gastrointest Endosc* 2001;53:514–515.

Castellanos G, Piñero A, Serrano A, Parrilla P. Infected pancreatic necrosis. Translumbar approach and management with retroperitoneoscopy. *Arch Surg* 2002;137:1060–1063.

Chambon J, Saudemont A, Porte H, Gambiez L, Quandalle P. Drenaje retroperitoneal lumboscópico para el tratamiento de las pancreatitis agudas necrotizantes. *Cir Laparosc Endosc* 1995;2:176–180.

Fagniez P, Rotman N, Kracht M. Direct retroperitoneal approach to necrosis in severe acute pancreatitis. *Br J Surg* 1989;76:264–267.

Halkic N, Pezzetta E, Abdelmoumene A, Corpataux JM. Indications and results of retroperitoneal laparostomy in the treatment of infected acute necrotizing pancreatitis. *Minerva Chir* 2003;58:97–99.

Nakasaki H, Tajima T, Fujii K, Makuuchi H. A surgical treatment of infected pancreatic necrosis: retroperitoneal laparotomy. *Dig Surg* 1999;16:506–511.

Van Vyve E, Reynaert M, Lengele B, Pringot J, Otte J, Kestens P. Retroperitoneal laparostomy: a surgical treatment of pancreatic abscesses after an acute necrotizing pancreatitis. *Surgery* 1992;111:369–375.

Villazón A, Villazón O, Terrazas F, Raña R. Retroperitoneal drainage in the management of the septic phase of severe acute pancreatitis. *World J Surg* 1991;15:103–108.

19 What should be done to prevent relapses of acute pancreatitis?

Karlheinz Kiehne and Ulrich R. Fölsch

Introduction

When discussing recurrent acute pancreatitis, it has to be considered that usually an extrapancreatic etiology is present that causes the relapses. The correct identification of an underlying cause may be easy or difficult, but proper treatment will almost certainly prevent recurrences of acute pancreatitis. Every time patients with acute pancreatitis experience a relapse there is a risk that they will suffer the general complications of the disease.

Relapses of acute pancreatitis need to be clearly distinguished from relapsing chronic pancreatitis, which is characterized by typical morphologic changes (dilated pancreatic duct and branches, duct stone, pseudocysts, calcifications, fibrous pancreatic tissue) and impaired pancreatic secretory function as documented by pancreatic function tests. Sometimes, repeated attacks progress to organ changes comparable to chronic pancreatitis, with reduced secretory capacity and pancreatic calcifications and scars.

Chronic pancreatitis often progresses even when the initiating causes have been eliminated. Acute episodes of chronic pancreatitis can be severe and dangerous and cannot be distinguished from a bout of acute pancreatitis, although on closer inspection the signs of chronic pancreatitis can be identified. Chronic pancreatitis in the Western Hemisphere is mainly caused by chronic alcohol abuse. Other reasons for chronic pancreatitis include mutations of cationic trypsinogen and serine protease inhibitor Kazal type 1 (*SPINK1*) genes (see Chapter 23) or abnormalities in pancreatic duct development. In this chapter, only the reasons for relapsing acute pancreatitis are discussed.

In the case of chronic pancreatitis, the episode of pain and inflammation can be envisaged as a reactivated chronic inflammatory process. It is a fact that in many cases the differences between relapses of acute pancreatitis and reactivation of chronic pancreatitis will never be clear. This chapter deals with issues and possible causes for recurrences of acute pancreatitis. Nevertheless, some of these causes for attacks of acute pancreatitis may also be present in a patient with chronic pancreatitis. If this is the case, chronic pancreatitis could be aggravated by the identified cause. The reasons for the current episode of pain and inflammation then have to be treated as they would in acute pancreatitis.

Acute pancreatitis is mainly triggered by extrapancreatic causes. An episode is most often induced by a biliary stone passing through the sphincter of Oddi or a single occurrence of alcohol excess. The clinical presentation is of the same kind, irrespective of the underlying causes. Edematous and necrotizing pancreatitis follow a general scheme of organ damage, inflammation, bacterial infection, and restitution. Complications arise from organ necrosis, infection, and general shock. If the patient is continuously exposed to the damaging event, a prolonged course follows and leads to a higher complication rate. There is also a generally increased risk for relapses if the damaging conditions are maintained. Thus, efforts have to be made to identify and eliminate the individual reasons for acute pancreatitis from the onset of clinical treatment. The course of therapy might be generally influenced if one or another pathophysiologically relevant condition is identified. Furthermore, the potential risk of relapses will certainly be eliminated after adequate treatment. Since acute pancreatitis is a heterogeneous disease with regard to pathophysiology, reliable data on the frequency of relapses by a defined cause are not available. However, it is assumed that about 5–10% of all patients with acute pancreatitis will have repeated attacks. Bearing in mind that edematous acute pancreatitis has a lethality of 1–3% and necrotizing acute pancreatitis a lethality of 10–15%, elimination of pathophysiologic risks is favorable for the patient's prognosis.

All patients with recurrent idiopathic acute pancreatitis are candidates for repeated and invasive diagnostic procedures and therapeutic interventions. The indications for some of these interventions (e.g., endoscopic sphincterotomy for biliary sludge) are based on studies demonstrating long-term benefit for patients undergoing the special therapy, whereas other procedures such as manometry of the biliopancreatic sphincter for the detection of sphincter dysfunction can cause pancreatitis iatrogenically. Patients with idiopathic recurrent acute pancreatitis are a special challenge for pancreatologists. Often these patients suffer from undetected biliary stones or microlithiasis. Sometimes, follow-up reveals chronic pancreatitis in some patients who were initially diagnosed as having idiopathic recurrent acute pancreatitis. Nevertheless, a thorough diagnostic evaluation of patients has to be planned after an attack of acute pancreatitis, but one has to remember that each intervention in or around the pancreas sometimes has a substantial risk for development of another attack of acute pancreatitis. The most important indication for an extended diagnostic work-up after an attack of acute pancreatitis is the suspicion of an otherwise poorly detectable biliary microlithiasis or a tumor in general.

General aspects after recovery from an attack of acute pancreatitis

After an attack of acute pancreatitis, patients need days to several weeks to recover from abdominal pain, bowel dysfunction, and weight loss. The recovery period begins when abdominal pain is grossly reduced and inflammatory parameters normalize. The first steps toward a normal life are the reduction of analgetic drugs and reuptake of oral food. Analgetics should be reduced when the patient reports continued improval of abdominal discomfort. However, oral food should first be given when the patient is almost free of pain and serum lipase levels are below twice the upper normal limits. Otherwise a relapse of pain is certain, which will almost double the hospital stay. When the patient is considered fit for oral food uptake, water or tea and biscuit or toast will be the first servings, the persistence of paralytic ileus having been excluded beforehand. If the food is well tolerated without pain relapse, then a stepwise addition of protein and fat content is ordered. Table 19.1 shows a proposed food plan after acute pancreatitis. The first steps contain only water and/or fat-free carbohydrates. Protein is added at step 4, fat at step 5. Total protein and fat contents should usually be low and the majority of calories based on carbohydrate intake. Although the patients have a reduced caloric uptake during the first days of oral feeding, progress toward a higher caloric diet should not be too fast. Parenteral nutrition appears to be useful if the patient's general condition suggests that oral feeding cannot be started after the first 3 days of hospital treatment. Jejunal enteral tube feeding is another way of administering food without stimulating the pancreas. It is feasible in patients with edematous or necrotizing pancreatitis if an ileus is not present. As in patients under parenteral nutrition, patients with jejunal tube feeding can begin with oral feeding when lipase is almost normalized and if they are largely free of pain (for details see Chapter 10).

Most patients experience a dramatic reduction in food tolerance and suffer early satiety after an attack of severe acute pancreatitis. When patients are overloaded with food, they will certainly have upper ab-

Table 19.1 Dietary recommendations after an attack of acute pancreatitis with stepwise increase of nutritional contents. The patient is usually given several servings (four to six) per day.

Step 1: nothing by mouth, parenteral nutrition (or jejunal tube feeding)
Step 2: tea, water
Step 3: biscuits, porridge
Step 4: toast without butter; jam, rice, cooked vegetables
Step 5: potatoes, fish, poultry

Avoid: large meals, alcoholic beverages, milk or high-fat milk products, meat with high fat content, grilled or fried food, eggs, smoked meat or fish, vinegar, chocolate, coffee

dominal pain. Only a renewed fasting period followed by a slower increase in food quantity will be of help. Patients generally tolerate six to eight small servings per day better than three or four larger ones. Alcohol in any form is prohibited. Other nutrients like beans, cabbage, sour juices, or cream are seldom tolerated by most patients. In addition, each patient will experience an individual pattern of intolerance for a variety of nutrients. If pancreatitis is completely healed, which can be assumed after 2–4 months, most patients regain their former nutritional habits. However, they should be advised to omit potential nutritional triggers for new pancreatitis attacks, such as large quantities of fat, fried food, or alcohol. Nutritional consultation is always helpful.

If the patient is unable to achieve a sufficient intake of calories or vitamins, nutritional support is indicated. If a deficit is documented, the fat-soluble vitamins A, D, E, and K often have to be administered parenterally because of impaired enteral absorption. Deficits of fat-soluble vitamins usually arise when steatorrhea is present, usually a sequel of chronic pancreatitis, but sometimes steatorrhea follows a single attack of acute pancreatitis when large parts of the pancreatic organ have become scar tissue.

Substitution with pancreatic enzymes is usually not necessary after acute pancreatitis, since patients regain their normal pancreatic function. After the first attack of acute pancreatitis about 10–30% of patients develop subclinical or clinical pancreatic exocrine insufficiency, a manifestation that has generated controversy about whether it represents progression of acute to chronic pancreatitis or presentation of the first clinical episode of chronic pancreatitis. If after recovery from acute pancreatitis patients continue to experience abdominal pain or discomfort or fail to regain their former body weight, substitution of pancreatic enzymes is recommended in order to improve digestion and reduce the pancreatic secretory demand. The common tubeless noninvasive pancreatic function test often shows regular pancreatic function in these patients. Because of the low sensitivity of all pancreatic function tests for mild to moderate exocrine pancreatic insufficiency, a trial period for a few weeks with pancreatic enzymes is recommended. Supporting the patient's digestion with pancreatic enzymes reduces the need for an otherwise larger food intake, which might itself be the cause for abdominal pain.

Biliary pancreatitis

Patients with cholecystolithiasis, microlithiasis, or even biliary sludge are at risk for biliary pancreatitis. Bile duct stones cause acute pancreatitis by permanent or short-term obstruction of the sphincter of Oddi. The diagnostic procedures used to identify biliary causes should include serum bilirubin and γ-glutamyltransferase levels, ultrasonography, and endosonography if available. If the attack of acute pancreatitis is most likely caused by a biliary stone, endoscopic biliary therapy is usually indicated. Since biliary material is the reason for acute pancreatitis in this group of patients, it has to be eliminated in order to treat the current attack and to prevent repeated attacks of pancreatitis. If the biliary system is not cleared of any material spontaneously, by endoscopy or surgery, then the patient has a persisting and increased risk for recurrence of acute pancreatitis.

Depending on the presence of continued biliary obstruction (elevated bilirubin levels and dilated bile duct) or even cholangitis in addition to acute pancreatitis, endoscopic retrograde cholangiopancreatography (ERCP) with papillotomy and stone extraction has to be performed more or less immediately. All other patients with suspected biliary pancreatitis should be stabilized and treated for their acute pancreatitis until they have generally improved. It is not until then that endoscopic examinations of biliary causes have to be performed. If available, endoscopic ultrasonography is the method of choice for detecting or excluding bile duct stones (Fig. 19.1). Endosonography has an accuracy as good as ERCP and has the advantage of being almost free of complications compared with ERCP and papillotomy. If endosonography detects bile duct stones, ERCP with papillotomy and stone extraction should follow. In the case where endosonography shows a normal common bile duct, no further diagnostic procedures are necessary. A flow chart is shown in Fig. 19.2 to help identify patients who are to be treated with ERCP immediately or after stabilization.

As a major site of stone formation, the gallbladder needs careful examination. Patients recovering after acute biliary pancreatitis with gallbladder stones treated without cholecystectomy have a significant risk (up to 20%) of another attack of pancreatitis. If sludge or stones are identified, cholecystectomy needs to be performed independent of biliary duct therapy with ERCP. However, a recent study has provided evidence that cholecystectomy is of value only if there are overt

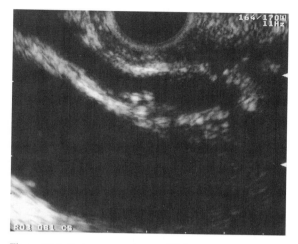

Figure 19.1 Endosonography: small biliary stones are detected in the common bile duct in a patient after an attack of acute pancreatitis.

manifestations of gallbladder disease, such as cholecystitis, gallbladder pain, or cystic duct obstruction. If these conditions are not present, endoscopic sphincterotomy alone is sufficient to prevent relapses of acute pancreatitis.

Even "idiopathic" recurrent pancreatitis might have been caused by biliary microlithiasis in up to 75% of patients initially classified as being free of biliary stones and in whom other causes of acute pancreatitis had been excluded. Microlithiasis was detected when the bile of these patients was collected after papillotomy and examined under a microscope. The patients remained free of acute pancreatitis recurrences after endoscopic papillotomy. However, performance of prophylactic endoscopic papillotomy after an attack of acute pancreatitis without direct evidence of biliary material is still intensely debated. Another study reported a significant benefit of pancreatic duct stenting in patients with idiopathic recurrent pancreatitis. Pancreatic duct stent therapy was continued for over 1 year. Despite the pathophysiologically unclear situation, this study provides some evidence that pancreatitis in a variety of patients seems to be caused by short-term

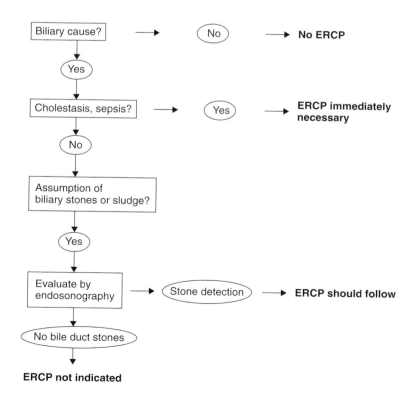

Figure 19.2 Flow chart for indication and timing of endoscopic retrograde cholangiopancreatography (ERCP).

papillary obstruction, thus supporting the hypothesis that stent therapy protects the pancreatic duct system from stasis and improves pancreatic drainage. Unfortunately, reliable longitudinal observations are not available. Studies of this kind lead pancreatologists to the conclusion that idiopathic pancreatitis is mainly a pancreatitis of undiagnosed biliary causes.

In elderly patients with underlying cholecystolithiasis or choledocholithiasis who appear to be unfit for cholecystectomy or who have bile duct stones that cannot be extracted endoscopically, papillotomy and insertion of plastic bile duct stents has been proved to be safe and effective in the treatment of complicated biliary stones. These stents have to be exchanged every 4–6 months to prevent stent occlusion and cholangitis, although a watch-and-wait tactic until complications occur has also been recommended for this group of patients.

Obstructive nonbiliary acute pancreatitis

In rare instances, acute pancreatitis is caused by anatomic variations of the pancreatic duct system itself or of neighboring organs. Pancreas divisum, pancreas anulare, aneurysm of the splenic artery or aorta, or duodenal diverticulosis are mentioned, but many other conditions exist (e.g., metastases, papillary tumors, retroperitoneal hematoma). Large controlled trials comparing the various treatment options for these rare situations are not available.

Another group of patients with recurrent attacks of acute pancreatitis are patients with sphincter of Oddi dysfunction. In this group of patients the papilla seems to react with prolonged and stronger contractions that are suspected of obstructing the biliary and pancreatic duct, finally leading to pancreatitis. Sphincter of Oddi dysfunction is diagnosed by the typical clinical symptoms of biliary pain, absence of biliary stones, and presence of pathologic sphincter of Oddi function tests (manometry and prolonged presence of contrast medium in the bile duct after endoscopic retrograde cholangiography). Despite controversies about the nature and diagnosis of sphincter of Oddi dysfunction, some pancreatologists describe improvement of patients after specific treatment of the papilla. Usually an endoscopic sphincterotomy is performed, which reduces significantly the incidence of acute pancreatitis and biliary pain. However, with regard to the poor study data, lack of knowledge about normal sphincter pressure, and the considerably increased complication rate in patients with suspected sphincter of Oddi dysfunction after ERCP or sphincter manometry, endoscopic therapy of sphincter of Oddi dysfunction remains experimental.

Pancreatic tumors also can cause acute pancreatitis. Benign and malignant tumorous lesions of the papillary region, such as papillary adenomas, leiomyomas, hamartomas, lymphomas, or choledochoceles, might cause obstruction of the ampulla or pancreatic duct. Usually, patients with these tumors present with obstructive jaundice but occasionally pancreatitis is the first sign of the disease. Thus, the tumor might be missed in early stages when patients with acute pancreatitis are not examined thoroughly. These conditions are sometimes detectable by sonography, but regular ERCP and/or endosonography is much more sensitive. If all patients with acute pancreatitis are evaluated by a structured diagnostic program including sonography, endosonography, and finally ERCP, almost any anatomic cause should be identified.

Aneurysms of the splenic artery, which in individual cases could cause acute pancreatitis, need to be surgically resected because of the risk of rupture. Acute pancreatitis in these cases might appear as a symptom of the aneurysm, and thus pancreatitis should be envisaged as an event leading to proper diagnosis. Aneurysm of the splenic artery or vascular malformations in the pancreas have been repeatedly reported to lead to a misdiagnosis of pancreatic cancer. Duplex sonography or CT angiography is extremely useful in identifying these vascular conditions and indicating an adequate therapy, which as a side effect will prevent further relapses of acute pancreatitis.

Nonneoplastic lesions, such as posttraumatic strictures, pseudocyst, and pancreaticobiliary malformations, are other potential but rare causes of recurrence of acute pancreatitis. Duodenal diverticulum is identified relatively often in elderly people, although it seldom leads to obstruction of the pancreatic duct. If so, a duodenal diverticulum that is believed to be the cause of relapsing acute pancreatitis needs to be treated by either papillotomy and stent insertion or resection. Pancreas divisum causes pancreatitis presumably by partial obstruction at the minor papilla, which in these patients is the orifice where the majority of pancreatic secretions pass. Because pancreas divisum is often diagnosed late in the history after several attacks of acute pancreatitis, patients may have developed chronic pancreatitis. However, large controlled studies have not confirmed pancreas divisum as a major risk for developing acute pancreatitis.

If a potential harmful anatomic situation has been identified, surgical or endoscopic therapy is usually recommended. In most cases of pancreatic duct compression, insertion of a pancreatic stent by ERCP is helpful and the least invasive therapy. If pancreas divisum is the underlying cause of acute pancreatitis, pancreatic duct stenting is also necessary, but the stent is placed through the minor papilla into the dorsal duct. Stents need to be exchanged after a few months to prevent occlusion. Over a total treatment period of about 1–2 years, the stenosis could resolve and stenting does not need to be continued. Overall in patients with pancreas divisum, stent therapy causes slight pain relief and significantly reduces the frequency of acute pancreatitis episodes. It remains currently unclear if the potential progression to chronic pancreatitis could be halted by long-term stent therapy.

Alcohol-induced acute pancreatitis

Alcohol is a potential cause for an attack of acute pancreatitis as well as the major reason for chronic pancreatitis in populations with significant alcohol consumption. Each type of alcohol consumption, occasional or chronic, may cause an episode of acute pancreatitis or another attack of chronic pancreatitis. There is no lower limit of daily alcohol intake that clearly excludes alcohol-induced pancreatitis. The pathophysiology of alcohol-induced pancreatitis remains largely unclear. Toxic metabolic products, decreased vitamin levels, decreased oxidative capacity, and uncontrolled pancreatic stimulation have been proposed as participating factors.

If the attack of acute pancreatitis is first caused by a single episode of alcohol excess, then there is a good prognosis that the pancreas will heal completely. However, most patients have chronic alcohol abuse so that their pancreas is considered to be relatively damaged before the first attack of pancreatitis. Often it remains unclear if the pancreatitis is a single attack of acute pancreatitis or is a manifestation of chronic pancreatitis.

The argument that alcoholic acute pancreatitis is partially caused by a nutritional deficit has led to proposals for preventing repeated attacks or for treatment during the acute illness. Among the suggested diverse

exotic medications are vitamins like B_1, B_6, and C or trace minerals such as selenium and zinc. However, there are no reliable studies which demonstrate that defined medications or nutritional components are effective in preventing further attacks of acute pancreatitis.

After acute pancreatitis each patient has to be advised to live strictly without alcohol, regardless of the cause for the recent attack. Any amount of alcohol could cause repeated attacks of pancreatitis, as clinical observations support. The shortest time period of alcohol abstinence is undefined, but patients appear to be well advised with recommendation for abstinence longer than 6 months. After this time, the pancreas is supposed to have completely recovered from the acute inflammation and regained its function. Progression of pancreatitis to chronic pancreatitis and its complications might even occur after a single attack of acute pancreatitis and immediate discontinuation of alcohol consumption. Patients with chronic alcohol abuse need professional help to control their alcohol abuse. Success rates are low and disappointing, but long-term alcohol abstinence rates are higher in the psychotherapeutic intervention group than in patients without further support.

Post-ERCP pancreatitis

ERCP is a significant cause of acute pancreatitis due to its frequent use. Despite its benefit for patients with acute biliary pancreatitis, about 2–15% of all patients undergoing ERCP develop a moderately severe acute pancreatitis. This variation in the incidence rate is related to the definition of acute pancreatitis (elevated pancreatic enzymes after ERCP or clinical symptoms with morphologic signs of pancreatitis) and, more importantly, to the experience of the endoscopist. Furthermore, patients themselves and the underlying pancreatic disease contribute to the risk of developing post-ERCP acute pancreatitis. Large studies have identified suspicion of sphincter of Oddi dysfunction and previous attacks of acute pancreatitis as major patient-related risks for the induction of post-ERCP pancreatitis. Procedure-related risks for pancreatitis include sphincter manometry, needle knife or precut sphincterotomy, repeated attempts, and difficult cannulation. All together, these procedure- and patient-related risks comprise about 10–20% of all ERCP interventions. As a consequence, the incidence of post-ERCP pancreatitis should be greatly reduced if patients with risk factors are investigated by the most experienced endoscopists and potentially harmful techniques are omitted. The development of alternative techniques for examination of the biliopancreatic system is therefore contributing greatly to the prevention of post-ERCP pancreatitis. The increasing use of magnetic resonance cholangiopancreatography as an alternative technique for examining the biliopancreatic system should lead to a decreased incidence of post-ERCP pancreatitis. In addition, endosonography is another valuable, reliable, and safe technique for studying the biliary system and the pancreatic parenchyma, and is gaining its place in the clinical routine.

If endoscopic interventions are necessary in patients at elevated risk of post-ERCP pancreatitis, placement of a short-term pancreatic duct stent has proved to be helpful in reducing the rate of post-ERCP pancreatitis. Pancreatic stents augment pancreatic drainage after the endoscopic procedure when manipulations at the papilla might cause swelling that leads to retainment of pancreatic juice. Pancreatic stenting is usually performed at the end of ERCP by placement of a short 5 or 7 French stent into the pancreatic duct. The stent remains in place for about 1 week, after which it is removed endoscopically. Some endoscopists promote the insertion of small stents without proximal flaps to allow spontaneous migration of the stent into the intestine, which occurs after several days to a few weeks.

There have been various attempts to prevent post-ERCP pancreatitis by infusion of theoretically protective drugs (e.g., aprotinin, somatostatin, octreotide). These drugs were earlier used for treatment of acute pancreatitis but failed to show clinical effects in large controlled trials. The rationale for the use of these drugs in the prevention of post-ERCP pancreatitis was as potential protective agents before ERCP. Protease inhibitors have been most intensively studied. Gabexate mesylate, a potent protease inhibitor, has a well-documented potential in the prevention of experimental pancreatitis. There are now a number of human studies reporting a significant decrease of post-ERCP pancreatitis in humans when gabexate is administered before ERCP. It is effective in patients at normal or increased risk for post-ERCP pancreatitis. The major concern about general use of gabexate is the considerable costs associated with the treatment frequency required to prevent one episode of post-ERCP pancreatitis. Thus, despite its documented potency, gabexate

is currently used only in clinical trials. Another promising medication in the prevention of post-ERCP pancreatitis might be diclofenac. A seminal study provided evidence that diclofenac given after a difficult ERCP resulted in significant reduction of post-ERCP pancreatitis. It would be of great benefit if this observation is confirmed by other groups because only those patients at risk for post-ERCP pancreatitis need to be treated and treatment is given after a difficult ERCP. Until then, the best way to prevent post-ERCP pancreatitis is not to use ERCP.

Hyperlipidemia

Severe hyperlipidemia, especially hypertriglyceridemia, might result in acute pancreatitis. The pathophysiology is poorly understood. Disturbances in local capillary blood flow by capillary occlusion with chylomicrons, changes in membrane fluidity, or disruption of the regulatory signalling of pancreatic exocrine secretion are the most suspected mechanisms. Patients with familiar hyperlipidemia with Frederikson classification type I, IV, or V are at special risk. The typical patient with hyperlipidemia-induced acute pancreatitis has a preexisting lipid abnormality and an additional event triggering the acute pancreatitis. Before the onset of acute pancreatitis, most patients report excessive food intake over a period of one or a few days. Alcohol abuse or poor control of diabetes, pregnancy, or hypothyroidism are other situations that can aggravate a preexisting lipid disorder and cause the induction of acute pancreatitis. Some of these patients also suffer from biliary stones, which makes the differentiation between biliary pancreatitis or pancreatitis due to hyperlipidemia difficult. When acute pancreatitis is caused by hyperlipidemia, serum triglycerides are usually greater than 500 mg/dL, and frequently above 2000 mg/dL. A serum triglyceride level above 1000 mg/dL is a relatively certain marker of hyperlipidemia-induced acute pancreatitis. Sometimes, acute pancreatitis is the first manifestation of diabetes or a metabolic syndrome, which then has to be included in further therapeutic plans. On the other hand, uncontrolled diabetes or pregnancy are sometimes identified as conditions leading to hyperlipidemia and acute pancreatitis, without the presence of a predisposing lipid disorder.

During the acute phase, lipid levels will fall after cessation of oral food intake. Care has to be taken when parenteral nutrition is given, and serum lipid levels have to be monitored much more strictly than in other patients. Sometimes, the elevated lipid levels do not respond to the general therapy for acute pancreatitis. In this case, lipid apheresis or plasmapheresis has to be started rapidly in order to disrupt the pathophysiologic sequence. If apheresis procedures are not available, then heparin and insulin could be tried since some case reports have showed a significant and rapid reduction of serum triglyceride levels with intravenous administration of heparin (controlled by coagulation tests) and insulin (controlled by blood glucose).

Since metabolic derangement precipitates acute pancreatitis, patients need strict dietary control after the acute phase. Food should be prepared largely from fat-free nutrients and high-fat nutrients are prohibited. Total dietary fat intake should be not more than 10% of the administered calories. Since the majority of patients are overweight, a reduction of body weight has to be attempted. Several small servings daily are better tolerated than two or three larger ones. Some nutrients may induce acute pancreatitis when consumed in larger quantities in predisposed patients, for example milk, oil, fried food, or meat with high fat content. The changes in dietary fat composition, such as the exchange of long-chain fatty acids for medium-chain fatty acids, appears to be of further benefit. A diet containing medium-chain triglycerides produces a much lower increase in postprandial triglyceride levels in patients with primary hypertriglyceridemia, although cholesterol levels often increase with this diet. A theoretical improvement of oxidative capacity by the administration of vitamins, trace minerals, or immunonutrients seems to have no measurable clinical effect on relapses of acute pancreatitis. The prescription of lipidemia-reducing drugs (usually fibrates; statins are less effective in reducing triglycerides) is recommended since dietary treatment alone is usually insufficient in reducing lipid levels. In general, fibrates are well tolerated. It has to be remembered that the combination of fibrates with statins is generally contraindicated due to the increased risk of severe adverse effects. Patients with hyperlipidemia often do not only have hypertriglyceridemia, which induces acute pancreatitis, but also display hypercholesterolemia and are at risk for atherosclerosis. If triglyceride levels in these hypercholesterolemic patients are not excessively high, statins might be preferred as lipid-lowering drugs be-

cause of their protective effect on atherosclerosis and coronary heart disease.

Identified metabolic disorders like diabetes or hypothyroidism need to be treated until sufficient metabolic control is achieved. Only very limited experience is available on the effects of long-term treatment with plasmapheresis and lipid apheresis in the prevention of repeated attacks of acute pancreatitis. Clinical experience and reports of small patient groups suggest that the compliant patient who adheres to the recommended diet, abstains from alcohol completely, shows control of triglyceride levels, and who eventually is successfully treated for associated metabolic disorders has a favorable prognosis with regard to prevention of repeated episodes of acute pancreatitis.

Hypercalcemia

Another rare but relatively easily treatable cause of acute pancreatitis is hypercalcemia, most often caused by primary hyperparathyroidism. Hyperparathyroidism by itself is not a direct cause of acute pancreatitis, but hypercalcemia of any cause leads to acute pancreatitis. Plasmacytoma, sarcoidosis, vitamin D intoxication, calcium supplementation, extensive bone metastases, and other even rarer conditions have to be considered. Despite the well-known association between hypercalcemia and acute pancreatitis, none of the theoretical pathophysiologic concepts are proven. It is assumed that hypercalcemia causes increased intracellular responsiveness to damaging events, increased trypsin activity, and disruption of the cellular architecture, all finally leading to intracellular activation of digestive enzymes.

The treatment of hypercalcemia-induced acute pancreatitis involves identification and treatment of the underlying disorder. Symptomatic control of hypercalcemia is only temporarily effective since regulatory mechanisms are rapidly activated that counteract the initiated therapy. Therefore, treatment of the underlying disorder, such as primary hyperparathyroidism, is mandatory, making surgery for example necessary. Some but not all of these conditions are treatable. If no causative therapy is available, symptomatic control of hypercalcemia, for example by infusion of bisphosphonates on a regular basis or diuretic therapy, will be at least partially effective and is helpful in palliative situations.

Drug-induced acute pancreatitis

A vast variety of drugs are accused of inducing acute pancreatitis, although actual instances are rare. Most suspected drugs are taken without any adverse effects, even when dosages above the recommendations are taken. Nothing is known about the special pathophysiologic processes involved in the action of comedications. Interaction with the cytochrome P450 system is assumed; furthermore, imbalance in the oxygen reductase system, action as a pancreatic secretagogue, interference with pancreatic blood flow, or disturbance of the prostaglandin system is also implicated. Potentially hazardous drugs are listed in Table 19.2.

If acute pancreatitis appears to be caused by a certain drug, one has to exclude the presence of other more frequent conditions first. However, during the acute phase of pancreatitis all potentially deleterious drugs should be omitted. Reexposure after complete recovery will eventually provide evidence that the accused drug was causing pancreatitis, but obtaining proof in this way is certainly far too dangerous. As documented by a variety of case reports, rechallenge of patients with the harmful medications often caused another rapid induction of acute pancreatitis. Generally, the patient should be treated by alternative therapies.

Summary

The prevention of relapses of acute pancreatitis starts with treatment of the present episode. Precipitating causes of acute pancreatitis need to be identified in order to allow effective current treatment and to avoid future risks. Biliary stones or sludge, hyperlipidemia, or hypercalcemia should be treated immediately. The majority of cases initially classified as idiopathic pancreatitis will presumably be reclassified as biliary pancreatitis after more intense investigations. Morphologic abnormalities and tumors also have to be excluded. Each identified risk factor has to be treated to prevent repeated attacks of acute pancreatitis.

After the acute phase, patients have to learn to adhere to a diet avoiding alcohol and nutrients with high fat content. They should have four to six small meals per day. Several months after the attack, patients could try a somewhat extended diet with increased fat content and grilled meat. Alcohol in any form should be avoided for as long as possible. Patients should be advised that a repeated attack of acute pancreatitis could be more severe and dangerous than the previous one, so that the required changes in lifestyle are hopefully easier to accept.

Table 19.2 Drugs known to potentially induce acute pancreatitis. (Modified from Gorelick 1995.)

Definite association between drug therapy and induction of acute pancreatitis
Azathioprine
Furosemide (frusemide)
Estrogens
Sulfonamides
Tetracycline
Valproic acid
Cytostatic agents (asparaginase, cisplatin, cytosine
  arabinoside)

Possible association with induction of acute pancreatitis
Chlorthalidone (chlortalidone)
Corticosteroids
Ethacrynic acid (etacrynic acid)

Selection of drugs that have been anecdotally associated with induction of acute pancreatitis
Amphetamines (amfetamines)
Ampicillin
Clofibrate
Enalapril
Ergotamine
Histamine
Indomethacin (indometacin)
Isoniazid
Metronidazole
Rifampicin
Trimethoprim

Recommended reading

Andriulli A, Clemente R, Solmi L *et al.* Gabexate or somatostatine administration before ERCP in patients at high risk for post-ERCP pancreatitis: a multicenter, placebo-controlled, randomized clinical trial. *Gastrointest Endosc* 2002;56:488–495.

Braganza JM. Towards a novel treatment strategy for acute pancreatitis. 1. Reappraisal of the evidence on aetiogenesis. *Digestion* 2001;63:69–91.

Braganza JM. Towards a novel treatment strategy for acute pancreatitis. 2. Principles and potential practice. *Digestion* 2001;63:143–162.

Fogel EL, Eversman D, Jamidar P, Sherman S, Lehman GA. Sphincter of Oddi dysfunction: pancreaticobiliary sphincterotomy with pancreatic stent placement has a lower rate of pancreatitis than biliary sphincterotomy alone. *Endoscopy* 2002;34:280–285.

Freeman ML, DiSario JA, Nelson DB *et al.* Risk factors for post-ERCP pancreatitis: a prospective, multicenter study. *Gastrointest Endosc* 2001;54:425–434.

Gorelick FS. Acute pancreatitis. In: T Yamada (ed.) *Textbook of Gastroenterology.* Philadelphia: Lippincott, 1995: 2064–2091.

Heyries L, Barthet M, Delvasto C, Zamora C, Bernard JP, Sahel J. Long-term results of endoscopic management of pancreas divisum with recurrent acute pancreatitis. *Gastrointest Endosc* 2002;55:376–381.

Jacob L, Geenen JE, Catalano MF, Geenen DJ. Prevention of pancreatitis in patients with idiopathic recurrent pancreatitis: a prospective nonblinded randomized study using endoscopic stents. *Endoscopy* 2001;33:559–562.

Kaw M, Al-Antably Y, Kaw P. Management of gallstone pancreatitis: cholecystectomy or ERCP and endoscopic sphincterotomy. *Gastrointest Endosc* 2002;56:61–65.

Kiehne K, Fölsch UR, Nitsche R. High complication rate of bile duct stents in patients with chronic alcoholic pancreatitis due to non compliance. *Endoscopy* 2000;32:377–380.

Lankisch PG. Chronic pancreatitis: development from acute pancreatitis? A physicians view. *Surg Clin North Am* 1999; 79:815–827.

Murray B, Carter R, Imrie C, Evans S, O'Suilelabhain C. Diclofenac reduces the incidence of acute pancreatitis after endoscopic retrograde cholangiopancreaticography. *Gastroenterology* 2003;124:1786–1791.

Nitsche R, Fölsch UR. Role of ERCP and endoscopic sphincterotomy in acute pancreatitis. *Baillieres Best Pract Res Clin Gastroenterol* 1999;13:331–343.

Ouest L, Lombard M. Pancreas divisum: opinio divisa. *Gut* 2000;47:317–319.

Steinberg WM. Should the sphincter of Oddi be measured in patients with idiopathic recurrent pancreatitis, and should sphincterotomy be performed if the pressure is high? *Pancreas* 2001;27:118–121.

Yadav D, Pitchumoni CS. Issues in hyperlipidemic pancreatitis. *J Clin Gastroenterol* 2003;36:54–62.

20 Treatment of acute pancreatitis in clinical practice: a global view

J. Enrique Domínguez-Muñoz

Most attacks of acute pancreatitis are mild, with recovery occurring within a few days of simple supportive therapy. Conversely, patients with severe pancreatitis are at high risk of developing pancreatic necrosis, organ failure, and septic complications, with death occurring in up to 25% of cases. The therapeutic goal in severe pancreatitis is to prevent development of complications. If these occur, early treatment is mandatory. Both in mild and severe pancreatitis, any potential etiologic factor should be corrected in order to prevent relapses.

Management of mild acute pancreatitis

Patients predicted to have mild pancreatitis are treated for a few days with simple supportive therapy consisting of nothing by mouth, intravenous fluids, and analgesics. Even in the presence of vomiting at onset, mild pancreatitis only exceptionally requires a nasogastric tube. Fluid replacement requires intravenous administration of 3–4 L of electrolyte fluids daily, which can be easily controlled by monitoring vital constants and urine output. Pain control in patients with mild pancreatitis can be achieved by regular intravenous administration of a nonopiate analgesic. Opiates (e.g., meperidine) may be additionally given on demand.

Once the patient is pain-free, gut peristalsis is present, and simple inflammatory markers (e.g., leukocytes) are becoming normal, oral nutrition can be progressively restarted. This occurs usually 2–4 days from onset of the disease. Finally, in cases of biliary etiology, patients should undergo cholecystectomy before hospital discharge.

Management of severe acute pancreatitis

Management of severe pancreatitis is based on four cornerstones:
- intensive monitoring and support of cardiac, pulmonary, renal, and hepatobiliary function;
- appropriate nutritional support;
- early treatment of biliary etiology;
- prevention of septic complications.

Acute pancreatitis is characterized by a narrow therapeutic window, which is most probably limited to the first 72 hours from onset of the disease. This is especially relevant in severe pancreatitis. Any therapeutic measure in severe acute pancreatitis should be applied early enough, within the time window of 72 hours from onset, in order to exert a positive effect on morbidity and mortality.

Intensive monitoring and systemic support

The principles of intensive monitoring and systemic support in severe acute pancreatitis are summarized in Table 20.1. Monitoring must include cardiac and respiratory frequency, arterial and central venous pressure, peripheral oxygen saturation, and urine output. Occasionally, monitoring of pulmonary capillary pressure is required.

Aggressive fluid resuscitation is particularly important in severe acute pancreatitis in order to prevent hypotension, acute tubular necrosis and, to some extent, pancreatic necrosis. Fluid requirements in severely affected patients may reach 6–10 L daily over the first days of disease. In these cases, plasma

Table 20.1 Basis of intensive management in severe acute pancreatitis.

Intensive invasive monitoring of vital constants
Analgesics (consider epidural analgesia if necessary)
Fluid resuscitation with monitoring of central venous pressure
   Electrolyte solutions
   Plasma expanders
Humidified oxygen administration
Catecholamines (dopamine, dobutamine)
Early nutritional support
Early treatment of systemic complications
   Mechanical ventilation with positive end-expiratory
     pressure
   Catecholamines (epinephrine)
   Hemofiltration, dialysis
   Insulin and calcium substitution

expanders are frequently required together with electrolyte solutions.

Respiratory insufficiency is the most frequent single organ failure in severe acute pancreatitis. Hypoxemia should be prevented by assuring the permeability of the airways and by additional humidified oxygen administration. Arterial oxygen saturation should be maintained above 95%. If respiratory insufficiency develops, mechanical ventilation with positive end-expiratory pressure is necessary.

Inotropic support with catecholamines should be used to prevent renal failure and shock. Low-dose dopamine (2–3 μg/kg per min), and better dobutamine, are useful for improving perfusion of abdominal organs. If shock develops, administration of other catecholamines such as epinephrine (adrenaline) is needed. If renal failure occurs, hemofiltration or dialysis should be started early in order to maintain adequate fluid resuscitation and nutrition.

Metabolic complications such as hyperglycemia and hypocalcemia should be treated by giving intravenous insulin and calcium.

Nutritional support

Severe acute pancreatitis is characterized by marked nutritional depletion. Thus, nutritional support is required with the goal of achieving a positive nitrogen balance. Since patients with severe acute pancreatitis may present with paralytic ileus and since maintaining pancreas at rest has been classically considered as mandatory, these patients have been typically fed parenterally. Parenteral nutrition is able to improve the evolution of severe pancreatitis, mainly if started within the first 72 hours of disease and if a positive nitrogen balance is obtained. The main disadvantage of parenteral nutrition in patients with severe acute pancreatitis is the risk of catheter sepsis.

Accumulated evidence over the last few years suggests that enteral feeding through a nasojejunal tube is not only safe but also effective in reducing the incidence of complications in patients with severe acute pancreatitis compared with parenteral feeding. This positive effect is probably achieved by the role of enteral nutrients on the maintenance of the intestinal barrier. Enteral feeding is also less expensive than parenteral nutrition and is now the preferred route of nutrition in severe acute pancreatitis. Recently, due to problems related to the placement of the nasojejunal tube, gastric nutrition through a nasogastric tube has been proposed as a safe and simpler alternative. If the volume of enteral nutrients tolerated by the patient is not enough to achieve nutritional goals, parenteral feeding should be instituted.

Early treatment of biliary etiology

Early endoscopic sphincterotomy in patients with severe acute biliary pancreatitis is associated with a lower incidence of complications and probably mortality secondary to the disease compared with the standard conservative treatment. This has been demonstrated in three relevant randomized controlled clinical trials and supported by a metaanalysis. As with other therapeutic measures, endoscopic sphincterotomy should be performed within the therapeutic window of acute pancreatitis, i.e., within 72 hours from onset of the disease.

There is no doubt that patients with acute pancreatitis and associated cholangitis or obstructive jaundice benefit from early endoscopic sphincterotomy. It seems to be also clear that early endoscopic sphincterotomy should not be performed in patients with mild pancreatitis. The question remains whether patients classified as suffering from severe biliary pancreatitis but without associated biliary sepsis or obstructive jaundice benefit from this endoscopic approach. This question was specifically addressed in a multicenter randomized clinical trial from Germany, although some important

177

methodologic limitations have hindered the relevance of the reported results.

From a practical point of view, patients with acute pancreatitis of suspected biliary etiology and classified as suffering from severe disease should undergo early endoscopic retrograde cholangiography; sphincterotomy should be performed where there is biliary sludge or stones within the common bile duct.

Prevention of septic complications

Infection of pancreatic necrosis is the most severe local complication and the leading cause of late death in patients with acute pancreatitis. In fact, mortality associated with acute necrotizing pancreatitis is significantly higher in infected than in sterile pancreatic necrosis. Because of this, prevention of infection of pancreatic necrosis is one of the major therapeutic goals in acute pancreatitis.

Translocation of bacteria from the gut is the main source of pancreatic infection. This is supported by several experimental studies as well as by analysis of the flora infecting pancreatic necrosis. Most of these organisms are enteric Gram-negative bacteria, basically *Escherichia coli*, as well as anaerobic organisms. Aerobic Gram-positive bacteria are also found, which proceed most probably from systemic foci (catheter sepsis, respiratory infections, etc.). As a consequence, any measure aiming to prevent infection of pancreatic necrosis should be effective against Gram-positive and Gram-negative aerobes as well as anaerobes.

Although infection of pancreatic necrosis becomes clinically evident from the third to fourth week of disease, contamination of the necrosis occurs much earlier, within the first 3–4 days from onset of disease. Therefore, measures to prevent infected pancreatic necrosis should be applied early, probably within the narrow therapeutic window of acute pancreatitis. In addition, extrapancreatic septic foci (e.g., catheter sepsis, pneumonia, urinary infection) should be treated early and efficiently in order to prevent bacteremia.

Together with enteral nutrition, which preserves the gut barrier, the risk of bacterial infection in acute necrotizing pancreatitis may be decreased by either selective decontamination of the gut or prophylactic systemic antibiotics. The effect of selective gut decontamination is unclear. A single clinical trial has shown a positive effect on morbidity and mortality, but a rather cumber-

some protocol was used and systemic antibiotics were additionally given.

Prophylactic systemic antibiotics are nowadays the procedure of choice to prevent infection of necrosis. Antibiotic prophylaxis is associated with a significant reduction of septic complications in acute necrotizing pancreatitis. Furthermore, a metaanalysis of eight controlled trials has shown that prophylactic antibiotics also reduce mortality.

The efficacy of antibiotic prophylaxis depends on two main factors.

- The beneficial effect is limited to patients with demonstrated necrotizing pancreatitis. Thus, the presence of necrosis should be demonstrated by dynamic computed tomography (CT) prior to antibiotic administration.
- Only broad-spectrum antibiotics capable of achieving therapeutic concentrations within the pancreas should be used. Among them, imipenem is probably the most appropriate. Imipenem is able to reduce the risk of septic complications in the context of acute necrotizing pancreatitis. Moreover, a comparative clinical trial showed a superior prophylactic effect of imipenem compared with fluoroquinolones. Finally, a recent randomized, double blind, placebo-controlled study found no positive effect of prophylactic administration of ciprofloxacin and metronidazole in preventing septic complications in severe acute pancreatitis.

From a practical point of view, dynamic CT should be performed between 48 and 72 hours from onset of the disease only in patients classified as suffering from severe acute pancreatitis (based on any of the prognostic markers mentioned in Chapter 6). If pancreatic necrosis is found, imipenem 500 mg q.i.d. should be administered intravenously for at least 14 days, and as long as failure of one or more organs persists. Because of the risk of fungal infection, prophylactic fluconazole is recommended for antibiotic administration that lasts for more than 2 weeks. If, despite prophylactic antibiotics, infection of pancreatic necrosis is suspected based on signs of sepsis or persistent organ failure, percutaneous fine-needle aspiration for Gram staining and culture is indicated. If bacterial infection is demonstrated, surgical necrosectomy is usually required.

Key messages for clinical practice

After assessment of the severity of the disease (see

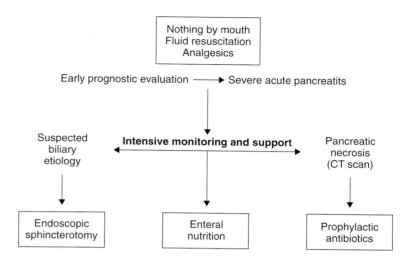

Figure 20.1 Approach to severe acute pancreatitis in clinical practice. CT, computed tomography.

Chapter 6), mild acute pancreatitis requires only adequate intravenous fluid substitution to avoid renal damage, analgesics, and nothing by mouth for 2–4 days. Severe acute pancreatitis should be managed in an intensive-care environment in order to apply intensive monitoring and systemic support. Together with this, three main therapeutic measures need to be applied: (i) early enteral nutrition, (ii) early endoscopic sphincterotomy for biliary etiology, and (iii) prophylactic antibiotics. This approach is summarized in Fig. 20.1.

Recommended reading

Al-Omram M, Groof A, Wilke D. Enteral versus parenteral nutrition for acute pancreatitis. *Cochrane Database of Systematic Reviews* 2003;1:CD002827.

Bassi C, Falconi M, Talamini G *et al.* Controlled clinical trial of pefloxacin versus imipenem in severe acute pancreatitis. *Gastroenterology* 1998;115:1513–1517.

Beger HG, Bittner R, Block S, Büchler M. Bacterial contamination of pancreatic necrosis. A prospective clinical study. *Gastroenterology* 1986;91:433–438.

Brown A, Baillargeon JD, Hughes MD, Banks PA. Can fluid resuscitation prevent pancreatic necrosis in severe acute pancreatitis? *Pancreatology* 2002;2:104–107.

Büchler M, Malfertheiner P, Friess H *et al.* Human pancreatic tissue concentration of bactericidal antibiotics. *Gastroenterology* 1992;103:1902–1908.

Dervenis C, Johnson CD, Bassi C *et al.* Diagnosis, objective assessment of severity and management of acute pancreatitis. Santorini consensus conference. *Int J Pancreatol* 1999;25:195–210.

Golub R, Siddiqi F, Pohl D. Role of antibiotics in acute pancreatitis: a meta-analysis. *J Gastrointest Surg* 1998;2:496–503.

Isenmann R, Runzi M, Kron M *et al.* Prophylactic antibiotic treatment in patients with predicted severe acute pancreatitis: a placebo-controlled, double-blind trial. *Gastroenterology* 2004;126:997–1004.

Kalfarentzos F, Kehagias J, Mead N *et al.* Enteral nutrition is superior to parenteral nutrition in severe acute pancreatitis: results of a randomized prospective trial. *Br J Surg* 1997; 84:1665–1669.

Luiten EJ, Hop WC, Lange JF, Bruining HA. Controlled clinical trial of selective decontamination for the treatment of severe acute pancreatitis. *Ann Surg* 1995;222:57–65.

Maraví-Poma E, Gener J, Alvarez-Lerma F, Olaechea P, Blanco A, Domínguez-Muñoz JE. Early antibiotic treatment (prophylaxis) of septic complications in severe acute necrotizing pancreatitis: a prospective, randomized, multicenter study comparing two regimens with imipenem–cilastatin. *Intensive Care Med* 2003;29:1974–1980.

Meier R, Beglinger C, Layer P *et al.* ESPEN guidelines on nutrition in acute pancreatitis. *Clin Nutr* 2002;21:173–183.

Sharma VK, Howden CW. Metaanalysis of randomized controlled trials of endoscopic retrograde cholangiography and endoscopic sphincterotomy for the treatment of acute biliary pancreatitis. *Am J Gastroenterol* 1999;94:3211–3214.

Windsor AC, Kanwar S, Li AG *et al.* Compared with parenteral nutrition, enteral feeding attenuates the acute phase response and improves disease severity in acute pancreatitis. *Gut* 1998;42:431–435.

21 Chronic pancreatitis: definition and classification for clinical practice

Peter Layer and Ulrike Melle

Introduction

Ideally, any definition and classification of chronic pancreatitis should be based on objective and reproducible criteria readily available during routine clinical workup. Clinical features should reflect corresponding underlying histopathologic changes, and both should be the common consequence of specific (or at least characteristic) etiopathogenic and pathophysiologic mechanisms. In particular, key clinical criteria and aspects (such as leading symptoms and signs as well as natural history, course, and prognosis) should be associated with distinctive diagnostic criteria as available from imaging and functional tests, and should translate into specific therapeutic approaches. Unfortunately, due to several reasons outlined below, definition and classification of chronic pancreatitis have remained difficult, and their current practical use does not meet these requirements.

The first accepted definition of chronic pancreatitis, based on clinical observations and surgical and pathologic findings, was suggested in 1946 by Comfort *et al.* They reported the chronic progressive and/or relapsing course of the disease, and commented on its association with long-standing alcoholic intake, its predominant onset in the third and fourth decades of life, and its typical complications.

The Symposium of Marseilles in 1963 defined and classified inflammatory pancreatic diseases in detail and created a coherent system that provided a workable clinical and scientific basis for the next two decades. It was primarily based on pathologic anatomy and on etiologic factors. Morphologically, chronic pancreatitis was characterized as irreversible irregular

sclerosis with destruction and loss of exocrine parenchyma. In contrast, acute pancreatitis was characterized as clinical and morphologic restitution of the pancreas if the cause of inflammation was eliminated, and was divided into an acute and a relapsing form. It was considered unusual for acute pancreatitis to develop into chronic pancreatitis. The Marseilles classification was focused primarily on alcohol-induced chronic pancreatitis, but also mentioned rarer forms of chronic pancreatitis, such as hereditary, vascular, endocrine, metabolic, and nutritional etiologies. The entity of obstructive chronic pancreatitis was grouped with chronic pancreatitis despite its potential reversibility. No attempts were made to correlate anatomic and functional changes, or to incorporate clinical course and severity.

During the following two decades, important pathogenetic, diagnostic, and therapeutic advances were made, including longitudinal studies on the natural course of the disease as well as the development of spectacular new imaging techniques such as ultrasound, computed tomography, and endoscopic retrograde cholangiopancreatography, and standardized functional tests. The resulting increased understanding of mechanisms and vastly improved diagnostic approaches made revision of the traditional classification system inevitable.

Hence, since the mid-1980s several symposia have reviewed the current level of knowledge of the disease processes from the standpoints of physicians, surgeons, radiologists, and pathologists, and revised the classification systems accordingly. Overall, although different approaches were taken, neither system incorporated the entire spectrum of criteria that had potential pathomechanistic and/or clinical relevance; a few major components are described below.

Histopathology

Chronic pancreatitis can be defined as continuing inflammatory disease of the pancreas with irreversible morphologic change in the gland's parenchymal as well as ductal system, which persists and/or progresses even if the primary cause or factors are eliminated, and results in functional loss. In this context, hemochromatosis and cystic fibrosis are not commonly classified as chronic pancreatitis. It has been emphasized that in obstructive chronic pancreatitis, characterized by dilatation of the ductal system, diffuse atrophy of the acinar parenchyma, fibrosis, and uncommonly calculi proximal to occlusion of the major duct, both structural and functional changes tend to improve when the obstruction is removed.

Morphologically, chronic pancreatitis was characterized by the Marseille classification as irregular sclerosis with destruction and/or loss of exocrine parenchyma (focal, segmental, or diffuse) irrespective of its etiology. It may be associated with varying degrees of dilatation of the duct system, which may be localized, and is usually (but not invariably) associated with strictures. The ducts may contain eosinophilic protein plugs and/or intraductal calcifications. Pseudocysts are common and usually communicate with the ductal system. All types of inflammatory cells as well edema, necrosis, or abscess formation can be found. Compared with the degree of acinar destruction, the islets of Langerhans are relatively well preserved.

Overall, the second Marseilles classification provided a clearer description of the morphologic changes and an emphasis on the irreversibility of all forms of chronic pancreatitis except obstructive chronic pancreatitis.

Nevertheless, tissue specimens are generally not available, because pancreatic biopsies are only of clinical importance in the case of pancreatic tumors, despite it being possible to obtain ultrasound-guided biopsies. Histopathologic specimens are often nonspecific for acute or chronic inflammation, and may reflect nonrepresentative sampling in cases of focal rather than diffuse inflammatory gland changes. Moreover, aging *per se* may induce histologic changes within the pancreas that are difficult to distinguish from chronic pancreatitis. Hence, for these reasons definition of chronic pancreatitis based on histology has never become clinically useful.

Etiology

The cause of pancreatitis should be elucidated whenever possible because of its potential implications for further management and prognosis.

In Western countries, 70–90% of all cases of chronic pancreatitis are related to alcohol ingestion. The risk of alcohol-induced pancreatitis increases logarithmically with increasing alcohol use without any threshold value. However, only 5–15% of heavy drinkers develop chronic pancreatitis, suggesting important cofactor(s), for example a diet high in fat and protein, deficiency in antioxidants or trace elements, and, last but not least, smoking.

There is convincing recent evidence that smoking is not only associated with alcohol use in the majority of patients but is also an independent etiologic and pathogenic factor, particularly for the formation of calcifications. It is still uncertain whether mutations in the genes for trypsinogen, serine protease inhibitor Kazal type 1 (*SPINK1*), or cystic fibrosis transmembrane conductance regulator (*CFTR*) are relevant cofactors in alcohol-induced chronic pancreatitis.

Tropical pancreatitis is the most common form of chronic pancreatitis in certain areas of India, Africa, Brazil, and Southeast Asia, and *SPINK1* mutations are crucially involved in its etiopathogenesis. Endocrine insufficiency is an inevitable consequence of the disease.

Hereditary pancreatitis is an autosomal dominant disorder associated with trypsinogen gene mutations that carries an 80% penetrance. It is a rare disease (about 1% of all cases of chronic pancreatitis) that presents typically in childhood or early adulthood.

Autoimmune pancreatitis is characterized by the presence of autoantibodies, elevated levels of immunoglobulins, enlargement and lymphocytic infiltration of the gland, and pancreatic duct strictures. It may be associated with other autoimmune diseases, such as Sjögren's syndrome, primary biliary cirrhosis, and primary sclerosing cholangitis. In the small number of patients reported, the disease has responded to glucocorticoid treatment. Immune mechanisms are also involved in pancreatitis associated with chronic inflammatory bowel diseases.

Obstruction of the main pancreatic duct by tumors,

scars, cysts, or stenosis of the papilla of Vater or minor papilla (e.g., in pancreas divisum) can produce pancreatitis in the parenchyma upstream of the obstruction. Obstructive chronic pancreatitis is a separate entity of chronic pancreatitis, because it tends to improve after removal of the obstruction.

Idiopathic chronic pancreatitis accounts for up to 10–25% of all cases of chronic pancreatitis, but some of these patients likely are mislabeled due to an underestimated alcohol input or undetected genetic abnormality. Based on age at onset of the clinical symptoms, the disease can be separated into two distinct entities: early- and late-onset idiopathic chronic pancreatitis. Early-onset disease becomes manifest in childhood or adolescence, usually with severe pain. Pancreatic calcifications and exocrine or endocrine insufficiency are rare at presentation, and develop slowly thereafter. There is evidence that *SPINK1* mutations may be involved in its genesis.

In contrast, late-onset disease presents with its first clinical symptoms following the fifth decade, and is associated less commonly with pain but more frequently with exocrine and endocrine insufficiency as the presenting symptom.

Clinical manifestations

The Marseille classification characterized the disease clinically by its recurrent or permanent abdominal pain and/or permanent loss of exocrine function.

Indeed, abdominal pain is considered the dominant clinical problem in patients with chronic pancreatitis. It is commonly described as boring, deep, penetrating, and localized in the epigastrium, often with radiation to the back. Pain may increase after a meal and often be associated with nausea and vomiting. Chronic severe pain impairs appetite and limits food intake, contributing to weight loss and malnutrition. In this way it leads to a reduction in the quality of life, and carries a potential for narcotic analgesic addiction.

The natural history of abdominal pain (character, timing, severity) is variable, but many studies have documented a decrease in pain ("burn out") over time in the majority of patients.

The strong reliance on pain as the crucial manifestation created a certain problem for the Marseille definition since a substantial group of patients with chronic pancreatitis may have primary painless disease, or only mild pain and the only morphologic evidence of an inflammatory process may be fibrosis indicating previous inflammation, with the clinical symptoms of steatorrhea and/or diabetes.

Nevertheless, the presence (or absence), degree, and course of pain counts among the principal clinical factors describing the disease.

Function

In most cases, exocrine pancreatic insufficiency occurs several years after the onset of chronic pancreatitis, mostly during the second decade of clinical disease, due to the substantial exocrine reserve capacity of the human pancreas. More than 90–95% of the secreting parenchyma need to be destroyed before malabsorption develops. In the case of exocrine pancreatic insufficiency, steatorrhea (often associated with malabsorption of the lipid-soluble vitamins A, D, E, and K) is generally more severe and occurs several years before clinical malabsorption of protein or carbohydrates, because the pancreatic synthesis and secretion of lipase is impaired more rapidly, its intraluminal survival is shorter due to its higher susceptibility to acidic and proteolytic denaturation, and its luminal digestive action is hardly compensated by nonpancreatic mechanisms. Weight loss may be absent or minimal, but patients with postprandial abdominal pain and nausea may lose weight due to fear of eating. Other patients may increase their caloric intake to compensate for maldigestion and stool losses. Endocrine pancreatic insufficiency (diabetes mellitus) is another consequence of long-standing destructive chronic pancreatitis.

Imaging

In contrast to the Marseille definition, the Cambridge classification incorporated the newer imaging tests into the heart of its diagnostic system and used them to grade disease severity. A grading system was developed for normal pancreas and equivocal, mild, moderate, and severe chronic pancreatitis for each of the imaging procedures (Table 21.1). This grading system has proved helpful to a certain extent in assessing or comparing disease manifestations clinically, although it has

Table 21.1 Grading of chronic pancreatitis by imaging methods.

	Endoscopic retrograde pancreatography	Ultrasound (US) or computed tomography (CT)
Normal	Good-quality study visualizing the whole gland without abnormal signs	Good-quality study visualizing the whole gland without abnormal signs
Equivocal	Less than three abnormal branches Normal main duct	One abnormal sign: main pancreatic duct 2–4 mm diameter
Mild	More than three abnormal branches Normal main duct	Two or more abnormal signs: Cyst < 10 mm Duct irregularity Focal acute pancreatitis Parenchymal heterogeneity Increased echogenicity of duct wall Contour irregularity of head/body
Moderate	As above with abnormal main duct	As above
Severe	All of the above with at least one of: Cyst > 10 mm Intraductal filling defects Calculi/pancreatic calcifications Duct obstruction (stricture) Severe duct dilatation or irregularity Contiguous organ invasion on US or CT	All of the above with at least one of: Cyst > 10 mm Intraductal filling defects Calculi/pancreatic calcifications Duct obstruction (stricture) Severe duct dilatation or irregularity Contiguous organ invasion on US or CT

remained uncertain whether it has therapeutic and prognostic implications. In particular, in many cases structural and functional changes are not associated, for example ductograms or scan may be normal in patients with proven disease and the presence of functional insufficiency or, conversely, abnormal images may be found but pancreatic function is unimpaired. Generally, the speed with which morphologic lesions and functional impairment develop, as well as the length of time before their detection by imaging and functional tests, differ widely among patients, and are only loosely correlated.

Imaging abnormalities that may be diagnostic include changes within the main pancreatic duct (dilatation, strictures, irregularity, pancreatic ductal stones), side branches of the pancreatic duct (dilatation, irregularity), or pancreatic parenchyma (lobularity, hyperechoic strands, enlargement or atrophy, and others). This has prompted a general classification of chronic pancreatitis as either "big-duct" or "small-duct" disease. "Big-duct" disease implies substantial abnormalities of the main pancreatic duct, is usually alcohol-induced, and is usually associated with functional abnormalities, whereas "small-duct" disease implies the absence of these findings and is less frequently associated with exocrine and endocrine pancreatic insufficiency. This distinction may have both diagnostic and therapeutic implications. The diagnosis of "big-duct" disease is simpler, and the treatment options may include endoscopic or surgical decompression of the dilated pancreatic duct. On the other hand, the diagnosis of "small-duct" disease may be more difficult: the roles of endosonographic ultrasound and functional magnetic resonance have not been defined satisfactorily in a prospective controlled fashion. Treatment may be restricted to medical therapy.

Chronic versus acute pancreatitis

The inability to clearly separate acute and chronic pancreatitis is generally considered to be a continuing major problem. In the early phases of alcohol-induced chronic pancreatitis, exacerbations closely resemble attacks of acute pancreatitis, and in clinical practice it may be impossible to distinguish the two entities. Moreover it is now generally recognized that alcohol-induced pancreatic disease may present both as acute pancreatitis and chronic pancreatitis with or without acute clinical bouts, but current routine diagnostic methods permit no distinction. Moreover, an important criterion of chronic pancreatitis is impairment of function, but following an acute attack decreased function may persist for a variable length of time and in varying degrees of severity, and may be irreversible.

On the other hand, in practical terms, prospective discrimination between acute pancreatitis and an acute attack of a future chronic pancreatitis may be irrelevant, in particular because initial clinical management is identical. Indeed, modern concepts such as the necrosis–fibrosis hypothesis postulate a common mechanism: chronic pancreatitis may be the result of repetitive attacks of focal necrotizing inflammation and subsequent scarring and fibrosis. Thus, it may be uncertain whether even typical acute and chronic pancreatitis are separate nosologic entities despite their different manifestations, but rather may be different syndromes of the same underlying disease.

Summary and suggestions

In any clinical setting suggestive of chronic pancreatitis, one should attempt to verify or exclude the diagnosis by utilizing available imaging and/or functional tests. In many cases, however, it may be difficult or even impossible to rely on a single test, and we suggest a combination of clinical, imaging, and functional criteria (Table 21.2). A substantial proportion of patients will not match these criteria, particularly in early disease stages prior to manifestation of coarse structural and/or functional defects, and until future development of more sensitive diagnostic techniques will have to be considered as "suspected" chronic pancreatitis and therefore, at least transiently, may escape diagnosis.

Once chronic pancreatitis is reasonably established, we suggest incorporating the following aspects into the diagnosis and description; these should be addressed in a standardized manner, independent of their presence or adequacy of information (Table 21.3).

1 Etiology of pancreatitis, as well as potential further pathogenic mechanisms.

Table 21.2 Diagnosis of chronic pancreatitis by scoring system.

Findings	Score
Pancreatic calcifications	4
Typical histologic changes	4
Characteristic findings on ERCP	3
Pancreatic exocrine insufficiency	2
Attacks of pancreatits and/or chronic upper abdominal pain	2
Diabetes mellitus	1

Diagnosis of chronic pancreatitis was established if a score of 4 or more was achieved

ERCP, endoscopic retrograde cholangiopancreatography.

2 Dominant clinical feature or status, particularly presence and grading of pain; presence, frequency, and severity of attacks.

3 Functional status, particularly presence and grading of exocrine and/or endocrine insufficiency.

4 Grading of morphologic changes on imaging, using the Cambridge classification (Table 21.1).

5 Presence and grading of complications.

A simple standardized structure for clinical classification is warranted for one particular reason: in contrast to most other major gastrointestinal diseases, chronic pancreatitis is characterized by a striking scarcity of large, controlled, prospective trials. As a result, we observe, with few exceptions, meager evidence for most therapeutic concepts and recommendations. A major reason for this unsatisfactory situation is the poor comparability and stratification of patient cohorts due to their nonstandardized classification (as an obvious result of the inherent problems outlined above). Thus, a rational, acceptable, and workable classification would greatly improve not only practical management but also the quality of future clinical research in the field of chronic pancreatitis.

Table 21.3 Diagnosis and classification of chronic pancreatitis.

Etiopathogenesis of chronic pancreatitis
Alcohol-induced
Mutations in *SPINK1*, trypsinogen, or *CFTR* genes?

Smoking

Hereditary
Trypsinogen gene mutations

Autoimmune

Metabolic/nutritional
Hypercalcemia
Hyperparathyroidism
Acquired or inherited hypertriglyceridemia

Tropical (SPINK1 mutations)
Tropical calcific pancreatitis
Fibrocalculous pancreatic diabetes

Idiopathic
Early-onset (*SPINK1* mutations)
Late-onset

Obstructive
Benign pancreatic duct obstruction
   Traumatic stricture
   Stricture after necrotizing pancreatitis
   Sphincter of Oddi stenosis
   Pancreas divisum (with inadequate accessory papilla)
   Sphincter of Oddi dysfunction?
   Stones
   Duodenal obstruction (diverticula, duodenal wall cysts)
Malignant pancreatic duct stricture
   Pancreatic, ampullary, or duodenal carcinoma

Clinical features
Grading of pain
Painless
Mild pain
Severe pain

Presence of pain
Continuous
Intermittent

Course of pain
Ameliorating
Persistent
Progressive

Grading of functional status
Exocrine insufficiency (steatorrhea)
No fecal fat excretion (< 7 g/day)
Mild fecal fat excretion (7–15 g/day)
Severe fecal fat excretion (> 15 g/day)

Endocrine insufficiency
None
Latent diabetes mellitus
Manifest diabetes mellitus

Grading of morphologic status by imaging (see Table 21.1)
Normal
Equivocal
Mild
Moderate
Severe

Complications
Cysts/pseudocysts with or without infections, abscesses
Portal hypertension caused by thrombosis of portal or splenic vein
Bleeding/pseudoaneurysms
Ascites
Obstruction/stricture of the ductus pancreaticus and/or choledochus
Pancreatic fistula
Duodenal stenosis
Pancreatic cancer

CFTR, cystic fibrosis transmembrane conductance regulator; SPINK1, serine protease inhibitor Kazal type 1.

Recommended reading

Ammann RW, Heitz PU, Kloppel G. The "two-hit" pathogenetic concept of chronic pancreatitis. *Int J Pancreatol* 1999;25:251.

Axon AT, Classen M, Cotton PB, Cremer M, Freeny PC, Lees WR. Pancreatography in chronic pancreatitis: international definitions. *Gut* 1984;25:1107–1112.

Bourliere M, Barthet M, Berthezene P, Durbec JP, Sarles H. Is tobacco a risk factor for chronic pancreatitis and alcoholic cirrhosis? *Gut* 1991;32:1392–1395.

Chari ST, Singer MV. The problem of classification and staging of chronic pancreatitis. Proposals based on current knowledge of its natural history. *Scand J Gastroenterol* 1994;29:949–960.

Horiuchi A, Kawa S, Akamatsu T *et al*. Characteristic pancreatic duct appearance in autoimmune chronic pancreatitis: a case report and review of the Japanese literature. *Am J Gastroenterol* 1998;93:260–263.

Imoto M, DiMagno EP. Cigarette smoking increases the risk of pancreatic calcification in late-onset but not early-onset idiopathic chronic pancreatitis. *Pancreas* 2000;21:115–119.

Kloppel G. Progression from acute to chronic pancreatitis. A pathologist's view. *Surg Clin North Am* 1999;79:801–814.

Lankisch PG, Assmus C, Maisonneuve P, Lowenfels AB. Epidemiology of pancreatic diseases in Luneburg County. A study in a defined German population. *Pancreatology* 2002;2:469–477.

Layer P, DiMagno EP. Early and late onset in idiopathic and alcoholic chronic pancreatitis. Different clinical courses. *Surg Clin North Am* 1999;79:847–860.

Layer P, Holtmann G. Pancreatic enzymes in chronic pancreatitis. *Int J Pancreatol* 1994;15:1–11.

Layer P, von der Ohe M, Gröger G, Dicke D, Goebell H. Luminal availability and digestive efficacy of substituted enzymes in pancreatic insufficiency. *Pancreas* 1992;7:745.

Layer P, Yamamoto H, Kalthoff L, Clain JE, Bakken LJ, DiMagno EP. The different courses of early- and late-onset idiopathic and alcoholic chronic pancreatitis. *Gastroenterology* 1994;107:1481–1487.

Layer P, Keller J, Lankisch PG. Pancreatic enzyme replacement therapy. *Curr Gastroenterol Rep* 2001;3:101–108.

Levy P, Mathurin P, Roqueplo A, Rueff B, Bernades P. A multidimensional case–control study of dietary, alcohol, and tobacco habits in alcoholic men with chronic pancreatitis. *Pancreas* 1995;10:231–238.

Lin Y, Tamakoshi A, Hayakawa T, Ogawa M, Ohno Y. Cigarette smoking as a risk factor for chronic pancreatitis: a case–control study in Japan. Research Committee on Intractable Pancreatic Diseases. *Pancreas* 2000;21:109–114.

Lowenfels AB, Maisonneuve P, Cavallini G *et al*. Prognosis of chronic pancreatitis: an international multicenter study. International Pancreatitis Study Group. *Am J Gastroenterol* 1994;89:1467–1471.

Pfutzer RH, Barmada MM, Brunskill AP *et al*. SPINK1/PSTI polymorphisms act as disease modifiers in familial and idiopathic chronic pancreatitis. *Gastroenterology* 2000;119:615–623.

Sarles H. Definitions and classifications of pancreatitis. *Pancreas* 1991;6:470–474.

Sarner M, Cotton PB. Classification of pancreatitis. *Gut* 1984;25:756–759.

Sarner M, Cotton PB. Definitions of acute and chronic pancreatitis. *Clin Gastroenterol* 1984;13:865–870.

Schneider A, Suman A, Rossi L *et al*. SPINK1/PSTI mutations are associated with tropical pancreatitis and type II diabetes mellitus in Bangladesh. *Gastroenterology* 2002;123:1026–1030.

Singer MV, Gyr K, Sarles H. Revised classification of pancreatitis. Report of the Second International Symposium on the Classification of Pancreatitis in Marseille, France, March 28–30, 1984. *Gastroenterology* 1985;89:683–685.

Standop J, Standop S, Itami A *et al*. ErbB2 oncogene expression supports the acute pancreatitis–chronic pancreatitis sequence. *Virchows Arch* 2002;441:385–391.

Truninger K, Witt H, Kock J *et al*. Mutations of the serine protease inhibitor, Kazal type 1 gene, in patients with idiopathic chronic pancreatitis. *Am J Gastroenterol* 2002;97:1133–1137.

Worning H. Alcoholic chronic pancreatitis. In: HG Beger, AL Warshaw, MW Büchler *et al*. (eds) *The Pancreas*. Oxford: Blackwell Science, 1998:672.

22 Epidemiology of chronic pancreatitis: an infrequent disease or an infrequently diagnosed disease?

Salvador Navarro and Antonio Soriano

Chronic pancreatitis is an inflammatory process that leads to the progressive and irreversible destruction of exocrine and endocrine glandular pancreatic tissue and its substitution by fibrotic tissue. As a result, a series of morphologic and functional alterations can be detected which are responsible for the characteristic symptoms of this disease.

This symptomatology appears according to the degree of morphologic change caused by various etiologic factors. At the onset, when these changes are less developed, clinical manifestations might be nonexistent or limited to purely dyspeptic symptoms. In contrast, when changes are fully established, they become morphologically and functionally evident and symptoms are clearly recognizable. Thus chronic pancreatitis undergoes transformation of various degrees from the onset through to the most developed stage, and this may be divided into four stages: an initial latent or subclinical period is followed by an early second stage with inflammatory complications; the third or late period shows exocrine pancreatic insufficiency and the fourth is identified as the advanced or painless stage.

1 The latent or subclinical period might last from 1 to 20 years, during which patients show no symptoms but have usually consumed large quantities of alcohol. At this stage two subperiods might be identified: an early stage where the small cellular alterations are reversible and a later period of irreversible histologic changes. Only when these histologic lesions, characteristic of chronic pancreatitis, have caused considerable damage do the symptoms of the disease become observable. During this latent period, sonography and even helical computed tomography (CT) may not guarantee a successful diagnosis. However, according to previous studies, endoscopic retrograde cholangiopancreatography (ERCP) may show the equivocal changes of the Cambridge classification. Exocrine pancreatic function may be normal or show a certain degree of hyperfunction.

2 The second period, the early stage involving inflammatory complications, lasts for 5 or 6 years after the first symptoms or until the development of severe exocrine pancreatic insufficiency. Pain and inflammatory complications like pseudocysts, stenosis of the biliary tract, and splenic vein thrombosis are frequent. Surgery is often needed. The histologic lesions harden and increase gland size in different areas and to varying degrees. Pseudocysts and focal fat necrosis occur often, whereas calculi appear less frequently. Exocrine function may show slight insufficiency or be normal. Gland lesions and related complications may be detected by imaging techniques.

3 The late period or period of exocrine pancreatic insufficiency appears some 8 years after the initial symptoms. Pain persists and exocrine function decreases, inducing steatorrhea. Surgery is required to relieve pain.

4 The advanced or painless period marks the final stage of the disease. Pain may have been relieved spontaneously or by surgery; the exocrine function of the pancreas has totally deteriorated and usually diabetes occurs.

In the Western world, 66–80% of cases of chronic pancreatitis are a result of high alcohol consumption. The remaining cases are not related to alcohol abuse but to genetic factors favoring its development in the early or later periods. Chronic pancreatitis may start earlier due to a dominant genetic mutation that enhances its development even in the absence of alcohol; in chronic pancreatitis starting later, the genetic mutation is less dominant. All these factors make us believe that the success of epidemiologic research depends primarily on the stage of the disease at examination, because patient selection depends on the examiner's degree of suspicion of the disease, its clinical manifestations, and the extent of morphologic and functional lesions.

Studies of chronic pancreatitis should therefore take into account that the disease does not always occur in chronic alcoholics and that only 5–15% of heavy consumers of alcohol develop it. The disease may appear at any moment in a patient's life and the lesions, depending on the stage of the disease, may be incipient and impossible to demonstrate since the available techniques lack sensitivity. Epidemiologic studies should thus address multiple questions, such as the following.

- Are all patients with a given pathology considered?
- When can patients be considered to be suffering from a determined pathology?
- When should the various examination techniques be used to obtain information about a given disease in a patient?
- Are available techniques of diagnosis sensitive enough to identify all patients?

In the context of chronic pancreatitis, and especially with regard to the role of alcohol as the most frequent etiology, one should consider that alcohol consumption might precede the symptoms by 10–20 years and only after a relatively long period of consumption do the first histologic alterations typical of the disease start to appear. In this relatively unknown time period, patients show no symptoms until the histologic alterations are sufficiently advanced. Initially, these may be limited to purely dyspeptic discomfort. At this stage, the investigator's degree of suspicion of the diagnosis is of utmost importance in initiating imaging and functional tests. However, in some difficult cases, confirmation of the initial suspicion remains impossible due to the fact that diagnostic methods lack sensitivity and specificity. In these and many other cases, the disease cannot be diagnosed until the symptoms are sufficiently evident (Fig. 22.1).

One might regard histologic changes as the gold standard for identification of a disease. In the case of chronic pancreatitis, the histologic alterations in pancreatic structure include fibrosis and inflammation, both of irregular distribution, and the progressive loss

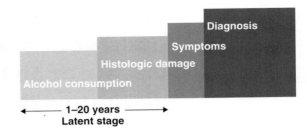

Figure 22.1 Evolutionary stages of chronic pancreatitis from initial alcohol consumption until diagnosis.

of acinar cells and islets. Using a combination of these phenomena, and their abundance, pathologists have proposed a classification that differentiates chronic pancreatitis into cases of minimum, moderate, and severe histologic changes. As expected, minimum alterations are typical of the initial phase of the disease and consist of loss of a small number of acini and their substitution by small areas of fibrosis. During the stage of moderate changes, loss of acini is more significant and fibrotic areas are more extensive and associated with lymphocyte and fibroblast infiltrates. The islets of Langerhans and intralobular ducts are relatively distorted. In the advanced phase of pancreatitis, the changes are severe and show an almost complete disappearance of the typical acinar picture and of the islets, which have been replaced by wide bands of fibrosis completely surrounding the nerve strands. Severe distortions of the pancreatic duct system may also be observed (Fig. 22.2).

However, this type of histologic classification has manifold shortcomings. On the one hand, we lack a well-established system that allows us to quantify the degree of tissue damage in a sufficiently objective way. On the other hand, the histologic changes are spread over different areas and to various degrees. Consequently, the nature of the histologic findings depends on the zone explored. Furthermore, the typically large areas of fibrotic tissue and its resulting toughness make it difficult for the method of fine-needle biopsy to extract a sample representative enough to allow a satisfactory medical report. Finally, the ethical aspects of these methods should be considered. How may the use of fine-needle biopsy be justified in patients who are asymptomatic or have unspecific symptoms? The risk involved may not be justified by an epidemiologic study

Figure 22.2 Development of the histologic lesions of chronic pancreatitis (hematoxylin and eosin). (a) In the central area, acini have disappeared and been replaced by fibrotic tissue and inflammatory cells typical of the onset of the disease. ×40. (b) Fibrotic zones surround the acini and islets of Langerhans. ×40. (c) Extensive areas of fibrosis have substituted zones of exocrine parenchyma. Pancreatic ductuli are large, containing protein substance (arrow). ×40. (d) In the central area, there is a hypertrophied nerve strand, completely surrounded by fibrotic tissue and an infiltrate of inflammatory cells on one of its edges (arrow), marking the final stage of chronic pancreatitis. ×100. (Courtesy of Dr Rosa Miguel, Department of Pathology, Hospital Clínic, Barcelona.)

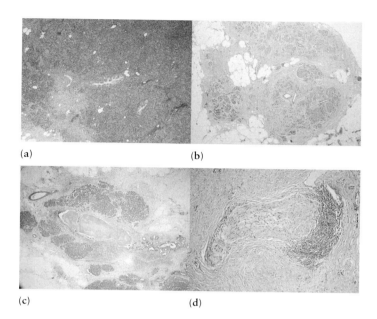

(a)　(b)　(c)　(d)

searching for a pathology that does not cause any discomfort and whose progressive lesions may not be avoidable, except by a recommendation to stop alcohol consumption, advice which should be given to any heavy drinker.

Nothing is yet known about the exact degree of histologic lesions necessary for the appearance of the morphologic and functional changes identified by current diagnostic techniques nor the degree of histologic change necessary for manifestation of the first symptoms of chronic pancreatitis. Consequently, epidemiologic research into chronic pancreatitis should take into account three types of history of the populations evaluated: asymptomatic, atypical, and typical chronic pancreatitis. This differentiation is of utmost importance for establishing criteria for suspected diagnosis in incidence studies designed to detect new cases of the disease, as well as for prevalence studies defining the population to be studied. Another interesting aspect is the definition of risk factors (alcohol consumption and genetic change) leading to patient selection and diagnosis, since not all alcoholics, as mentioned above, develop chronic pancreatitis and not every case is alcohol-induced.

The final key aspect is evaluation of the value and applicability of the different methods used for diagnosis of chronic pancreatitis. It is essential to evaluate the cost–benefit relation of the various techniques and if the discovery of chronic pancreatitis before the first clinical manifestations benefits the patient. Helical CT may be used as the initial imaging test for diagnosis and determination of the severity of chronic pancreatitis, since it is noninvasive and its sensitivity allows identification of the disease in moderate and severe stages. It reveals the existence of pancreatic calcifications, dilation of the Wirsung duct, presence of cavities, and atrophy of parenchyma. In addition, previous studies show good correlation between data obtained by CT and degree of histologic change. ERCP is another technique that allows differentiation between moderate and severe stages of the disease, although it is sometimes very difficult to establish criteria for the mild stage. Magnetic resonance cholangiopancreatography (MRCP) is a noninvasive technique that does not require systematic sedation and provides resolution of up to 1 mm. It produces results that can be combined with those from CT of the parenchyma and those from ERCP of the pancreatic duct. Nevertheless, small changes in the secondary ducts are not easily detected and MRCP lacks the therapeutic potential of ERCP. Endoscopic ultrasonography plays an important role in the diagnosis of pancreatic pathology. It has good sensitivity (resolution 1 mm), the advantage of avoiding ionized radiation, and allows the extraction of tissue and pancreatic juice, and is therefore a very useful technique especially since its results can be combined with results from imaging, pancreatic function tests, histology, and molecular markers. Unfortunately, it depends entirely on the experience of the examiner.

The above-mentioned tests are clearly acceptable in cases of patients with suspected chronic pancreatitis. However, their use in incidence and prevalence studies of asymptomatic populations remains questionable since the use of diagnostic methods and imaging techniques such as helical CT and MRCP are expensive and lack discriminative sensitivity. In addition, endoscopic ultrasonography is invasive and ERCP is not free of complications. Abdominal ultrasonography is the only feasible technique from an economic point of view but its diagnostic power with regard to chronic pancreatitis is very limited in the initial stage. When examining the methods for testing exocrine function, the same criteria of diagnostic performance and cost should be taken into account. The secretin–cerulein test permits early diagnosis but, despite being the most sensitive technique, remains difficult to apply in population studies due to its invasiveness and high cost. A further drawback is the enormous difference in the standardization of technique and of normality and abnormality. Also, the secretin–cerulein test should only be applied in cases where there is a reasonable suspicion of the diagnosis. However, incidence and prevalence studies should include populations with little or no symptomatology. Among noninvasive modalities, the pancreaolauryl test and determination of fecal elastase may be used for screening of suspect chronic pancreatitis populations since they have been very useful in cases of severe pancreatic exocrine insufficiency and are reasonably sensitive in moderate stages of the disease. However, their efficiency remains doubtful in detection of the initial stages.

This complex situation, involving patients generally asymptomatic or with atypical symptoms, and diagnostic methods with serious limitations, results in a lack of sufficiently reliable and veracious epidemiologic information. The literature on incidence and prevalence studies of chronic pancreatitis is not very abundant. A study in the Copenhagen area in the 1970s states an incidence of 6.9–10 new cases per 100 000 inhabitants per year. It should be mentioned that the researchers had to make a distinction between verified and possible chronic pancreatitis since they regarded more than half of the cases as not plainly verified. In the

Cantabria region of Spain between 1981 and 1991, De las Heras found an incidence of 14/100 000 and a prevalence of 18.3 /100 000, 80% alcohol-induced, constituting one of the highest incidences worldwide. More recent studies have observed clear geographic differences, ranging from 1.6 new cases per 100 000 per year in Switzerland, 7.9 /100 000 per year in the Czech Republic (very similar to Denmark and Germany), to 23/100 000 per year in Finland. Some studies have found an important increase in the number of patients with chronic pancreatitis admitted to hospitals. In the UK, this increase came to 100% during the period 1989–90 to 1999–2000. Japan also registered an increase, from 32 000 in 1994 to 42 000 in 1999, figures which represent an increase in prevalence from 28.5 to 32.9/100 000 and in incidence from 5.4 to 5.7/100 000. This increase in diagnosis may have happened for two reasons: (i) the development of new diagnostic methods and improvement of existing techniques (refinement of equipment and growing experience of examiners); and (ii) higher alcohol consumption.

Prevalence may also vary according to population characteristics. Banciu *et al.* identified chronic pancreatitis in 41% of cases by performing abdominal ultrasonography on alcoholic patients who were originally examined for other clinical reasons. On the other hand, a Spanish study in the Mediterranean region evaluating sonography and CT of 105 alcoholic patients belonging to a rehabilitation program and who never displayed any pancreatic symptoms found that only 3.5% showed morphologic changes of mild chronic pancreatitis. Nevertheless, a pancreolauryl test assessing exocrine pancreatic function showed that 26% of patients were afflicted with moderate exocrine insufficiency and 9% with steatorrhea. However, if population studies consist of autopsy material, the percentage may be completely different, as shown in a report by Suda *et al*. In this study, 33 of 46 patients (72%) with verified alcohol dependence, but who died of different causes than alcoholism, showed major histologic changes of the pancreatic gland, especially proliferation of fibrotic tissue, despite never having displayed a symptomotology that would have led to the suspected diagnosis of chronic pancreatitis.

These examples reinforce the view that one should pay special attention to the existence of a latent period, where morphologic and/or functional alterations occur that may remain inconspicuous and not lead to the symptomatology of chronic pancreatitis, thus preventing a suspected diagnosis. Consequently, cases of diagnosed chronic pancreatitis may only be the tip of the iceberg, mainly because there might be an invisible but numerous population of alcoholic individuals with pancreatic lesions but no symptomotology and who therefore have been neither examined nor diagnosed. Because of this, one should always be on the lookout for the appearance of any of the possible symptoms which might lead to the manifestation of chronic pancreatitis, especially since the examiner's suspicion will determine an early diagnosis and put an end to chronic pancreatitis as an infrequently diagnosed disease.

Recommended reading

Andersen BN, Pedersen NT, Scheel J, Worning H. Incidence of alcoholic chronic pancreatitis in Copenhagen. *Scand J Gastroenterol* 1982;17:247–252.

Aparisi L, Navarro S, Pérez-Mateo M, Bautist D. Prevalencia de la disfunción pancreática y de la desnutrición en pacientes alcohólicos en programa de deshabituación. *Med Clin (Barc)* 2000;114:444–448.

Banciu T, Susan L, Jovin G, Sporea I, Vacariu V. Prevalence of chronic (latent) pancreatitis in hospitalized chronic consumers of alcohol. *Rom J Intern Med* 1991;29:49–53.

Boeck WG, Adler G, Gress ThM. Pancreatic function tests: when to choose, what to use. *Curr Gastroenterol Rep* 2001;3:95–100.

Chari ST, Singer MV. The problem of classification and staging of chronic pancreatitis. Proposals based on current knowledge of its natural history. *Scand J Gastroenterol* 1994;29:949–960.

De las Heras G, Pons F. Epidemiología y aspectos etiopatogénicos de la pancreatitis alcohólica crónica. *Rev Esp Enferm Dig* 1993;84:253–258.

Dite P, Stary K, Novotny I *et al*. Incidence of chronic pancreatitis in the Czech Republic. *Eur J Gastroenterol* 2001; 13:749–750.

Dominguez-Muñoz E, Hieronymus C, Sauerbruch T, Malfertheiner P. Fecal elastase test: evaluation of a new non-invasive pancreatic function test. *Am J Gastroentrerol* 1995;90:1834–1837.

Etemad B, Whitcomb DC. Chronic pancreatitis: diagnosis, classification, and new genetic developments. *Gastroenterology* 2001;120:682–707.

Lankisch PG. Progression from acute to chronic pancreatitis: a physician's view. *Surg Clin North Am* 1999;79:815–827.

Lankisch PG, Assmus C, Maisonneuve P, Lowenfels AB. Epidemiology of pancreatic diseases in Luneburg County. A study in a defined German population. *Pancreatology* 2002;2:469–477.

Otsuki M. Chronic pancreatitis in Japan: epidemiology, prognosis, diagnostic criteria, and future problems. *J Gastroenterol* 2003;38:315–326.

Sarner M, Cotton PB. Classification of pancreatitis. *Gut* 1984;25:756–759.

Suda K, Shiotsu H, Nakamura T, Akai J, Nakamura T. Pancreatic fibrosis in patients with chronic alcohol abuse: correlation with alcoholic pancreatitis. *Am J Gastroenterol* 1994;89:2060–2063.

Thuluvanth PJ, Imperio D, Nair S, Cameron JL. Chronic pancreatitis. Long-term pain relief with or without surgery, cancer risk, and mortality. *J Clin Gastroenterol* 2003;36: 159–165.

Tinto A, Lloyd DA, Kang JY *et al*. Acute and chronic pancreatitis-diseases on the rise: a study of hospital admissions in England 1989/90–1999/2000. *Aliment Pharmacol Ther* 2002;16:2097–2105.

Wallace MB, Hawes RH. Endoscopic ultrasound in the evolution and treatment of chronic pancreatitis. *Pancreas* 2001;23:26–35.

23 Etiopathogenesis of chronic pancreatitis: a genetic disease with some precipitating factors?

Georgios I. Papachristou and David C. Whitcomb

Chronic pancreatitis constitutes a major source of morbidity worldwide. Less than a decade ago, chronic pancreatitis was considered an "enigmatic process of uncertain pathogenesis, unpredictable clinical course, and unclear treatment." However, remarkable progress is being made in the understanding of the etiopathogenesis of the chronic pancreatitis syndrome. The breakthrough for this advancement came with the application of molecular genetics to a rare inherited form of acute and chronic pancreatitis known as hereditary pancreatitis. These studies provided the framework for understanding the complex genetic, environmental, and immunologic factors associated with susceptibility to acute pancreatitis and the initiation and progression toward chronic pancreatitis.

Etiology

Until recently, the etiology of chronic pancreatitis was divided into three categories: alcohol, idiopathic, and "other." Excessive alcohol consumption was thought to be the most common cause, accounting for 70–80% of all cases in the Western world. About 20% of cases were considered idiopathic pancreatitis, while the remaining 10% was categorized as "other" and included cases associated with hyperparathyroidism, hypertriglyceridemia, duct obstruction, trauma, pancreas divisum, autoimmune pancreatitis, and hereditary pancreatitis. With the discovery of pancreatitis-associated gene mutations and the recognition that alcohol alone seldom causes chronic pancreatitis, a new classification system was needed.

TIGAR-O risk factor classification

In 2001, the TIGAR-O classification system was published. This system is based on the mechanism of injury and addresses the risk, etiology, and complexity of chronic pancreatitis. Multiple lines of evidence now suggest that chronic pancreatitis is a complex disorder that may involve the interaction of two or more environmental or genetic factors. The TIGAR-O model addresses this potential synergistic role of multiple risk factors in a single individual with chronic pancreatitis, and allows one to organize and assess the level of contribution of each of the interacting risk factors. In this way, risk-reduction strategies and specific therapies can be instituted. Although the critical information about different forms of chronic pancreatitis is not fully available, the TIGAR-O system lays the foundation for further advancement in the field. The major categories include toxic–metabolic (T), idiopathic (I), genetic (G), autoimmune (A), recurrent severe acute pancreatitis-associated (R), and obstructive (O) mechanisms. The TIGAR-O classification also organizes the etiologies, in general, by prevalence.

Toxic and metabolic factors

Alcohol An association between alcohol and chronic pancreatitis was first described by Comfort and colleagues more than 50 years ago. There is a general logarithmic relationship between the risk of chronic pancreatitis and the amount of alcohol consumed. However, there is no apparent threshold value below which the disease does not occur. This makes it difficult to distinguish between low-threshold alcohol-induced pancreatitis and idiopathic chronic pancreatitis. The duration of alcohol consumption is also important. In general, prolonged alcohol intake is required for the development of chronic pancreatitis. In most patients, the onset of alcoholic chronic pancreatitis occurs after alcohol intake that exceeds 150 g/day for at least 10–15 years.

It is observed that only a minority (~ 5%) of heavy drinkers ultimately develop chronic pancreatitis. Therefore, alcohol consumption is not an independent risk factor for chronic pancreatitis. Rather, it appears to be a cofactor associated with pancreatitis only in conjunction with a specific trigger, or other additional predisposing genetic or environmental factors whose identity currently eludes us. Based on epidemiologic studies, there is evidence of a genetic basis in alcoholic pancreatitis. However, studies of mutations in the major alcohol-metabolizing genes (e.g., aldehyde dehydrogenase), cationic trypsinogen gene, cystic fibrosis transmembrane conductance regulator (CFTR) gene, and human leukocyte antigen (HLA) failed to identify an alcoholic pancreatitis-associated gene mutation.

The relationship between acute and chronic alcoholic pancreatitis has been debated. Clinically, there is usually an initial period of recurrent acute attacks lasting for several years, followed by the development of chronic pain and functional insufficiencies. It was believed, based on studies of natural history, that at the time of the initial attack of acute alcoholic pancreatitis there is already histologic evidence of chronic disease. However, the studies of Ammann and associates, as well as the observations in families with hereditary pancreatitis, provide strong evidence that recurrent attacks of acute alcoholic pancreatitis precede chronic disease.

Tobacco smoking The independent causative effect of tobacco smoking on chronic pancreatitis has been confirmed in research studies, with odds ratios ranging from 7.8 to 17.3. The exact mechanism is unknown, although tobacco smoking inhibits pancreatic bicarbonate secretion in humans. The effects of tobacco smoking may also be potentiated by polymorphisms in the gene for uridine 5′-diphosphate (UDP) glucuronosyltransferase (UGT1A7) (see below), especially the UGT1A7*3 haplotype. The risk of pancreatitis in patients with the UGTA7*3 genotype was reported to be associated with alcohol drinking, but since the majority of these subjects smoked, it was not possible to determine which of these environmental factors was responsible. However, this family of enzymes is responsible for detoxifying complex products of tobacco smoke, so an association with tobacco smoking is more likely.

Idiopathic chronic pancreatitis
Idiopathic chronic pancreatitis is reported to account for 10–30% of all cases of chronic pancreatitis. The category of idiopathic chronic pancreatitis includes a number of well-described symptoms and also cases where an associated factor cannot be identified. As new genetic, environmental, and metabolic factors are discovered, the number of patients in this category is expected to diminish. Nonalcoholic chronic pancreatitis has pathologic characteristics distinct from those of alcoholic chronic pancreatitis, including T-lymphocytic infiltrates around interlobular ducts resulting in ductal obstruction and destruction and acinar atrophy and fibrosis.

Idiopathic chronic pancreatitis shows a bimodal pattern regarding age of onset. Early-onset idiopathic pancreatitis has a mean age of onset of around 20 years. Pain is the predominant feature of this disease, occurring in 96% of patients, whereas pancreatic calcifications, exocrine insufficiency, or endocrine insufficiency are extremely rare at presentation (< 10%). Late-onset idiopathic pancreatitis has a mean age of onset of 56 years. It tends to follow a comparatively painless course associated with the frequent development of pancreatic calcifications and exocrine and endocrine insufficiency. Pfützer and associates recently found mutations in the gene for the serine protease inhibitor Kazal type 1 (SPINK1) in about 25% of patients with idiopathic chronic pancreatitis, mainly related with early-onset disease.

Minimal-change chronic pancreatitis refers to the syndrome of severe abdominal pain, which is presumed to be pancreatic in origin with minimal changes on imaging studies. Minimal-change chronic pancreatitis is most often seen in middle-aged women.

Tropical pancreatitis is considered a type of idiopathic chronic pancreatitis occurring in tropical areas. It is the most common form of chronic pancreatitis in certain areas of India and is generally a disease of youth and early adulthood. It is subgrouped into tropical calcific pancreatitis, characterized by severe abdominal pain and extensive pancreatic calcifications, and fibrocalculous pancreatic diabetes, characterized by diabetes mellitus as the first clinical sign. The exact etiology of tropical pancreatitis remains unknown.

Rossi was the first to identify an excess of the *SPINK1* N34S haplotype in tropical pancreatitis, suggesting that excess trypsinogen activation was associated with a component of the injury process. This was confirmed in all forms of tropical pancreatitis, including fibrocalculous pancreatic diabetes, tropical calcific pancreatitis, and a subset of cases of non-insulin-dependent diabetes mellitus, with the latter group possibly representing pancreatic injury without calcification. Further major insights into the two forms of tropical pancreatitis are likely in the near future.

Genetic predispositions

The mutations associated with acute recurrent or chronic pancreatitis that have been identified will be discussed in detail later. It is important to understand that genetic disorders can occur through mutations in different disease-associated gene classes. Disease-causing genes refer to dominant mutations in a single allele that cause the disease (gain-of-function mutations, e.g., R122H mutation in hereditary pancreatitis) or to recessive mutations in both alleles of a single gene (ΔF508 deletion in typical cystic fibrosis). These mutations result in mendelian patterns of inheritance within families. Susceptibility genes are genes with mutations that alone are not disease-causing, but increase the risk of disease and confer unique phenotypic features (*SPINK1* mutations in chronic pancreatitis). Finally, modifier of response genes refer to mutations that alone are not disease-causing but which alter the course of an established disease by determining the severity and complications (mutations in key genes of inflammatory pathways that drive chronic inflammation and fibrosis yet to be identified). Some modifier gene mutations may represent relatively common polymorphisms that under special conditions contribute to the overall phenotypic features of pancreatitis.

Autoimmune chronic pancreatitis

Autoimmune chronic pancreatitis is a distinct entity characterized by the presence of autoantibodies, elevated levels of immunoglobulins, and unique pathologic features comprising a dense lymphocytic infiltrate and ductal destruction with acinar atrophy. In 60% of cases, it is associated with other autoimmune diseases, such as primary sclerosing cholangitis, primary biliary cirrhosis, autoimmune hepatitis, Sjögren's syndrome, and other immune-mediated inflammatory disorders. It is important for the clinician to promptly make the

diagnosis of autoimmune chronic pancreatitis because it seems to respond to glucocorticosteroid treatment.

Recurrent and severe acute pancreatitis

As previously mentioned, the association between recurrent acute and chronic pancreatitis is well established nowadays. Evidence suggests that recurrent acute pancreatitis leads to chronic pancreatitis. The etiologies of recurrent acute pancreatitis and chronic pancreatitis are impressively similar. Therefore, several disorders characterized as causing acute pancreatitis may lead to progression to chronic pancreatitis.

Obstructive chronic pancreatitis

Obstructive chronic pancreatitis refers to a distinct entity produced by a usually single dominant narrowing of the main pancreatic duct. It is characterized by upstream ductal dilation, acinar cell atrophy, and diffuse fibrosis. A number of distinct causes can produce obstructive chronic pancreatitis, such as trauma, sphincter of Oddi dysfunction, pancreas divisum, and sequelae of acute pancreatitis. With prompt and early treatment of the obstructive process, histologic and functional pancreatic changes are partially or fully reversible.

Pathogenesis

The mechanism of development of chronic pancreatitis has been debated for decades. Multiple disease concepts have been developed through the years, with acceptance waxing and waning. In 1946, Comfort and colleagues concluded that chronic pancreatitis was the result of recurrent episodes of acute pancreatitis by studying tissue specimens of patients with chronic relapsing pancreatitis. The consensus from the 1963 Marseille meeting supported the notion that acute pancreatitis could not be the cause of chronic pancreatitis and that they represent different entities. Sarles and other experts proposed, based on morphologic features of pancreatic tissue, the hypothesis of ductal obstruction. Chronic alcohol consumption was predicted to lead to secretion of pancreatic juice rich in protein and low in bicarbonate concentration and volume. This favors the precipitation of protein and calcium crystals. Proteinaceous plugs are one of the earliest findings in the evolution of chronic pancreatitis. Protein plugs are thought to obstruct ductules and cause ductal and parenchymal damage upstream of the obstruction. This hypothesis focused on lithostathine, a protein that was proposed to inhibit calcium crystal formation in the pancreatic juice. Although the above concept has been abandoned, it is likely that ductal plugging contributes to the progression of chronic pancreatitis. However, it is not known whether the protein precipitates and ductal stones are causing pancreatic injury or if they are markers of the underlying pathophysiologic events.

Bordalo and colleagues suggested the toxic–metabolic hypothesis for alcoholic pancreatitis. They proposed that alcohol and its toxic metabolites result in alterations of intracellular lipid metabolism and lead to fatty regeneration of the pancreatic acini. Increased membrane lipid peroxidation and free radical production are seen in both animal models and human chronic alcoholic pancreatitis. Braganza postulated the cause of acute pancreatitis to be oxidative stress. Products of hepatic "detoxification," such as lipid peroxidation products, toxic epoxides, and free radicals, are excreted in bile, reflux into the pancreatic duct, and induce pathologic changes by damaging the acinar cell membranes. Ongoing oxidative stress will subsequently lead to chronic pancreatitis.

Klöppel and associates revisited the hypothesis of Comfort and proposed the concept of necrosis–fibrosis. On the basis of histologic findings from pancreatic resection specimens, it was suggested that recurrent episodes of acute pancreatitis affect intrapancreatic fat deposits, resulting in areas of focal necrosis. During the healing process, necrotic tissue is replaced by fibrosis that eventually leads to chronic pancreatitis. This theory had significant supporting evidence from some natural history studies showing that the higher the severity and frequency of acute attacks of alcoholic pancreatitis, the more often they lead to chronic pancreatitis.

Sentinel acute pancreatitis event hypothesis

In 1999, Whitcomb introduced the sentinel acute pancreatitis event (SAPE) hypothesis that allowed many of the key elements of divergent previous concepts and hypotheses to be unified. The SAPE hypothesis recognizes the need for a sentinel event of acute pancreatitis to initiate the inflammatory process. Furthermore, multiple risk factors are needed to sustain the inflammatory response that leads to progressive fibrosis.

The SAPE model was based on several observations in alcoholic chronic pancreatitis, and later hereditary pancreatitis. In chronic alcohol-consuming subjects the acinar cells appear to be under metabolic and oxidative stress. A number of factors are also commonly identified that injure the cell, including toxic products of alcohol metabolism and fatty acid ethyl esters. They result in membrane and mitochondrial injury and release of a variety of proinflammatory cytokines. Despite all these proinflammatory events, close study of animals exposed to long-term alcohol treatment, as well as most of the alcoholic patients, does not reveal significant pancreatic fibrosis. Thus, continued oxidative stress cannot cause chronic pancreatitis by itself under otherwise normal conditions. Second, some patients with expression of the hereditary pancreatitis gene, as well as most patients with SPINK1 mutations, do not develop acute or chronic pancreatitis until some point that may be years after birth. In both cases the susceptibility is present, but a critical sentinel event appears to be necessary to "trigger" the processes causing acute and chronic pancreatitis.

Third, a "trigger" may also be necessary to activate stellate cells, attract T lymphocytes and monocytes, with the latter becoming long-term resident tissue macrophages, and promote the antiinflammatory process. There is a strong association between injury, chronic inflammation, and fibrosis. Pancreatic fibrosis, the hallmark of chronic pancreatitis, is a result of stimulation and proliferation of pancreatic stellate cells. Fibrosis appears to be promoted by transforming growth factor (TGF)-β and other antiinflammatory cytokines. TGF-β is an antiinflammatory cytokine that most likely constitutes response to preexisting proinflammatory events. A significant amount of TGF-β originates from resident macrophages, which are present in response to recurrent pancreatic stress, possibly aiming to suppress proinflammatory macrophages. Areas of necrosis–fibrosis would provide a significant proinflammatory event, to be followed by an antiinflammatory process, leading to fibrosis and scarring. Nonetheless, the necrosis–fibrosis concept cannot explain how some patients can progress to chronic pancreatitis with little or no evidence of pancreatic necrosis.

At some point in time, an episode of acute pancreatitis is initiated. This is called the "sentinel" event since it foresees the progression to chronic pancreatitis. The SAPE results in activation of stellate cells and recruitment of active lymphocytes and monocytes into the pancreas that constitute the early proinflammatory phase. Under normal conditions, acute pancreatitis resolves, and the pancreas recovers. However, the antiinflammatory cells remain in the pancreatic parenchyma for a long time. If there is not chronic stress present, such as in a case of single-episode biliary pancreatitis, the long-term resident tissue macrophages remain quiescent and progressively diminish in number.

If, on the contrary, chronic stress persists (i.e., the patient continues to consume alcohol) or recurrent pancreatitis develops, the stellate cells will remain in a state of metabolic stress, continuing to release proinflammatory cytokines and other signals. The residual antiinflammatory macrophages and activated stellate cells, which constitute the later antiinflammatory phase, have receptors that respond to the above signals and release TGF-β. This results in continuous synthesis and deposition of collagen, fibronectin, and other matrix proteins, leading to widespread fibrosis and chronic pancreatitis. The role of genetic factors in this process seems to be very important. Genetically predisposed individuals, such as persons carrying specific *SPINK1/CFTR* mutations or mutations in key genes in the inflammatory pathways, will have a more prominent and sustained inflammatory response and also will be much more susceptible to the antiinflammatory cascade and therefore progress faster to fibrosis.

Thus, the SAPE hypothesis includes elements of several divergent historical theories of the etiopathogenesis of chronic pancreatitis. The toxic–metabolic hypothesis, the oxidative stress hypothesis, the necrosis–fibrosis hypothesis, even elements of the primary intraductal obstruction concept, are introduced within the SAPE hypothesis in an understandable sequence. In addition, the definition of chronic pancreatitis, as an overriding syndrome of different etiologies that can converge through ongoing long-standing inflammation to a similar end point, is logically explained. If future evidence strengthens the SAPE model further, the sentinel event may also have clinical utility, by alerting the clinician to initiate as yet undeveloped therapies targeted to delay or prevent progression to chronic pancreatitis.

Genetic variations associated with chronic pancreatitis

In 1996, hereditary pancreatitis was discovered as a gain-of-function, single-point mutation in the cationic

trypsinogen gene. Hereditary chronic pancreatitis is a genetic disorder with high disease penetrance (80%). Hereditary pancreatitis usually presents in childhood with recurrent episodes of acute pancreatitis. These episodes are clinically similar to acute pancreatitis caused by other causes. Following repeated episodes of acute pancreatitis about half the patients progress to chronic pancreatitis. Studies on families with hereditary pancreatitis, and subsequent studies in other types of pancreatitis, suggest that trypsin is central to the process of pancreatic injury and initiation of the inflammatory process, but that frequency, severity, and duration of injury and the rate of progression to fibrosis and other complications fall into the domain of environmental factors and altered immunologic responses. These latter two domains remain an area of active research.

Mutations increasing susceptibility to recurrent acute pancreatitis

Trypsinogen (PRSS1) *mutations*

The cationic trypsinogen gene, also called protease serine 1 (*PSSR1*), has been extensively studied and found to have a central role in hereditary pancreatitis. An arginine (R) to histidine (H) (CGC→CAG) substitution was identified in 1996. In the initial reports, this mutation was called R117H using the chymotrypsinogen numbering system. Subsequently, the term "R122H" has been accepted, based on the codon numbering system. The R122H mutation does not seem to affect the tertiary structure of trypsin nor alter its catalytic activity or interfere with trypsin inhibitor binding, since the three-dimensional position of R122 is located on the opposite surface of the trypsin molecule to the catalytic and trypsin inhibitor binding sites. It was proposed that the R122H mutation eliminates a "failsafe" mechanism for the inactivation of trypsin. Codon 122 arginine is the initial site of hydrolysis of trypsin by trypsin itself. Substitution of histidine for arginine at this site eliminates this initial hydrolysis site, rendering trypsin resistant to failsafe autolysis. The discovery of an autolysis-resistant trypsinogen molecule in hereditary pancreatitis associated with acute, and later chronic, pancreatitis offers the strongest support yet in favor of the necrosis–fibrosis hypothesis.

A second mutation in cationic trypsinogen, numbered N21I, was detected shortly afterwards. N21I mutation results in a clinical syndrome of hereditary pancreatitis with a slightly delayed age of onset and less severe clinical features in comparison to R122H mutation. An A→T transversion results in an asparagine (N) to isoleucine (I) (AAC→ATC) substitution in codon 21. The exact molecular mechanism underlying this mutation is not yet fully clarified. It is suggested that the substitution will place a hydrophobic isoleucine on the surface of cationic trypsinogen. This will alter the secondary structure of the protein in such a way that the critical autolysis site at codon 122 cannot be attacked by trypsin. These two mutations are found in approximately two-thirds of the families with classical hereditary pancreatitis and currently are the only mutations for which genetic testing is recommended. They are identified uncommonly and do not seem to constitute a major pathogenic factor in patients with common causes of chronic pancreatitis, such as alcoholic or idiopathic pancreatitis.

No mutations have been identified in any other pancreatic digestive enzyme genes, including anionic trypsinogen or mesotrypsinogen, that lead to hereditary pancreatitis. This should not be of great surprise. Hereditary pancreatitis is an autosomal dominant disorder and it therefore occurs only with mutations that involve a critical regulatory part of the gene product and result in a gain-of-function mechanism. Surprisingly, some individuals with the same PRSS1 mutation will never develop acute pancreatitis at all, whereas others progress rapidly to chronic pancreatitis. The incomplete disease penetrance (80%) likely reflects the effect of environmental and other genetic modifiers and supports the complex nature of pancreatitis.

Several new mutations have been reported within the cationic trypsinogen gene that are associated with acute recurrent and chronic pancreatitis, such as K23R (22) and A16V. The growing number of pancreatitis-associated mutations identified in the cationic trypsinogen gene illustrates the important role of trypsinogen in acute recurrent and chronic pancreatitis.

Pancreatic secretory trypsin inhibitor (SPINK1) mutations

An association between mutations in the SPINK1 gene and idiopathic chronic pancreatitis was first reported in 2000. SPINK1, also called pancreatic secretory trypsin inhibitor (PSTI), appears to play a key role in protecting the pancreas from prematurely activated trypsin. It is a 56-amino acid peptide that specifically inhibits trypsin by directly blocking the active catalytic site. A lysine carboxyl group of SPINK1 forms a reversible covalent bond with the catalytic serine residue of trypsin. It has been estimated that SPINK1 is only capable of neutralizing about 20% of potential activated trypsinogen. Since both cationic trypsinogen and SPINK1 are synthesized within the pancreatic acinar cells, SPINK1 most likely provides the first line of defense against prematurely activated trypsinogen.

The SPINK1 N34S and P55S are the most commonly found mutations, being present in about 1–2% of the general population. This means that these mutations are many times more prevalent than chronic pancreatitis (0.006% of the general population). Therefore the risk of chronic pancreatitis in an asymptomatic individual with a heterozygous SPINK1 mutation alone is low (~ 1%). Unlike patients with cationic trypsinogen R122H and N21I mutations, patients with SPINK1 mutations and pancreatic disease can present with a variety of phenotypes. Furthermore, the severity of pancreatitis appears to be similar between subjects with heterozygous, homozygous, or compound heterozygous genotypes, suggesting that the genetics is complex. The incidence of SPINK1 mutations is 15–25% in children with idiopathic chronic pancreatitis but is reduced to 5–10% in adults with idiopathic or alcoholic chronic pancreatitis. SPINK1 mutations are also associated with alcoholic pancreatitis (6%) and occur in a high percentage of patients with fibrocalculous pancreatic diabetes, a subtype of tropical pancreatitis.

SPINK1 mutations cause SPINK1 loss of function and result in elevated trypsin levels within the pancreas. However, if the trypsin R122H autolysis mechanism remains intact, the trypsin activation process will fail to progress beyond the failsafe trypsin autolysis phase. Therefore, SPINK1 mutations alone are not sufficient to cause pancreatic disease. Modeling and familial clustering suggest that SPINK1 mutations result in proteins with loss of function. They possibly act as susceptibility genes by lowering the threshold for initiating pancreatitis and by interacting with other disease genes such as CFTR mutations. Another suggestion is that SPINK1 mutations are disease-modifying mutations and act by worsening the severity of pancreatitis caused by other genetic or environmental factors.

CFTR mutations

The CFTR gene is divided into 24 exons that code for a single protein of 1480 amino acids. The protein forms a cyclic adenosine monophosphate (cAMP)-dependent anion channel for chloride, to a lesser degree for bicarbonate, and other ion channels. CFTR is a critical molecule in the proper functioning of the pancreatic duct cells and other anion-secreting epithelial cells. Loss of function results in inability to hydrate mucus and other macromolecules, leading to accumulation of viscid material and inspissated glands. In the pancreas, CFTR is located on the luminal membrane of the pancreatic duct cell, conducts both chloride and bicarbonate, and controls the bulk of pancreatic fluid excretion.

CFTR mutations were initially identified in 1989. Cystic fibrosis (CF) is the most common lethal genetic disorder of white populations, inherited as an autosomal recessive disorder. Major mutations in both alleles of the *CFTR* gene result in complete loss of CFTR function and the typical CF phenotype, presenting in childhood with progressive pulmonary disease and a cystic fibrotic pancreas. Among CF patients, two-thirds have a 3-bp deletion of codon 508 (ΔF508) that codes for phenylalanine. Approximately 1000 other mutations and sequence variations have been identified. The *CFTR* polymorphisms have been classified based on their functional impact on the CFTR protein. Classes 1–3 yield little or no functional protein and are considered severe mutations. Classes 4 and 5 retain more than 1% of CFTR function, are considered mild, and are often associated with pancreatic sufficiency or atypical CF. Class 6 does not affect chloride conductance but rather the ability of CFTR to regulate other channels. There are numerous silent mutations, intronic and exonic polymorphisms, and sequence variations with unknown significance.

In 1998, two studies demonstrated the strong association between *CFTR* mutations and idiopathic chronic pancreatitis. They showed approximately six times increased frequency of *CFTR* mutations in patients with idiopathic chronic pancreatitis who had no other evidence of CF. The *CFTR* mutations identified in the above reports may actually underestimate their frequency in the setting of pancreatitis since only limited genetic screening of the most severe *CFTR* mutations was performed.

Subsequent studies involving complete DNA sequencing of more than 800 known *CFTR* mutations reported that one-third of all patients with idiopathic chronic pancreatitis have *CFTR* mutations. The observed genotypes were combinations of severe and mild *CFTR* mutations rather than mild and mild or severe and severe combinations. In contrast to typical CF, mild mutations, such as R117H or intron 8 "5T allele" variant, when combined with a severe mutation such as ΔF508, result in a subclinical pancreatic-sufficient form of CF. These individuals appear to be at increased risk of developing recurrent acute and chronic pancreatitis (around 80 times), but the majority with this genotype do not develop pancreatitis. *CFTR* mutations seem to act as susceptibility genes. CFTR-associated chronic pancreatitis appears to be a complex disease with additional genetic or environmental risk factors involved that are yet to be identified. Furthermore, as with *SPINK1* mutations, there are likely multiple different CFTR-associated mechanisms contributing to the disease.

Hyperlipidemia syndromes

Acute and chronic recurrent pancreatitis have been reported in patients with a variety of inborn errors of metabolism, including hyperlipidemia syndromes, as well as various disorders of branched-chain amino acid degradation, homocystinuria, hemolytic disorders, acute intermittent porphyria, and several amino acid transporter defects. Some of these disease entities are exceedingly rare. In most of these disorders, pancreatitis is not very common and, with the exception of lipoprotein lipase and apolipoprotein C-II deficiency, is not the most distressing clinical manifestation of the underlying metabolic defect.

The association of hypertriglyceridemia (> 500 mg/dL) and recurrent acute pancreatitis is well documented. Both lipoprotein lipase and apolipoprotein C-II deficiencies cause chronic hypertriglyceridemia and bouts of pancreatitis that segregate with the disease gene. Furthermore, there is evidence of their association with chronic pancreatitis in an extended Dutch kindred with genetically deficient lipoprotein lipase catalytic activity and in a kindred with apolipoprotein C-II deficiency. It appears that in the most severe and prolonged cases of hyperlipidemia dominated by recurrent acute pancreatitis, chronic pancreatitis can develop rarely.

Hypercalcemia syndromes

Calcium appears to play a central role in trypsinogen secretion and trypsin stabilization. The trypsin molecule contains a calcium-binding pocket near the R122 position. As the intracellular concentration of calcium increases, calcium binds with trypsin within the binding pocket. This results in formation of a bond with

R122 that subsequently limits the exposure of R122 to other trypsin molecules and inhibits hydrolysis.

Hypercalcemia is associated with acute pancreatitis. Another event should precede that results in pancreatic stimulation. Only after trypsinogen is activated to trypsin will the high calcium concentrations stabilize and protect the trypsin molecules from autolysis. Subsequently, pancreatic autodigestion by trypsin and pancreatic inflammation (pancreatitis) will follow.

The association between familial hyperparathyroidism and chronic pancreatitis has been described, mainly in cases of long-standing untreated hyperparathyroidism. Nowadays hypercalcemia is considered a rare but accepted factor for chronic pancreatitis.

Mutations increasing acinar cell toxicity

UPD glucuronosyltransferase gene mutations

UDP glucuronosyltransferases (UGTs) are a superfamily of proteins that represent major biochemical factors in cellular defense. UGTs act as phase II detoxifying enzymes capable of inactivation of dietary byproducts, endogenous metabolites, as well as tobacco-borne toxicants. One of the ten major isoforms, the UGT1A7 gene is the only one expressed in high levels in the pancreas. The UGT1A7 gene is known to have five common polymorphisms, which are linked as three polymorphic UGT1A7 alleles. Recently, the role of UGT1A7 gene polymorphisms in pancreatic diseases was investigated. An increased risk for chronic pancreatitis was found in patients with the polymorphic allele UGT1A7*3. The UGT1A7*3 haplotype results in a low detoxification activity of UGT1A. UGT1A7*3 was significantly more common in the subgroup of patients with alcoholic pancreatitis, of whom almost 90% were smokers. There was also a trend toward chronic pancreatitis in the nonalcoholic subjects who were negative for SPINK1 N34S. Thus, the low-detoxification-activity UGT1A7*3 allele could represent a novel risk factor for pancreatic diseases, defining the interaction of genetic predisposition and environmentally induced oxidative injury.

Glutathione S-transferase null genotype

Glutathione S-transferases (GSTs) play critical roles in providing protection against electrophiles and products of oxidative stress, by catalyzing the formation of glutathione conjugates and by eliminating peroxides. The most important polymorphisms encode a partial gene deletion in GSTM1 and GSTT1 (null genotypes), resulting in complete absence of GSTM1 and GSTT1 and are found in 50% and 20% of the Caucasian population respectively. A recent study investigated whether polymorphisms in GST genes modified the risk of chronic pancreatitis. GSTM1 null genotypes were found significantly less commonly in alcoholic chronic pancreatitis patients, especially young females. This might suggest that the GSTM1 null genotype provides protection against chronic pancreatitis in alcohol users, particularly female alcoholics under the age of 50 years.

Mutations altering the proinflammatory or antiinflammatory response

HLA-DRB1 0401 allele

The role of the major histocompatibility complex genes as a genetic background in chronic pancreatitis was recently investigated. Among the HLA-DRB1 genes, DRB1*04 was found to be significantly more frequent in chronic pancreatitis patients. This might suggest a role of HLA-DRB1*04 as a susceptibility factor in the development of chronic pancreatitis.

Conclusions

The discovery of the genetic basis of hereditary pancreatitis has emerged as a new model for understanding pancreatic diseases. Premature intrapancreatic activation of trypsin with subsequent pancreatic digestion has been established as the molecular mechanism of acute pancreatitis. Furthermore, the above discovery supports the progressive link between acute and chronic pancreatitis. Chronic pancreatitis arises from acute pancreatitis-initiated inflammation.

The proposed SAPE hypothesis combines modern features from genetic and immunologic advances with important aspects of previous concepts on pancreatic disease pathogenesis. The new risk factor classification system (TIGAR-O) accommodates a risk-assessment approach and provides the framework for future advancements in pathogenesis and potential treatment.

Indeed, chronic pancreatitis is a syndrome encompassing several complex disease mechanisms. Multiple factors, including genetic factors (mutations in SPINK1, CFTR, possibly UGT1A, HLA-DRB1, and other yet-to-be-identified genes) and environmental factors (alcohol intake, smoking tobacco), are often required for the development of chronic pancreatitis. These factors can have a disease-causative, disease-susceptibility, or disease-modifying role. More data are slowly emerging and are updating the gaps in the framework of the TIGAR-O risk classification and SAPE model. New methods for early diagnosis and early genetic prognosis, as well as pathway-specific preventative and therapeutic strategies, are needed.

Recommended reading

Ammann RW. A clinically based classification system for alcoholic chronic pancreatitis: summary of an international workshop on chronic pancreatitis. *Pancreas* 1997;14: 215–221.

Bordalo O, Goncalves D, Noronha M *et al*. Newer concept for the pathogenesis of chronic alcoholic pancreatitis. *Am J Gastroenterol* 1977;68:278–285.

Cavestro GM, Frulloni L, Neri TM *et al*. Association of HLA-DRB*0401 allele with chronic pancreatitis. *Pancreas* 2003;26:388–391.

Cohn JA, Friedman KJ, Noone PG *et al*. Relation between mutations of the cystic fibrosis gene and idiopathic pancreatitis. *N Engl J Med* 1998;339:653–658.

Comfort M, Gambill E, Baggenstoss A. Chronic relapsing pancreatitis. *Gastroenterology* 1946;6:239–285.

Durie PR. Pancreatitis and mutations of the cystic fibrosis gene. *N Engl J Med* 1998;339:687–688.

Etemad B, Whitcomb DC. Chronic pancreatitis: diagnosis, classification, and new genetic developments. *Gastroenterology* 2001;120:682–707.

Gorry MC, Gabbaizedeh D, Furey W *et al*. Mutations in the cationic trypsinogen gene are associated with recurrent acute and chronic pancreatitis. *Gastroenterology* 1997; 113:1063–1068.

Guy O, Robles-Diaz G, Adrich Z *et al*. Protein content of precipitates present in pancreatic juice of alcoholic subjects and patients with chronic calcifying pancreatitis. *Gastroenterology* 1983;84:102–107.

Homma T, Harada H, Koizumi M. Diagnostic criteria for chronic pancreatitis by the Japan Pancreas Society. *Pancreas* 1997;15:14–15.

Kloppel G, Maillet B. A morphological analysis of 57 resection specimens and 9 autopsy pancreata. *Pancreas* 1991;6:266–274.

Ockenga J, Vogel A, Teich N *et al*. UDP glucuronosyltransferase (UGT1A7) gene polymorphisms increase the risk of chronic pancreatitis and pancreatic cancer. *Gastroenterology* 2003;124:1802–1808.

Pfutzer RH, Barmada MM, Brunskill AP *et al*. SPINK1/PSTI polymorphisms act as disease modifiers in familial and idiopathic chronic pancreatitis. *Gastroenterology* 2000; 119:615–623.

Sarles H. Definitions and classifications of pancreatitis. *Pancreas* 1991;6:470–474.

Schneider A, Whitcomb DC. Hereditary pancreatitis: a model for inflammatory diseases of the pancreas. *Best Pract Res Clin Gastroenterol* 2002;16:347–363.

Schneider A, Suman A, Rossi L *et al*. SPINK1/PSTI mutations are associated with tropical pancreatitis and type II diabetes mellitus in Bangladesh. *Gastroenterology* 2002;123: 1026–1030.

Whitcomb DC. Hereditary pancreatitis: new insights into acute and chronic pancreatitis. *Gut* 1999;45:317–322.

Whitcomb DC, Gorry MC, Preston RA *et al*. Hereditary pancreatitis is caused by a mutation in the cationic trypsinogen gene. *Nat Genet* 1996;14:141–145.

Witt H, Luck W, Hennies HC *et al*. Mutations in the gene encoding the serine protease inhibitor, Kazal type 1 are associated with chronic pancreatitis. *Nat Genet* 2000;25: 213–216.

Witt H, Luck W, Becker M *et al*. Mutation in the SPINK1 trypsin inhibitor gene, alcohol use, and chronic pancreatitis. *JAMA* 2001;285:2716–2717.

24 Pathophysiology of chronic pancreatitis

Frank Ulrich Weiss and Markus M. Lerch

Introduction

Chronic pancreatitis is an inflammatory condition characterized by fibrosis that leads to the destruction of exocrine and endocrine tissue in the pancreas. Most patients present clinically with pain and the disease later progresses to exocrine and endocrine insufficiency, calcification, and duct dilatation. In developed countries the disease is most commonly associated with excessive consumption of alcohol over many years (approximately 60–70% of cases). Alcohol is therefore regarded as the most common cause of chronic pancreatitis. However, the factors that predispose some but not all heavy drinkers to chronic pancreatitis remain poorly understood. In 10–30% of patients with chronic pancreatitis the disease cannot be attributed to known causative factors and these patients are labeled as having idiopathic chronic pancreatitis. Idiopathic chronic pancreatitis occurs in two distinct subgroups of patients: (i) early-onset individuals, aged 15–30 years; and (ii) late-onset individuals, aged 50–70 years. These two subgroups have been shown to differ in severity and course of disease progression. A less common form of idiopathic chronic pancreatitis that begins in young children in some areas of Africa and Asia is termed "tropical pancreatitis." It has been subclassified either as tropical calcific pancreatitis or as fibrocalculous pancreatic diabetes, in which diabetes is the first major clinical symptom. In a minority of patients, germline mutations in the genes for cationic trypsinogen, cystic fibrosis transmembrane conductance regulator (CFTR), and pancreatic secretory trypsin inhibitor (PSTI) have been associated with familial or hereditary forms of pancreatitis.

While the diverse designation of chronic pancreatitis as idiopathic, familial, tropical, alcoholic, or hereditary points to multifaceted triggering events, the clinical phenotype and disease process are remarkably similar. As the diagnosis of pancreatitis in a clinical setting is normally delayed beyond the initiating steps of the disease, a comprehensive analysis of the initiating mechanisms and the subsequent inflammatory response is more than difficult and only limited data on the molecular mechanisms of human disease development are presently available. Instead, experimental animal models have been developed that attempt to simulate some, if not all, characteristics of the human disease. It appears that chronic pancreatitis is the result of a process that is based on individual genetic predisposition, greatly affected by nutritional and environmental factors and contributed to by the patient's individual inflammatory and defensive responses.

Etiology

Various predisposing factors for chronic pancreatitis have been identified in the past, but their impact on etiology and natural disease course is still a matter of debate. According to the TIGAR-O classification, the risk factors for chronic pancreatitis can be categorized into (i) toxic–metabolic, (ii) idiopathic, (iii) genetic, (iv) autoimmune, (v) recurrent and severe acute pancreatitis, and (vi) obstructive pancreatitis (Fig. 24.1).

Alcohol

In industrialized countries, long-term alcohol abuse

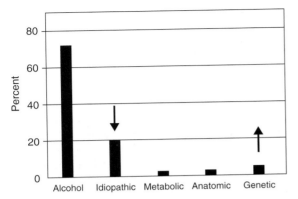

Figure 24.1 Causes of chronic pancreatitis: due to recent progress in the identification and diagnosis of genetic factors for chronic pancreatitis, the number of patients classified as having idiopathic chronic pancreatitis is decreasing.

accounts for approximately 70% of patients with chronic pancreatitis, with a mortality rate approaching 50% within 20–25 years due to malnutrition, severe infections, diabetes, alcohol- and nicotine-related diseases and, most commonly forgotten, fatal accidents. Bordalo and colleagues initially suggested that alcoholic chronic pancreatitis is caused by the direct toxic effects of ethanol and its metabolites and that these would interfere with intracellular lipid metabolism and lead to fatty degeneration of pancreatic acinar cells. The pathologic effects of alcohol on the pancreas are, however, difficult to study in humans. In experimental studies, ethanol and its metabolites appear to have complex short-term and long-term effects on acinar cell physiology. They can cause damage to cell membranes and affect cellular signaling pathways. Animal models, which have been frequently used to investigate the effect of ethanol *in vivo*, have demonstrated that the pancreatic injury induced by ethanol exposure is likely to be multifactorial. The mechanisms seem to include some degree of ductal hypertension, decreased pancreatic blood flow, oxidative stress, direct acinar cell toxicity, changes in protein synthesis, an enhanced inflammatory response, or the stimulation of fibrosis. Acute administration of alcohol in the rat results in increased injury during pancreatitis induced by a combination of pancreatic duct obstruction and hormonal hyperstimulation. Rats under chronic ethanol feeding have also more severe pancreatitis. While the generation of oxygen free radicals has been clearly demonstrated in the

pancreas of rats under continuous ethanol feeding, ethanol alone, i.e., without an additional disease-inducing stimulus, does not cause pancreatitis. Generation of free radicals has been shown to cause depletion of intracellular antioxidants, such as glutathione, and accounts for subsequent oxidative damage to lipids, proteins, and nucleic acids. Some of the toxic effects of ethanol may therefore be secondary to its effect on lipid metabolism and other metabolic pathways.

There is a clear dose-related risk for the development of alcoholic pancreatitis but the disease process appears to be very extended, with an interval between the start of continuous alcohol consumption and the clinical manifestation of alcohol-induced chronic pancreatitis of as long as 15–20 years. Recurrent episodes of subclinical acute pancreatitis may lead, over time, to chronic inflammation and fibrosis. Other observations suggest that chronic pancreatitis may also arise independently of acute disease recurrences. Interestingly, the correlation between alcohol consumption and chronic pancreatitis is not strict and less than 5% of alcoholics develop pancreatitis as a consequence of excessive ethanol consumption. Why the pancreas of some individuals is more susceptible to alcohol than that of others and why the development of alcoholic pancreatitis appears to follow different patterns in individual alcoholics has prompted investigators to study genetic predisposition in patients with pancreatitis. Candidate genes that have been studied include aldehyde dehydrogenase polymorphisms, *CFTR*, cationic trypsinogen, HLA antigens and others, but none of these were found to predispose to alcoholic pancreatitis. While the mechanisms involved in alcoholic pancreatitis are still being explored, much progress has been made in elucidating the role of gallstones in the pathophysiology of pancreatitis.

Gallstone-induced pancreatitis

About 150 years ago Claude Bernard discovered that bile can cause pancreatitis when it is injected into the pancreatic duct of laboratory animals. Since that time many studies have been performed to elucidate the underlying pathophysiologic mechanisms. Today it is firmly established that the passage of a gallstone from the gallbladder through the biliary tract can initiate pancreatitis, whereas gallstones that remain in the gallbladder do not cause pancreatitis. The various hypotheses that were proposed to explain this association are mostly contradictory. In 1901 Eugene Opie postulated that an impairment of the pancreatic outflow due to obstruction of the pancreatic duct causes pancreatitis. This initial "duct obstruction" hypothesis was somewhat forgotten when Opie published his second "common channel" hypothesis during the same year. This later hypothesis predicts that an impacted gallstone at the papilla of Vater creates a communication between the pancreatic and the bile duct (the said "common channel") through which bile flows into the pancreatic duct and thus causes pancreatitis.

From a mechanistic point of view, Opie's common channel hypothesis seems rational and has become one of the most popular theories in the field; however, considerable experimental and clinical evidence is incompatible with its assumptions. Anatomic studies have shown that the communication between the pancreatic duct and the common bile duct is much too short (< 6 mm) to permit biliary reflux into the pancreatic duct. Therefore an impacted gallstone would most likely obstruct both the common bile duct and the pancreatic duct. Even in the event of an existing anatomic communication, pancreatic juice would be expected to flow into the bile duct rather than bile into the pancreatic duct due to the higher secretory pressure of pancreatic juice exceeding biliary pressure. Late in the course of pancreatitis when necrosis is firmly established, a biliopancreatic reflux due to a loss of barrier function in the damaged pancreatic duct may well explain the observation of a bile-stained necrotic pancreas at the time of surgery. However, this should not be regarded as evidence for the assumption that reflux of bile into the pancreas is a triggering event for disease onset.

Based on these inconsistencies of the common channel hypothesis, it was proposed that the passage of a gallstone might damage the duodenal sphincter in such a way that sphincter insufficiency results. In turn, this could permit duodenal content, including bile and activated pancreatic juice, to flow through the incompetent sphincter into the pancreatic duct and induce pancreatitis. However, this hypothesis was shown not to be applicable to the human situation, in which sphincter stenosis rather than sphincter insufficiency results from the passage of a gallstone through the papilla, and flow of pancreatic juice into the bile duct, rather than flow of duodenal content into the pancreas, is the consequence. Finally, another argument against the common channel hypothesis is that perfusion of bile through the pancreatic duct is completely harmless. Only an influx of infected bile, which might occur after prolonged obstruction at the papilla when the pressure gradient between the pancreatic duct (higher) and the bile duct (lower) is reversed, may represent an aggravating factor for the course of pancreatitis.

Taken together, the initial pathophysiologic events that occur during the course of gallstone-induced pancreatitis are believed to affect the acinar cell and are triggered, in accordance with Opie's initial hypothesis, by obstruction or impairment of flow from the pancreatic duct. Bile reflux into the pancreatic duct, either through a common channel created by an impacted gallstone or through an incompetent spincter caused by the passage of a gallstone, is neither required nor likely to occur during the initial course of pancreatitis.

Molecular aspects during pancreatic duct obstruction

In an animal model based on pancreatic duct obstruction the cellular events involved in gallstone-induced pancreatitis were investigated in rodents. Intracellular calcium release in response to hormonal stimuli was investigated in addition to a morphologic and biochemical characterization. Under physiologic resting conditions most cell types, including the acinar cells of the exocrine pancreas, maintain a Ca^{2+} gradient across the plasma membrane, with low intracellular Ca^{2+} concentrations (nanomolar range) facing high extracellular Ca^{2+} concentrations (millimolar range). Many of these cells use rapid Ca^{2+} release from intracellular stores in response to external and internal stimuli as a signaling mechanism that regulates diverse biological events, such as growth, proliferation, locomotion, contraction, or the regulated secretion of exportable proteins. An impaired capacity to maintain the Ca^{2+} gradient across the plasma membrane represents a common pathophysiologic characteristic of vascular hypertension, malignant tumor growth, and cell damage in response to some toxins. Ligation of the pancreatic duct in rats and mice, a condition that mimics gallstone-induced pancreatitis in humans, induced leukocytosis, hyperamylasemia, pancreatic edema, and granulocyte immigration into the lungs, all of which were not observed in bile duct-ligated controls. It also led to significant intracellular activation of pancreatic proteases such as trypsin, an event we discuss in more detail in the next paragraph. Whereas the resting $[Ca^{2+}]_i$ in isolated acini rose by 45% to 205 ± 7 nmol/L, the acetylcholine- and cholecystokinin-stimulated calcium peaks as well as amylase secretion declined. However, neither the $[Ca^{2+}]_i$ signaling pattern nor the amylase output in response to the Ca^{2+}-ATPase inhibitor thapsigargin, nor secretin-stimulated amylase release, were impaired by pancreatic duct ligation. At the single-cell level, pancreatic duct ligation reduced the percentage of cells in which physiologic secretagogue stimulation was followed by a physiologic response (i.e., Ca^{2+} oscillations) and increased the percentage of cells with a pathologic response (i.e., peak-plateau or absent Ca^{2+} signal). Moreover, it reduced the frequency and amplitude of Ca^{2+} oscillations as well as the capacitative Ca^{2+} influx in response to secretagogue stimulation.

To test whether these prominent changes in intra-acinar calcium signaling not only parallel pancreatic duct obstruction but are also directly involved in the initiation of pancreatitis, animals were systemically treated with the intracellular calcium chelator BAPTA-AM. As a consequence, both the parameters of pancreatitis as well as intrapancreatic trypsinogen activation induced by duct ligation were found to be significantly reduced. These experiments suggest that pancreatic duct obstruction, the critical event involved in gallstone-induced pancreatitis, rapidly changes the physiologic response of the exocrine pancreas to a pathologic Ca^{2+}-signaling pattern. This pathologic Ca^{2+} signaling is associated with premature digestive enzyme activation and the onset of pancreatitis, both of which can be prevented by administration of an intracellular calcium chelator.

Autoactivation of pancreatic proteases

The exocrine pancreas, which synthesizes more protein than any other exocrine organ, secretes digestive proenzymes called zymogens that require proteolytic cleavage of an activation peptide to become fully active. After entering the small intestine, the pancreatic zymogen trypsinogen is first activated to trypsin by an intestinal protease called enterokinase (enteropeptidase). Activated trypsin is subsequently able to proteolytically process other pancreatic enzymes to their active forms. Under physiologic conditions, pancreatic proteases thus remain inactive during synthesis, intracellu-

lar transport, secretion from acinar cells, and transit through the pancreatic duct. Activation only occurs when they reach the lumen and brush border of the small intestine. About a century ago, the pathologist Hans Chiari suggested that the pancreas of patients who had died during episodes of acute necrotizing pancreatitis "had succumbed to its own digestive properties," and he created the term "autodigestion" to describe the underlying pathophysiologic disease mechanism. Many attempts have been made since then to prove or disprove the role of premature intracellular zymogen activation as an initial or initiating event in the course of pancreatitis. Only recent advances in biochemical and molecular techniques have allowed investigators to address some of these questions conclusively.

There are several reasons why many of these studies have been performed on animal or isolated cell models and have not been gained directly from human pancreas or patients with pancreatitis.

1 Because of its anatomic localization, the pancreas is rather inaccessible and biopsies of human pancreas are difficult to obtain for ethical and medical reasons.

2 When patients present to hospital with the first symptoms of acute pancreatitis, the initial stages of the disease, where triggering events could be studied, have already passed.

3 Investigations that address initiating pathophysiologic events are disturbed by the autodigestive process. Mechanisms of premature protease activation have therefore mostly been studied in animal and cell models that can be experimentally controlled and which are highly reproducible.

Pathophysiologic significance of digestive protease activation

Early hypotheses concerning the question of where and how pancreatitis starts were based on autopsy studies of patients who had died during the course of pancreatitis. One of these early theories suggested that peripancreatic fat necrosis represents the initial event from which all later alterations arise. This hypothesis implicated pancreatic lipase, which is secreted from acinar cells in its active form, as the culprit for pancreatic necrosis. Another hypothesis suggested that periductal cells represented the site of initial damage and that extravasation of pancreatic juice from the ductal system is responsible for initiating the disease. However, controlled studies subsequently demonstrated that the acinar cell is the initial site of morphologic damage. It is important to note that pancreatitis begins in exocrine acinar cells, as opposed to the pancreatic ducts or some poorly defined extracellular space, because it represents a shift from earlier mechanistic and histopathologic interpretations of the disease onset.

Trypsinogen and other pancreatic proteases are synthesized by acinar cells as inactive proenzyme precursors and stored in membrane-bound zymogen granules. After activation in the small intestine, trypsin converts other pancreatic zymogens, such as chymotrypsinogen, proelastase, procarboxypeptidase, or prophospholipase A_2, to their active forms. Although small amounts of trypsinogen are probably activated within the pancreatic acinar cell under physiologic conditions, two protective mechanisms normally prevent cell damage from proteolytic activity.

1 PSTI, the product of the gene for serine protease inhibitor Kazal type 1 (SPINK1), is cosecreted with pancreatic zymogens and may inhibit up to 20% of cellular trypsin activity in humans. Mutations in the SPINK1 gene have been found associated with certain forms of human pancreatitis, indicating that this protective mechanism may play a role in pancreatic pathophysiology.

2 Cell biological experiments using living rodent acini provided evidence that trypsin limits its own activity by autodegradation under conditions that mimic pancreatitis (see below). An important discovery was that the specific cationic trypsinogen mutations that have been found associated with human hereditary pancreatitis seem to stabilize trypsin against autolysis, suggesting that autodegradation might play a protective role against excess intrapancreatic trypsin activity.

Although experimentally not demonstrated as yet, other pancreatic proteases might participate in a similar protective mechanism, and a different trypsin isoform, mesotrypsin, has been labeled a candidate for this function in humans. This minor trypsin isoform constitutes less than 5% of total secreted trypsinogens and, due to a Gly→Arg substitution at position 198 (Gly→Arg at position 193 in chymotrypsin numbering), is poorly inhibited by PSTI. However, mesotrypsin is grossly defective not only in inhibitor binding but also in cleaving protein substrates. A pathophysiologic role of mesotrypsin in intracellular protease degradation and a protective function in pancreatitis is therefore rather unlikely.

Theoretically, premature activation of large amounts of trypsinogen could overwhelm these protective mechanisms, rupture the zymogen-confining membranes, and release activated proteases into the cytosol. Moreover, the release of large amounts of calcium from zymogen granules into the cytosol might activate calcium-dependent proteases such as calpains which, in turn, would contribute to cell injury.

The apparent role of prematurely activated digestive enzymes in the pathogenesis of pancreatitis is supported by the following observations:

1 the activity of both pancreatic trypsin and elastase increases early in the course of experimental pancreatitis;

2 the activation peptides of trypsinogen and carboxypeptidase A_1 are cleaved early in the course of acute pancreatitis from the respective proenzyme and are released into either the pancreatic tissue or the serum;

3 pretreatment with a serine protease inhibitor (gabexate mesylate) reduces the incidence of endoscopic retrograde cholangiopancreatography (ERCP)-induced pancreatitis;

4 serine protease inhibitors reduce injury in experimental pancreatitis;

5 mutations in the cationic trypsinogen gene that have been found associated with hereditary pancreatitis render trypsinogen either more prone to premature activation or more resistant to degradation by other proteases;

6 mutations in the SPINK1 gene which might render PSTI a less effective protease inhibitor are associated with certain forms of chronic pancreatits.

In clinical and experimental studies it was found that zymogen activation occurs very early in the disease course and one study reported a biphasic pattern of trypsin activity that reached an early peak after 1 hour and a later second peak after several hours. This observation is interesting because it suggests that more than one mechanism may be involved in the activation of pancreatic zymogens and the second peak may require the infiltration of inflammatory cells into the pancreas. In patients who underwent ERCP, an interventional medical procedure that requires cannulation of the pancreatic duct and is associated with a significant complication rate for pancreatitis, the prophylactic administration of a low-molecular-weight protease inhibitor reduced the incidence of pancreatitis. While protease inhibitors have not been found to be effective when used therapeutically in patients with clinically established pancreatitis, the result of the prophylactic study supports the conclusion that activation of pancreatic proteases is an inherent feature of disease onset. Taken together these observations represent compelling evidence that premature intracellular zymogen activation plays a critical role in the early pathophysiologic events of pancreatitis.

Subcellular site of initial protease activation

Identification of the subcellular site where pancreatitis begins is critical for understanding the pathophysiologic mechanisms involved in premature intrapancreatic protease activation. By using a fluorogenic trypsin-specific substrate, trypsinogen activation after secretagogue stimulation could be clearly localized to the secretory compartment within acinar cells. When subcellular fractions containing different classes of secretory vesicles were subjected to density gradient centrifugation, it was found that trypsinogen activation does not initially arise in mature zymogen granules but in membrane-bound vesicles of lesser density that most likely correspond to immature condensing secretory vacuoles. These data indicate that mature zymogen granules in which digestive proteases are highly condensed are not necessarily the primary site of this activation. The first trypsin activity in acinar cells following a pathologic stimulus is clearly detectable in membrane-bound secretory vesicles in which trypsinogen, as well as lysosomal enzymes (see below), are both physiologically present.

Cathepsin B

Several lines of evidence have suggested a possible role for the lysosomal cysteine protease cathepsin B in the premature and intrapancreatic activation of digestive enzymes. Observations that would support such a role of cathepsin B include the following: (i) cathepsin B can activate trypsinogen *in vitro*; (ii) during experimental pancreatitis, cathepsin B is redistributed from its lysosomal compartment to a zymogen granule-enriched subcellular compartment; and (iii) lysosomal enzymes such as cathepsin D colocalize with digestive zymogens in membrane-bound organelles during the early course of experimental pancreatitis. Although the cathepsin hypothesis seems attractive from a cell biological point of view, it has received much criticism because some experimental observations that partly made use of lysosomal protease inhibitor appeared to be incompatible with its assumptions. In view of the limited specificity and bioavailability of the existing inhibitors for lysosomal hydrolases, the cathepsin hypothesis was addressed in cathepsin B-deficient animals.

The most dramatic change during experimental pancreatitis in these animals was a more than 80% reduction in premature intrapancreatic trypsinogen activation over the course of 24 hours. This observation can be regarded as the first direct experimental evidence for a critical role of cathepsin B in intracellular premature protease activation during the onset of pancreatitis. Surprisingly, the decrease in trypsinogen activation is not paralleled by a dramatic prevention of pancreatic necrosis, and the systemic inflammatory response during pancreatitis is not affected at all. This observation, and the fact that cathepsin B can activate pancreatic digestive zymogens other than trypsinogen, raises two important questions: (i) is trypsin activation itself, which is clearly cathepsin B-dependent, directly involved in acinar cell damage, and (ii) does cathepsin B-induced activation of other digestive proteases ultimately cause pancreatic necrosis?

Cathepsin B is clearly present in the subcellular secretory compartment of the healthy human pancreas and in the pancreatic juice of controls and pancreatitis patients. A redistribution of cathepsin B into the secretory compartment of the exocrine pancreas may therefore not be required for interaction between trypsinogen and cathepsin B because both classes of enzymes are already colocalized under physiologic conditions in the human pancreas. On the other hand, the capacity of cathepsin B to activate trypsinogen is not affected by the most common trypsinogen mutations found in association with hereditary pancreatitis. While the onset of human pancreatitis may well involve mechanisms that depend on cathepsin B-induced protease activation, the cause of hereditary pancreatitis cannot be easily reduced to an increased cathepsin-B induced activation of mutant trypsinogen.

Role of trypsin in premature digestive protease activation

In isolated pancreatic acini and lobules, experiments using a specific cell-permeant and reversible trypsin inhibitor established that complete inhibition of trypsin activity does not prevent, nor even reduce, the conversion of trypsinogen to trypsin. On the other hand, a cell-permeant cathepsin B inhibitor prevented trypsinogen activation completely. Inhibitor washout experiments determined that following hormone-induced trypsinogen activation, 80% of the active trypsin is immediately and directly inactivated by trypsin itself. These experiments suggest that trypsin activity is neither required nor involved in trypsinogen activation and that its most prominent role is apparently its own auto-degradation. This, in turn, suggests that intracellular trypsin activity might have a role in the defense against other, potentially more harmful digestive proteases. Consequently, structural alterations that impair the function of trypsin in hereditary pancreatitis would eliminate a protective mechanism rather than generate a triggering event for pancreatitis. Whether these experimental observations obtained from rodent pancreatic acini and lobules have any relevance to human hereditary pancreatitis is presently unknown because human cationic trypsinogen may have different activation and degradation characteristics *in vivo*.

How structural changes in the cationic trypsinogen gene caused by germline mutations can lead to the onset of hereditary pancreatitis has also been a matter of debate. Trypsin is one of the oldest known digestive enzymes able to activate several other digestive proteases in the gut and *in vitro*. Because pancreatitis is regarded as a disease caused by proteolytic autodigestion of the pancreas, it seemed reasonable to assume that pancreatitis is caused by a trypsin-dependent protease cascade within the pancreas itself. Trypsinogen mutations found in association with hereditary pancreatitis should therefore confer a gain of enzymatic function in such a way that either mutant trypsinogen would be more readily activated inside acinar cells or, alternatively, that active trypsin would become less rapidly degraded. Both events would increase or extend enzymatic action of trypsin within the cellular environment. From a statistical point of view, however, most hereditary disorders, including most autosomal dominant diseases, are associated with loss-of-function mutations that render a specific protein defective or impair its intracellular processing or targeting. Moreover, a total of 16 mutations in the cationic trypsinogen protein, scattered over various regions of the molecule, have been reported to be associated with pancreatitis or hereditary pancreatitis. It seems therefore unlikely that such a great number of mutations located in entirely different regions of the protease serine 1 (*PRSS1*) gene

would all have the same effect on trypsinogen and result in a gain of enzymatic function. A loss of enzymatic function *in vivo* would, accordingly, be a much simpler and consistent explanation for the pathophysiologic role of hereditary pancreatitis mutations. On the other hand, several *in vitro* studies found that either facilitated trypsinogen autoactivation or extended trypsin activity can result under defined experimental conditions. Whether these *in vitro* conditions reflect the highly compartmentalized situation under which intracellular protease activation begins *in vivo* is presently unknown, but these findings would favor a gain of trypsin function as a consequence of several trypsinogen mutations.

Some recently reported kindreds with hereditary pancreatitis that carry a novel R122C mutation are very interesting with respect to a loss-of-function concept. The single nucleotide exchange in these families is located within exactly the same codon as in the most common variety of hereditary pancreatitis (R122C vs. R122H). Biochemical studies revealed that enterokinase-induced activation, cathepsin B-induced activation, and autoactivation of Cys122 trypsinogen are significantly reduced by 60–70% compared with the wild-type proenzyme. Cys122 trypsinogen seems to form mismatched disulfide bridges under intracellular *in vivo* conditions, resulting in a dramatic loss of trypsin function that cannot be compensated for by increased autoactivation. Indeed, if this scenario reflects the *in vivo* conditions within the pancreas, it would represent the first direct evidence from a human study for a "loss-of-function" mutation and therefore for a potential protective role of trypsin activity in the pancreas. Whether the gain-of-function hypothesis or the loss-of-function hypothesis correctly explains the pathophysiology of hereditary pancreatitis presently cannot be completely resolved, short of direct access to living human acini from carriers of *PRSS1* mutations or a transgenic animal model into which the human *PRSS1* mutations have been introduced.

Trypsinogen isoforms in human pancreatitis

The human pancreas secretes three isoforms of trypsinogen, encoded by the *PRSS* genes 1, 2, and 3. On the basis of their relative electrophoretic mobility, the three trypsinogen species are commonly referred to as cationic trypsinogen, anionic trypsinogen, and mesotrypsinogen. Normally the cationic isoform constitutes about two-thirds of the total trypsinogen content, while anionic trypsinogen makes up approximately one-third.

A characteristic feature of human pancreatic diseases as well as chronic alcoholism is the relatively selective upregulation of anionic trypsinogen secretion. Even though the two major human isoforms of trypsinogen are about 90% identical in their primary structure, their properties with respect to autocatalytic activation and degradation differ significantly. Anionic trypsinogen (and trypsin) exhibits a markedly increased propensity for autocatalytic degradation in comparison with cationic trypsinogen (and trypsin). Furthermore, acidic pH stimulates autoactivation of cationic trypsinogen, whereas it inhibits autoactivation of anionic trypsinogen. The distinctly different behavior of the two trypsinogen isoforms suggests that changes in their ratio should have profound effects on the overall stability of the pancreatic trypsinogen pool and its susceptibility to autoactivation.

Biochemical analysis of mixtures of the two trypsinogens at different ratios and in pH and calcium conditions indicative of physiologic or pathologic situations have provided evidence that upregulation of anionic trypsinogen in pancreatic disorders does not affect physiologic trypsinogen activation but significantly limits trypsin generation under potentially pathologic conditions. It seems that anionic trypsinogen plays a protective role in pancreatic physiology. As a defensive mechanism, acinar cells increase secretion of the anionic isoform in pancreatic diseases or under toxic conditions, thereby decreasing the risk for premature trypsinogen activation inside the pancreas while maintaining adequate trypsin function in the duodenum. On the other hand, the decreased ability of intrapancreatic trypsinogen to autoactivate can be regarded as a "loss of trypsin function" which, in this context, may play a disease-causing instead of a safeguarding role (see discussion on the possible role of loss of trypsin function in the onset of pancreatitis).

While these interpretations assume that total trypsinogen levels remain constant and that only the ratio of the two isoforms changes, in reality this is rarely the case. In chronic pancreatitis, trypsinogen secretion is generally decreased whereas in chronic alcoholism total trypsinogen secretion can be significantly elevated. As a consequence of increased trypsinogen synthesis the pancreas could be more susceptible to inappropriate zymogen activation, and becomes so

despite the protective effects of anionic trypsinogen. In this context, it is noteworthy that the rare pancreatitis-associated E79K mutation in human cationic trypsinogen results in a loss of function as far as autoactivation is concerned. However, the mutant enzyme activates anionic trypsinogen with twofold greater efficiency than wild-type cationic trypsin. The unusual mechanism of action of this mutant underscores the potential importance of an interaction between the two human trypsinogen isoforms in the pathogenesis of pancreatitis.

Role of calcium in pancreatic protease activation

Calcium is a critical intracellular second messenger in the regulated exocytosis of digestive enzymes from the apical pole of the acinar cell. On the other hand, calcium can also directly affect the activation and stability of trypsinogen and other proteases. These two aspects of calcium function are both involved in the onset of pancreatitis.

In vitro, Ca^{2+} is not required for trypsinogen activation by enterokinase or cathepsin B but stimulates autocatalytic activation of bovine cationic, rat anionic, or human anionic trypsinogen that usually requires high millimolar Ca^{2+} concentrations (2–10 mmol/L). In contrast, autoactivation of human cationic trypsinogen is stimulated in the submillimolar concentration range, while concentrations above 1 mmol/L inhibit autoactivation. The trypsinogen activation peptide (TAP) contains a negatively charged tetra-aspartate motif (Asp19-Asp20-Asp21-Asp22), which together with Lys23 forms the enterokinase recognition site. The negative charges of the aspartate carboxylates are believed to inhibit trypsin-induced (auto)activation, and high Ca^{2+} concentrations may shield these charges by binding to the tetra-aspartate sequence, which is also referred to as the low-affinity Ca^{2+}-binding site of trypsinogen. In the case of human cationic trypsinogen, stimulation of autoactivation already at low Ca^{2+} concentrations ($EC_{50} \sim 15\ \mu mol/L$) appears to be a consequence of Ca^{2+} binding to a different high-affinity binding site (see below). The mechanism whereby high-affinity Ca^{2+} binding facilitates autoactivation of cationic trypsinogen is unclear at present.

Ca^{2+} is also essential for the structural integrity of trypsinogen and trypsin. This effect of Ca^{2+} is mediated by the high-affinity Ca^{2+} binding site ($K_D \sim 20\ \mu mol/L$ for human cationic trypsin, as judged by protection against autolysis), which is located between Glu75 and Glu85. Binding of Ca^{2+} to this site is believed to induce conformational changes that reduce the proteolytic accessibility of surface-exposed Arg and Lys residues that are targets of trypsinolytic degradation. Differences in surface exposure of conserved Lys and Arg side-chains may further contribute to a trypsin isoform's specific sensitivity to autocatalytic degradation.

In acinar cells, Ca^{2+} is also a critical intracellular second messenger for the regulated exocytosis of digestive enzymes. Endocrine diseases associated with clinical hypercalcemia are known to predispose patients to develop pancreatitis, presumably by decreasing the threshold level for the onset of pancreatitis or by induction of morphologic alterations equivalent to pancreatitis. An elevation of acinar cytosolic free Ca^{2+} should be regarded as the most probable common denominator for the onset of various clinical varieties of acute or chronic pancreatitis. While the requirement for calcium in protease activation is undisputed and high intracellular Ca^{2+} concentrations are thought to represent a prerequisite for premature protease activation, Ca^{2+} alone seems to be insufficient to trigger this process.

Role of pH in pancreatic protease activation

Changes in pH also have a profound impact on autoactivation and autodigestion of trypsinogen. It is assumed that the pH within the lysosomal compartment is held between 4.5 and 5.5, whereas it is maintained between 6 and 7 in the secretory compartment. Some cytoplasmic vacuoles that arise during pancreatitis also appear to be acidic. Pancreatic zymogens, as opposed to cathepsins, are stable at very acidic pH (3.0 or 3.5) and neither autoactivation nor autodegradation occur to any significant degree. When pH is raised, autoactivation becomes more rapid up to a maximum at pH 5–6. At neutral or slightly alkaline pH and in the absence of Ca^{2+}, the rate of autoactivation declines while autodegradation becomes prevalent. In the presence of Ca^{2+} (see above), autoactivation is maximal at slightly alkaline pH with minimal autodegradation. Inside the acinar cell the pH is regulated in a much more narrowly controlled range than used in *in vitro* experiments. Maximal as well as supramaximal stimulation of pancreatic acinar cells leads to a slight increase (0.1–0.3) in intracellular pH but this process is again dependent on the presence of intracellular Ca^{2+}. In studies in which the acidic pH inside the vesicular compartments of acinar cells was neutralized by exposure to weak cell-permable bases, premature protease activation was found to be blocked. On the other hand, when the same agents were used to neutralize the acinar cell compartments *in vivo*, experimental pancreatitis was still found to occur and neither its onset nor its course were affected. This indicates that the role of intracellular pH in premature zymogen activation is complex. A shift of intracellular pH to conditions less favorable for premature activation of procarboxypeptidase and trypsinogen by trypsin may optimize the conditions for premature activation by cathepsin B. In this context it is noteworthy that activation of human cationic trypsinogen by cathepsin B exhibits a very sharp pH dependence in the acidic range. Between pH 4.0 and 5.2 a 100-fold decrease in activity was observed, suggesting that minor changes in intravesicular pH can have profound effects on cathepsin B-mediated trypsinogen activation in acinar cells. Which of these mechanisms plays the critical role in the onset or subsequent course of acute clinical pancreatitis will require additional studies.

Pancreatic secretory trypsin inhibitor gene (*SPINK1*)

PSTI, a 56-amino acid SPINK1, is synthesized in acinar cells as a 79-amino acid single-chain polypeptide precursor that is subsequently processed to the mature peptide, stored in zymogen granules, and secreted into pancreatic ducts. It is regarded as a first-line defense system that is capable of inhibiting up to 20% of total trypsin activity which may result from accidental premature activation of trypsinogen to trypsin within acinar cells. First studies on the role of *PSTI* mutations in chronic pancreatitis patients reported that some of these patients had a point mutation in exon 3 of the *PSTI* gene that leads to the substitution of an asparagine by serine at position 34 (N34S). Analysis of intronic sequences showed that the N34S mutation is in complete linkage disequilibrium with four additional sequence variants: IVS1–37TC, IVS2+268AG, IVS3–604GA, and IVS4–69insTTTT. Whether the N34S amino acid exchange or its association with these intronic mutations, which may confer splicing abnormalities, are causative in the context of PSTI pathophysiology is not clear at the moment. In a number of studies further mutations and polymorphisms have been detected in *PSTI*, including a methionine to threonine exchange that destroys the start codon of *PSTI* (1MT), a leucine to proline exchange in codon 14 (L14P), an aspartate to glutamine exchange in codon 50 (D50E), and a proline to serine exchange in codon 55 (P55S). Few studies have reported the frequencies of these mutations and they seem to be fairly low in comparison to the N34S mutation. N34S is present at a low level (0.4–2.5%) in the normal healthy population, but appears to be accumulated in selected groups of chronic pancreatitis patients. As a result of inconsistent selection criteria, different groups have reported N34S mutations in 6%, 19%, 26%, or even 86% of alcoholic, hereditary, or familial idiopathic pancreatitis patient groups. The considerable differences in these study results may be related not only to the absence of a generally accepted terminology for "familial" or "hereditary" and "idiopathic" pancreatitis, but could also be explained by the fact that determination of frequencies in some cases may involve several family members whereas other studies counted unrelated patients only. Independent of different reports about the strength of this association with chronic pancreatitis, the prevalence of N34S mutations appears to be increased in pancreatitis but does not follow a clear-cut recessive or complex inheritance trait. In hereditary pancreatitis associated with mutations in the cationic trypsinogen gene, studies have demonstrated that the additional presence of *SPINK1* mutations affects neither penetrance nor disease severity nor the onset of secondary diabetes mellitus. While this does not rule out that *SPINK1* is a "weak" risk factor for the onset of pancreatitis in general, it makes a modifier role in the onset of hereditary pancreatitis associated with "strong" *PRSS1* mutations very unlikely.

In studies that analyzed the association of PSTI with tropical pancreatitis, an endemic variety of pancreatitis in Africa and Asia, several groups have reported a strong association of N34S in populations in India and Bangladesh. Tropical pancreatitis is a type of idiopathic chronic pancreatitis of unknown etiology that can be categorized by its clinical manifestations into either tropical calcific pancreatitis or fibrocalculous pancreatic diabetes. While frequencies of the N34S mutation in the normal control population are comparable to previous reports from Europe and North America (1.3%), the mutation was found in 55% and 29% of patients with fibrocalculous pancreatic diabetes and in 20% and 36% of those with tropical calcific pancreatitis in Bangladesh and South India respectively.

Mutations in the *PSTI* gene may define a genetic predisposition for pancreatitis and apparently lowers the threshold for pancreatitis caused by other factors. However, a biochemical analysis of the protease-inhibiting activity of PSTI by Kuwata *et al.* reported unchanged trypsin-inhibiting function of N34S-PSTI under both alkaline and acidic conditions. At pH values between 5 and 9 recombinant N34S protein had the same inhibitory activity for trypsin as wild-type PSTI and also a variation of calcium concentrations revealed no differences of N34S function. The pathophysiology of N34S mutations may therefore follow mechanisms other than decreased protease inhibitory activity due to a conformational change. Instead the predisposition to pancreatitis in N34S patients may be caused by differences in PSTI expression levels possibly due to splicing defects. An analysis of PSTI protein expression levels in N34S patients will have to clarify this issue.

Cystic fibrosis transmembrane conductance regulator

In the general population a large number of different, relatively severe mutations are commonly found within the *CFTR* gene. Some of these mutations involve a single allele, whereas others are combinations of severe and mild mutations and additional 5T alleles in intron 8, that further reduce the amount of functional CFTR. The gene encodes a cyclic adenosine monophosphate-sensitive chloride channel essential for normal bicarbonate secretion and which is expressed in epithelial cells, such as those in the lung, biliary tract, pancreas, and vas deferens. Typical cystic fibrosis (CF) is an autosomal recessive inherited disease that results from severe mutations (e.g., Δ508) in both alleles of the *CFTR* gene. Besides chronic pulmonary disorders, CF shows multiorgan involvement and is the most common inherited disease of the pancreas. Children with *CFTR* mutations are often born with a severely damaged fibrotic pancreas and pancreatic insufficiency. Observations in chronic pancreatitis patients of abnormally increased sweat electrolyte levels and pancreatic ductal plugging comparable to findings in CF further suggested that CFTR may play a role in chronic pancreatitis as well. Several studies on patients with idiopathic chronic pancreatitis subsequently confirmed an increased *CFTR* mutation rate, which was elevated above the expected 5% carrier frequency normally observed in Caucasian populations. Genotypes that reduce CFTR protein function to 1% of its normal value cause typical CF, characterized by pulmonary disorders, pancreatic insufficiency, congenital bilateral absence of vas deferens, and sweat test alteration. Genotype–phenotype studies indicate that mutations that cause severe loss of CFTR function (<2% residual function) are linked to pancreatic insufficiency, whereas mutations that cause a milder loss of CFTR function (~5% residual function) are classified as pancreatic-sufficient, even though they still cause CF. Disease manifestation appears to depend on the amount of preserved CFTR function and also on a presumably (pancreatic) tissue-specific threshold level. To date, while more than 1000 *CFTR* mutations are known, commercial tests generally detect only a few severe mutations known to cause classical CF. Comprehensive *CFTR* gene testing in patients with idiopathic chronic pancreatitis will have to clarify whether the combination of specific severe/mild or of mild/mild *CFTR* mutations in a compound heterozygous state (and eventually also in combination with T5 alleles) represents a genetic predisposition to chronic pancreatitis.

Autoimmune chronic pancreatitis

Autoimmune pancreatitis represents a distinct form of chronic pancreatitis. The distinction of autoimmune pancreatitis from other forms is important because these patients respond very well to steroid therapy. Autoimmune pancreatitis may be occasionally observed in association with Sjögren's syndrome, primary biliary cirrhosis, primary sclerosing cholangitis, Crohn's disease, ulcerative colitis, or other immune-mediated disorders. Histologic features consist of destruction of the duct and fibrotic atrophy of the acinar tissue without calcifications. Ectors and colleagues noted a unique pattern of inflammation that particularly involved the ducts and resulted in duct obstruction and sometimes duct destruction. Histopathologically, an infiltration with lymphocytes, plasma cells, and fibrosis can be found.

Multiple autoantibodies have been detected in autoimmune pancreatitis, including those against nuclear structures, lactoferrin, carbonic anhydrase II, smooth muscle cells, and rheumatoid factor. The numbers of CD8+ and CD4+ cells are increased in the peripheral blood, suggesting a Th1-type immune response.

Inflammatory cells in chronic pancreatitis

Chronic inflammation is one of the characteristics of chronic pancreatitis. Mediators involved in the recruitment of inflammatory cells to the site of tissue injury are known as chemotactic factors and are produced in large quantities at the inflammatory site. These mediators, such as tumor necrosis factor-α, cytokines, and proinflammatory and antiinflammatory interleukins, regulate pancreatic tissue infiltration of mast cells, neutrophils, lymphocytes, and monocytes and initiate and control the subsequent healing process. This inflammatory response, which in some cases may lead to incomplete recovery from episodes of acute pancreatitis, presumably represents the key in a disease mechanism that controls the course of pancreatitis progression from the acute to the chronic state. In 1999, the so-called sentinel acute pancreatitis event (SAPE) hypothesis was introduced by David Whitcomb. This hypothesis is based on an initial "sentinel" event that indicates an episode of acute pancreatitis apparently due to any triggering event. Subsequent progression to a chronic disease state may then depend on the persistent presence of antiinflammatory cells (macrophages and activated stellate cells) that remain in the pancreatic tissue for a substantial period of time and which normally are important in limiting the inflammatory reaction and starting the healing process. Continued challenge of acinar cells by alcohol or other stresses during this period will provoke acinar cells to release cytokines and other mediators that are then able to induce, in still resident antiinflammatory cells, the production and deposition of collagen and extracellular matrix proteins characteristic of the fibrotic processes. As a consequence, the severity of recurrent episodes of acute pancreatitis may be tempered by the antiinflammatory response, yet the process of fibrosis is started, as seen in hereditary pancreatitis. While acute or chronic cellular stresses generally influence acinar cells to produce cytokines, it is the presence of macrophages and activated stellate cells, which may persist in pancreatic tissue only after a first "sentinel" event, that determines disease progression according to the SAPE hypothesis.

Recurrent and severe pancreatitis

For a long time the relationship between acute and chronic pancreatitis has been controversial and, under the Marseille definition, they were thought to represent two distinct entities assuming that acute pancreatitis would not progress to chronic pancreatitis. However, evidence from patients with frequent attacks of alcoholic acute pancreatitis revealed that progression to alcoholic chronic pancreatitis can happen rapidly and it appears that, in at least a subset of patients, progression from acute pancreatitis to chronic pancreatitis occurs. Indeed, it is now well established that an association between acute and chronic pancreatitis exists and in hereditary pancreatitis the majority of cases begin as recurrent acute pancreatitis. Several entities of chronic pancreatitis may therefore manifest in the early stage as recurrent episodes of acute pancreatitis and eventually evolve over years into a painless stage dominated by progressive pancreatic dysfunction and pancreatic calcification. The SAPE hypothesis currently provides a first explanation of how subsequent progression to a chronic disease state may depend on the persistent presence and modulating activity of antiinflammatory cells that remain in the pancreatic tissue for a substantial period of time.

Conclusions

Recent advances in cell biological and molecular techniques have permitted investigators to address intracellular pathophysiology in a much more direct manner than was previously considered possible. Initial studies that have employed these techniques have delivered a number of surprising results that appear to be incompatible with long-standing dogmas and paradigms of pancreatic research. Some of these insights will lead to new and testable hypotheses that will bring us closer to understanding the pathophysiologic mechanisms of pancreatitis. Only progress in elucidating the intracellular and molecular mechanisms involved in disease onset and progression will permit the development of effective strategies for the prevention and cure of this debilitating and still somewhat enigmatic disease.

Recommended reading

Cohn JA, Bornstein JD, Jowell PS. Cystic fibrosis mutations and genetic predisposition to idiopathic chronic pancreatitis. *Med Clin North Am* 2000;84:621–631, ix.

Etemad B, Whitcomb DC. Chronic pancreatitis: diagnosis, classification, and new genetic developments. *Gastroenterology* 2001;120:682–707.

Halangk W, Lerch MM, Brandt-Nedelev B *et al*. Role of cathepsin B in intracellular trypsinogen activation and the onset of acute pancreatitis. *J Clin Invest* 2000;106:773–781.

Halangk W, Kruger B, Ruthenburger M *et al*. Trypsin activity is not involved in premature, intrapancreatic trypsinogen activation. *Am J Physiol* 2002;282:G367–G374.

Hanck C, Schneider A, Whitcomb DC. Genetic polymorphisms in alcoholic pancreatitis. *Best Pract Res Clin Gastroenterol* 2003;17:613–623.

Hernandez CA, Lerch MM. Sphincter stenosis and gallstone migration through the biliary tract. *Lancet* 1993;341:1371–1373.

Howes N, Lerch MM, Greenhalf W *et al*. European Registry of Hereditary Pancreatitis and Pancreatic Cancer (EUROPAC). Clinical and genetic characteristics of hereditary pancreatitis in Europe. *Clin Gastroenterol Hepatol* 2004;2:252–261.

Kukor Z, Toth M, Sahin-Toth M. Human anionic trypsinogen. *Eur J Biochem* 2003;270:2047–2058.

Lerch MM, Saluja AK, Runzi M, Dawra R, Saluja M, Steer ML. Pancreatic duct obstruction triggers acute necrotizing pancreatitis in the opossum. *Gastroenterology* 1993;104:853–861.

Mooren FC, Hlouschek V, Finkes T *et al*. Early changes in pancreatic acinar cell calcium signaling after pancreatic duct obstruction. *J Biol Chem* 2003;278:9361–9369.

Okazaki K, Uchida K, Ohana M *et al*. Autoimmune-related pancreatitis is associated with autoantibodies and a Th1/Th2-type cellular immune response. *Gastroenterology* 2000;118:573–581.

Pfutzer RH, Barmada MM, Brunskill AP *et al*. SPINK1/PSTI polymorphisms act as disease modifiers in familial and idiopathic chronic pancreatitis. *Gastroenterology* 2000;119:615–623.

Sahin-Toth M. The pathobiochemistry of hereditary pancreatitis: studies on recombinant human cationic trypsinogen. Pancreatology 2001;1:461–465.

Sahin-Toth M, Toth M. Gain-of-function mutations associated with hereditary pancreatitis enhance autoactivation of human cationic trypsinogen. *Biochem Biophys Res Commun* 2000;278:286–289.

Schoenberg MH, Buchler M, Pietrzyk C *et al*. Lipid peroxidation and glutathione metabolism in chronic pancreatitis. *Pancreas* 1995;10:36–43.

Simon P, Weiss FU, Sahin-Toth M *et al*. Hereditary pancreatitis caused by a novel PRSS1 mutation (Arg-122 → Cys) that alters autoactivation and autodegradation of cationic trypsinogen. *J Biol Chem* 2002;277:5404–5410.

Teich N, Mossner J, Keim V. Screening for mutations of the

cationic trypsinogen gene: are they of relevance in chronic alcoholic pancreatitis? *Gut* 1999;44:413–416.

Teich N, Ockenga J, Keim V, Mossner J. Genetic risk factors in chronic pancreatitis. *J Gastroenterol* 2002;37:1–9.

Truninger K, Malik N, Ammann RW *et al*. Mutations of the cystic fibrosis gene in patients with chronic pancreatitis. *Am J Gastroenterol* 2001;96:2657–2661.

Truninger K, Kock J, Wirth HP *et al*. Trypsinogen gene mutations in patients with chronic or recurrent acute pancreatitis. *Pancreas* 2001;22:18–23.

Whitcomb DC. Hereditary pancreatitis: a model for under-standing the genetic basis of acute and chronic pancreatitis. *Pancreatology* 2001;1:565–570.

Whitcomb DC, Gorry MC, Preston RA *et al*. Hereditary pancreatitis is caused by a mutation in the cationic trypsinogen gene. *Nat Genet* 1996;14:141–145.

Witt H. Chronic pancreatitis and cystic fibrosis. *Gut* 2003;52(Suppl 2):ii31–41.

Witt H, Luck W, Hennies HC *et al*. Mutations in the gene encoding the serine protease inhibitor, Kazal type 1 are associated with chronic pancreatitis. *Nat Genet* 2000;25:213–216.

25 What is clinically relevant about the genetics of cystic fibrosis?

Harry Cuppens

Clinical aspects of cystic fibrosis

Cystic fibrosis (CF) is a common autosomal recessive disorder usually found in populations of white Caucasian descent. The disease is characterized by progressive lung disease, pancreatic dysfunction, elevated sweat electrolytes, and male infertility. However, wide variability in clinical expression is found among patients. Up to 20% of affected infants present at birth with intestinal obstruction and inspissated meconium (meconium ileus). Other patients are diagnosed with various modes of presentation from birth to adulthood, with considerable variability in the severity and rate of disease progression.

Although progressive lung disease is the most common cause of mortality in CF, there is great variability in age of onset and severity of lung disease in different age groups. The extent of pancreatic disease also varies. Most affected individuals suffer from pancreatic insufficiency, but up to 15% of patients possess sufficient exocrine pancreatic function to permit normal digestion and are called pancreatic sufficient. Symptoms of recurrent acute or chronic pancreatitis develop in approximately 2% of CF patients diagnosed on clinical grounds. It appears, however, that the latter symptoms first occur in adolescence or adulthood and only in patients with pancreatic sufficiency. Presumably, patients with pancreatic insufficiency are free of these complications because functional acinar tissue is lost *in utero* or soon after birth.

Variability is also found in male infertility. Almost all male CF patients are infertile due to congenital bilateral absence of the vas deferens (CBAVD); occasionally, however, fertile male patients have been reported.

Cystic fibrosis transmembrane conductance regulator

CF is caused by mutations in the cystic fibrosis transmembrane conductance regulator (*CFTR*) gene. The *CFTR* gene spans about 190 kb at the genomic level and contains 27 exons. Several alternatively spliced transcripts have been found, the most important being one that lacks exon 9 sequences. The CFTR protein is a glycosylated transmembrane protein that functions as a chloride channel. CFTR is expressed in epithelial cells of exocrine tissues, such as the lungs, pancreas, sweat glands, and vas deferens. Apart from its chloride channel function CFTR also functions as a regulator of, and is regulated by, other proteins: it regulates the outwardly rectifying chloride channel, inhibits the amiloride-sensitive epithelial sodium channel, and influences extracellular ATP delivery and HCO_3^- transport.

Individuals inherit one *CFTR* gene from their father and one *CFTR* gene from their mother; both genes are called *CFTR* alleles. Since CF is inherited in a recessive way, CF will develop when deleterious mutations are found on both *CFTR* alleles. When a deleterious mutation is found on only one *CFTR* allele, the individual is called a CF carrier. About 1 in 25 Caucasians is a CF carrier and therefore about 1 in 2500 newborns have CF.

Before the identification of the *CFTR* gene, it was generally expected that less then 10 mutations would occur in the gene causing CF. However, more than 1000 CF-causing *CFTR* mutations have been identified (http://genet.sickkids.on.ca/cgi-bin/WebObjects/MUTATION). Most mutations are point mutations, i.e., only one nucleotide is mutated in a *CFTR* gene. A CF patient can carry either an identical mutation on both *CFTR* alleles or two different mutations on both *CFTR* alleles and is then called compound heterozygous for two *CFTR* mutations. The distribution of *CFTR* mutations differs between different ethnic populations. The most common mutation, F508del, reaches frequencies of about 70% in northern European populations, whereas lower frequencies are observed in southern European populations. Besides F508del, other common mutations exist in most populations, each reaching frequencies of about 1–2%. Examples include the G542X, G551D, R553X, W1282X, and N1303K mutations. Finally, for a given ethnic population, ethnic-specific mutations that reach frequencies of about 1–2% might exist. For most populations, all these common mutations cover about 85–95% of all mutant *CFTR* genes. The remaining group of mutant *CFTR* genes in a particular population comprises rare mutations, some of them only found in a single family. CF-causing *CFTR* mutations are found in 95–99% of the *CFTR* genes derived from northern European CF patients; however, in southern European CF patients the mutation detection rate is only about 90–95%.

Depending on the effect at the protein level, *CFTR* mutations can be divided into at least five classes (Fig. 25.1). Class I mutations result in no CFTR synthesis because of mutations affecting splice sites, nonsense mutations resulting in truncated CFTR proteins that are mostly unstable and therefore degraded, and mutations shifting the coding frame in the gene (frameshift deletions and insertions). Class II mutations, such as the most common mutation F508del, result in CFTR proteins that fail to mature and which are degraded. Class III mutations result in CFTR proteins that mature and therefore reach the apical membrane of the cell, but which result in abnormal regulatory properties of the chloride channel. Class IV mutations result in CFTR channels with abnormal conductive properties because of mutations in the conductivity pore. Finally, class V mutations result in some functional CFTR protein. Class I, II, and III mutations are severe mutations, whereas class IV and V mutations are mild mutations.

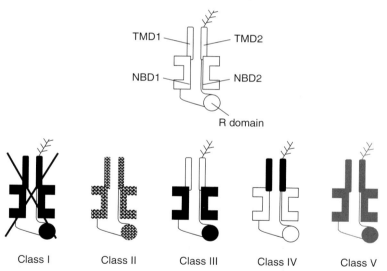

Figure 25.1 The different classes of *CFTR* mutations. The CFTR protein is a glycosylated transmembrane protein composed of two nucleotide-binding domains (NBD1 and NBD2), a regulatory (R) domain, and two transmembrane domains (TMD1 and TMD2). Class I mutations result in no CFTR synthesis; class II mutations result in CFTR proteins that fail to mature and which are degraded so that the glycosylated form is not observed; class III mutations result in CFTR proteins that mature but which result in abnormal regulatory properties of the chloride channel; class IV mutations result in CFTR channels having abnormal conductive properties; and class V mutations result in some functional CFTR protein.

Modifiers of CF disease

There is a good correlation between *CFTR* genotype and CF phenotype with regard to pancreatic disease. Most individuals homozygous for a severe mutation on both *CFTR* genes are pancreatic insufficient. However, the pulmonary phenotype can be quite variable, even between individuals with an identical *CFTR* genotype, and even between CF sibs. Other genetic factors and environmental factors affect the phenotype. Given the fact that the lungs are in direct contact with the environment, a higher number of factors influence lung disease compared with pancreatic disease. Other genetic factors that affect lung disease are, for example, the mannose-binding lectin protein and transforming growth factor-β_1. Nutrition, exposure to bacteria, and therapy are examples of environmental factors affecting disease.

CF-related diseases

Since identification of the gene that is defective in CF, *CFTR* has also been found to be involved in other diseases that share some of the symptoms seen in CF patients, such as CBAVD, disseminated bronchiectasis, and chronic pancreatitis.

Neonatal screening programs, using measurement of immunoreactive trypsinogen concentration (IRT), allow the detection of CF newborns. However, the IRT test produces rather high false-positive and false-negative results. In fact, in extensive retrospective studies of neonates having a false-positive IRT test (i.e., positive IRT without a CF diagnosis), an increased frequency of *CFTR* mutations is found and a considerable number of these patients are compound heterozygous for a severe and mild *CFTR* mutation. Although they do not present with CF, they might present with CF-related diseases eventually.

While in the majority of CF patients a mutation is found on both *CFTR* genes, a lower proportion of patients with CF-related diseases are found to carry a mutation on both *CFTR* genes. Disease-causing mutations are found in about 79% of the *CFTR* genes derived from CBAVD patients, in about 30% of the *CFTR* genes derived from patients with disseminated bronchiectasis, and in about 20% of chronic pancreatitis patients. The involvement of *CFTR* in the latter diseases is therefore more complex, multifactorial (i.e.,

involvement of other genetic and environmental factors), and far from unraveled.

In patients with two mutant *CFTR* genes, at least one will be a mild class IV or V mutation. The most frequent mutation conferring a mild phenotype found in these patients is the T5 polymorphism. In the Caucasian population, the T5 polymorphism is found in about 21% of the *CFTR* genes derived from CBAVD patients, whereas it is only found in about 5% of the *CFTR* genes derived from control individuals. T5 is one of the alleles found at the polymorphic T_n locus in intron 8 of the *CFTR* gene. A stretch of 5, 7, or 9 thymidine residues is found at this locus, hence the alleles T5, T7, and T9 (Fig. 25.2). A less-efficient splicing will occur when a lower number of thymidines is found, resulting in *CFTR* transcripts that lack exon 9 sequences (Fig. 25.3). Alternatively spliced *CFTR* transcripts lacking

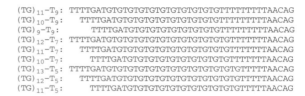

Figure 25.2 TG_m/T_n haplotype sequences at the end of intron 8 of the *CFTR* gene.

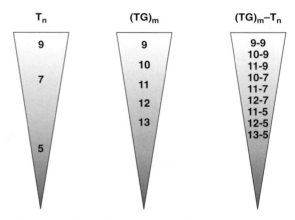

Figure 25.3 Effect of particular alleles on the amount of functional CFTR. For different polymorphic loci (T_n and TG_m) or haplotypes (TG_m-T_n), the effect of each allele/haplotype on the amount of CFTR chloride channel activity is shown. Decreasing amounts of functional CFTR are obtained (shown by the triangles narrowing from top to bottom).

exon 9 sequences are found in any individual, but the extent varies depending on the alleles present at the T_n locus. In individuals homozygous for a T5 allele, up to 90% of the *CFTR* transcripts lack exon 9. *CFTR* transcripts that lack exon 9 sequences result in CFTR proteins that do not mature. When T5 is found in compound heterozygosity with a severe *CFTR* mutation, or even T5, pathology such as CBAVD might be observed. However, not all male individuals who are compound heterozygous for a severe *CFTR* mutation and T5 develop CBAVD, such as some fathers of CF children. The T5 polymorphism was therefore classified as a disease mutation with partial penetrance. The partial penetrance can be explained by another genetic factor, namely the polymorphic TG_m locus in front of the T_n locus. Different alleles can be found depending on the number of TG repeats that are found (Fig. 25.2). The higher the number of TG repeats, the less efficient exon 9 splicing will be (Fig. 25.3). The T5 polymorphism can be found in combination with a TG11, TG12, or TG13 allele (11, 12, or 13 TG repeats respectively). In CBAVD patients, the milder TG11-T5 allele is hardly found, while the TG12-T5 is most frequently found. TG13-T5 is rarer but also found in CBAVD patients. It might even result in pancreatic-sufficient CF, possibly because of additional polymorphisms that affect *CFTR* such as V470. In individuals who are compound heterozygous for a severe mutation and the T5 allele, such as fathers of CF patients, T5 is associated with the milder TG11 allele. The fact that the allele found at the polymorphic TG_m locus determines whether the T5 polymorphism is pathologic or benign has been confirmed in a large international study. Frequent, apparently innocent, polymorphisms can in particular combinations result in mutant *CFTR* genes. Such mutant *CFTR* genes have been named polyvariant mutant *CFTR* genes.

The spectrum and distribution of *CFTR* mutations differ between patient groups and even control individuals. For example, the F508del mutation is found at a higher frequency in CF patients compared with patients having CBAVD, disseminated bronchiectasis, or chronic pancreatitis. The opposite is true for other mutations, such as the class IV mutation R117H. The spectrum and distribution of mutations found in CF patients are not suitable for calculating the frequencies of these mutations in the general population or other CFTR-related diseases.

It should be noted that in commercial genetic *CFTR* tests, the majority of mutations tested are severe mutations causing CF, such that mild mutations may not be detected.

Idiopathic chronic pancreatitis

In the majority of patients with chronic pancreatitis, the causative factor is long-term alcohol abuse. In 10–30% of these patients, the etiology remains unknown and this category has been labeled idiopathic chronic pancreatitis (ICP). Rare hereditary, obstructive, or autoimmune processes may be involved in ICP.

The observation that pancreatic lesions of CF develop *in utero* and closely resemble those of chronic pancreatitis stimulated two research groups to explore a possible relationship between *CFTR* mutations and chronic pancreatitis. This led to the important finding that about 20% of ICP patients carry at least one severe (CF-causing) *CFTR* mutation, whereas in the control population only 3–4% of individuals carry one CF-causing *CFTR* mutation.

In the original studies, only the most common *CFTR* mutations were screened. In a French study, the complete coding region and exon–intron junctions of the *CFTR* genes of 39 patients with ICP were studied. Here, also, about 20% of ICP patients carry one CF-causing (severe) *CFTR* mutation. Since each individual carries two *CFTR* genes, a severe mutation is found on about 10% of the *CFTR* genes derived from ICP patients. If milder mutations are included, a mutation is found on 33% of the *CFTR* genes derived from ICP patients. About 15% of ICP patients are compound heterozygous for two mutations, one of the two being a mild mutation. Some of these ICP patients who are compound heterozygous for two *CFTR* mutations may even show a positive sweat test, but without presentation of CF-related pulmonary symptoms. Besides the *CFTR* gene, the pancreatic secretory trypsin inhibitor (*PSTI*) gene and the cationic trypsinogen (*PRSS1*) gene have also been found to be associated with chronic pancreatitis. Mutations in *PSTI* appear at a detection rate of about 10% in ICP patients, and mutations in *PRSS1* are occasionally found.

The fact that *CFTR* mutations can cause pancreatic insufficiency in CF patients or pancreatitis only in pancreatic-sufficient CF patients might be explained by the multiple functions of CFTR. It might be that the different properties of CFTR are responsible for the two disease entities. In this regard it is interesting to note that CFTR is also involved in HCO_3^- transport. Ductal obstruction due to inspissated secretions is generally regarded as the initiating event in both CF and chronic pancreatitis. However, this theory is undermined by several observations, as well as by histologic evidence to the contrary. Sharer *et al.* proposed an alternative explanation wherby the acinar cell is a direct target and the damage is amplified when bicarbonate-producing epithelium is affected in a manner that reduces the pH within the intraacinar space and the lumen of ductules.

CF remains a clinical diagnosis

Once the defective CF gene was found, it was expected that DNA tests would make the diagnosis and screening of CF straightforward. This was based on the belief that only a limited number of mutations would exist. However, more than 1200 mutations have been identified in the *CFTR* gene, which in many cases makes a diagnosis on the basis of a genetic test too laborious and expensive. In routine genetic tests only the most common severe *CFTR* mutations are screened; these tests detect about 90% of the CF-causing *CFTR* mutations. Whenever a patient harbors mutations on both *CFTR* genes and which are detected in these routine DNA tests, a CF diagnosis can be easily made. The remaining group of mutant *CFTR* genes in a particular ethnic population comprises rare mutations, some of them only found in a single family. Moreover, when one of the more common mutations is not found, it is likely that a mutation is present that has never previously been detected in that given ethnic population. It is therefore very hard to establish a strategy for general screening of *CFTR* mutations that allows sensitivities close to 100%, even in a well-characterized ethnic population. The remaining mutations (10%) can only be screened by assays that analyze the complete coding region and exon–intron junctions of the *CFTR* gene, but they are too laborious and too expensive in a routine setting.

Moreover, in some cases, a mutation cannot be identified in any *CFTR* gene from a patient. Particular mutations may not be detected because of the limitations of the screening assays (e.g., deep intronic regions and promoter regions, which are not screened in current assays because of their huge size). The frequency of *CFTR* genes in which no mutation can be identified is

about 1–2% in northern European populations but up to 10% in southern European populations. Moreover, CF-like disease not caused by CFTR has been reported, and therefore it is possible that another gene might be involved in some CF patients. Furthermore, there is the problem of "atypical" CF patients (i.e., patients who have only a borderline abnormal sweat test and in whom no mutation is found on at least one *CFTR* gene), which also complicates the diagnosis based on current DNA tests. Finally, the disease phenotype, especially the pulmonary phenotype, is very variable, even between patients with the same *CFTR* genotype. This variability is explained by other genes as well as environmental factors. This in turn makes the interpretation of genetic tests for the phenotypic outcome of the disease very complex. It can thus be expected that in CF-related diseases and the more common adult multifactorial diseases in general, genetic tests and the interpretation of their results will be even more complicated than in CF.

Despite the sophisticated molecular technology available in genetic laboratories, CF therefore remains a clinical diagnosis, based on the typical clinical symptoms of CF, being a relative of a CF patient, and/or having a positive sweat test. The diagnosis can then be easily confirmed by DNA tests if the patient harbors common mutations on both *CFTR* genes. However, *CFTR* genetic tests allow better genetic counseling, such as determination of the carrier status of relatives of CF patients, prenatal diagnosis, or determination of the carrier status of female partners of CBAVD patients for *CFTR* mutations since such couples have an increased risk for CF children in intracytoplasmic sperm injection (ICSI) programs. As the human genome is further unraveled and with improving technologies, it is expected that DNA tests will allow quicker and more accurate diagnosis of disease phenotypes in the future.

Recommended reading

Arkwright PD, Laurie S, Super M *et al.* TGF-β_1 genotype and accelerated decline in lung function of patients with cystic fibrosis. *Thorax* 2000;55:459–462.

Audrezet MP, Chen JM, Le Marechal C *et al.* Determination of the relative contribution of three genes—the cystic fibrosis transmembrane conductance regulator gene, the cationic trypsinogen gene, and the pancreatic secretory trypsin inhibitor gene—to the etiology of idiopathic chronic pancreatitis. *Eur J Hum Genet* 2002;10:100–106.

Castellani C, Benetazzo MG, Tamanini A, Begnini A, Mastella G, Pignatti P. Analysis of the entire coding region of the cystic fibrosis transmembrane regulator gene in neonatal hypertrypsinaemia with normal sweat test. *J Med Genet* 2001;38:202–205.

Chillón M, Casals T, Mercier B *et al*. Mutations in the cystic fibrosis gene in patients with congenital absence of the vas deferens. *N Engl J Med* 1995;332:1475–1480.

Choi JY, Muallem D, Kiselyov K, Lee MG, Thomas PJ, Muallem S. Aberrant CFTR-dependent HCO_3^- transport in mutations associated with cystic fibrosis. *Nature* 2001; 410:94–97.

Chu C-S, Trapnell BC, Curristin S, Cutting GR, Crystal RG. Genetic basis of variable exon 9 skipping in cystic fibrosis transmembrane conductance regulator mRNA. *Nat Genet* 1993;3:151–156.

Claustres M, Guittard C, Bozon D *et al*. Spectrum of CFTR mutations in cystic fibrosis and in congenital absence of the vas deferens in France. *Hum Mutat* 2000;16:143–156.

Cohn JA, Friedman KJ, Noone PG, Knowles MR, Silverman LM, Jowell PS. Relation between mutations of the cystic fibrosis gene and idiopathic pancreatitis. *N Engl J Med* 1998;339:653–658.

Cuppens H, Lin W, Jaspers M *et al*. Polyvariant mutant cystic fibrosis transmembrane conductance regulator genes: the polymorphic (TG)m locus explains the partial penetrance of the T5 polymorphism as a disease mutation. *J Clin Invest* 1998;101:487–496.

Delaney SJ, Rich DP, Thomson SA *et al*. Cystic fibrosis transmembrane conductance regulator splice variants are not conserved and fail to produce chloride channels. *Nat Genet* 1993;4:426–431.

Dumur V, Gervais R, Rigot J-M *et al*. Abnormal distribution of CF F508del allele in azoospermic men with congenital aplasia of epididymis and vas deferens. *Lancet* 1990;336: 512.

Egan M, Flotte T, Afione S *et al*. Defective regulation of outwardly rectifying Cl⁻ channels by protein kinase A corrected by insertion of CFTR. *Nature* 1992;358:581–584.

Garred P, Pressler T, Madsen HO *et al*. Association of mannose-binding lectin gene heterogeneity with severity of lung disease and survival in cystic fibrosis. *J Clin Invest* 1999;104:431–437.

Groman JD, Meyer ME, Wilmott RW, Zeitlin PL, Cutting GR. Variant cystic fibrosis phenotypes in the absence of CFTR mutations. *N Engl J Med* 2002;347:401–407.

Groman JD, Hefferon TW, Casals T *et al*. Variation in a repeat sequence determines whether a common variant of the cystic fibrosis transmembrane conductance regulator gene is pathogenic or benign. *Am J Hum Genet* 2004;74: 176–179.

Pignatti PF, Bombieri C, Marigo C, Benetazzo M, Luisetti M. Increased incidence of cystic fibrosis gene mutations in adults with disseminated bronchiectasis. *Hum Mol Genet* 1995;4:635–639.

Reisin IL, Prat AG, Abraham EH *et al*. The cystic fibrosis transmembrane conductance regulator is a dual ATP and chloride channel. *J Biol Chem* 1994;269:20584–20591.

Riordan JR, Rommens JM, Kerem B-S *et al*. Identification of the cystic fibrosis gene: cloning and characterization of complementary DNA. *Science* 1989;245:1066–1073.

Santis G, Osborne L, Knight RA, Hodson ME. Independent genetic determinants of pancreatic and pulmonary status in cystic fibrosis. *Lancet* 1990;336:1081–1084.

Sharer N, Schwarz M, Malone G *et al*. Mutations of the cystic fibrosis gene in patients with chronic pancreatitis. *N Engl J Med* 1998;339:645–652.

Strong TV, Wilkinson DJ, Mansoura MK *et al*. Expression of an abundant alternatively spliced form of the cystic fibrosis transmembrane conductance regulator (CFTR) gene is not associated with a cAMP-activated chloride conductance. *Hum Mol Genet* 1993;2:225–230.

Stutts MJ, Canessa CM, Olsen JC *et al*. CFTR as a cAMP-dependent regulator of sodium channels. *Science* 1995;269: 847–850.

Welsh MJ, Smith AE. Molecular mechanisms of CFTR chloride channel dysfunction in cystic fibrosis. *Cell* 1993; 73:1251–1254.

Welsh MJ, Tsui L-C, Boat TF, Beaudet AL. Cystic fibrosis. In: CR Scriver, AL Beaudet, WS Sly, D Valle (eds) *The Metabolic and Molecular Bases of Inherited Disease*, 7th edn. New York: McGraw-Hill, 1995: 3799–3876.

Wilschanski M, Zielenski J, Markiewicz D *et al*. Correlation of sweat chloride concentration with classes of the cystic fibrosis transmembrane conductance regulator gene mutations. *J Pediatr* 1995;127:705–710.

26 How does alcohol damage the pancreas?

Tomas Hucl, Alexander Schneider, and Manfred V. Singer

Alcohol and pancreatitis

It is generally accepted that excessive alcohol consumption can lead to acute and chronic pancreatitis. Although the relationship between alcohol abuse and pancreatic disease has been supported by many studies, the exact mechanisms underlying the disease are not yet fully understood. This chapter summarizes the pathophysiologic effects of alcohol on the pancreas.

Several retrospective and prospective studies have investigated the incidence of alcohol-induced pancreatitis in cohorts of patients with acute and chronic pancreatitis in industrialized countries. These investigations demonstrated that alcohol abuse accounts for 38–94% of all cases of chronic pancreatitis. The varying results may reflect the difficulties in establishing the diagnosis of chronic pancreatitis and in identifying the underlying alcohol abuse. One prospective study of patients with alcoholic chronic pancreatitis demonstrated an incidence of 8.2 cases per year and an overall prevalence of 27.4 cases per 100 000 individuals.

Further information regarding the frequency of pancreatic damage in patients with excessive alcohol consumption was obtained in autopsy studies. These revealed that chronic alcohol abuse does not always lead to the clinical manifestation of pancreatic disease but may result only in histologic changes suggestive of chronic pancreatitis in up to 30% of individuals with chronic alcohol abuse. Thus, chronic pancreatitis may develop frequently in alcoholic individuals, but the pancreatic damage often remains asymptomatic.

The epidemiologic data clearly suggest that alcohol consumption represents an important factor for the development of chronic pancreatitis. Most patients with alcoholic chronic pancreatitis have a long history of heavy alcohol consumption. In 1997 an international conference on alcoholic chronic pancreatitis agreed to define the disease as chronic pancreatitis which occurs after a daily intake of ethanol equal to or greater than 80 g/day for several years. It usually requires 13–21 years of continuous alcohol abuse to develop alcohol-induced chronic pancreatitis. One study demonstrated that the risk of alcoholic chronic pancreatitis increases logarithmically with higher amounts of alcohol consumption. However, there appears to be no precise threshold of toxicity below which alcoholic pancreatitis does not occur. In general, the individual susceptibility makes it difficult to correlate the various levels of alcohol ingestion with disease risk. The kind of alcoholic beverage appears not to play a major role in predisposing to the disease.

Several observations suggest that there are as yet unidentified cofactors that must be present for the development of alcoholic pancreatitis. It remains unclear why only up to 10% of heavy alcohol drinkers ever develop clinically recognized pancreatic inflammation. Some alcoholics develop alcoholic pancreatitis, but more present with alcoholic liver disease, and only a few develop both conditions. Thus, the relationship between alcohol consumption and the resulting end-organ damage appears unpredictable. The clinical course of pancreatic disease demonstrates marked variability. Racial susceptibility may play a role, since black patients are two to three times more likely to be hospitalized for pancreatitis than white patients. Finally, factors such as gender, diet, nutritional status, tobacco smoking, hypertriglyceridemia, anatomy of the biliary and pancreatic ducts, bacterial or viral infections, and genetic predispositions may also have significant impact on the development of the disease.

The majority of patients with alcoholic chronic pancreatitis are diagnosed between 35 and 40 years of age. Alcoholic chronic pancreatitis usually presents with an early phase of recurrent attacks of acute pancreatitis that may last for several years, followed by the late phase of the disease characterized by the development of chronic pain, pancreatic calcifications, and exocrine and endocrine insufficiency.

The relationship between acute and chronic alcoholic pancreatitis remains controversial. Studies in patients with an initial episode of acute alcoholic pancreatitis revealed that these patients already demonstrated histologic changes of chronic pancreatitis. In contrast, several long-term clinical studies, autopsy studies, recent experimental studies, and investigations in patients with hereditary pancreatitis provide strong evidence that recurrent attacks of acute pancreatitis may also lead to chronic pancreatitis. Indeed, one autopsy study showed that acute alcoholic pancreatitis represented the first manifestation of chronic pancreatitis in only about half of 247 alcoholic patients who died of acute pancreatitis, but not in the other half who demonstrated no signs of chronic pancreatic damage.

Mechanisms of ethanol-induced pancreatic damage

Animal models of acute and chronic ethanol administration have been developed in order to study the effects of ethanol on the pancreas. Unfortunately, none of them have been successful in producing acute or chronic pancreatitis with alcohol administration alone. Protein plugs and sclerosis of the pancreas developed in animals after prolonged ethanol feeding in one study. However, these results were not reproducible by others, and the same changes occurred even spontaneously in control animals. Therefore, ethanol exposure has been combined with other factors and interesting results have been demonstrated regarding the specific effects of ethanol on pancreatic exocrine secretion, pancreatic blood flow, pancreatic duct permeability, zymogen activation, intracellular signaling, oxidative stress generation, and the interaction of ethanol and its metabolites with recently identified pancreatic stellate cells (Tables 26.1–26.4).

Table 26.1 Major effects of acute ethanol administration on pancreatic exocrine secretion in studies on humans and ethanol-fed animals.

Oral and intragastric ethanol administration increases pancreatic bicarbonate and protein secretion

Intravenous ethanol administration reduces basal and hormonally stimulated pancreatic bicarbonate and protein secretion

Nonalcoholic constituents of beer may increase pancreatic secretion

Table 26.2 Major effects of chronic ethanol administration on pancreatic exocrine secretion in studies on humans and ethanol-fed animals.

Human alcoholics
Basal pancreatic enzyme secretion is increased
Viscosity of the pancreatic juice is enhanced
Pancreatic juice contains a higher concentration of proteins
Pancreatic bicarbonate secretion is decreased
Enhanced ratio of trypsinogen levels to pancreatic secretory trypsin inhibitor levels is present in pancreatic juice

Ethanol-fed animals
Diet rich in fat and protein increases the concentrations of enzymes in pancreatic juice

Table 26.3 Major effects of acute ethanol administration on pancreatic morphology in studies using animal models.

Ethanol administration (intragastrically, intraperitoneally, intravenously) with physiologic stimulation (cholecystokinin, secretin) and obstruction of the pancreatic duct results in acute pancreatitis

Ethanol administration enhances the vulnerability of the pancreas to acute pancreatitis and limits pancreatic regeneration from acute pancreatitis

Ethanol administration selectively reduces pancreatic blood flow and microcirculation

Cigarette smoke enhances ethanol-induced pancreatic ischemia

Ethanol administration increases free oxygen radical generation in the pancreas

Ethanol metabolites directly damage the pancreas

Table 26.4 Major effects of chronic ethanol administration on pancreatic morphology in studies using animal models.

Dietary fat potentiates ethanol-induced pancreatic injury

Ethanol administration increases free oxygen radical generation in the pancreas

Ethanol administration increases pancreatic acinar cell expression and glandular content of digestive and lysosomal enzymes

Ethanol administration decreases the number of muscarinic receptor sites

Ethanol administration limits pancreatic regeneration after temporary obstruction of the pancreatic duct and further aggravates the pancreatic damage already induced

Ethanol administration sensitizes pancreatic acinar cells to endotoxin-induced injury

Ethanol administration enhances the vulnerability of the pancreas to pancreatitis caused by cholecystokinin octapeptide

---

Pancreatic blood flow

The influence of acute ethanol application on pancreatic blood flow has been investigated in several studies. Ethanol administration may result in pancreatic hypoxia, increased capillary permeability, and induction of oxidative stress. A reduction of pancreatic blood flow was achieved by intravenous infusion of ethanol in dogs. In cats, pancreatic damage resembling human chronic pancreatitis was created by partial pancreatic duct ligation. In the operated animals, basal pancreatic blood flow was reduced to 51% of normal. Acute ethanol administration led to a decrease in pancreatic blood flow in all animals. However, the magnitude and duration of diminished blood flow after ethanol administration was greater in the cats with chronic pancreatitis induced by partial pancreatic duct ligation. In ethanol-treated rats, pancreatic hemoglobin oxygen saturation was significantly decreased and remained depressed for over an hour, whereas pancreatic hemoglobin content remained unaffected. Since these parameters remained unchanged in the stomach and kidney, a possible link between ethanol-induced ischemia and pancreas-specific organ damage was suggested. Of note, a marked reduction in pancreatic microcirculation has been shown in human alcoholic chronic pancreatitis as well.

Pancreatic duct obstruction and pancreatic duct pressure

The interaction between oral ethanol ingestion, physiologic stimulation of the gland with cholecystokinin (CCK) and secretin, and obstruction of the pancreatic duct led to acute pancreatitis in rats. Only the combination of all three factors induced pancreatic damage. This experimental model demonstrates the importance of pancreatic duct obstruction in the development of alcoholic pancreatitis.

Indeed, obstruction of the small pancreatic ducts is a frequent finding in human chronic pancreatitis. In another model, incomplete pancreatic duct obstruction was achieved by surgical intervention in dogs. Ethanol-fed dogs without pancreatic duct obstruction demonstrated no pancreatic injury, whereas ethanol-fed animals with pancreatic duct obstruction showed reduced exocrine pancreatic function and histologic damage comprising fibrosis, parenchymal cell loss, and chronic inflammatory cell infiltration. In rats, obstruction of the pancreatic duct was achieved with Ethibloc application, a tissue adhesive that is subsequently completely decomposed by the organism. Changes such as extensive fibrosis, inflammatory cell infiltration, and acinar cell degeneration caused by application of Ethibloc alone were reversible after its decomposition. Interestingly, further prolonged alcohol administration in these rats via an intragastric cannula inhibited the recovery and resulted frequently in parenchymal calcifications. Pancreatic regeneration was less pronounced in ethanol-fed animals, and the calcifications remained in some animals. Thus, these data support the importance of pancreatic duct obstruction during the progression of chronic pancreatitis.

Pancreatic duct pressure is influenced by the viscosity of pancreatic fluid, the rate of pancreatic secretion, and the resistance to outflow within the pancreatic duct. Sphincter of Oddi dysfunction, pancreatic duct stones, and pancreatic strictures may increase the resistance to pancreatic outflow and the pressure in the pancreatic duct. Two studies revealed increased basal sphincter of Oddi and pancreatic duct pressures in patients with alcoholic chronic pancreatitis. However, these studies included only few patients, and the significance of sphincter dysfunction in alcoholic chronic pancreatitis remains unclear.

Nutrition in alcoholic chronic pancreatitis

The failure of most animal models of chronic alcohol consumption to cause pancreatitis may result from the administration of relatively less alcohol than that usually observed in humans with chronic alcohol abuse. Thus, feeding protocols have been developed to allow independent control over ethanol and nutrient intake using implanted gastrostomy catheters. These models were used to administer higher doses of alcohol. Using this experimental approach, rats were fed continuously with ethanol and a liquid diet containing different amounts of fat. Sustained blood ethanol levels were achieved, and after 1–5 months pancreatic tissue was examined. In animals that received no ethanol or were fed ethanol together with a low-fat diet, pancreatic histology was either unremarkable or showed only mild pancreatic damage such as steatosis. In rats receiving ethanol together with a high-fat diet, pancreatic damage was observed, such as hypogranulation and apoptosis of acinar cells, focal lesions of chronic pancreatitis such as fat necrosis, mononuclear cell infiltration, fibrosis, acinar atrophy, and ductal dilatation. Intraductal plugs were present in up to 30% of the animals. It was suggested that dietary fat potentiates ethanol-induced pancreatic injury. In a similar study, rats were fed with ethanol and either saturated or unsaturated fat. The dose of ethanol was gradually increased as tolerance toward ethanol developed, thereby allowing the administration of a higher dosage of alcohol. After 4 weeks, acinar cell atrophy, fatty infiltration of pancreatic acinar and islet cells, infiltration of inflammatory cells, and focal necrosis were observed in rats from the high-dose ethanol group that were also fed unsaturated fat. After 8 weeks, focal fibrosis developed in this group, and radical adducts were also significantly increased. The effects were blunted by administration of dietary saturated fat. The authors concluded that the total amount of ethanol consumption and the type of dietary fat represent important factors for pancreatic damage. Further studies with regard to nutrition are clearly necessary in human alcoholics.

Pancreatic exocrine secretion

Many studies have focused on the effects of ethanol administration on pancreatic exocrine function. These investigations have suggested that the resulting changes in protein and bicarbonate output cause premature activation of zymogens or protein plug formation and subsequent obstruction of the duct system, thereby leading to the development of pancreatitis. The results of these studies support both an increase and a decrease in digestive enzyme secretion. This contradictory evidence is probably due to different experimental conditions. The exact mechanisms by which ethanol administration alters pancreatic exocrine secretion have not been fully revealed. The following sections provide a short overview of the interaction of ethanol with pancreatic exocrine secretion in the setting of acute and chronic ethanol exposure (Tables 26.1 and 26.2).

Acute effects of ethanol

The acute effects of ethanol *in vitro* have been studied by several groups. One group showed increased basal amylase release after ethanol exposure (0.3–1.3 mol), and ethanol (0.6 mol) also induced inhibition of CCK-stimulated amylase release. Later, similar findings were observed by other groups and the inhibition of CCK-stimulated amylase release was explained by the inhibition of CCK-stimulated Ca^{2+} efflux. Another study also demonstrated that ethanol alone increased pancreatic amylase secretion, but inhibited the sustained phase of amylase release that was stimulated by CCK. In this study ethanol increased the Ca^{2+} rise caused by CCK and inhibited the CCK-stimulated Ca^{2+} outflux. Changes in the Ca^{2+} content suggested that ethanol may affect the calcium stimulus–secretion coupling pathway. The precise mechanism of ethanol action on amylase release remains to be determined.

In humans, cats, and pigs, oral or intragastric administration of ethanol has been shown to cause weak stimulation of pancreatic bicarbonate and protein output when the gastric content is allowed to enter the duodenum. Without alcohol entering the duodenum, instillation of ethanol inhibits or does not affect pancreatic exocrine secretion in humans, dogs, and rats. These data suggest a modifying role for ethanol-induced gastric acid secretion in changes of pancreatic secretion. However, it later turned out that this mechanism was most probably only true in dogs. In humans, intragastric application of ethanol does not cause significant gastric acid output and gastrin release.

The modifications of pancreatic secretion caused by ethanol ingestion in combination with a meal have been studied in a few experiments. In one study, inhibition of postprandial enzyme secretion was observed with intragastric application of ethanol. However, another study reported a mild decrease in the early postprandial period followed by a significant increase in enzyme secretion.

Intravenous administration of ethanol appears to be the most reliable method for investigating the direct effects of alcohol on pancreatic cells *in vivo*. With this route of administration, ethanol leads to a dose-dependent inhibition of the basal and hormonally stimulated pancreatic bicarbonate and enzyme output in humans and in different animal species. Although the inhibitory action of ethanol on pancreatic secretion has been suggested to be a consequence of cholinergic mediation, this mechanism has never been proven in humans. Thus, the exact mechanism remains unclear. Two studies investigated the effects of ethanol after premedication with atropine, and demonstrated that ethanol had no further inhibitory effects on pancreatic amylase output in this setting.

Acute effects of alcoholic beverages

Alcoholic beverages contain several nonalcoholic constituents that may also affect pancreatic secretion. Intragastric administration of beer in a dose (250 mL) that does not alter plasma ethanol concentrations caused a significant stimulation of basal pancreatic enzyme output. It was proposed that the stimulatory effect might be mediated by the hormones CCK and gastrin. The intragastric administration of ethanol in concentrations similar to the ethanol content of beer (4% v/v) has no effect on pancreatic enzyme output. Therefore, the nonalcoholic constituents might be responsible for the stimulatory effect of beer on pancreatic secretion in humans and the alcoholic fermentation of glucose might be the important event that generates the stimulatory substances in beer.

In a similar study, pancreatic enzyme output was determined after intragastric administration of beer (850 mL) or wine (400 mL) in a dose that elevated plasma ethanol concentrations. Since the basal pancreatic enzyme output remained unchanged, it was suggested that the direct inhibitory effect of the circulating ethanol in the blood may have neutralized the stimulatory effect of the nonalcoholic components.

Meal-stimulated pancreatic enzyme output has been shown to be inhibited by intragastric application of beer, white wine, and gin. Plasma levels of ethanol were elevated in these studies. Therefore, the circulating ethanol in the blood may have again neutralized the possible stimulatory effect of beer and wine on pancreatic secretion.

Chronic effects of ethanol

The effects of chronic alcohol consumption on pancreatic gene expression and glandular content of pancreatic enzymes have been studied in rats. Messenger RNA levels for lipase, trypsinogen, chymotrypsinogen, and cathepsin B were elevated in ethanol-fed rats, suggesting that chronic ethanol consumption increases the capacity of the pancreatic acinar cell to synthesize digestive and lysosomal enzymes and that these changes might lead to an elevated susceptibility of the pancreas to enzyme-related damage. Interestingly, an enhanced ratio of trypsinogen levels to pancreatic secretory trypsin inhibitor levels was found in the pancreatic juice of alcohol-abusing humans. This distortion of the normal ratio in favor of trypsinogen may facilitate premature activation of pancreatic proenzymes within the pancreas. These studies suggest that chronic alcohol consumption leads to changes in pancreatic enzyme synthesis that may increase the risk of premature zymogen activation.

Basal pancreatic enzyme output was increased in human alcoholics compared with nonalcoholics. The enhanced viscosity of the pancreatic juice was correlated with increased concentrations of proteins. Pancreatic bicarbonate secretion was significantly lower in human alcoholics than in nonalcoholics. Since the volume of pancreatic juice was similar in control individuals and in subjects with chronic alcohol abuse, a true hypersecretion of pancreatic proteins may exist in patients with excessive alcohol consumption. The basal plasma concentrations of secretin, CCK, and gastrin remained unchanged in alcoholic and nonalcoholic subjects.

In an experimental setting, the administration of a diet rich in fat and protein resulted in an increase of the pancreatic juice concentrations of enzymes in dogs and rats that were fed ethanol for a prolonged period of time. A decreased flow rate of pancreatic juice together with protein plug formation was found in some of these dogs.

Studies of the effects of chronic alcohol intake on the hormonally stimulated pancreatic secretion have revealed that pancreatic bicarbonate secretion remains unaffected. However, patients with chronic alcohol abuse demonstrated an increase in the enzyme secretion response on exogenous administration of CCK. As already mentioned, an enhanced ratio of trypsinogen levels to pancreatic secretory trypsin inhibitor levels was found in the pancreatic juice from humans with chronic alcohol abuse. This distortion of the normal ratio between trypsinogen and its inhibitor may contribute to the premature activation of pancreatic proenzymes within the pancreas, with an increased risk of subsequent pancreatic autodigestion.

In summary, ethanol-induced alterations in pancreatic secretion may contribute to the development of alcoholic pancreatitis.

Zymogen activation and CCK

It has been demonstrated that supraphysiologic or hyperstimulatory doses (i.e., doses greater than those that cause maximal secretion of digestive enzymes by the pancreatic acinar cell) of CCK and its analogs such as cerulein cause intrapancreatic zymogen activation and pancreatitis. Supraphysiologic concentrations of CCK also lead to retention of the active enzymes within the acinar cells. CCK-induced pancreatitis is mild, rapid in onset, and uniform across the gland. It enables researchers to investigate the role of CCK in zymogen activation and in the inflammatory response associated with the subsequent cell injury. The transcriptional factor NF-κB, which plays a crucial role in cytokine production and cellular death, has been shown to be activated in the early phase of CCK-induced pancreatitis.

Thus, several studies have investigated the effects of ethanol administration on plasma levels of CCK. However, conflicting results have been generated. Plasma levels of CCK remained unchanged after administration of ethanol. In contrast, when rats were exposed to intravenous and intragastric ethanol, it resulted in a significant but transient increase in the rate of digestive enzyme secretion and an increase in plasma CCK levels. Administration of a specific CCK-A receptor antagonist inhibited ethanol-stimulated amylase secretion. When the action of CCK-releasing peptide was prevented by either instillation of trypsin in the duodenum or lavage of the duodenum with saline, the increase in plasma CCK levels and amylase secretion in response to ethanol administration was inhibited. This observation suggested a role for CCK-releasing peptide in the ethanol-induced changes in amylase secretion.

In vitro and in vivo models have recently shown that ethanol sensitizes the pancreas to CCK-induced activation of zymogens. Physiologically relevant concentrations of ethanol sensitized the acinar cells to physiologic concentrations of CCK. In an in vivo model, rats that received an ethanol diet for 2–6 weeks developed morphologic and biochemical signs of acute pancreatitis after administration of CCK in a dose which by itself did not cause pancreatitis in control animals.

Although the sensitizing effect of ethanol on CCK-induced pancreatitis has been clearly established, the exact mechanisms are not fully understood. Since it is known that CCK is a potent activator of NF-κB, the effects of ethanol on the NF-κB signaling pathway were studied. Incubation of acinar cells with ethanol and acetaldehyde decreased basal NF-κB activity, but potentiated the activation of NF-κB stimulated by both maximal and supramaximal doses of CCK.

The relationship between the structure of an alcohol and its ability to sensitize the acinar cells to CCK has also been investigated. A direct relationship between sensitization and chain length of alcohol was demonstrated. The mechanism of this sensitization and its relevance to the development of pancreatitis remains unclear.

Toxicity of ethanol metabolites

Ethanol metabolism occurs via two major pathways: the oxidative pathway, generating acetaldehyde, and the nonoxidative pathway, generating fatty acid ethyl esters (FAEEs). The oxidation of ethanol to acetaldehyde is catalyzed by alcohol dehydrogenese, cytochrome P4502E1 (CYP2E1), and catalase. The nonoxidative pathway is catalyzed by FAEE synthases and involves the esterification of ethanol with fatty acids to form FAEEs. In vitro studies show that in the pancreas the rate of oxidative metabolism of ethanol is higher than that of nonoxidative metabolism. The metabolism of ethanol by pancreatic acinar cells and pancreatic stellate cells, with subsequent generation of toxic metabolites, may play an important role in the development of ethanol-induced pancreatic injury and has been a topic of recent research.

Acetaldehyde can cause morphologic damage to the pancreas of rats and dogs. Acetaldehyde inhibits stimulated enzyme secretion from isolated pancreatic acini, which may be explained by interference with the binding of secretagogues to their receptors and by microtubular dysfunction affecting exocytosis from acinar cells. The oxidation of ethanol to acetaldehyde and acetate alters the release of hydrogen ions and the intracellular redox state of the cell, which may lead to a number of metabolic alterations that could contribute to pancreatic acinar cell injury.

Interestingly, FAEEs have been shown to induce pancreatic injury *in vivo* and *in vitro*. Intravenous infusion of FAEEs was followed by an increase in pancreatic edema formation, pancreatic trypsinogen activation, and acinar cell vacuolization. These observations suggest an organ-specific toxic effect of FAEEs. An *in vitro* model demonstrated destabilization of lysosomes within pancreatic acinar cells. The toxicity of FAEEs may be caused by their direct interaction with cellular membranes, by a release of free acids through their hydrolysis, and by promotion of cholesteryl ester synthesis.

New insights have been gained into the specific signaling pathways that may be influenced by toxic metabolites of ethanol. Recent observations have suggested that the metabolism of ethanol to acetaldehyde may be responsible for downregulation of NF-κB activity following CCK administration, whereas the metabolism of ethanol by the nonoxidative pathway may be responsible for the stimulatory effect of ethanol on NF-κB activation.

All aerobic organisms generate reactive oxygen species, such as superoxide ion, hydrogen peroxide, and hydroxyl radical, during the normal metabolism of oxygen. Although low levels of these oxygen intermediates are indispensable for normal cellular function, high levels are potentially toxic to cells and may lead to protein modification, cellular membrane disruption, destruction of nucleic acids within DNA, and mitochondrial damage. Therefore, it has been hypothesized that the tissue damage during pancreatitis may also result from uncontrolled free radical activity. Of note, ethanol consumption results in increased free radical generation. This pathway of alcohol toxicity is well established in the research on alcoholic liver disease. The mechanisms responsible for oxidative stress secondary to ethanol exposure include acetaldehyde-induced depletion of reduced glutathione and the increased generation of free radicals during the metabolism of ethanol via the CYP2E1 pathway.

Increased lipid peroxidation products have been detected in pancreatic tissue from patients with chronic pancreatitis. Patients with hereditary, idiopathic, and alcoholic chronic pancreatitis revealed a decreased antioxidative capacity. Limited placebo-controlled studies in patients with chronic pancreatitis further support the assumption of an important role of oxidative stress in chronic pancreatitis.

The possible role of oxidative stress in the development of chronic pancreatitis has also been addressed in studies of acute and chronic ethanol feeding in rats. In one study, histologic examination of pancreatic tissue revealed only mild acinar steatosis after long-term ethanol administration, but an increase of free radical adducts was demonstrated in pancreatic fluid secretion. In other experimental investigations, elevation of oxidative stress markers was found in pancreatic tissue after ingestion of alcohol. Since histologic pancreatic damage was not observed in these studies, it was suggested that the elevation of oxidative stress markers occurs as a primary phenomenon rather than as part of an inflammatory response. Thus, oxidative stress may represent an important factor in alcoholic pancreatitis that needs to be studied in future research protocols.

Pancreatic stellate cells

In the past decade, the identification of pancreatic stellate cells has provided important insights into the development of pancreatic fibrosis. Fibrosis represents a key feature of chronic pancreatitis, which is generally characterized by a pathologic change in the composition and amount of extracellular matrix within the tissue. Recent investigations have demonstrated a central role of pancreatic stellate cells in pancreatic fibrogenesis. These cells have similar characteristics to hepatic stellate cells, which are of central importance in fibrosis of the liver. They are situated at the base of the pancreatic acinar cells and in a quiescent state can be identified by the presence of vitamin A-containing lipid droplets in the cytoplasm. Pancreatic stellate cells represent the main cellular source of extracellular matrix proteins, such as collagens I and III, fibronectin, and laminin. Recently it has been shown that stellate cells also secrete the enzymes known to degrade extracellular matrix, suggesting their role in the maintenance of normal tissue architecture. Pancreatic stellate cells may be activated by ethanol. The mechanisms that cause pancreatic stellate cell activation by ethanol include direct effects of ethanol and its metabolites such as acetaldehyde, effects of proinflammatory cytokines released during ethanol-induced inflammation (platelet-derived growth factor, transforming growth factor-β, tumor necrois factor-α, interleukins 1 and 6), and effects of oxidative stress. Pancreatic stellate cells have been shown to metabolize ethanol by the oxidative pathway. The inhibition of alcohol dehydrogenese by its specific inhibitor abolished pancreatic stellate cell activation, suggesting a role for acetaldehyde in the activation process. Exposure of stellate cells to both ethanol and acetaldehyde caused oxidative stress within the cultured cells and their subsequent activation. This activation was prevented by vitamin E.

Genetic susceptibility to alcoholic pancreatitis

The discovery of the genetic cause of hereditary pancreatitis renewed interest in possible genetic predisposition to alcoholic chronic pancreatitis. The most important pancreatitis-associated gene mutations are found in the cationic trypsinogen (PRSS1) gene, the pancreatic secretory trypsin inhibitor Kazal type 1 (SPINK1) gene, and the cystic fibrosis transmembrane conductance regulator (CFTR) gene. Further genes that have been hypothesized as associated with alcoholic chronic pancreatitis represent alcohol-metabolizing enzymes and the human leukocyte antigen (HLA) locus.

The cationic trypsinogen mutations R122H and N29I (in older nomenclature R117H and N21I) cause the majority of cases of hereditary pancreatitis. The presence of a mutation may lead to inappropriate activation of pancreatic zymogens within the pancreas. Several studies have screened patients with alcoholic chronic pancreatitis for cationic trypsinogen gene mutations but have failed to demonstrate an association. These results exclude hereditary pancreatitis-associated trypsinogen mutations as a dominant factor for the development of alcoholic chronic pancreatitis.

In the mechanistic models of pancreatic acinar cell protection, the pancreatic secretory trypsin inhibitor SPINK1 specifically inhibits trypsin by blocking the active site of the molecule. SPINK1 is thought to act as the first line of defense against prematurely activated trypsinogen. In 2000, mutations in the SPINK1 gene were found to be associated with familial and idiopathic chronic pancreatitis. The most frequent mutation in the SPINK1 gene is the N34S mutation in exon 3 that changes the amino acid sequence (asparagine to serine). Therefore several groups have investigated the frequency of the SPINK1 N34S mutation in patients with alcoholic pancreatitis. In one study, the N34S mutation was detected in 5.8% (16/274) of patients with alcoholic pancreatitis and in 0.8% (4/540) of the control population. Although the frequency was only slightly elevated in patients compared with controls, the difference was statistically significant. The other studies reported about similar frequencies of the N34S mutation in alcoholic patients. However, so far only one study has compared the clinical course of the disease in two patients with the N34S mutation with the course of the disease in patients without the mutation, but significant differences were not found. Thus, at present the SPINK1 N34S mutation appears not to be associated with a different clinical phenotype of alcoholic pancreatitis.

An association with CFTR gene mutations has been shown in patients with idiopathic chronic pancreatitis, thus raising the possibility that CFTR mutations may also increase the risk of pancreatitis after exposure to alcohol. Several studies have investigated the incidence of CFTR mutations among patients with alcoholic pancreatitis. By screening a subset of CFTR mutations, an association between abnormal CFTR alleles and alcoholic chronic pancreatitis has not been demonstrated in most of these studies. However, recent preliminary reports have revealed an increased frequency of abnormal CFTR alleles in patients with alcoholic pancreatitis by screening the entire CFTR gene Thus, further investigations of the entire CFTR gene in patients with alcoholic chronic pancreatitis are clearly necessary.

Summary

Although it is generally accepted that chronic excessive alcohol consumption represents a major risk factor for the development of pancreatic inflammation, the exact mechanisms involved in alcohol-induced pancreatic damage are not yet fully clarified. Since only a subset of heavy alcohol drinkers present with clinically recognized acute or chronic pancreatitis, alcohol alone probably does not cause pancreatitis. It is likely that several other factors act together and increase the risk of developing alcoholic pancreatitis. Several specific effects of ethanol or its metabolites on the pancreas are known and may play a role in the pathogenesis of pancreatitis.

Acute ethanol administration selectively reduces pancreatic blood flow and microcirculation. In animal models, obstruction of the pancreatic duct results in morphologic changes similar to human obstructive chronic pancreatitis, and further alcohol application suppresses pancreatic regeneration. Therefore, the development of pancreatic duct plugs within the course of alcoholic chronic pancreatitis may contribute to the progression of the disease.

The changes in pancreatic exocrine secretion and the distortion of the normal ratio between trypsinogen and its inhibitor may facilitate the premature activation of pancreatic proenzymes within the pancreas. Chronic ethanol administration increases the expression of digestive and lysosomal enzymes within the pancreatic acinar cells and increases the glandular content of these enzymes. Chronic ethanol consumption significantly decreases pancreatic bicarbonate secretion. In addition, chronic ethanol consumption increases basal pancreatic enzyme output, protein concentration, and viscosity of the pancreatic juice. Acute and chronic exposure to ethanol have been been shown to sensitize the pancreas to CCK-induced activation of zymogens and the development of pancreatitis. Thus, changes in pancreatic exocrine secretion patterns may contribute to the development of pancreatic damage.

Ethanol and its metabolites, such as acetaldehyde and FAEEs, have direct toxic effects on pancreatic tissue. Several specific metabolic alterations caused by toxic metabolites of ethanol have been described. Ethanol administration results in the generation of reactive oxygen species, and oxidative stress may play a central role in development of acute and chronic pancreatitis.

Pancreatic stellate cells represent the main source of extracellular matrix in pancreatic fibrosis and are activated directly by ethanol and its metabolite acetaldehyde, growth factors, inflammatory cytokines, and oxidative stress.

Recent genetic findings have revealed major insights into the development of nonalcoholic chronic pancreatitis. Therefore, genetic studies are important for understanding individual susceptibility to alcoholic chronic pancreatitis.

Acknowledgment

Tomas Hucl was supported by a scholarship from DAAD (A/03/09379).

Recommended reading

Ammann R, Heitz P, Klöppel G. Course of alcoholic chronic pancreatitis: a prospective clinicomorphological long-term study. *Gastroenterology* 1996;111:224–231.

Bachem MG, Schneider E, Gross H *et al*. Identification, culture, and characterization of pancreatic stellate cells in rats and humans. *Gastroenterology* 1998;115:421–432.

Gukovskaya AS, Mouria M, Gukovsky I *et al*. Ethanol metabolism and transcription factor activation in pancreatic acinar cells in rats. *Gastroenterology* 2002;122:106–118.

Haber PS, Apte MV, Applegate TL *et al*. Metabolism of ethanol by rat pancreatic acinar cells. *J Lab Clin Med* 1998;132:294–302.

Niebergall-Roth E, Harder H, Singer MV. A review: acute and chronic effects of ethanol and alcoholic beverages on the pancreatic exocrine secretion *in vivo* and *in vitro*. *Alcohol Clin Exp Res* 1998;22:1570–1583.

Norton ID, Apte MV, Lux O. Chronic ethanol administration causes oxidative stress in the rat pancreas. *J Lab Clin Med* 1998;131:442–446.

Pandol SJ, Periskic S, Gukovsky I. Ethanol diet increases the sensitivity of rats to pancreatitis induced by cholecystokinin octapeptide. *Gastroenterology* 1999;117:706–716.

Schneider A, Whitcomb DC, Singer MV. Animal models in alcoholic pancreatitis: what can we learn? *Pancreatology* 2002;2:189–203.

Schneider A, Pfutzer RH, Barmada MM. Limited contribution of the SPINK1 N34S mutation to the risk and severity of alcoholic chronic pancreatitis: a report from the United States. *Dig Dis Sci* 2003;48:1110–1115.

Singer MV, Goebell H. Acute and chronic actions of alcohol on pancreatic exocrine secretion in humans and animals. In: HK Seitz, B Kommerell (eds) *Alcohol-related Diseases in Gastroenterology*. Berlin: Springer-Verlag, 1985:376–414.

Singer MV, Gyr KE, Sarles H. Revised classification of pancreatitis. *Gastroenterology* 1985;89:683–690.

Whitcomb DC, Gorry MC, Preston RA. Hereditary pancreatitis is caused by a mutation in the cationic trypsinogen gene. *Nat Genet* 1996;14:141–145.

Why is chronic pancreatitis so difficult to detect? Key clinical aspects for an early diagnosis

Paul G. Lankisch and Bernhard Lembcke

Introduction

The time interval between the onset of symptoms and the diagnosis of chronic pancreatitis is unacceptably long. There are only two studies addressing this problem. In the Denmark study, which took place between 1970 and 1979, it was found that for alcoholics, the time interval was 30 months. In our study, we found that the diagnosis, after the onset of symptoms, was delayed for 62 months. With an average delay of 55 months, the disease was detected earliest in alcoholics and patients with pseudocysts. However, the delay was significantly longer for nonalcoholics (81 months) and it took a further 8–9 months to discover the disease in patients with calcifying rather than noncalcifying pancreatitis. There was no gender bias. Similar or even longer delays in diagnosis have also been found in other benign gastrointestinal diseases, such as celiac disease and Crohn's disease.

Although there are no recent data available for chronic pancreatitis, we have found that the delay has not been significantly reduced, even though morphologic procedures such as ultrasound, endoscopic ultrasound, computed tomography (CT), and nuclear magnetic resonance investigations have been introduced or have improved in quality.

In our experience, although there are no clear evidence-based data, we believe that the diagnosis of chronic pancreatitis is delayed because it is difficult to detect. Key clinical aspects would be useful for early diagnosis and subsequent treatment. This would help to prevent or ameliorate pain and prevent the complications of the disease.

This chapter is divided into statements that ask why it is difficult to detect the disease and which suggest ways of improving the development of key clinical aspects.

Statement 1: it is difficult to detect alcohol- induced chronic pancreatitis because the answers given by alcoholics can be misleading

The increased frequency of chronic pancreatitis in the industrialized countries parallels a marked increase in alcohol consumption. A linear relationship between alcohol consumption and the logarithmic risk for chronic pancreatitis has been demonstrated. Neither the type of alcoholic beverage nor the frequency of consumption (daily or only weekends) appears to influence the development of the disease. In contrast to the liver, the pancreas has no threshold for alcohol toxicity, although pancreatic sensitivity to alcohol seems to be greater in women than in men.

Although there is no doubt that alcohol is the major etiologic factor behind chronic pancreatitis, it is still unclear why the majority of heavy drinkers do not develop the disease. It has been hypothesized that a diet high in fat and protein predisposes persons with a high alcohol consumption to pancreatitis. Both a high (≥ 100 g/day) and a low (≤ 85 g/day) consumption of fat have been reported to be risk factors, but this has not been confirmed in France, the USA, or Australia.

We have found that when a patient is asked how much alcohol is consumed, the amount given is rarely correct. Patients from the more affluent classes tend to feel embarrassed about their intake and will give lower amounts. Those from poorer backgrounds may be unaware of how much alcohol they are drinking. In each case, even when we know the correct amount, information about the time when drinking started and whether it fluctuated in intensity are rarely correct. Unlike the measurement of hemoglobin (Hb)A_{1c} in diabetes mellitus, which helps to control the treatment of the disease, there is no reliable laboratory parameter for measuring the amount of alcohol consumed.

Statement 2: it is difficult to detect idiopathic chronic pancreatitis in nonalcoholics

In the absence of alcohol abuse, idiopathic chronic pancreatitis is especially difficult to diagnose, as we may not link the signs and symptoms we observe to the disease. This form of the disease is frequent and found in 10–30% of patients with chronic pancreatitis. The course is different: exocrine pancreatic insufficiency and calcifications develop more slowly.

Furthermore, other difficulties arise because two subgroups of chronic pancreatitis have been reported, a juvenile and a senile form, and the courses for these differ from alcohol-induced chronic pancreatitis. At the onset of symptoms, the juvenile form is characterized by a mean age of about 25 years with equal sex distribution. It has a painful clinical course. Several other reports also seem to indicate that juvenile chronic pancreatitis is unusual. Manifestation of the senile form does not become clinically evident until around the age of 62 years. Men predominate, the clinical course is usually painless, and vascular disease is often present.

About 10 years ago, the Mayo Clinic group found that patients with early-onset pancreatitis suffer a long course of severe pain, slowly developing morphologic and functional pancreatic damage, whereas patients with late-onset pancreatitis have a mild and often painless course. Both forms are said to differ from alcoholic pancreatitis, with equal gender distribution and a much slower rate of calcification.

Finally, it is not clear whether low alcohol consumption may increase the risk of chronic pancreatitis. Those patients who developed the disease after the age of 35 and who had a low alcohol intake (< 50 g/day, definition of a low intake) frequently had more pain, developed calcifications, and had more complications.

Thus, it is necessary to identify the amount of alcohol that may affect the pancreas and to consider whether all cases of idiopathic chronic pancreatitis may have a genetic basis that was then aggravated by environmental toxins. Future studies that include genetic analysis in the clinical work-up may support a genetic basis for chronic pancreatitis and its diagnosis.

Statement 3: it is difficult to detect painless chronic pancreatitis when only exocrine and/or endocrine insufficiency are present

In a large study by our group on 335 patients with chronic pancreatitis, we found that 7% of patients were without pain. In these cases, it is especially difficult to suspect chronic pancreatitis when there are only two other major manifestations of the disease, i.e., exocrine and endocrine pancreatic insufficiency. Thus, in each case where there is a sudden onset of diabetes mellitus or steatorrhea, staging procedures for the imaging of the pancreas should be performed for the detection of pancreatic calcifications, which are not infrequent in this form of the disease. A direct or indirect pancreatic function test for the detection of exocrine pancreatic insufficiency is also necessary. This is important, as enzyme substitution may prevent further complications of chronic pancreatitis, especially osteoporosis.

Statement 4: it is difficult to detect drug-induced chronic pancreatitis

Although many different drugs are thought to induce acute pancreatitis but only a few that induce chronic pancreatitis, drug-induced chronic pancreatitis has to be considered in those patients who are on routine medication. There are some case reports on patients who have been treated with phenacetin, antihypertensive drugs, and anticonvulsant drugs. These reports indicate that the drugs may initiate the disease. Therefore, we need to consider the drugs taken for the treatment of gastrointestinal and nongastrointestinal diseases by patients who have proven chronic pancreatitis. This will help us to establish whether there are more drugs that may induce the disease and this knowledge can then be applied to those patients who have unexplained abdominal pain.

Statement 5: it is difficult to detect chronic pancreatitis in patients who have had radiotherapy

It has been shown in animal experiments that irradiation of the pancreas leads to histologic changes and progressive exocrine pancreatic insufficiency, compatible with the findings of chronic pancreatitis. Radiation-induced chronic pancreatitis was recognized 80 years ago, when atrophy of the acini and degeneration and necrosis of the duct cells of the pancreas were described in patients who had experienced hepatic radiation injury. Pancreatic fibrosis has been described in young men who received high-dose radiation for testicular tumors. More recently, there have been reports of additional patients with chronic pancreatitis probably due to radiation therapy. Radiotherapy for tumors in the same area as the pancreas is thought to affect the vascular process of the organ and this is regarded as the underlying pathogenetic mechanism.

We are used to thinking of damage to the small and large intestine following radiation therapy. However, we do not consider, when patients present with abdominal pain years after radiation therapy, that there may be damage to the pancreas. This approach should be changed.

Statement 6: it is difficult to detect chronic pancreatitis because the signs and symptoms are unspecific

Pain

Abdominal pain is the most common symptom of chronic pancreatitis. However, it is difficult to differentiate between pain caused by pancreatic inflammation and that caused by other abdominal conditions. Pain may be in the left or middle upper abdomen. It sometimes radiates around the abdomen like a girdle or is localized in the back (Fig. 27.1).

Pain may occur independently of meals or within 30 min after a meal, thereby resembling abdominal angina caused by celiac or mesenteric artery stenosis. In patients with this syndrome, a high incidence of isolated duct stenosis and slightly impaired pancreatic function have been found. In this group of patients,

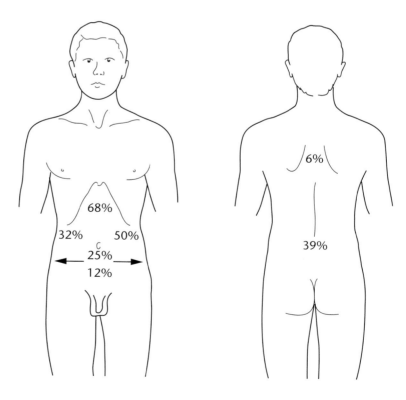

Figure 27.1 Major sites of pain in 311 patients with painful chronic pancreatitis.

weight loss may be an early symptom, indicating that patients are avoiding food in order to prevent pain.

In chronic pancreatitis, pain is often severe and tends to be prolonged but is less intense than in acute pancreatitis. In some studies, about half of the patients described their pain as severe, while the other half described it as moderate or mild. Few studies have been carried out using pain scores and/or quality-of-life measures.

Radiation of pain to other parts of the body is poorly understood. Some authors have used electrical stimuli to localize the pain and the direction of its radiation. Stimulation of the tail of the gland, for example, usually induced pain in the left upper abdomen, whereas stimulation of the head usually induced it on the right.

The association between alcohol consumption and pain in chronic pancreatitis is also unclear. Some patients drink alcohol in an effort to relieve the pancreatic pain; others experience a painful attack after having consumed alcohol. In South Africa, it has been observed that painful attacks of pancreatitis usually start about 12–48 hours after a drinking bout, i.e., the "morning after the night before."

In chronic pancreatitis, pain may result not only from inflammation of the gland but also from complications of the disease, such as the incomplete or even complete inflammatory stenosis of the duodenum, the common bile duct, or the colon. The incidence of duodenal stenosis may be as high as 20% and may even require pancreaticoduodenectomy. The incidence of stenosis of the common bile duct varies from 10 to 46%, whereas the incidence of colonic stenosis was 14% in one series.

Pancreatic pseudocysts can cause pain, but in acute pancreatitis about 40% of them resolve spontaneously. This rarely happens in chronic pancreatitis and never when pancreatic calculi are present. Contrary to popular belief, gallstones play no part in the development of chronic pancreatitis, although this has been questioned recently. However, it should be noted that gallstones are found in 6% of patients with chronic pancreatitis and these may cause pain.

The incidence of (painful) peptic ulceration in chronic pancreatitis varies from 6 to 38%. Patients with pancreatitis and relapsing abdominal pain should therefore have a gastroscopy. In contrast, chronic pancreatitis should be suspected when alcoholics have peptic ulcerations. Therefore, abdominal pain can indicate peptic ulcerations.

Diabetes mellitus

Diabetes-related symptoms occur more frequently in idiopathic than in alcoholic pancreatitis. They are not specific for chronic pancreatitis.

Weight loss

Weight loss is a frequent symptom. It may be due to a reduced oral intake because of fear of postprandial pain or to severe exocrine pancreatic insufficiency. A reduction in lipase secretion will lead to diarrhea and steatorrhea. In one-third of patients, the causes of unexplained weight loss are found in the gastrointestinal tract and many involve the pancreas. Thus, in any patient with unexplained weight loss, ultrasound of the pancreas for the detection of chronic pancreatitis and fecal fat analysis for the detection of steatorrhea are useful and should be considered.

When patients present for physical examination during a painful attack of chronic pancreatitis, they frequently, as in the case of acute pancreatitis, try to relieve their pain by flexing the spine, by sitting forward with the knees flexed against the chest, by squatting and clasping the knees to the chest, or by lying on one side with the knees flexed. Therefore, although this is not a specific sign, chronic pancreatitis should be considered when a patient reports that these positions relieve pain.

Skin signs are not characteristic, although erythema ab igne (redness of the skin caused by application of hot water bottles or electric pads to relieve pain) may be observed on the abdominal wall or on the back (Fig. 27.2). However, this sign is seen in both chronic pancreatitis and pancreatic cancer.

Finally, during an asymptomatic period, the standard physical examination does not help to establish the diagnosis.

Statement 7: it is difficult to detect chronic pancreatitis because function tests are inadequate and unreliable

To some extent, exocrine pancreatic insufficiency is present in all cases of chronic pancreatitis. However, this is not the only cause of exocrine pancreatic insufficiency (Table 27.1). Other reasons, especially a pancreatic carcinoma obstructing the pancreatic duct, have to be considered.

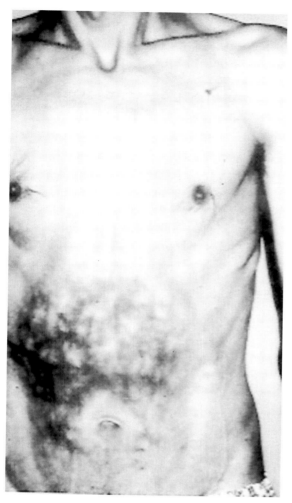

Figure 27.2 Patient with chronic pancreatitis and erythema ab igne.

Table 27.1 Causes of exocrine pancreatic insufficiency.

Overall reduction of enzyme formation or delivery due to
Chronic pancreatitis
Acute pancreatitis (mostly short-term insufficiency)
Carcinoma obstructing the pancreatic duct
Major pancreatic resection
Pancreatic trauma (mostly short-term insufficiency)
Primary sclerosing cholangitis
Kwashiorkor
Hereditary disorders or congenital abnormalities
Cystic fibrosis
Shwachman's syndrome

Isolated deficiency in the following enzymes
Lipase
Trypsin
Amylase

Failure of enzyme activation of the small intestine due to enterokinase insufficiency

It is not the purpose of this review to summarize all the advantages and disadvantages of the direct and indirect function tests used for diagnosing exocrine pancreatic deficiency. They may be found elsewhere. Generally speaking, the direct pancreatic function tests, especially the gold standard, the secretin–cholecystokinin test and its modifications, are time-consuming, invasive, and expensive and are only used in gastroenterologic centers. Indirect pancreatic function tests, such as serum pancreatic isoamylase and immunoreactive trypsin, urine tests like the pancreolauryl test and bentiromide test, or fecal enzyme estimations such as fecal elastase-1 and chymotrypsin, are neither specific nor sensitive enough to detect early chronic pancreatitis or mild to moderate exocrine pancreatic insufficiency. This is a major diagnostic problem. None of these tests are sufficiently reliable to distinguish between pancreatogenic and nonpancreatogenic steatorrhea, which presents another diagnostic problem. Therefore, the simpler, less expensive tests are also less specific and less sensitive. A gold standard test for diagnosing mild to moderate chronic exocrine pancreatic insufficiency still has to be developed.

Steatorrhea occurs only when stimulated lipase secretion is reduced to 10% or less of normal. At this stage, it is generally believed that patients with chronic pancreatitis have diarrhea and steatorrhea. This could imply that fecal weight determination can replace the unpopular and costly fecal fat estimation for diagnosing steatorrhea. However, this is not the case. A large study on fecal weight and fat estimations in 625 patients who were being investigated for malabsorption showed that about 22% had steatorrhea but did not have diarrhea (normal stool weight). Furthermore, steatorrhea cannot be reliably diagnosed by inspection. Thus, unpleasant fecal fat estimation is still necessary.

Statement 8: it is difficult to detect chronic pancreatitis because morphologic procedures are not always a reliable aid

It is not the purpose of this review to summarize the reliability of morphologic examinations performed using endoscopic retrograde cholangiopancreatography (ERCP), magnetic resonance cholangiopancreatography, CT, and endoscopic ultrasound. It should be stated that the diagnosis is highly dependent on the experience of the investigator. Pancreatic calcifications can be found with any procedure and these help confirm the diagnosis of chronic pancreatitis. However, calcifications can appear in the early or later stages of the disease and may disappear during the course of the disease. They do not indicate severe exocrine pancreatic insufficiency requiring pancreatic enzyme substitution. At least for ERCP, CT, and ultrasound, there is the clear-cut Cambridge classification for diagnosing equivocal, mild, moderate, and severe changes. However, this classification is not widely used.

It must also be noted that, after acute pancreatitis, exocrine pancreatic insufficiency may return to normal. However, morphologic findings may persist and these can be misinterpreted as an indicator for chronic pancreatitis. In the case of acute pancreatitis, an exocrine pancreatic function test plus an imaging procedure is recommended. This will clarify whether there has been a full recovery or whether the patient will develop chronic pancreatitis.

Recommended reading

Introduction

Andersen BN, Thorsgaard Pedersen N, Scheel J, Worning H. Incidence of alcoholic chronic pancreatitis in Copenhagen. *Scand J Gastroenterol* 1982;17:247–252.

Lankisch PG, Peiper M, Löhr-Happe A, Otto J, Seidensticker F, Stöckmann F. Delay in diagnosing chronic pancreatitis. *Eur J Gastroenterol Hepatol* 1993;5:713–714.

Statement 1

Lankisch PG, Banks PA. *Pancreatitis*. Berlin: Springer-Verlag, 1998.

Statement 2

Ammann RW, Buehler H, Muench R, Freiburghaus AW,

Siegenthaler W. Differences in the natural history of idiopathic (nonalcoholic) and alcoholic chronic pancreatitis. A comparative long-term study of 287 patients. *Pancreas* 1987;2:368–377.

Lankisch PG, Banks PA. *Pancreatitis*. Berlin: Springer-Verlag, 1998.

Lankisch MR, Imoto M, Layer P, DiMagno EP. The effect of small amounts of alcohol on the clinical course of chronic pancreatitis. *Mayo Clin Proc* 2001;76:242–251.

Statement 3

Lankisch PG, Löhr-Happe A, Otto J, Creutzfeldt W. Natural course in chronic pancreatitis. Pain, exocrine and endocrine pancreatic insufficiency and prognosis of the disease. *Digestion* 1993;54:148–155.

Statement 4

Hangartner PJ, Bühler H, Münch R, Zaruba K, Stamm B, Ammann R. Chronische Pankreatitis als wahrscheinliche Folge eines Analgetikaabusus. *Schweiz Med Wochenschr* 1987;117:638–642.

Pezzilli R, Billi P, Melandri R, Broccoli PL, Fontana G. Anticonvulsant-induced chronic pancreatitis. A case report. *Ital J Gastroenterol* 1992;24:245–246.

Statement 5

Lévy P, Menzelxhiu A, Paillot B, Bretagne JF, Fléjou JF, Bernades P. Abdominal radiotherapy is a cause for chronic pancreatitis. *Gastroenterology* 1993;105:905–909.

Mitchell CJ, Simpson FG, Davison AM. Losowsky MS. Radiation pancreatitis: a clinical entity? *Digestion* 1979;19:134–136.

Sarles H. Chronic pancreatitis and main pancreatic duct stricture following cobalt therapy. *Eur J Gastroenterol Hepatol* 1992;4:509–510.

Statement 6

Aranha GV, Prinz RA, Esguerra AC, Greenlee HB. The nature and course of cystic pancreatic lesions diagnosed by ultrasound. *Arch Surg* 1983;118:486–488.

Bradley EL. Parapancreatic biliary and intestinal obstruction in chronic obstructive pancreatitis. Is prophylactic bypass necessary? *Am J Surg* 1986;151:256–258.

Lankisch PG. Diagnosis of abdominal pain. How to distinguish between pancreatic and extrapancreatic causes. *Acta Chir Scand* 1990;156:273–278.

Lankisch PG, Andrén-Sandberg Å. Standards for the diagnosis of chronic pancreatitis and for the evaluation of treatment. *Int J Pancreatol* 1993;14:205–212.

Lankisch PG, Banks PA. *Pancreatitis*. Berlin: Springer-Verlag, 1998.

Lankisch PG, Creutzfeldt W. Erythema ab igne (Livedo reticularis e calore): ein Hautzeichen für chronische Pankreaserkrankungen. *Z Gastroenterol* 1986;24:119–120.

Lankisch PG, Gerzmann M, Gerzmann J-F, Lehnick D. Unintentional weight loss: diagnosis and prognosis. The first prospective follow-up study from a secondary referral centre. *J Intern Med* 2001;249:41–46.

Marks IN, Bank S. Chronic pancreatitis. Etiology, clinical aspects, and medical management. In: JE Berk (ed.) *Bockus Gastroentrology*, Vol 5. Philadelphia: Saunders, 1985: 4020–4040.

Miyake H, Harada H, Kunichika K, Ochi K, Kimura I. Clinical course and prognosis of chronic pancreatitis. *Pancreas* 1987;2:378–385.

Statement 7

DiMagno EP, Go VLW, Summerskill WHJ. Relations between pancreatic enzyme outputs and malabsorption in severe pancreatic insufficiency. *N Engl J Med* 1973;288:813–815.

Lankisch PG. Function tests in the diagnosis of chronic pancreatitis. Critical evaluation. *Int J Pancreatol* 1993;14: 9–20.

Lankisch PG, Banks PA. *Pancreatitis*. Berlin: Springer-Verlag, 1998.

Lankisch PG, Lembcke B, Wemken G, Creutzfeldt W. Functional reserve capacity of the exocrine pancreas. *Digestion* 1986;35:175–181.

Lankisch PG, Dröge M, Hofses S, König H, Lembcke B. Steatorrhoea: you cannot trust your eyes when it comes to diagnosis. *Lancet* 1996;347:1620–1621.

Lankisch PG, Dröge M, König H, Lehnick D, Lembcke B. Fecal weight determination can unfortunately not replace unpopular and costly fecal fat estimation in the diagnosis of steatorrhea. *Int J Pancreatol* 1999;25:71–72.

Statement 8

Ammann RW, Muench R, Otto R, Buehler H, Freiburghaus AU, Siegenthaler W. Evolution and regression of pancreatic calcification in chronic pancreatitis. A prospective long-term study of 107 patients. *Gastroenterology* 1988;95: 1018–1028.

Lankisch PG, Otto J, Erkelenz I, Lembcke B. Pancreatic calcifications: no indicator of severe exocrine pancreatic insufficiency. *Gastroenterology* 1986;90:617–621.

Sarner M, Cotton PB. Classification of pancreatitis. *Gut* 1984;25:756–759.

Seidensticker F, Otto J, Lankisch PG. Recovery of the pancreas after acute pancreatitis is not necessarily complete. *Int J Pancreatol* 1995;17:225–229.

28 Role of imaging methods in diagnosing, staging, and detecting complications of chronic pancreatitis in clinical practice: should MRCP and MRI replace ERCP and CT?

Carmen Villalba-Martín and J. Enrique Domínguez-Muñoz

Introduction

Chronic pancreatitis is defined as a chronic inflammatory disease that results in irreversible morphologic and functional changes within the pancreas. In the context of this inflammatory process, there is progressive damage and loss of pancreatic parenchyma, which is replaced by fibrotic tissue. Although diagnosis of chronic pancreatitis is easy in late stages of the disease using currently available diagnostic methods, diagnosis of early or mild chronic pancreatitis before the development of severe morphologic changes is a difficult task. The absence of a simple and internationally available gold standard is still a problem. Although chronic pancreatitis is well defined on a histopathologic basis, histologic confirmation is not available in the vast majority of patients. The diagnosis is thus usually based on the demonstration of morphologic and functional abnormalities of the gland by means of imaging studies and pancreatic function tests. Imaging modalities also play a primary role in the management of chronic pancreatitis. Appropriate imaging not only confirms the diagnosis and defines the severity of the disease, but it also detects potential complications and assists in selecting the most appropriate treatment among available therapeutic alternatives.

Transabdominal ultrasound (TUS) is frequently used as the first imaging method for the evaluation of patients who suffer from abdominal pain, jaundice, or even unspecific abdominal symptoms. The sensitivity reported for TUS in chronic pancreatitis ranges from 48 to 96%. This variation reflects the morphologic spectrum of chronic pancreatitis, ranging from normal in early or mild disease to grossly abnormal in severe disease. Although the sensitivity of TUS is quite low, it may detect some severe pancreatic changes and may be useful for identifying the need for subsequent images using more expensive and accurate methods.

Endoscopic retrograde cholangiopancreatography (ERCP) and computed tomography (CT) have long been considered the main imaging modalities in the evaluation of patients with suspected chronic pancreatitis. The severity of the disease has been classified according to the morphologic changes within the pancreatic parenchyma and ducts, as defined by the Cambridge classification (Table 28.1). However, some discrepancies exist between the clinical severity of the inflammatory process, the degree of functional exocrine and endocrine impairment, and the morphologic changes detected by CT and ERCP.

Early diagnosis and accurate staging of chronic pancreatitis require accurate cross-sectional imaging with careful protocols. Development of faster imaging systems with improved contrast resolution have enhanced the role of magnetic resonance imaging (MRI) in the assessment of the pancreas and, nowadays, MRI and magnetic resonance cholangiopancreatography (MRCP) after secretin administration (S-MRCP), both of which may be performed in a single session, could replace CT and diagnostic ERCP. MRI and MRCP are thus increasingly accepted as the primary imaging modalities for the diagnosis of chronic pancreatitis. MRI combines the advantages of cross-sectional imaging techniques, such as ultrasound and CT, with the ability to visualize the pancreatic duct when MRCP is performed (Fig. 28.1).

MRI techniques in the setting of suspected chronic pancreatitis include evaluation of the pancreatic

Table 28.1 Grading of chronic pancreatitis by imaging methods: the Cambridge classification 1983.

	Endoscopic retrograde pancreatography	Ultrasound (US) or computed tomography (CT)
Normal	Good-quality study visualizing the whole gland without abnormal signs	Good-quality study visualizing the whole gland without abnormal signs
Equivocal	Less than three abnormal branches	One of the following: Main pancreatic duct 2–4 mm diameter Gland one to two times normal
Mild	More than three abnormal branches	Two or more abnormal signs: Cyst < 10 mm Duct irregularity Focal acute necrosis Parenchymal heterogeneity Increased echogenicity of duct wall Contour irregularity of head/body
Moderate	As above with abnormal main duct	As above
Severe	All of the above plus one or more of: Cyst > 10 mm Intraductal filling defects Calculi/pancreatic calcification Duct obstruction (stricture) Severe duct dilatation or irregularity Contiguous organ invasion on US or CT	All of the above plus one or more of: Cyst > 10 mm Intraductal filling defects Calculi/pancreatic calcification Duct obstruction (stricture) Severe duct dilatation or irregularity Contiguous organ invasion on US or CT

parenchyma before and after intravenous administration of gadolinium, evaluation of the ductal system by MRCP before and after intravenous secretin administration, and the semiquantitative evaluation of exocrine pancreatic function by measuring duodenal fluid volume after secretin stimulation.

MRI of the pancreas is optimally performed with a high-performance gradient system (23 mT/m), using phased-array torso coils to improve the signal-to-noise ratio with a smaller field of view and thin slice profile. The high-performance gradient system allows the use of faster sequences. These technologic advances allow breath-hold pancreatic imaging in all sequences for evaluation of both pancreatic parenchyma and the pancreatic duct system.

Imaging methods that evaluate the pancreatic duct system: ERCP versus MRCP

ERCP is still considered the gold standard for the morphologic diagnosis and staging of chronic pancreatitis.

Side-branch ectasia is the earliest feature of the disease. Other findings are multifocal dilatations, strictures and irregular contours of the main duct and side branches, filling defects from calculi, mucinous plugs or debris, and pseudocysts. The severity of these changes allows staging of the disease (Table 28.1).

Although ERCP has been considered as the most sensitive imaging method for detecting the early changes of chronic pancreatitis, it is operator-dependent, expensive, and invasive. The reported morbidity rate of ERCP ranges from 1 to 7% and the mortality rate is 0.2%, although complications are clearly less frequent in experienced hands. Other disadvantages are that ERCP requires routine sedation, successful cannulation is obtained in only 70–91% of patients, and opacification of areas proximal to obstructions is usually limited. These problems may be overcome by the use of MRI-based exploration of the pancreatic duct system.

MRCP has emerged as an accurate noninvasive method for evaluating the pancreatic duct. MRCP takes advantage of the long T2 relaxation time of pancreatic secretions, bile, or cystic lesions. Heavily T2-weighted sequences show pancreatic secretions as a

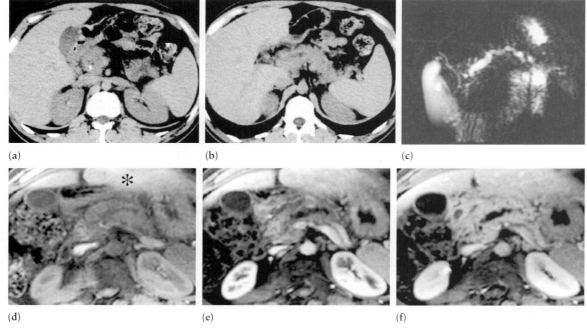

(a)　　　　　　　　　　　(b)　　　　　　　　　　(c)

(d)　　　　　　　　　　　(e)　　　　　　　　　　(f)

Figure 28.1 Idiopathic severe chronic pancreatitis in a 27-year-old man. (a) Unenhanced CT at the level of uncinate process demonstrates a stone within the distal pancreatic duct. (b) Unenhanced CT at the level of pancreatic body shows a dilated main pancreatic duct. (c) MRCP in coronal plane shows an irregular dilated main pancreatic duct and upstream dilated side branches. (d) Unenhanced, T1-weighted, fat-suppressed MRI demonstrates decreased signal intensity of pancreatic parenchyma compared with normal signal intensity of the liver (asterisk). (e) Heterogeneous and decreased enhancement of pancreatic parenchyma during the arterial phase of contrast-enhanced dynamic MRI. (f) Fibrosis-related increased enhancement of the pancreatic parenchyma during the delayed phase of contrast-enhanced dynamic MRI. The peak of enhancement occurs at this delayed phase.

signal of very high intensity over a background of low intensity (Fig 28.2). Because MRCP is a relatively new imaging technique and because of ongoing advances in software and coils, the technique is still evolving and thus differences among institutions may occur.

Multiple magnetic resonance techniques have been used to evaluate the pancreatic duct. Current MRCP techniques use breath-hold single-shot turbo spin-echo (SSTSE) T2-weighted sequences. In this context, both two-dimensional thick-collimation (single section) RARE (rapid acquisition with relaxation enhancement) and three-dimensional thin-collimation (multisection) HASTE (half-Fourier acquisition single-shot turbo spin-echo) sequences are obtained. Because of anatomic variability, MRCP thick-collimation acquisitions should be obtained at various angles to allow optimal visualization of the bile and pancreatic ducts. In addition, three-dimensional reconstruction is possible by using a maximum-intensity projection (MIP) algorithm on the thin-collimation source images. Although the thick-collimation and three-dimensional MIP images more closely resemble conventional cholangiopancreatograms, spatial resolution is degraded due to volume-averaging effects, so the source images, which provide greater spatial resolution, must be carefully analyzed in order to detect every filling defect and stricture.

The normal pancreatic duct measures 2–3 mm in diameter, increasing from the tail to the head, and shows smooth margins. Complete visualization of a dilated pancreatic duct, as in patients with chronic pancreatitis, is possible by MRCP in 100% of cases. However, the normal progressive tapering of the duct toward the tail is lost in these patients. Visualization of this alter-

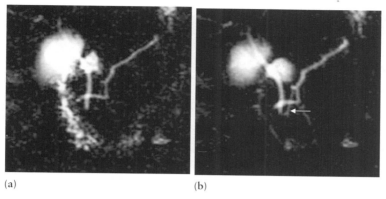

(a)　　　　　　　　　　　(b)

Figure 28.2 Improved visualization of the Santorini duct in a patient suffering from an early form of chronic pancreatitis. (a) MRCP before secretin stimulation is concordant with a pancreas divisum. (b) MRCP after secretin stimulation demonstrates a peculiar duct of Wirsung draining into major papilla (arrow), a finding that indicates persistent duct of Santorini instead of pancreas divisum. Loss of normal progressive tapering of the duct toward the tail can also be seen.

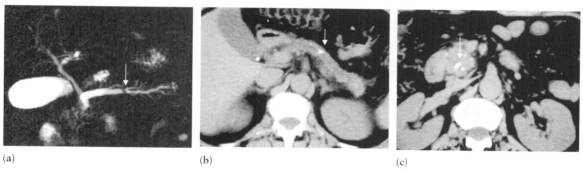

(a)　　　　　　　　　　　(b)　　　　　　　　　　　(c)

Figure 28.3 MRCP and CT features in a patient with calcifying chronic pancreatitis. (a) Coronal, two-dimensional, single-shot turbo spin-echo (RARE) image shows atrophy of pancreatic gland, dilated main pancreatic duct and side branches, and a ductal filling defect in the pancreatic duct (arrow). Unenhanced CT images at the level of the pancreatic body (b) and the uncinate process (c) demonstrate the ductal filling defect to be a stone in the pancreatic duct (arrow) and a calculus in the distal part of the duct. See also the parenchymal calcification in the uncinate process (arrow).

ation in duct morphology may be improved by secretin administration (Fig. 28.2). When the pancreatic duct is not dilated, it can be visualized by MRCP in the head and body in 97% of cases and in the tail in 83% of cases. Secretin stimulation of pancreatic secretion significantly increases these figures. Finally, pancreatic side branches are not seen on MRCP unless dilated.

Imaging features of chronic pancreatitis shown by MRCP are similar to those obtained by ERCP and include segmental dilatation of the pancreatic duct, ductal strictures, dilatation of side branches, ductal filling defects representing calculi, proteinaceous plaques or mucinous casts, pseudocysts, and biliary duct dilatation (Figs 28.1c, 28.3a, and 28.4b). In severe cases, the marked dilation of the duct has a "chain of lakes" appearance.

Accuracy for detection of changes of chronic pancreatitis

Comparisons between MRCP and ERCP in cases of chronic pancreatitis have revealed agreement of

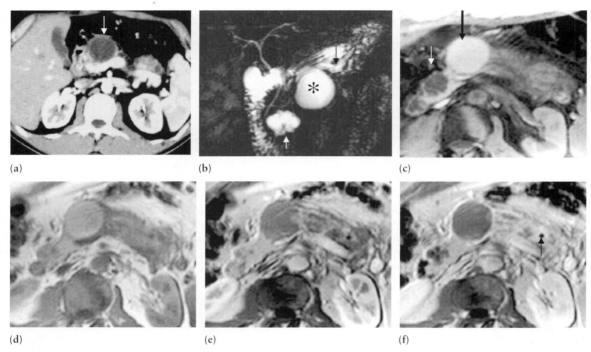

(a) (b) (c)

(d) (e) (f)

Figure 28.4 CT, MRCP, and dynamic MRI in a 34 year-old patient with pancreas divisum and severe chronic pancreatitis. (a) Venous-phase contrast-enhanced CT shows a pseudocyst in the neck of the pancreas (arrow). (b) Coronal RARE image depicts main pancreatic duct entering at the minor papilla, a pseudocyst in the body of the pancreas (asterisk) that produces dilatation of the duct in the tail (black arrow), and a pseudocyst at the uncinate process (white arrow). (c) Axial T1-weighted fat-suppressed image shows focal enlargement and significant decreased signal of pancreatic parenchyma in the body and tail compared with the normal size and signal intensity of parenchyma in the pancreatic head. Note the high signal intensity of the pseudocyst in the pancreatic neck (black arrow) due to debris and proteinaceous contents (confirmed at surgery) compared with the hypointensity of the pseudocyst located in the uncinate process (white arrow). (d–f) Dynamic MRI. (d) Unenhanced axial T1-weighted image shows the difference in signal intensity between head and body–tail of the pancreas. (e) On arterial-phase contrast-enhanced dynamic MRI, the dorsal pancreas shows heterogeneous and less enhancement than normal in the pancreatic head. (f) On delayed-phase contrast-enhanced dynamic MRI, the dorsal pancreas demonstrates an increased and heterogeneous enhancement related to inflammatory fibrosis. A small cyst can also be seen (arrow).

83–100% for identification of ductal dilation, 70–92% for identification of narrowing, and 92–100% for identification of filling defects. In cases of ductal obstruction, MRCP but not ERCP is able to explore the duct on both sides of the obstruction.

The overall sensitivity of MRCP in the detection of chronic pancreatitis increases from 77 to 89% and the overall negative predictive value from 84 to 98% with the intravenous administration of secretin (S-MRCP). This is due to the increase of stationary fluid volume into the pancreatic ducts after secretin stimulation. S-MRCP is performed with dynamic, breath-hold, two-dimensional, thick-collimation RARE in the coronal plane (Fig. 28.2). To eliminate the overlapping fluid-containing organs, a negative oral contrast agent is given before dynamic imaging. A set of MRCP images must be acquired before the administration of secretin in order to select the optimal image section. After intravenous administration of secretin (1 U/kg body weight), acquisition of the optimal section is repeated every 15–30 s for 10–15 min. Physiologically, the main pancreatic duct dilates immediately after a bolus injection of secretin, reaches a maximum diameter after 2–5 min, and recovers gradually. The whole main pancreatic duct and the side branches are visualized in 100% of cases by S-MRCP compared with 91% and 71% respectively by MRCP. In patients with functional or organic papillary stenosis, either at the major or at the accessory papilla, the caliber of the pancreatic duct increases dramatically and remains enlarged even after 10 min.

Simultaneous exploration of exocrine pancreatic function

In contrast with ERCP, S-MRCP provides information about exocrine pancreatic function, which may be of interest in patients with suspected chronic pancreatitis. Assessment of pancreatic secretory function by S-MRCP is based on the volume of fluid output in the duodenum. The duodenal filling volume has been graded as follows: grade 0, no fluid observed; grade 1, filling remains limited to the duodenal bulb; grade 2, fluid fills the duodenal bulb and partially fills the duodenum up to the second duodenal knee; grade 3, the duodenum is largely filled beyond the second duodenal knee. Exocrine function is defined as reduced when the duodenal filling grade is less than 3.

Exocrine pancreatic function assessed by S-MRCP may be normal in patients with abnormal ERCP findings and vice versa, with discordant results in 27% of cases. Follow-up of patients with abnormal S-MRCP function test but normal ERCP findings has shown evolution to overt chronic pancreatitis. These findings suggest that the S-MRCP function test may be of help in the diagnosis of chronic pancreatitis. Therefore, S-MRCP could be more useful than ERCP since it allows evaluation of both morphologic and functional changes during a single noninvasive procedure.

Imaging methods that evaluate pancreatic parenchyma: CT versus MRI

Computed tomography

Spiral CT is the most widely used modality for imaging inflammatory and neoplastic diseases of the pancreas. This technology permits scanning of the entire pancreas during a single breath-hold.

A routine abdominal spiral CT without contrast media, and after contrast injection in portal venous phase, is commonly used for patients with known or suspected pancreatitis. Dual-phase scanning is performed when evaluating a suspected pancreatic neoplasm and in cases where a careful evaluation of peripancreatic arterial anatomy is required. Arterial-phase imaging with contiguous thin overlapping slices can be crucial for detecting small and subtle noncontour-deforming neoplasms.

Three-dimensional reconstructions using multiplanar techniques, including MIP, shaded surface display, and volume rendering, provide comprehensive additional information about the relationship and possible involvement of vascular structures in the vicinity of focal pancreatic lesions and the degree and level of dilation of pancreatic and biliary ducts.

Diagnostic criteria of chronic pancreatitis using CT are shown in Table 28.1. Although the early changes of chronic pancreatitis are difficult to recognize on CT, the features of advanced disease are readily recognized and include dilation of the main pancreatic duct and its side branches, focal or diffuse parenchymal atrophy or enlargement, pancreatic calcifications, biliary ductal dilation, alteration in peripancreatic fat or fascia, and pseudocysts (Figs 28.1a,b, 28.3b,c, and 28.4a). While diffuse enlargement is common in acute pancreatitis, this finding is rare in chronic pancreatitis and parenchymal atrophy is more frequently observed. Occasionally, pancreatic enlargement can occur due to extensive interlobular and periductal fibrosis.

These diagnostic criteria are the same for TUS, but CT is less operator-dependent and shows the best diagnostic accuracy for pancreatic calcifications, a specific sign of advanced chronic pancreatitis. Reported sensitivity of CT for chronic pancreatitis ranges from 60 to 95% depending on the severity of the disease. A normal-appearing gland on CT is frequently found in patients with early stages of chronic pancreatitis.

Rather than diagnosis, the main role of CT in patients with chronic pancreatitis is the detection of complications such as inflammatory masses or pseudocysts (Fig. 28.4a).

Magnetic resonance imaging

T1-weighted sequences with fat suppression images before and after gadolinium administration are the key sequences for evaluating the pancreatic parenchyma by MRI. Three-dimensional, volumetric, contrast-enhanced dynamic imaging with fat suppression allows further three-dimensional reconstructions in MIP, and in multiple planes, which is very useful for showing the relationship between the main vascular structures and the pancreatic gland in cases of suspected pancreatic malignancy or for preoperative planning in patients with chronic pancreatitis. For gadolinium-DTPA-enhanced MRI (0.1 mmol/kg), at least three-phase (arterial, portal, and delayed) imaging should be performed.

The normal pancreas is of intermediate signal intensity, similar to the liver, and surrounded by retroperitoneal fat, which has high signal intensity on in-phase T1-weighted sequences. On opposed-phase T1-weighted sequences, a hypointense rim surrounding the pancreas is observed in the fat–parenchyma borders. On the fat-suppressed T1-weighted images, the relative signal intensity of the pancreas increases dramatically, which allows the detection of pathologic conditions with low signal intensity, such as fibrosis, cysts, or malignancies. The pancreas shows a clear enhancement during the earlier arterial phase after intravenous gadolinium administration, remains highly enhanced during the portal phase and over the first 3 min, and diminishes in signal intensity as the gadolinium is washed out.

Morphologic findings of chronic pancreatitis on MRI are analogous to those seen on CT and include atrophy or diffuse enlargement of the gland, focal enlargement, changes in signal intensity of pancreatic parenchyma, irregular dilation of the pancreatic duct, pancreatic calcifications seen as focal signal voids, and chronic pseudocysts (Figs 28.1, 28.4, and 28.5).

In patients with moderate to severe chronic pancreatitis, the pancreatic parenchyma tends to show a decreased signal on fat-suppressed unenhanced T1-weighted images. In addition, the gland shows an abnormal enhancement after gadolinium administration, consisting of decreased enhancement in the arterial phase and increased enhancement in the late venous phase. In this regard, measurement of pancreatic signal intensity on gadolinium chelate dynamic MRI may be helpful for the diagnosis of mild chronic pancreatitis, before morphologic or signal intensity changes develop. The presence of a signal intensity ratio (enhanced/unenhanced) less than 1.7 in the arterial phase and/or delayed peak enhancement after contrast administration has a sensitivity of 79% and a specificity of 75% for early chronic pancreatitis, which is significantly higher than the sensitivity of 50% obtained by the analysis of morphologic abnormalities (Figs 28.1, 28.4 and 28.5).

Complications of chronic pancreatitis: MRI/MRCP versus CT

Both MRI and CT can detect most complications of chronic pancreatitis, including vascular complications, such as splenic vein thrombosis or arterial pseudoaneurysm, pseudocysts, or biliary dilation.

MRI seems to be better than CT in evaluating pancreatic pseudocysts. Differences in the signal intensity and homogeneity of T1-weighted images allow the differentiation of pus, blood, necrosis, and pancreatic fluid (Fig. 28.4). Furthermore, MRI has demonstrated its ability to discriminate between noninfected and infected cysts that contain solid debris, thus identifying drainability. When pancreatic pseudocysts penetrate the thoracic cavity, massive effusions in the mediastinum or the pleural space can occur. MRCP is able to identify the connection between the thoracic cyst and the pancreatic duct.

Due to the underlying fibrosis in chronic pancreatitis, the intrapancreatic common bile duct may be narrowed at the head of the pancreas. Although CT detects biliary dilation, MRCP shows better detail of the smooth and tapered appearance of the distal bile duct and mild proximal duct dilatation in cases of chronic pancreatitis, as compared with the more severe dilation usually seen in pancreatic malignancy (Fig. 28.6).

Vascular complications in chronic pancreatitis are associated with high morbidity and mortality rates. Venous complications include splenic or portal vein thrombosis. Chronic pancreatitis accounts for 65% of cases of splenic vein thrombosis, and it can lead to varices in short gastric veins and the gastroepiploic vein. Pseudoaneurysms, mainly involving the pancreaticoduodenal or splenic arteries, result from vessel wall inflammatory involvement, and are mostly located near to the pancreatic head or splenic hilus. The identification of an aneurysm or a pseudoaneurysm is based classically on angiography. However, MRI is more accurate in delineating the size of aneurysms, and when dynamic MRI is performed using fat-suppressed, three-dimensional, T1-weighted images, it is able to differentiate an artery-to-pancreatic duct fistula from an aneurysm in cases of hemosuccus pancreaticus.

Of particular interest is the differentiation between the presence of an inflammatory mass and a superimposed pancreatic adenocarcinoma in a patient with chronic pancreatitis. Because the risk of pancreatic

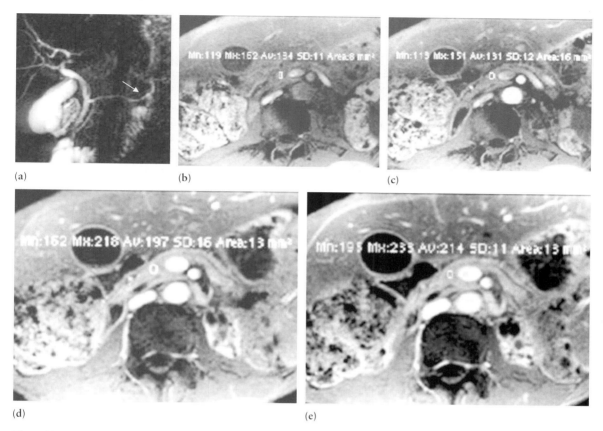

(a) (b) (c)

(d) (e)

Figure 28.5 Early chronic pancreatitis on MRI in a patient with normal imaging on TUS and CT. (a) Coronal pancreatogram after secretin stimulation depicts subtle irregularity and dilatation of pancreatic duct tail (arrow). (b) Axial-oblique unenhanced T1-weighted fat-suppressed image shows pancreatic atrophy. (c–e) T1-weighted fat-suppressed contrast-enhanced dynamic MRI during the arterial phase demonstrates (c) a signal intensity enhanced/unenhanced ratio less than 1.7; the peak of pancreatic parenchymal enhancement takes place during the delayed phase (e). This pattern of enhancement reflects a significant histologic component of fibrosis in pancreatic parenchyma.

cancer in all forms of chronic pancreatitis is increased from 3.8 to approximately 16 times that in the general population, focal enlargement becomes a diagnostic challenge. Inflammatory pancreatic mass, which is seen as a focal enlargement of the pancreas, has been reported to occur in 20% of cases of chronic pancreatitis and typically involves the pancreatic head. It often mimics a pancreatic malignancy and differentiation is often difficult with any imaging method.

When chronic pancreatitis and pancreatic carcinoma occur together in the same patient, it may be very difficult to make the correct diagnosis. Moreover, tumors are hard to differentiate from focal areas of chronic pancreatitis. The presence of ductal calculi or parenchymal calcification is suggestive of a benign lesion. Regression of calcifications in a patient previously diagnosed with chronic pancreatitis may be a sign of a superimposed carcinoma. The sensitivities of ultrasound and CT in the differentiation of chronic pancreatitis and pancreatic carcinoma are 98% and 94% respectively, with specificities of 90% and 95% respectively. These figures are markedly lower when the diagnosis of pancreatic cancer over chronic pancreatitis is considered.

On CT and MRI, chronic pancreatitis and pancreatic carcinoma show abnormal pancreatic enhancement

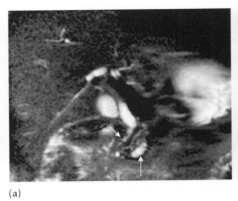
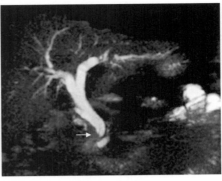

(a)   (b)

Figure 28.6 Encroached common bile duct: different appearance in encroaching by fibrosis or tumor. (a) Tapered stenosis of common bile duct secondary to severe chronic pancreatitis. Coronal half-Fourier single-shot turbo spin-echo (HASTE) MRCP shows tapered stenosis of distal main bile duct (short arrow). See also the pseudocyst in the uncinate process (long arrow). (b) Coronal half-Fourier single-shot turbo spin-echo (HASTE) MRCP demonstrates abrupt stenosis of the common bile duct encroached by a cancer in the uncinate process (arrow).

because of the presence of fibrosis. The decreased signal intensity and contrast enhancement patterns of the inflammatory mass on MRI are similar to those of pancreatic malignancy (Fig. 28.4). Fat-suppressed, high-resolution, T1-weighted images acquired 10 min after administration of mangafodipir trisodium (Mn-DPDP) (5 μmol/kg) in a slow bolus over 1–2 min are useful for detection of lesions in some equivocal cases.

S-MRCP may also help in differentiating between inflammatory and malignant mass of the pancreas. The finding of a smoothly stenotic or normal main pancreatic duct penetrating through the tumor is frequently seen in inflammatory pancreatic mass and is a useful sign for differentiating this entity from pancreatic malignancies.

Should MRCP and MRI replace ERCP and CT in the morphologic evaluation of chronic pancreatitis?

MRI is increasingly considered a major method for the morphologic diagnosis of chronic pancreatitis due to the development of improved techniques for MRI-based visualization of the pancreas, the association of intravenous administration of contrast media (i.e., gadolinium), and the possibility of accurate visualization of the pancreatic duct system by secretin stimulation. Together with the usual evaluation of morphologic changes within the parenchyma, the combination of S-MRCP with analysis of signal intensity of the gland, both in unenhanced conditions as well as with gadolinium enhancement, provides MRI with a high efficacy for the diagnosis of even mild forms of chronic pancreatitis. The simultaneous analysis of secretin-stimulated pancreatic outflow gives useful additional information on exocrine pancreatic function in these patients.

Although ERCP has long been considered the gold standard for the morphologic diagnosis of chronic pancreatitis, the wide and accurate information provided by S-MRCP and MRI, which are both performed during the same procedure and without any risk to the patient, has relegated ERCP to cases in which endoscopic therapy is required. A similar conclusion can be drawn with regards to CT. CT is clearly unable to detect chronic pancreatitis unless marked morphologic changes have already developed. Nevertheless, CT still plays an important role in detecting complications of the disease, aiding the diagnosis of malignant transformation, and providing surgeons with a clear map of the gland in cases where surgical therapy is considered.

Recommended reading

Calvo MM, Bujanda L, Calderon A *et al*. Comparison between magnetic resonance cholangiopancreatography and

ERCP for evaluation of the pancreatic duct. *Am J Gastroenterol* 2002;97:347–353.

Cappeliez O, Delhaye M, Debiere J *et al*. Chronic pancreatitis: evaluation of pancreatic exocrine function with MR pancreatography after secretin stimulation. *Radiology* 2000;215:358–364.

Del Frate C, Zanardi R, Mortele K *et al*. Advances in imaging for pancreatic disease. *Curr Gastroenterol Rep* 2002;4: 140–148.

Elmas N. The role of diagnostic radiology in pancreatitis. *Eur J Radiol* 2001;38:120–132.

Etemad B, Whitcomb DC. Chronic pancreatitis: diagnosis, classification, and new genetic developments. *Gastroenterology* 2001;120:682–707.

Freeny PC. Pancreatic imaging: new modalities. *Gastroenterol Clin North Am* 1999;28:723–744.

Fulcher AS, Turner MA, Capps GW *et al*. Half-Fourier RARE MR cholangiopancreatography: experience in 300 subjects. *Radiology* 1998;207:21–32.

Hellerhoff KJ, Helmberger H III, Rosch T *et al*. Dynamic MR pancreatography after secretin administration: image quality and diagnostic accuracy. *Am J Roentgenol* 2002;179: 121–129.

Ichikawa T, Nitatori T, Hachiya J *et al*. Breath-held MR cholangiopancreatography with half-averaged single-shot hybrid rapid acquisition with relaxation enhancement sequence: comparison of fast GRE and SE sequences. *J Comput Assist Tomogr* 1996;20:798–802.

Ichikawa T, Haradome H, Sou H *et al*. MR duct-penetrating sign on MR cholangiopancreatography (MRCP): a convenient sign for differentiating inflammatory pancreatic mass (IPM) from pancreatic malignancy. *Proc Int Soc Magn Reson Med* 2000;8:1475.

Irie H, Honda H, Tijima T *et al*. Optimal MR cholangiopancreatography sequence and its clinical application. *Radiology* 1998;206:379–387.

Ito K, Koike S, Matsunaga N. MR imaging of pancreatic diseases. *Eur J Radiol* 2001;38:78–93.

Johnson PT, Outwater EK. Pancreatic carcinoma versus chronic pancreatitis: dynamic MR imaging. *Radiology* 1999;212:213–218.

Kalra MK, Maher MM, Sahani DV, Subharao D, Saini S. Current status of imaging in pancreatic diseases. *J Comput Assist Tomogr* 2002;26:661–675.

Kim T, Murakami T, Takamura M *et al*. Pancreatic mass due to chronic pancreatitis: correlation of CT and MR imaging features with pathologic findings. *Am J Roentgenol* 2001; 177:367–371.

Koizumi J, Inoue S, Yonekawa H *et al*. Hemosuccus pancreaticus: diagnosis with CT and MRI and treatment with transcatheter embolization. *Abdom Imaging* 2002;27: 77–81.

Manfredi R, Costamagna G, Brizi MG *et al*. Severe chronic pancreatitis versus suspected pancreatic disease: dynamic MR cholangiopancreatography after secretin stimulation. *Radiology* 2000;214:849–855.

Matos C, Metens T, Deviere J *et al*. Pancreatic duct: morphologic and functional evaluation with dynamic MR pancreatography after secretin stimulation. *Radiology* 1997;203: 435–441.

Miyazaki T, Yamashita Y, Tsuchigame T *et al*. MR cholangiopancreatography using HASTE (half-Fourier acquisition single-shot turbo spin-echo) sequences. *Am J Roentgenol* 1996;166:1297–1303.

Morgan DE, Baron TH, Smith JK *et al*. Pancreatic fluid collections prior to intervention: evaluation with MR imaging compared with computed tomography and US. *Radiology* 1997;203:773–778.

Murcia NM, Jeffrey BR, Beaullieu FC *et al*. Multidetector CT of the pancreas and bile duct system: value of curved planar reformations. *Am J Roentgenol* 2001;173:689–693.

Reinhold C. Magnetic resonance imaging of the pancreas in 2001. *J Gastrointest Surg* 2002;6:133–135.

Remer EM, Baker ME. Imaging of chronic pancreatitis. *Radiol Clin North Am* 2002;40:1229–1242.

Sica GT, Braver J, Cooney MJ *et al*. Comparison of endoscopic retrograde cholangiopancreatography with MR cholangiopancreatography in patients with pancreatitis. *Radiology* 1999;210:605–610.

Sica GT, Miller FH, Rodriguez G, McTavish J, Banks PA. Magnetic resonance imaging in patients with pancreatitis: evaluation of signal intensity and enhancement changes. *J Magn Reson Imaging* 2002;15:275–284.

Soto JA, Barish MA, Yucel EK *et al*. Pancreatic duct: MR cholangiopancreatography with a three-dimensional fast spin-echo technique. *Radiology* 1995;196:459–464.

Takehara Y, Ichijo K, Yooyama N *et al*. Breath-hold MR cholangiopancreatography with a long-echo-train fast spin-echo sequence and a surface coil in chronic pancreatitis. *Radiology* 1994;192:73–78.

Zhang XM, Shi H, Parker L, Dohke M, Holland GA, Mitchell DG. Suspected early or mild chronic pancreatitis: enhancement patterns on gadolinium chelate dynamic MRI. *J Magn Reson Imaging* 2003;17:86–94.

29 The place of endoscopic ultrasound in the diagnosis of chronic pancreatitis

Stefan Kahl and Peter Malfertheiner

Introduction

Chronic pancreatitis is diagnosed by imaging procedures. Endoscopic retrograde cholangiopancreatography (ERCP) is considered the gold standard because of a consensus among pancreatologists since 1984. Endoscopic ultrasound (EUS), initially introduced in the 1980s to improve imaging of the pancreas, has added significantly to the diagnosis of pancreatic cancer and chronic pancreatitis.

Value of different imaging procedures

The criteria for diagnosis of chronic pancreatitis using ultrasonography, computed tomography (CT), and ERCP are listed in Table 29.1. An important drawback of ultrasonography is its limited sensitivity for the diagnosis of early stages of chronic pancreatitis. CT is more expensive but less dependent on the investigator's skill and experience. It has probably the highest accuracy in detecting pancreatic calcifications as a specific sign of advanced chronic pancreatitis. ERCP is considered the gold standard for diagnosis and staging of chronic pancreatitis in the absence of histology. If the main pancreatic duct and side branches are displayed in high detail, well-defined abnormalities of pancreatograms can be considered highly specific findings of chronic pancreatitis. The accuracy of ERCP is superior to that of transabdominal ultrasound and CT, but the technique is invasive and needs specialized training. The crucial point is that the available imaging methods are focused either on the ductal system (ERCP) or on the pancreatic parenchyma (ultrasound, CT). The gap-

ing hole between these imaging modalities is filled by EUS.

In standard EUS, the transducer located at the tip of an endoscope is placed into the third portion of the duodenum and then withdrawn to allow transduodenal and transgastric visualization of the entire pancreas. Two different EUS systems are available, both offering perfect visualization of the pancreas. Mechanical probes contain an engine-driven rotating transducer offering a 360° ultrasound image. The latest electronic sector-scanning probes with 150° sector images offer several additional features, like Doppler, color, and power Doppler tools or the opportunity to take EUS-guided fine needle biopsies. The ultrasound images obtained with electronic sector-scanning probes fits exactly the known appearance of the transabdominal ultrasound view. The close proximity of the pancreas, together with the absence of any intervening structures (fat, bowel, gas), allows the use of high-frequency transducers (up to 20 MHz). Therefore high-resolution imaging of the pancreas is obtained that can detect even subtle abnormalities in the parenchyma as well as in the pancreatic ductal system.

Features of chronic pancreatitis on EUS

The characteristic findings detectable by EUS in patients with chronic pancreatitis were first systematically described by Wiersema (Table 29.2). Several studies have extended our knowledge of the ductal and parenchymal features indicative of chronic pancreatitis. Parenchymal features include changes in gland size (mostly atrophic organ), cysts (Fig. 29.1), hypoechoic

Table 29.1 Cambridge criteria of chronic pancreatitis.

Stage	Typical changes on ERCP	Typical changes on CT and US
Normal	Normal appearance of side branches and main pancreatic duct	Normal gland size, shape; homogeneous parenchyma
Equivocal	Dilatation/obstruction of less than three side branches; normal main pancreatic duct	Normal main pancreatic duct; heterogeneous parenchyma
Mild	Dilatation/obstruction of side branches (more than three); normal main pancreatic duct	Normal main pancreatic duct; heterogeneous parenchyma, slide gland enlargement
Moderate	Additional stenosis and dilatation of main pancreatic duct	Small cysts (< 10 mm in diameter), increased echogenicity of the main pancreatic duct wall, dilatation of the main pancreatic duct
Severe	Additional obstructions, cysts, stenosis of main pancreatic duct; calculi	Cysts (> 10 mm in diameter), stenosis of main pancreatic duct with prestenotic dilatation; calculi

CT, computed tomography; ERCP, endoscopic retrograde cholangiopancreatography; US, ultrasound.

Table 29.2 Endoscopic ultrasound criteria of chronic pancreatitis.

Parenchymal features
Gland size, cysts
Echo-poor lesions (focal areas of reduced echogenicity)
Echo-rich lesions (> 3 mm diameter)
Accentuation of lobular pattern

Ductal features
Increased duct wall echogenicity
Narrowing, dilatation (main pancreatic duct, side branches)
Calculi

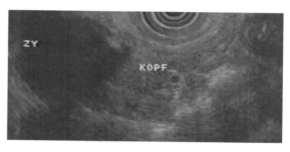

Figure 29.1 Cystic lesion (ZY) with a diameter of 20 mm adjacent to the head of the pancreas (KOPF). The echotexture of the visible pancreatic parenchyma shows additional features of chronic pancreatitis (echo-rich strands, lobulation).

lesions (Fig. 29.2), hyperechoic, i.e., echo-rich, foci (Fig. 29.3a,b), and strands (fibrosis), fibrosis (Fig. 29.3c) or calcifications (with shadowing) and accentuation of the lobular pattern, i.e., echo-poor normal parenchyma surrounded by hyperechoic strands (fibrosis) (Fig. 29.4). Ductal changes comprise dilatation of the main pancreatic duct (Fig. 29.5) or side branches, increased duct wall echogenicity (Fig. 29.6), and calcifications (Fig. 29.5). Calcifications are generally judged to have the highest predictive value in the diagnosis of chronic pancreatitis. Many authors have introduced a threshold number of EUS features for diagnosing chronic pancreatitis.

Threshold number of EUS features for diagnosing chronic pancreatitis

There is discussion about whether the total number of changes is more predictive than an individual criterion. It is well accepted that in cases without any of the above-mentioned criteria, chronic pancreatitis is unlikely, whereas in the presence of at least five features, chronic pancreatitis is likely even though other imaging modalities may be normal. If less than five features are detectable, the clinical significance of these findings is unresolved.

A given threshold influences the sensitivity and

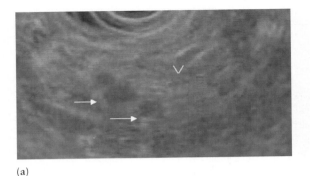

(a)

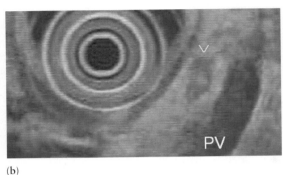

(b)

Figure 29.2 (a) Echo-rich pancreatic parenchyma with three echo-poor lesions (arrows), sharply demarcated from the surrounding parenchyma. The main pancreatic duct is slightly dilated, with an echo-rich duct wall (V). (b) Echo-poor lesion (V) within the echo-rich pancreatic parenchyma. This lesion corresponds to a necrosis detected during an acute bout of chronic pancreatitis 3 months prior to EUS examination. PV, portal vein.

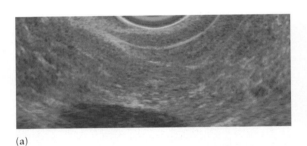

(a)

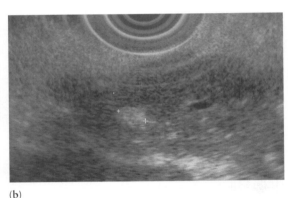

(b)

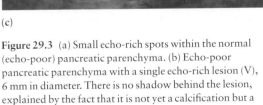

(c)

Figure 29.3 (a) Small echo-rich spots within the normal (echo-poor) pancreatic parenchyma. (b) Echo-poor pancreatic parenchyma with a single echo-rich lesion (V), 6 mm in diameter. There is no shadow behind the lesion, explained by the fact that it is not yet a calcification but a fibrous plaque, which will develop into a calcified plaque. (c) Inhomogeneous pancreatic parenchyma with several echo-rich (fibrotic) strands but without accentuation of the lobular pattern.

specificity of EUS compared with other imaging procedures, although selection of this threshold depends on the purpose of the examination. In a normal population with an average pretest probability of chronic pancreatitis of around 50%, a low threshold (one to two criteria) will lead to a high sensitivity by lowering the specificity. If in the same population a higher threshold is used (more than five criteria), the sensitivity will de-

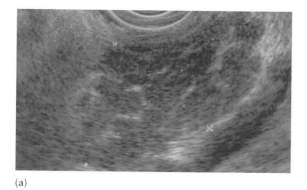

(a)

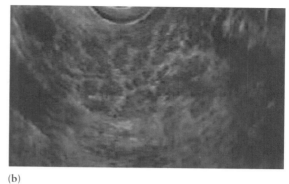

(b)

Figure 29.4 (a) Accentuation of the lobular pattern: echo-poor pancreatic parenchyma surrounded by echo-rich strands. This figure is the counterpart to the normal ERCP shown in Fig. 29.7a. (b) More advanced lobular pattern corresponding to a decreasing volume of normal (echo-poor) pancreatic parenchyma but an increase in fibrous strands (visible as echo-rich areas).

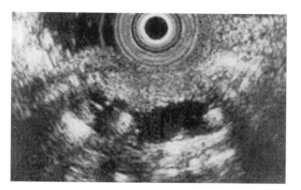

Figure 29.5 Dilatated main pancreatic duct (diameter 9 mm) with calcification in the duct.

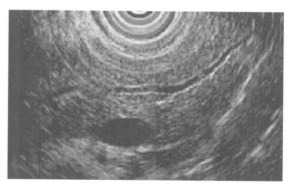

Figure 29.6 Main pancreatic duct is not yet dilated, but the duct wall has increased echogenicity (visible as echo-rich, i.e., white, lines at the border of the main pancreatic duct).

crease but will be combined with an increasing specificity. As EUS should be focused mainly on patients highly likely to have chronic pancreatitis based on clinical data and the patient's history, the pretest probability of chronic pancreatitis in this group is high (75–80%). In this setting it is possible to lower the threshold (to one feature) without any loss of specificity.

Once established, chronic pancreatitis is a lifelong disease, but it is unknown when the first symptoms occur. The majority of patients present with more than three EUS features at the first examination. However, there is a small group of patients with typical symptoms and clinical history who present with less than three features on EUS, probably in an early stage of the dis-

ease. In some of these patients even other imaging modalities are still normal (Fig. 29.7a). This population with high test probability will profit from high-resolution imaging by EUS.

In the early stages of chronic pancreatitis, the ductal system remains normal but the parenchymal changes can be detected by EUS. The necrosis–fibrosis sequence as the crucial event in the pathogenesis of chronic pancreatitis explains when and how focal necrosis is replaced by fibrotic tissue. This typically affects the parenchyma earlier than the ductal system. Crucially, this sequence leads to accentuation of the lobular pattern (Fig. 29.4a) of the pancreas: hypoechoic areas (representing inflamed pancreatic parenchyma)

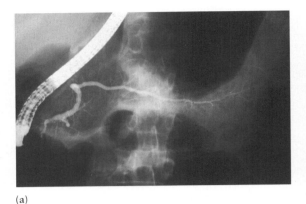

(a)

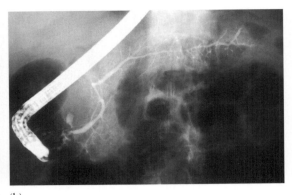

(b)

Figure 29.7 (a) Normal ERCP in a 38-year-old man with known history of alcohol abuse (this figure is the counterpart to the EUS image shown in Fig. 29.4a). (b) ERCP obtained 21 months later showing ductal changes of chronic pancreatitis involving main pancreatic duct and main duct branches in the body and tail of the pancreas.

surrounded by hyperechoic septae (fibrotic strands). This is by far the most frequent detectable feature of chronic pancreatitis on EUS. The accentuation of the lobular pattern has been described by several authors.

Age-related changes in the pancreas may affect the diagnostic threshold in older patients (diameter of the main pancreatic duct increases in older subjects). A possible solution, suggested by several authors, could be a scoring system that factors in the effects of aging. The practice now is to adapt the threshold according to the patient's age: a higher threshold for older individuals than for younger ones. The optimal cut-off for the diagnosis of chronic pancreatitis therefore depends on several factors:
• pretest probability (average pretest probability vs. high pretest probability);
• age of the patient;
• purpose of the examination (exclude vs. establish the diagnosis of chronic pancreatitis).

Reference standards

The ability of EUS to detect subtle parenchymal changes has raised the question of how reference standards for chronic pancreatitis should be defined. There is no accepted agreement on an appropriate reference standard to evaluate the EUS diagnosis of chronic pancreatitis. This is a major problem, especially in early stages of the disease when only minimal changes are de-

tectable and other imaging methods are still normal. Histology, ERCP, or natural history seem to be candidates for reference standards.

Several studies have compared results of EUS with subsequent evaluation of histology specimens after pancreatic resection or with the findings of EUS-guided fine needle aspiration (FNA). The major drawback of this approach is the focal distribution of chronic pancreatitis within the pancreas, which would probably lead to false-negative results. Although in published series EUS-guided FNA increased the negative predictive value of EUS to 100% and the specificity to 64%, biopsies for histologic or cytologic examination are currently restricted to scientific purposes and are not established in clinical routine.

EUS findings correlate extremely well with the severity of chronic pancreatitis according to the Cambridge classification at ERCP (Table 29.1). The problem is that there may be a number of patients with normal ERCP but abnormal EUS. Especially in patients with a high pretest probability of chronic pancreatitis, ERCP may underdiagnose chronic pancreatitis due to the absence of ductal findings in early stages. The evidence for this comes from studies including natural history as the reference standard. Natural history is the most relevant reference standard for early chronic pancreatitis for scientific purposes and clinical routine as well. Unfortunately, there are only limited data on the long-term natural history of "mild" chronic pancreatitis diagnosed by EUS.

Our clinical strategy involves surveillance of patients

positive on EUS but with normal ERCP findings (Fig. 29.7a,b). In a recently published paper, we assessed the sensitivity of EUS in patients with high clinical suspicion of chronic pancreatitis (based on clinical data). Among 38 patients with normal ERCP but a clinical history suggestive of chronic pancreatitis, EUS detected parenchymal changes attributable to chronic pancreatitis in 84%. Confirmation that the EUS abnormalities were related to chronic pancreatitis was obtained by the finding of abnormalities with ERCP during a median follow-up period of 1.5 years.

Methods to improve diagnostic accuracy

Additional techniques for enhancing the diagnostic accuracy of EUS have been developed, but most of them are only used under very restricted circumstances. Contrast agents or secretin stimulation may help improve the diagnostic yield but they are far from clinical routine and may probably never reach this level.

One of the newest developments is EUS imaging with miniprobes that can be passed through the accessory channel of a standard duodenoscope and then further inserted into the main pancreatic duct. They provide excellent high-resolution (20–30 MHz) images of the main pancreatic duct and small lesions within the parenchyma. The use of these probes is increasingly under investigation, but their role in clinical routine has not been established yet. Initial results appear promising, especially in differentiating chronic pancreatitis from pancreatic adenocarcinoma and for more precise evaluation of pancreatic duct abnormalities (irregularities, stenoses) depicted by ERCP.

Differentiation between benign and malignant pancreatic tumors

In patients with pancreatic tumors and chronic pancreatitis, EUS has difficulty in distinguishing benign from malignant lesions. Pancreatic tumors can be mimicked by focal inflammation due to acute bouts of chronic pancreatitis (Fig. 29.8). It is impossible to reliably differentiate between benign and malignant lesions in these cases. Several authors have attempted to find reliable criteria for differentiation.

Clinical role of EUS in the diagnosis of chronic pancreatitis

EUS is highly sensitive and specific for detecting chronic pancreatitis. EUS is as good as ERCP in diagnosing chronic pancreatitis in advanced stages. In early stages of the disease, when the ductal system

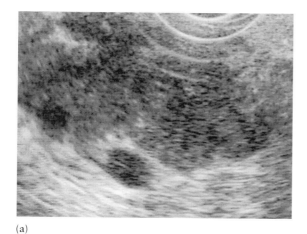

(a)

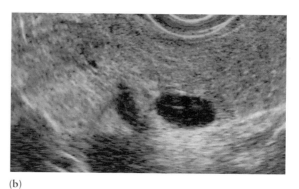

(b)

Figure 29.8 (a) Three weeks after acute pancreatitis: echo-poor enlargement of the pancreatic head. Differentiation between a solid, suspected malignant, mass and an inflammatory tumor is impossible by only factoring the EUS images. (b) Four months later the tumor disappeared.

remains normal, EUS is the most sensitive of the currently available imaging procedures for the diagnosis of chronic pancreatitis. EUS should be used in patients with a high pretest probability (due to known chronic alcohol use and typical symptoms of chronic pancreatitis).

Recommended reading

Axon AT, Classen M, Cotton PB, Cremer M, Freeny PC, Lees WR. Pancreatography in chronic pancreatitis: international definitions. *Gut* 1984;25:1107–1112.

Buscail L, Escourrou J, Moreau J *et al*. Endoscopic ultrasonography in chronic pancreatitis: a comparative prospective study with conventional ultrasonography, computed tomography, and ERCP. *Pancreas* 1995;10:251–257.

Catalano MF, Geenen JE. Diagnosis of chronic pancreatitis by endoscopic ultrasonography. *Endoscopy* 1998;30(Suppl 1):A111–A115.

Glasbrenner B, Kahl S, Malfertheiner P. Modern diagnostics of chronic pancreatitis. *Eur J Gastroenterol Hepatol* 2002;14:935–941.

Kahl S, Glasbrenner B, Leodolter A, Pross M, Schulz HU, Malfertheiner P. EUS in the diagnosis of early chronic pancreatitis: a prospective follow-up study. *Gastrointest Endosc* 2002;55:507–511.

Kloppel G, Maillet B. Chronic pancreatitis: evolution of the disease. *Hepatogastroenterology* 1991;38:408–412.

Kloppel G, Maillet B. The morphological basis for the evolution of acute pancreatitis into chronic pancreatitis. *Virchows Arch A* 1992;420:1–4.

Lees WR. Endoscopic ultrasonography of chronic pancreatitis and pancreatic pseudocysts. *Scand J Gastroenterol* (Suppl.) 1986;123:123–129.

Wiersema MJ, Hawes RH, Lehman GA, Kochman ML, Sherman S, Kopecky KK. Prospective evaluation of endoscopic ultrasonography and endoscopic retrograde cholangiopancreatography in patients with chronic abdominal pain of suspected pancreatic origin. *Endoscopy* 1993;25:555–564.

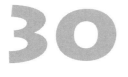

30

Should histology and/or cytology be the gold standard for the diagnosis of chronic pancreatitis in clinical practice?

Dale E. Bockman

The ideal method for diagnosing chronic pancreatitis would be a single, reliable, noninvasive test that exhibited 100% sensitivity and specificity. The test would necessarily be able to detect early changes, which might be subtle and heterogeneous. It should be able to differentiate between chronic pancreatitis and other changes in the pancreas, especially pancreatic cancer. It would be desirable if it could recognize chronic pancreatitis associated with pancreatic cancer in the same gland.

There is, of course, no such test available. In the absence of a single test, multiple diagnostic tools and techniques combined with clinical symptoms are used to determine that a patient suffers from chronic pancreatitis. The techniques improve constantly, especially with the increased resolution experienced with imaging techniques. The resolution available for examination of histologic specimens far surpasses any of the other techniques currently available. The morphology of all the components of the pancreas can be determined in detail by histology and electron microscopy. The specimens are available for immunocytochemical investigation for the detection of specific macromolecules. Histology is therefore a reasonable technique to use as a baseline for confirming the presence of chronic pancreatitis, and therefore as a gold standard against which other techniques may be compared.

A problem with using a histologic specimen for diagnosis is that histologic observation is usually possible only late in the disease when chronic pain and/or other complications have led to surgery. Clinical decisions must be made based on the experience of experts using the results from other diagnostic techniques.

Chronic pancreatitis is a progressive disease that is considered to be irreversible

The pathologic changes associated with chronic pancreatitis eventually affect all elements of the pancreas. The exocrine pancreas is altered more at first, but the islets eventually succumb as well. Acinar cells are lost or transdifferentiate. Duct cells may be lost. Extracellular fibers and substances increase. Frequently the fibrosis is sufficient to increase the size of the pancreas, although the epithelial elements are decreased significantly. The degenerative changes of chronic pancreatitis are generally considered to be irreversible. Treatment is directed toward alleviation of pain and providing substitution of pancreas-derived enzymes and hormones as they become deficient. However, some hope that epithelial recovery might be possible comes from the observations that cells in acini from patients with chronic pancreatitis are able to divide. Therefore, regeneration might be possible if causative factors could be controlled.

The earliest changes that signal the beginning of chronic pancreatitis are uncertain. They presumably would differ somewhat depending on the etiologic factors involved. Genetic factors have been identified, but the process by which they lead to development of chronic pancreatitis remains to be determined. The early changes that occur when alcohol is an etiologic factor have so far only been suggested. Convincing evidence has been advanced to support the progression of acute pancreatitis to chronic pancreatitis, that necrosis due to severe acute pancreatitis precedes the fibrosis that constitutes one of the typical characteristics of chronic pancreatitis. Cellular changes and fibrosis consistent with the changes observed in chronic pancreatitis may be observed after obstruction of the duct system, for example by a tumor expanding in proximity to the main duct.

Well-developed chronic pancreatitis is easier to diagnose than the earlier stages

It is of interest that despite the etiologic factors and the earliest changes that might occur, the pancreas tends to display the same pathologic picture when chronic pancreatitis is fully developed. Some of the later changes in the pancreas proper or in associated structures are not difficult to observe. Characteristic "pancreatic pain" accompanied by the presence of pancreatic stones detected by X-ray provides strong diagnostic evidence. The presence of pancreatic pseudocysts detectable by a number of techniques provides significant evidence.

The gold standard for detecting chronic pancreatitis in the clinical setting has been endoscopic retrograde pancreatography. Alterations in the main and accessory pancreatic ducts and in tributaries of these ducts are frequently detectable in the early and intermediate stages of chronic pancreatitis.

Variations in the echoes generated through ultrasonography are detectable when fibrosis is well developed and the parenchyma of the gland has been significantly affected. Endoscopic ultrasonography may offer enhanced resolution useful in the detection of alterations. However, early changes tend not to be uniform throughout the pancreas, and the relative quantity of parenchyma and intervening connective tissue may not be sufficient to produce reliable diagnostic information.

Regressive changes involving epithelial cells are a characteristic of chronic pancreatitis

Histologic sections of well-developed chronic pancreatitis commonly exhibit duct-like strands or groups of epithelial cells that exist within a sea of connective tissue (Fig. 30.1). This represents a great change from the normal pancreas in which the epithelial component is dominant whereas the connective tissue is limited to

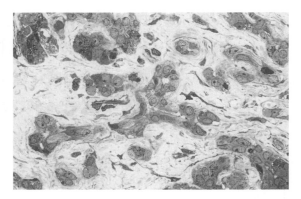

Figure 30.1 Histologic section from the pancreas of a patient with chronic pancreatitis. Although the disease is well advanced, the epithelial component continues to degrade. Some of the parenchyma seems, at first glance, to be ductules composed solely of ductal cells. Upon closer examination, however, it is obvious that acinar cells are being altered and are a part of the tubule. Clusters of altering acini are present in the upper left and lower right of the picture. These epithelial structures exist within a vastly expanded connective tissue. Fibrosis characteristically progresses as chronic pancreatitis progresses.

miniscule quantities separating acini, with larger quantities around interlobular and large ducts as well as larger blood vessels. Much of this epithelial component is composed of altered acinar cells and of cells that resemble ductular cells. It is not unusual for pancreatic islets, surrounded by connective tissue, to exist separately from acinar and ductular tissue.

The histologic picture of chronic pancreatitis is produced by the loss of exocrine epithelium plus the transdifferentiation of acinar cells to ductular cells. Some acinar cells die by apoptosis. Other acinar cells continue to live, but their morphology and function is altered. The continuity of the lumens that begin within the acinar unit and continue into ducts is lost, sealing off segments of the lobules. The acinar cells are unable to maintain their fully differentiated state. They lose the ability to synthesize and store zymogen granules. The height of acinar cells lessens, and there is a concomitant increase in the diameter of acinar lumens. Acinar cells therefore take on the characteristics of ductular cells. The result is the appearance of tubular complexes, which are collections of tubules composed of redifferentiated acinar cells plus preexisting ductular and centroacinar cells. These collections have been erroneously interpreted as resulting from ductular proliferation, unlikely in this regressive disease.

Fibrosis develops progressively, frequently increasing the size of the pancreas

Collagen fibers, fibroblasts, and myofibroblasts are major elements that comprise the fibrosis. Myofibroblasts, which differentiate from fibroblasts and pancreatic stellate cells as part of the fibrotic process, are detectable by immunohistologic localization of the smooth muscle α-actin that accumulates in their cytoplasm (Fig. 30.2).

There is considerable evidence that transforming growth factor (TGF)-β is involved directly in fibrosis, causing increased production of collagen and other extracellular products while inhibiting the breakdown of the extracellular matrix. Some inflammatory cells are sources of TGF-β, demonstrating an intimate relationship between two of the major characteristics of chronic pancreatitis. TGF-β is elevated in chronic

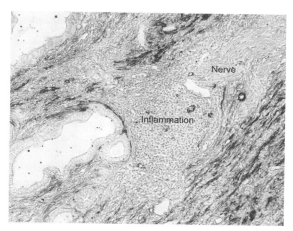

Figure 30.2 Histologic section of the pancreas from a patient with chronic pancreatitis. Some of the characteristics of chronic pancreatitis, including epithelial changes, inflammation, and fibrosis, are demonstrated. The section has been processed to localize smooth muscle a-actin, identifying myofibroblasts, which appear black. Production of myofibroblasts is part of the process of fibrosis. A collection of chronic inflammatory cells (inflammation) is close to altered epithelium and a pancreatic nerve. The normal morphology of the pancreas is lost.

pancreatitis. It is present primarily in ductules and centroacinar cells in normal pancreas but in chronic pancreatitis is present in all ducts and ductules, and in some acinar cells. TGF-β plays a key role in the modulation of fibroblasts or stellate cells into myofibroblasts.

TGF-β precursor is detected in inflammatory cells in chronic pancreatitis. Latent TGF-β may be activated by the increased amounts of plasmin produced by the activation of plasminogen. Transgenic mice overexpressing TGF-β in β cells of the islets of Langerhans have massive fibrosis of the pancreas, characterized by enhanced proliferation of fibroblasts and progressive accumulation of extracellular matrix.

The end result of TGF-β activity is increased deposition of extracellular matrix, including collagen, inhibited epithelial cell proliferation, and decreased activity of matrix metalloproteases, which degrade collagen. Fibrosis thus results from the net effect of increased production of collagen fibers coupled with a decrease in their breakdown. The laying down of collagen and associated compounds may be mediated by connective tissue growth factor.

Inflammation is present as chronic pancreatitis develops

Inflammation is part of the pathologic process and likely causes some of the changes in addition to reacting to them. Chronic inflammation is a common characteristic of chronic pancreatitis (Figs 30.2 and 30.3). Lymphoid cells predominate, but macrophages, plasma cells, and granulocytes are usually present as well. Inflammation and fibrosis (and perhaps proliferation and redifferentiation) are intimately linked. Macrophages, lymphoid cells, and platelets are sources of molecules that regulate cells and influence the composition of the extracellular matrix. CD8+CD103+ T cells analogous to intestinal intraepithelial lymphocytes infiltrate the pancreas in chronic pancreatitis. Sources of the fibrosis-promoting factor TGF-β include T cells and natural killer cells in addition to macrophages and platelets. Upregulation of messenger RNA encoding collagen type I and TGF-β occurs parallel to infiltration of mononuclear cells in experimentally induced pancreatitis in rats. In the pancreas of transgenic mice overexpressing TGF-β, macrophages and neutrophils invade the pancreas and acinar cell proliferation is inhibited.

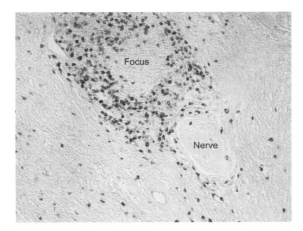

Figure 30.3 Inflammatory foci are sometimes closely associated with pancreatic nerves in patients with chronic pancreatitis. In this histologic section from a patient with chronic pancreatitis, a nerve is surrounded by fibrosis. Normal pancreatic parenchyma is missing. A focus of chronic inflammatory cells lies adjacent to the nerve. The section has been stained to identify natural killer cells, which appear black. The perineurial barrier, which normally provides a specialized microenvironment for the nerve fibers inside, may be damaged by the inflammatory process, as may the nerve fibers. It has been proposed that this is one of the mechanisms for generation of chronic pain in chronic pancreatitis.

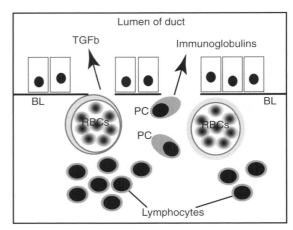

Figure 30.4 Major pancreatic ducts may be damaged in chronic pancreatitis. The normally continuous epithelial barrier is interrupted, allowing exchange of a number of products between the lumen and the underlying extracellular matrix. Groups of epithelial cells are lost, and the basal lamina (BL) is breached. Enlarged blood vessels contain packed erythrocytes (RBCs). Inflammatory cells populate the subepithelial connective tissue. The most populous are lymphocytes, but plasma cells (PC) and granulocytes are also found. These alterations are correlated with increased immunoglobulins and TGF-b in pancreatic juice. Inflammatory cells may enter the lumen and be contained in pancreatic juice.

Large pancreatic ducts lose their integrity

Pancreatic ducts are constructed in such a way as to form a barrier between the contents of the lumen and the surrounding structures. A continuous layer of epithelial cells joined by tight junctions borders the lumen. A continuous basal lamina parallels the basal surfaces of the epithelial cells. Beneath the basal lamina, in nonpathologic ducts, an extracellular matrix with scattered microvasculature forms an outer wall.

Ducts from patients with chronic pancreatitis frequently display significant changes. Epithelial cells are damaged and areas of the epithelial layer may be missing (Fig. 30.4), diminishing the barrier function. Basal lamina is missing in some areas. In these areas the barrier between lumen and underlying connective tissue is completely absent. Inflammatory cells, including plasma cells, are concentrated in the connective tissue wall. Inflammatory cells sometimes migrate into the lumen and may be collected from pancreatic juice.

Capillaries are increased in number and size. They are packed with erythrocytes and inflammatory cells.

These changes provide clear explanations for the increase in immunoglobulins and other substances, such as lactoferrin and TGF-β, in the pancreatic juice of patients with chronic pancreatitis. TGF-β is detectable in pure pancreatic juice from a majority of patients with chronic pancreatitis, whereas it is unusual in those without the disease.

Pancreatic nerves increase in number and size

Pain is a common symptom of chronic pancreatitis. Histologic specimens from patients with well-developed chronic pancreatitis commonly contain prominent nerves running through the fibrosis. The nerves are more obvious than in the normal pancreas because they have enlarged individually and there are more of them.

Collections of inflammatory cells are isolated in fibrotic areas and located adjacent to pancreatic parenchyma and nerves (Fig. 30.3). In some cases the inflammatory process has clearly affected the integrity of nerves. Pancreatic nerves are mixed, mainly unmyelinated nerves that are isolated from the surrounding tissue by a perineurium. This arrangement provides a specialized microenvironment for the multiple nerve fibers contained within. The inflammatory process sometimes damages the perineurium, eliminating the specialized microenvironment and allowing biologically active materials to penetrate into the nerve. Nerve fibers may be damaged. Inflammatory cells invade the nerve. It is logical that this chronic inflammation is one of the mechanisms for the generation of chronic pain in patients with chronic pancreatitis. This pathologic damage to the nerve is more severe than other methods by which nerve impulses might be generated. The presence of biologically active material and noxious substances produced by the inflammatory process can stimulate nerves without physically damaging them.

Percutaneous biopsy of the pancreas can detect chronic pancreatitis

Percutaneous biopsy is an alternate to study of histologic sections acquired by biopsy through a laparotomy. Cytology or microhistology may be used to study the retrieved specimens. The quantity of cells or tissue available for examination varies with the size of the needle and the number of times the percutaneous biopsy is taken from each pancreas. This quantity will obviously be less than in a routine surgical biopsy.

The needle can be guided with the help of ultrasound or computed tomography. Collecting data from both the biopsy and the guiding technology improves the diagnostic capability. As with other techniques, the early and intermediate stages are more difficult to detect with certainty.

The heterogeneous nature of the early stages of chronic pancreatitis, combined with the reduced sampling volume of a needle biopsy, reduce the likelihood that the requisite cytologic or histologic criteria are found. However, combinations of this technique have been used successfully by a number of investigators with positive results.

Finding cytologic evidence of pancreatic cancer is quite possible using this approach, providing an impor-

tant diagnosis. On the other hand, lack of evidence of cancer would not rule it out, even if histologic characteristics of chronic pancreatitis were evident.

Until a histologic specimen is available, multiple techniques aid diagnosis

It is generally easier to reach agreement about the diagnosis of chronic pancreatitis using histologic sections than using imaging techniques such as magnetic resonance imaging or ultrasonography. Histologic procedures and histopathologic expertise are generally more widely available than endoscopic ultrasound or direct pancreatic function tests. In the absence of a histologic/cytologic specimen, clinical observations and tests must be used.

Clinical criteria are detectable at different stages of the disease, and the presence of multiple symptoms or results enhance confidence in the diagnosis. Pain is a frequent first indication to the patient and is a common symptom. Steatorrhea and diabetes are late indicators. A variety of imaging techniques can detect complications such as pseudocysts, pancreatic stones, and duodenal obstruction.

The traditional clinical gold standard for the initial diagnosis of chronic pancreatitis is endoscopic retrograde pancreatography because it has been more sensitive than computed tomography or ultrasonography. Duct strictures and dilatation are detected. Endoscopic retrograde pancreatography is especially useful for detecting mild to moderate changes, indicating that the duct system may be affected relatively early in the disease. For the present, however, the histologic specimen must remain the ultimate gold standard with which the results of other techniques are compared.

Recommended reading

Bachem MG, Schneider E, Gross H *et al.* Identification, culture, and characterization of pancreatic stellate cells in rats and humans. *Gastroenterology* 1998;115:421–432.

Bockman DE. Toward understanding pancreatic disease: from architecture to cell signaling. *Pancreas* 1995;11: 324–329.

Bockman DE, Büchler M, Malfertheiner P, Beger HG. Analysis of nerves in chronic pancreatitis. *Gastroenterology* 1988;94:1459–1469.

Bockman DE, Müller M, Büchler MW, Friess H, Beger HG.

Pathological changes in pancreatic ducts from patients with chronic pancreatitis. *Int J Pancreatol* 1997;21:119–126.

Clain JE, Pearson RK. Diagnosis of chronic pancreatitis. Is a gold standard necessary? *Surg Clin North Am* 1999;79:829–845.

di Mola FF, Friess H, Martignoni ME *et al.* Connective tissue growth factor is a regulator for fibrosis in human chronic pancreatitis. *Ann Surg* 1999;230:63–71.

Di Stasi M, Lencioni R, Solmi L *et al.* Ultrasound-guided fine needle biopsy of pancreatic masses: results of a multicenter study. *Am J Gastroenterol* 1998;93:1329–1333.

Ebert MP, Ademmer K, Muller-Ostermeyer F *et al.* CD8⁺CD103⁺ T cells analogous to intestinal intraepithelial lymphocytes infiltrate the pancreas in chronic pancreatitis. *Am J Gastroenterol* 1998;93:2141–2147.

Emmrich J, Weber I, Nausch M *et al.* Immunohistochemical characterization of the pancreatic cellular infiltrate in normal pancreas, chronic pancreatitis, and pancreatic carcinoma. *Digestion* 1998;59:192–198.

Etemad B, Whitcomb DC. Chronic pancreatitis: diagnosis, classification, and new genetic developments. *Gastroenterology* 2001;120:682–707.

Freeny PC. Radiology. In: HG Beger, AL Warshaw, MW Büchler, DL Carr-Locke, JP Neoptolemos, C Russell, MG Sarr (eds) *The Pancreas*. Oxford: Blackwell Science, 1998:728–739.

Friess H, Cantero D, Graber H *et al.* Enhanced urokinase plasminogen activation in chronic pancreatitis suggests a role in its pathogenesis. *Gastroenterology* 1997;113:904–913.

Fritscher-Ravens A, Brand L, Knöfel WT *et al.* Comparison of endoscopic ultrasound-guided fine needle aspiration for focal pancreatic lesions in patients with normal parenchyma and chronic pancreatitis. *Am J Gastrenterol* 2002;97:2768–2775.

Hollerbach S, Klamann A, Topalidis T, Schmiegel WH. Endoscopic ultrasonography (EUS) and fine-needle aspiration (FNA) cytology for diagnosis of chronic pancreatitis. *Endoscopy* 2001;33:824–831.

Imdahl A, Nitzsche E, Krautmann F *et al.* Evaluation of positron emission tomography with 2-[¹⁸F]fluoro-2-deoxy-D-glucose for the differentiation of chronic pancreatitis and pancreatic cancer. *Br J Surg* 1999;86:194–199.

Jaskiewicz K, Nalecz A, Rzepko R, Sledzinski Z. Immunocytes and activated stellate cells in pancreatic fibrogenesis. *Pancreas* 2003;26:239–242.

Kasbay K, Tarnasky PR, Hawes RH, Cotton PB. Increased TGF beta in the pure pancreatic juice in pancreatitis. *Gastroenterology* 1999;116:A1136–A1137.

Lee MS, Gu DL, Feng LL *et al.* Accumulation of extracellular-matrix and developmental dysregulation in the pancreas by transgenic production of transforming growth-factor-beta-1. *Am J Pathol* 1995;147:42–52.

Malfertheiner P, Büchler M. Correlation of imaging and function in chronic pancreatitis. *Radiol Clin North Am* 1989;27:51–64.

Mallery JS, Centeno BA, Hahn PF, Chang Y, Warshaw AL, Brugge WR. Pancreatic tissue sampling guided by EUS, CT/US, and surgery: a comparison of sensitivity and specificity. *Gastrointest Endosc* 2002;56:218–224.

Mori T, Kawara S, Shinozaki M *et al.* Role and interaction of connective tissue growth factor with transforming growth factor-beta in persistent fibrosis: a mouse fibrosis model. *J Cell Physiol* 1999;181:153–159.

Müller MW, McNeil PL, Büchler MW, Friess H, Beger HG, Bockman DE. Membrane wounding and early ultrastructural findings. In: MW Büchler, W Uhl, H Friess, P Malfertheiner (eds) *Acute Pancreatitis: Novel Concepts in Biology and Therapy*. Oxford, Berlin: Blackwell Science, 1999:27–34.

Qi Z, Atsuchi N, Ooshima A, Takeshita A, Ueno H. Blockade of type beta transforming growth factor signaling prevents liver fibrosis and dysfunction in the rat. *Proc Natl Acad Sci USA* 1999;96:2345–2349.

Sanvito F, Nichols A, Herrera PL *et al.* TGF-beta-1 overexpression in murine pancreas induces chronic-pancreatitis and together with TNF-alpha, triggers insulin-dependent diabetes. *Biochem Biophys Res Commun* 1995;217:1279–1286.

Slater SD, Williamson RC, Foster CS. Expression of transforming growth factor-beta(1) in chronic pancreatitis. *Digestion* 1995;56:237–241.

Sparchez Z. Ultrasound-guided percutaneous pancreatic biopsy. Indications, performance and complications. *Rom J Gastroenterol* 2002;11:335–341.

Sparmann G, Merkord J, Jaschke A *et al.* Pancreatic fibrosis in experimental pancreatitis induced by dibutyltin dichloride. *Gastroenterology* 1997;112:1664–1672.

Van Laethem J-L, Deviere J, Resibois A *et al.* Localization of transforming growth factor β-1 and its latent binding protein in human chronic pancreatitis. *Gastroenterology* 1995;108:1873–1881.

Van Laethem JL, Robberecht P, Resibois A, Deviere J. Transforming growth factor beta promotes development of fibrosis after repeated courses of acute pancreatitis in mice. *Gastroenterology* 1996;110:576–582.

Vogelmann R, Ruf D, Wagner M *et al.* Development of pancreatic fibrosis in a TGFβ1 transgenic mouse. *Gastroenterology* 1999;116:A1174.

Werz O, Brungs M, Steinhilber D. Purification of transforming growth factor beta 1 from human platelets. *Pharmazie* 1996;51:893–896.

Yamanaka Y, Friess H, Büchler, Beger HG, Gold LI, Korc M. Synthesis and expression of transforming growth factor beta-1, beta-2, and beta-3 in the endocrine and exocrine pancreas. *Diabetes* 1993;42:746–756.

Zech CJ, Helmberger T, Wichmann MW, Holzknecht N, Diebold J, Reiser MF. Large core biopsy of the pancreas under CT fluoroscopy control: results and complications. *J Comput Assist Tomogr* 2002;26:743–749.

31

Pancreatic function tests for diagnosis and staging of chronic pancreatitis, cystic fibrosis, and exocrine pancreatic insufficiency of other etiologies: which tests are necessary and how should they be performed in clinical routine?

J. Enrique Domínguez-Muñoz

Because histology is usually not available for the diagnosis of chronic pancreatitis, this is based on the demonstration of the morphologic and/or functional changes that typically develop over time in the course of the disease. Exocrine pancreatic function is impaired progressively as chronic pancreatitis develops. Thus, exocrine pancreatic dysfunction refers to a mild, moderate, or severe reduction of exocrine pancreatic function. Finally, pancreatic function becomes insufficient to maintain normal digestive processes. Exocrine pancreatic insufficiency thus refers to the presence of maldigestion and malabsorption of nutrients as a consequence of primarily and/or secondarily impaired exocrine pancreatic function. Thus the terms "exocrine pancreatic insufficiency" and "severe exocrine pancreatic dysfunction" are synonymous.

Exocrine pancreatic dysfunction is a frequent finding not only in chronic pancreatitis but also in most other diseases of the exocrine and endocrine pancreas, i.e., cystic fibrosis, pancreatic tumors, after acute necrotizing pancreatitis and insulin-dependent diabetes mellitus. In addition, secondary exocrine pancreatic dysfunction frequently develops after gastrointestinal surgery (partial or total gastrectomy, duodenectomy).

Functional evaluation of the exocrine pancreas may be important for supporting the diagnosis of pancreatic disease in cases of inconclusive morphologic findings on imaging methods. However, the most relevant role for functional evaluation of the pancreas is the detection of primary or secondary pancreatic insufficiency in patients with known pancreatic disease or after gastrointestinal surgery in order to aid in the indication of enzyme substitution therapy and to control the efficacy of this therapy.

Exocrine pancreatic function may be evaluated by means of direct methods requiring duodenal intubation and noninvasive indirect methods (Table 31.1). The clinical usefulness of each of the available methods is related to factors like diagnostic accuracy, applicability to clinical routine, and cost. Direct pancreatic function tests, mainly the secretin–cholecystokinin test, are the gold standard for evaluation of exocrine pancreatic function. However, these tests are invasive, cumbersome, time-consuming, and expensive and thus limited to some specialized centers. Indirect pancreatic function tests are more easily applicable to clinical routine and therefore more widely used. Among these are oral and breath tests that, together with fecal fat quantification, evaluate the digestive ability of the exocrine pancreas, and fecal tests that measure the activity or concentration of pancreatic enzymes in feces. The sensitivity and specificity of these indirect tests are variable and lower than those of the direct tests. Since the information provided by each test is different, it is important to select the optimal test to be performed in each clinical situation.

In patients with clinical suspicion of chronic pancreatitis but normal imaging, only the secretin–cerulein test is sufficiently sensitive to support the diagnosis of the disease. The development of endoscopic ultrasonography, which has a very high sensitivity for the diagnosis of chronic pancreatitis, has further limited

Table 31.1 Pancreatic function tests.

Direct tests
Secretin–cholecystokinin test
Endoscopic test

Indirect tests
Fecal fat quantification
Fecal levels of pancreatic enzymes
NBT-PABA test
Pancreolauryl test
Amino acid consumption test
Breath tests (^{13}C-labeled substrates)

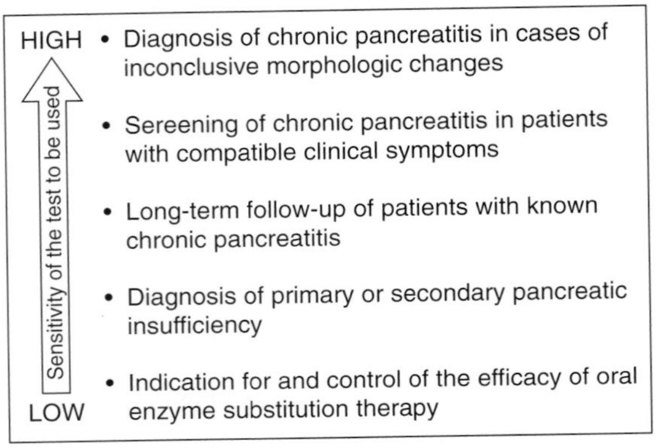

HIGH • Diagnosis of chronic pancreatitis in cases of inconclusive morphologic changes

• Sereening of chronic pancreatitis in patients with compatible clinical symptoms

• Long-term follow-up of patients with known chronic pancreatitis

• Diagnosis of primary or secondary pancreatic insufficiency

LOW • Indication for and control of the efficacy of oral enzyme substitution therapy

(vertical axis label) Sensitivity of the test to be used

Figure 31.1 Indications for evaluation of exocrine pancreatic function. The sensitivity of the function test to be used varies according to the indication.

the clinical usefulness of direct pancreatic function tests. Conversely, the diagnosis of primary or secondary exocrine pancreatic insufficiency and, in this context, the indication for or control of the efficacy of enzyme substitution therapy require a test able to detect maldigestion. It is easy to understand that in these two clinical situations the test to be used should have a very different sensitivity, highest in the former case, lowest in the latter (Fig. 31.1). In transitional situations, tests with an intermediate sensitivity may be useful for the screening of chronic pancreatitis in patients with a compatible clinical picture and for the long-term follow-up of patients with known chronic pancreatitis (Fig. 31.1).

Direct tests

Invasive pancreatic function tests are based on the direct measurement of pancreatic enzymes and bicarbonate output in samples of duodenal juice obtained after stimulation of the gland by intravenous administration of secretin and cholecystokinin (CCK) or cerulein (secretin–cholecystokinin test). Simple stimulation by intravenous secretin (secretin test) is used in the so-called endoscopic test, which is based on the measurement of bicarbonate concentration in endoscopy-guided aspirates of duodenal juice (see below). Finally, endogenous stimulation by a test meal (Lundh test) is no longer used because of a lower diagnostic accuracy.

Since direct pancreatic function tests are invasive, cumbersome, time-consuming, nonstandardized, and expensive, and since the development of novel sensitive imaging methods (i.e., endoscopic ultrasonography) has markedly improved the diagnosis of chronic pancreatitis, the usefulness of the secretin–cholecystokinin test is nowadays limited to its use as gold standard in the validation of new pancreatic function tests.

Secretin–cholecystokinin test

Method
The secretin–cholecystokinin test protocol differs among centers. A double-lumen nasoduodenal tube should be placed for constant aspiration of gastric juice and complete and fractionated collection of duodenal juice on ice during continuous intravenous infusion of secretin and CCK or cerulein. The protocol recommended by our group is summarized in Fig. 31.2. Despite duodenal juice being continuously aspirated, collection may be incomplete. The amount of juice lost toward the jejunum may be calculated by constant duodenal perfusion of a nonabsorbable dilution marker, usually polyethylene glycol. However, this requires a triple-lumen tube and further complicates the performance of the test.

An additional problem is the variable inactivation of pancreatic enzymes within the collected duodenal juice despite the use of antiproteases and collection on ice. This may be overcome by the single quantification of zinc instead of bicarbonate and enzymes. Zinc secretion is linked to pancreatic proteases; it is easily quantifiable and very stable in duodenal juice. Our group has recently demonstrated that the secretin–cerulein test based on single quantification of zinc output is as

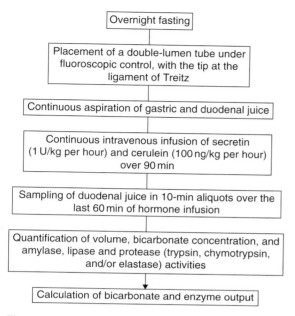

Figure 31.2 Secretin–cerulein test protocol.

Table 31.2 Severity of exocrine pancreatic dysfunction based on the secretin–cholecystokinin test.

Normal	Normal output of enzymes and bicarbonate
Mild dysfunction	Secretion of enzymes and bicarbonate ≥ 75% of the lower limit of normal
Moderate dysfunction	Secretion of enzymes and bicarbonate 30–75% of the lower limit of normal
Severe dysfunction	Secretion of enzymes and bicarbonate < 30% of the lower limit of normal

Table 31.3 Mean accuracy of exocrine pancreatic function tests for the diagnosis of chronic pancreatitis.

	Sensitivity (%)	Specificity (%)
Secretin–cholecystokinin test	90	94
Fecal chymotrypsin	57	88
Fecal elastase	70	85
Optimized serum pancreolauryl test	82	90

accurate as the test based on quantification of bicarbonate and enzymes for evaluation of exocrine pancreatic function.

Interpretation

The secretin–cholecystokinin test allows classification of the severity of exocrine pancreatic dysfunction (Table 31.2). The sensitivity and specificity of this test for the diagnosis of chronic pancreatitis both exceed 90% (Table 31.3).

Endoscopic test

The endoscopic pancreatic function test has been developed in order to avoid the problems associated with the secretin–cholecystokinin test, i.e., intubation, duration, and clinical applicability. It is based on the measurement of bicarbonate concentration and/or pancreatic enzyme activity in samples of duodenal juice obtained during upper gastrointestinal endoscopy after intravenous secretin stimulation.

Method

The protocol for the endoscopic pancreatic function test is based on the following four steps.

1 Standard endoscopy to the descending duodenum with the patient under conscious sedation.
2 Intravenous administration of secretin (1 U/kg or 0.2 mg/kg).
3 Endoscopic duodenal fluid collection at 0, 15, 30, 45, and 60 min after secretin injection. A short version of the test is based on the collection of duodenal juice for only 10 min.
4 Fluid analysis for bicarbonate concentration and/or pancreatic enzyme activity.

Interpretation

The peak bicarbonate concentration over 60 min is lower in patients with advanced chronic pancreatitis than in those with abdominal pain of extrapancreatic origin. Measurement of lipolytic activity in duodenal juice collected for 10 min after intravenous secretin is also significantly lower in patients with chronic pancreatitis compared with patients with normal pancreas, but it is not accurate enough for routine clinical use.

261

Although the endoscopic pancreatic function test is a promising procedure, it is far from being the current standard. Whether the peak bicarbonate concentration, instead of output over time, is a reliable marker of exocrine pancreatic function is questionable. In fact, most experts in this field support bicarbonate and enzyme output and not concentration as the most reliable marker of exocrine pancreatic function. This is due to the inverse relationship between bicarbonate concentration and rate of juice secretion in response to secretin. In addition, the endoscopic pancreatic function test requires the endoscope to be maintained in the duodenum for 1 hour, which is at least as uncomfortable for patients as nasoduodenal tubing. Because of this, pharmacologic conscious sedation is required in the context of the endoscopic test, although the effect of these drugs on exocrine pancreatic function has not been specifically evaluated. All these facts hinder the clinical usefulness of the endoscopic pancreatic function test.

Indirect tests

Indirect tests evaluate exocrine pancreatic function by quantifying either the digestive ability of the gland or levels of pancreatic enzymes in feces (Table 31.1). From a methodologic point of view, these tests can thus be classified as oral tests and fecal tests. In oral tests, a substrate is orally given together with a test meal. Pancreatic enzymes hydrolyze the substrate within the duodenum; the released metabolites are absorbed from the gut and can then be measured in serum, urine, or breath. Oral tests include the pancreolauryl test and different breath tests, mainly using ^{13}C-labeled substrates. Other tests like the NBT-PABA test and the amino acid consumption test are no longer commercially available and/or have insufficient diagnostic accuracy to be recommended for clinical use.

Several extrapancreatic factors are known to limit the accuracy of oral pancreatic function tests, mainly those interfering with normal digestion (slow gastric emptying rate, decreased bile acid secretion) and intestinal absorption (intestinal diseases) as well as those affecting the elimination of digestion products (renal insufficiency). Variability in gastric rate can be avoided to some extent by administration of metoclopramide or any other prokineticum in the context of the test. The potential negative role of renal disturbances is avoided

by the quantification of digestion products in serum instead of urine.

Fecal tests are based on the quantification of pancreatic enzyme concentration (elastase) or activity (chymotrypsin) in feces. Enzymes are deactivated and diluted or concentrated to a variable degree during intestinal passage, which must be taken into account when interpreting test results. Exocrine pancreatic function can also be measured indirectly in feces by means of fecal fat quantification. The amount of fat eliminated within the feces indirectly reflects fat digestion and therefore pancreatic lipase secretion.

Fecal tests

Fecal fat quantification
Fecal fat quantification using the classical Van de Kamer test is the gold standard for the diagnosis of steatorrhea. However, this test has several important disadvantages that limit its clinical applicability. Patients must eat a standard diet containing 80–120 g of fat daily for five consecutive days. This is an important handicap since the majority of patients with chronic pancreatitis are alcoholics and thus have limited compliance. Furthermore, patients should collect the total amount of feces produced over the last 3 days of the diet. Again this is not easy for alcoholic patients. A 3-day collection is needed to reduce errors and variability that may occur if a shorter collection period is used.

Patient compliance is not the only limitation of fecal fat quantification; so is the handling of stool samples in the laboratory. Stool samples collected over 3 days must be first homogenized and then processed manually, making this test unpleasant and cumbersome. A new methodology based on near-infrared reflectance analysis (NIRA) has greatly simplified the quantification of fat in stool and thus could make feasible the wide application of this test in clinical routine. Nevertheless, the difficulties associated with patient compliance remain the same.

Method In our laboratory, patients are instructed to eat a diet containing 92 g of fat for 5 days. Stool from the last three consecutive days is collected in three different containers. The daily amount of fat excreted (g/day) is quantified based on fat concentration measured by NIRA (g/100 g stool) and the total weight of the stool on each day. The mean of the three values obtained is considered as the result.

Interpretation Following the test protocol described above, a fecal fat excretion below 7.5 g/day is considered normal. Fat maldigestion indicating exocrine pancreatic insufficiency is defined by a fecal fat excretion greater than 7.5 g/day. Interpretation of the test may be improved by keeping a record of all dietary intake over the 5-day period. In this way, fat intake can be determined and thus the fractional fat absorption can be calculated. It should be noted that fecal fat quantification is a nonspecific pancreatic function test since any other cause of maldigestion (i.e., obstructive jaundice) or malabsorption (i.e., sprue, Crohn's disease) may also induce abnormal fecal fat excretion.

Fecal chymotrypsin activity

Quantification of fecal chymotrypsin is a simple test and easy to apply to the clinical routine. This test is based on the enzymatic quantification of chymotrypsin activity in an isolated small stool sample. Because of this, fecal chymotrypsin has been widely introduced in clinical routine as an exocrine pancreatic function test. However, chymotrypsin is variably inactivated during intestinal passage in such a way that fecal chymotrypsin activity does not accurately reflect pancreatic secretion of the enzyme. In addition, dilution of the enzyme in patients with diarrhea of any etiology will also decrease the fecal activity of the enzyme.

Because of this, and in order to maintain adequate specificity of the test, a low cut-off (3 U/g of stool) is generally accepted as the definition of an abnormal test. Patients with fecal chymotrypsin activity of less than 3 U/g of stool are thus considered as suffering from exocrine pancreatic dysfunction, although the sensitivity obtained with the test is too low to recommend it for clinical practice. In fact, the test is not able to detect a single case of mild exocrine pancreatic dysfunction, and can only detect slightly more than half of those patients with moderate or severe dysfunction (Table 31.3).

Last but not least, orally administered exogenous pancreatic enzymes as a treatment for exocrine pancreatic insufficiency interact with the determination of chymotrypsin in stool and thus this therapy should be interrupted for at least the 48 hours preceding stool sample collection. This is not always easy to accomplish for patients with exocrine pancreatic insufficiency.

In conclusion, and after taking into consideration all the aspects mentioned above, fecal chymotrypsin quantification should no longer be considered adequate for evaluating exocrine pancreatic function in clinical routine.

Fecal elastase concentration

Compared with chymotrypsin, pancreatic elastase is highly stable during gastrointestinal transit and the fecal concentration of this enzyme correlates significantly with the amount of enzyme secreted by the exocrine pancreas. Furthermore, since the methodology used to quantify this enzyme is based on human-specific monoclonal antibodies, oral enzyme substitution therapy does not interfere with the test. Therefore, interruption of this therapy previous to stool collection is not needed, which is an important advantage.

Method Quantification of fecal elastase is performed in a single small stool sample by a specific enzyme immunoassay.

Interpretation A fecal elastase concentration higher than 200 μg/g is considered normal. Concentrations lower than 50 μg/g are related to exocrine pancreatic insufficiency. Although fecal elastase quantification is not sensitive enough to detect patients with mild exocrine pancreatic dysfunction, its sensitivity in cases of moderate to severe dysfunction is very high, reaching values close to 100%. The specificity of fecal elastase is also high, only limited by dilution in cases of watery diarrhea.

Fecal elastase based on the use of human-specific monoclonal antibodies is therefore an excellent test for the diagnosis of exocrine pancreatic dysfunction in the context of chronic pancreatitis. Since this test is easy to apply to the clinical routine, it may be used as a first step in the study of patients with clinically suspected chronic pancreatic disease and for the follow-up of patients with known chronic pancreatitis. In situations of secondary exocrine pancreatic dysfunction (i.e., after gastrointestinal surgery), fecal elastase is useful for evaluating pancreatic secretion but not for detecting maldigestion.

Oral tests

Pancreolauryl test

Fluorescein dilaurate is administered orally together with a standardized breakfast. A pancreas-specific cholesterol ester hydrolase acts on this compound and water-soluble fluorescein is released and absorbed from the gut. Fluorescein can thus be measured in serum or urine after renal excretion. The advantage of this test is that it is easily applicable to the clinical routine and can be used not only for supporting the diagnosis of chronic pancreatitis but also for the follow-up of patients with this disease. The major disadvantages of the test are the limiting factors of oral tests described above and a limited sensitivity for the early diagnosis of chronic pancreatitis.

Method The standard test requires collection of urine over 10 hours after the ingestion of the standard breakfast and fluorescein dilaurate. The diuresis should be increased by the ingestion of at least 1500 mL of water during the test. In order to compensate for the variable intestinal absorption and renal excretion of the substrate, the test should be repeated 3 days later by giving fluorescein sodium as substrate. On both test days, urine fluorescein concentration is measured.

Repetition of the test is not necessary if fluorescein concentration is measured in serum. Our group has optimized the serum pancreolauryl test by administering intravenous metoclopramide just after the ingestion of the test meal in order to avoid potential problems related to gastric emptying. In addition, intravenous administration of secretin just before ingestion of the test meal significantly increases the sensitivity of the test by inducing a washout of stored pancreatic enzymes accumulated overnight. Finally, we have optimized the measurement of serum fluorescein concentration. The optimized serum pancreolauryl test protocol is summarized in Fig. 31.3. Potential adverse effects of metoclopramide and secretin present very rarely after a single dose. In our experience, transient mouth dryness is observed occasionally after metoclopramide administration. A few patients suffer from nausea after secretin, which can be prevented by slow injection of the drug (over 2–3 min).

Interpretation Results of the urine pancreolauryl test are expressed as the quotient between the urine fluorescein concentration at day 1 (when fluorescein dilaurate is given as substrate) and that at day 2 (when fluorescein sodium is given as substrate). A quotient is considered as normal if higher than 30 and abnormal if lower than 20. Values between 20 and 30 are inconclusive.

The peak serum fluorescein concentration is considered as the result of the serum test. A peak greater than

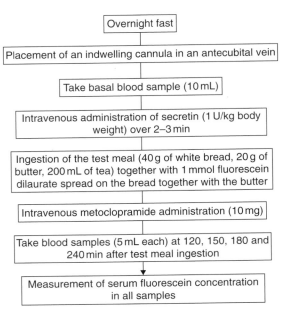

Figure 31.3 Optimized serum pancreolauryl test protocol.

4.5 μg/mL indicates normal exocrine pancreatic function. Mild to moderate exocrine pancreatic dysfunction is defined by a peak between 2.5 and 4.5 μg/mL. A result below 2.5 μg/mL is observed in patients with severe pancreatic dysfunction.

The accuracy of the optimized serum pancreolauryl test is much higher than the accuracy of the standard test in urine (Table 31.3). The sensitivity of the optimized serum test for the diagnosis of mild exocrine pancreatic dysfunction is 75%, and for moderate or severe dysfunction is 100%. False-positive results can be obtained in patients with gastrointestinal extrapancreatic diseases leading to maldigestion of fluorescein dilaurate (e.g., partial gastric resection with Billroth II anastomosis, obstructive jaundice) or to malabsorption of released fluorescein (e.g., sprue).

^{13}C-substrate breath tests

Several substrates, mainly ^{13}C-labeled, have been used to evaluate exocrine pancreatic function by means of breath tests. In these tests, the labeled substrate is given orally together with a test meal. After intraduodenal hydrolysis of the substrate by specific pancreatic enzymes, ^{13}C-marked metabolites are released, absorbed from the gut, and metabolized within the liver. As a consequence of hepatic metabolism, $^{13}CO_2$ is released and

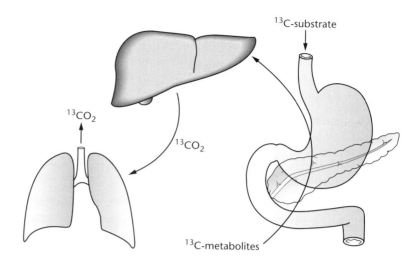

^{13}C-substrate

$^{13}CO_2$

$^{13}CO_2$

Figure 31.4 Basis of pancreatic function breath tests.

^{13}C-metabolites

thereafter eliminated with expired air (Fig. 31.4). The amount of $^{13}CO_2$ expired, which indirectly reflects exocrine pancreatic function, can be measured by means of mass spectrometry or infrared analysis.

Most substrates used in breath tests, among them mixed ^{13}C-triglyceride, cholesteryl ^{13}C-octanoate, ^{13}C-hiolein, and ^{13}C-triolein, are hydrolyzed by pancreatic lipase. In this way pancreatic function breath tests should be seen as fat digestion tests and thus considered as an alternative to fecal fat quantification.

The only breath test that has been optimized is the mixed ^{13}C-triglyceride (^{13}C-MTG) breath test. In our experience, this is the optimal substrate for the diagnosis of fat maldigestion and thus the ^{13}C-MTG breath test has been developed as a simple alternative to fecal fat quantification.

Method According to the protocol developed by our group, a total of 250 mg of ^{13}C-MTG is spread on a solid test meal containing 16 g of fat. Before the meal (basal sample) and in 30-min intervals for 6 hours after ingestion of the meal, breath samples are collected in 10-mL tubes. A single dose of a prokineticum (i.e., metoclopramide) is given orally 20–30 min before the meal in order to avoid potential problems related to gastric emptying. The amount of $^{13}CO_2$ in breath samples is measured by mass spectrometry. The result of the test is expressed as the total amount of recovered $^{13}CO_2$ over the 6 hours.

Interpretation A $^{13}CO_2$ below 58% indicates the presence of fat maldigestion, with a sensitivity and specificity higher than 90%. The test is also highly accurate for the diagnosis of maldigestion in clinical situations of secondary exocrine pancreatic insufficiency, such as partial or total gastrectomy or duodenectomy.

The ^{13}C-MTG breath test is a simple, noninvasive, and accurate method for the diagnosis of exocrine pancreatic insufficiency. It is easily applicable to the clinical routine and can be repeated as often as necessary. In this way, the utility of the test is not only limited to the diagnosis of exocrine pancreatic insufficiency but can also be extended to control of the efficacy of oral enzyme substitution therapy in these patients. Therefore, the ^{13}C-MTG breath test may play a relevant role in the management of patients with maldigestion secondary to chronic pancreatitis, cystic fibrosis, pancreatic cancer, and after acute necrotizing pancreatitis or gastric or duodenal surgery.

Summary

A wide variety of tests are nowadays available for the evaluation of exocrine pancreatic function. The secretin–cholecystokinin test is still the gold standard, but its use is presently limited to the evaluation of new function tests in specialized centers. Quantification of pancreatic zinc output as a single marker may simplify the clinical applicability of this direct test.

The optimized serum pancreolauryl test is the most sensitive tubuless pancreatic function test and probably the most appropriate for the screening of chronic pancreatitis in patients with clinical suspicion of the disease. The urine pancreolauryl test can no longer be recommended because of its low sensitivity and the need to repeat the test twice three days apart.

Fecal elastase quantification is the most adequate fecal test. It is clearly more accurate than fecal chymotrypsin for evaluation of exocrine pancreatic function and is easy to apply to the clinical routine. Therefore, fecal elastase may be applied as a first step in the study of patients with suspected chronic pancreatitis and to aid in the differential diagnosis of chronic diarrhea. Fecal chymotrypsin activity is a nonsensitive pancreatic function test and can no longer be considered for clinical routine.

The ^{13}C-MTG breath test appears to be an accurate alternative to fecal fat quantification for the diagnosis of maldigestion of any etiology. This is a simple and noninvasive method, easily applicable to the clinical routine, that can be repeated as frequently as needed and that is useful for the diagnosis of maldigestion as well as for optimization of enzyme substitution therapy in patients with primary or secondary exocrine pancreatic insufficiency.

Recommended reading

DiMagno EP, Go VLW, Summerskill HJ. Relations between pancreatic enzyme outputs and malabsorption in severe pancreatic insufficiency. N Engl J Med 1973;288:813–815.

Domínguez-Muñoz JE. Noninvasive pancreatic function tests. In: MW Büchler, H Friess, W Uhl, P Malfertheiner (eds) Chronic Pancreatitis: Novel Concepts in Biology and Therapy. Oxford, Berlin: Blackwell Publishing, 2002: 225–232.

Domínguez-Muñoz JE, Malfertheiner P. Optimized serum pancreolauryl test for differentiating patients with and without chronic pancreatitis. Clin Chem 1998;44:869–875.

Domínguez-Muñoz JE, Pieramico O, Büchler M, Malfertheiner P. Clinical utility of the serum pancreolauryl test in diagnosing and staging of chronic pancreatitis. Am J Gastroenterol 1993;88:1237–1241.

Domínguez-Muñoz JE, Hyeronimus C, Sauerbruch T, Malfertheiner P. Fecal elastase test: evaluation of a new noninvasive pancreatic function test. Am J Gastroenterol 1995;90:1834–1837.

Domínguez-Muñoz JE, Martínez S, Leodolter A, Malfertheiner P. Quantification of pancreatic zinc output as pancreatic function test: making the secretin–caerulein test applicable to clinical practice. Pancreatology 2004;4:57–62.

Gullo L. Value and clinical role of intubation tests in chronic pancreatitis. In: HG Beger, M Buchler, H Ditschuneit, P Malfertheiner (eds) Chronic Pancreatitis. Berlin: Springer-Verlag, 1990: 287–290.

Lembcke B. Present and future of breath test in the diagnosis of pancreatic insufficiency. In: P Malfertheiner, JE Dominguez-Muñoz, HU Schulz, H Lippert (eds) Diagnostic Procedures in Pancreatic Disease. Berlin: Springer-Verlag, 1997: 261–271.

Lembcke B, Grimm K, Lankish PG. Raised fecal fat concentration is not valid indicator of pancreatic steatorrhea. Am J Gastroenterol 1987;82:526–531.

Lembcke B, Braden B, Caspary WF. Exocrine pancreatic insufficiency: accuracy and clinical value of the uniformly labeled ^{13}C-hiolein breath test. Gut 1996;39:668–74.

Leodolter A, Kahl S, Domínguez-Muñoz JE, Gerard C, Glasbrenner B, Malfertheiner P. Comparison of two tubeless function tests in the assessment of mild to moderate exocrine pancreatic insufficiency Eur J Gastroenterol Hepatol 2000;12:1335–1338.

Löser C, Möllgaard A, Fölsch UR. Faecal elastase 1: a novel, highly sensitive and specific tubeless pancreatic function test. Gut 1996;39:580–586.

Löser C, Brauer C, Aygen S, Hennemann O, Fölsch UR. Comparative clinical evaluation of the ^{13}C-mixed triglyceride breath test as an indirect pancreatic function test. Scand J Gastroenterol 1998;33:327–334.

Malfertheiner P, Büchler M. Correlation of imaging and function in chronic pancreatitis. Radiol Clin North Am 1989;27:51–64.

Stein J, Purschian B, Bieniek U, Caspary WF, Lemcke B. Near-infrared reflectance analysis (NIRA): a new dimension in the investigation of malabsorption syndromes. Eur J Gastroenterol Hepatol 1994;6:889–894.

Stein J, Jung M, Sziegoleit A, Zeuzem S, Caspary F, Lembcke B. Immunoreactive elastase 1: clinical evaluation of a new noninvasive test of pancreatic function. Clin Chem 1996; 42:222–226.

Vantrappen GR, Rutgeerts PJ, Ghoos YF, Hiele MI. Mixed triglyceride breath test: a noninvasive test of pancreatic lipase activity in the duodenum. Gastroenterology 1989; 96:1126–1134.

Ventrucci M, Cipolla A, Ubalducci GM, Roda A, Roda E. ^{13}C-labelled cholesteryl octanoate breath test for assessing pancreatic exocrine insufficiency. Gut 1998;42:81–87.

32 Follow-up of patients with chronic pancreatitis: what to do and which complications can be expected

Lucio Gullo and Raffaele Pezzilli

In the initial stages of chronic pancreatitis, which generally last about 5 or 6 years, the disease is characterized by attacks of abdominal pain that recur at variable intervals during which the patient is pain-free. When the disease is more advanced, the pain tends to disappear, either spontaneously or following surgery, but other symptoms or complications may develop that can alter the course of the disease. In this chapter we discuss the role of the physician in management of this disease, particularly as regards follow-up and complications.

What to do in the follow-up

The clinical onset of chronic pancreatitis most commonly occurs when the patient is in his thirties or forties. A typical patient with chronic pancreatitis is a male who is employed in a job that requires heavy labor and who generally (70–80% of cases) drinks alcohol to excess. In Italy, alcohol is by far the most frequent etiologic factor, present in 75–80% of patients with chronic pancreatitis who have an average daily consumption of 120–140 g of pure alcohol. Thus, the first and most important task for the physician is to convince the patient to stop drinking alcohol, informing him that if he does not do so there is little or no chance that his condition will improve, and that he may well also develop unpleasant complications. It should also be explained that if he ceases to drink, the attacks may become less frequent and eventually disappear. Unfortunately, not all patients quit drinking, some resuming once a painful attack has subsided (Table 32.1).

A majority of individuals with chronic pancreatitis also smoke, and so another duty of the physician is to persuade the patient to quit this habit as well, even though it has not been clearly demonstrated that smoking has a pathogenetic role in chronic pancreatitis or that it can negatively influence progression of the disease.

Pain, the most important symptom in chronic pancreatitis, particularly in its initial stage, must be carefully assessed and monitored in each patient. If the frequency and intensity of the painful attacks are reduced by cessation of alcohol ingestion, the attacks are likely to eventually disappear, generally within the first 5 or 6 years of the disease; for these patients, surgical intervention is not indicated. Among our patients, roughly 50% fall into this category. If, on the contrary, the frequency and intensity of the painful attacks increase or remain high, surgery or, for a few selected patients, endoscopic intervention should certainly be considered, which is the case for about 50% of our patients. For most of the patients who undergo surgery, this generally occurs within 5 or 6 years of clinical onset.

It is important to study exocrine and endocrine pancreatic function from the initial stages of the disease, both to support the clinical diagnosis of chronic pancreatitis and to guide its treatment. In studies that utilized duodenal intubation and prolonged maximal pancreatic stimulation, we showed that exocrine pancreatic function is impaired in almost all patients with chronic pancreatitis, starting in the initial stages of the disease, at which point the functional impairment is generally mild or moderate. Although duodenal intubation is the more sensitive means of assessing exocrine pancreatic function, it is time-consuming and troublesome and is no longer used in clinical practice. At pre-

Table 32.1 What to do in follow-up.

Ascertain whether the patient has stopped drinking

In nonalcoholic forms, determine the cause and eliminate it

Evaluate pain; if the attacks are frequent, consider surgery or, in select patients, endoscopy

Assess exocrine and endocrine pancreatic function; if impaired, treat accordingly

Assess for complications and treat accordingly

Activity limitations and dietetic rules: this is pertinent mainly to patients with severe steatorrhea or advanced diabetes

Arrange for check-up visits at least every 6–12 months, when possible, with a specialist in pancreatic diseases

sent, it has been substituted by indirect tests of pancreatic function that often show normal results when the chronic pancreatitis is mild. We now use the fecal elastase test, which has good sensitivity particularly in patients who have moderate or severe pancreatic insufficiency.

Patients who have mild or moderate pancreatic insufficiency do not have steatorrhea and therefore do not require the use of pancreatic extracts. However, some authors have advocated the use of extracts in patients with mild to moderate insufficiency as well, for the purpose of preventing attacks of pain. In this regard, various studies have been carried out but the results have been conflicting, possibly due to the different types of enzyme preparations that have been used. The preparations that seemed to be useful in preventing attacks of pain were those administered in tablet form.

Endocrine pancreatic function is generally normal in the initial phases of chronic pancreatitis and clinically evident diabetes usually appears in the advanced stages of the disease, generally 8–10 years after onset. Thus, in the early stages of the disease blood glucose determination and a glucose tolerance test every 6–12 months are generally sufficient for monitoring endocrine function.

For optimal management of patients with chronic pancreatitis, especially in the initial stages of the disease, it is essential to have frequent follow-up visits, at least once every 6 or 12 months. This serves to monitor the frequency of episodes of pain as well as the appearance of other disturbances, and especially to determine whether the patient has stopped drinking. Many patients quit drinking alcohol and these same individuals generally keep their appointments for follow-up visits. Others, who are typically heavier drinkers and who do not stop drinking, often do not keep their scheduled appointments but may show up only after an attack of severe pain.

In the nonalcoholic forms of chronic pancreatitis (about 20–30% of cases), the most important measure is to determine the cause of the disease and to eliminate it, which usually leads to improvement in the clinical picture. With regard to the follow-up, the measures are essentially the same as those for alcoholic pancreatitis.

The patient with advanced chronic pancreatitis, who has had the disease for longer than 5 or 6 years, generally presents with different clinical problems. In the majority of studies on chronic pancreatitis, it is reported that pain, the principal clinical manifestation in the early stages of the disease, is generally no longer present in the more advanced stages. The patient may have had surgery for the pancreatitis, or the pain may have resolved on its own. Those for whom pain continues to be a significant problem are generally either those who continue to drink, and for these patients it is difficult to find a definitive solution for the pain, or they are patients who have developed a complication, most often a pseudocyst. We should mention, however, that in one study pain has been reported to be frequent even in advanced stages of the disease.

In the advanced stages of chronic pancreatitis, generally after 8–10 years from clinical onset, exocrine pancreatic insufficiency may become severe (< 10% of normal enzyme production) and steatorrhea develops, necessitating the administration of pancreatic extracts. It is very important to establish the correct daily dose of the extracts, which must be adequate to prevent the loss of fat in the feces; a dose of 30 000 U per meal is generally sufficient. If steatorrhea does not disappear completely, this dose can be increased. In patients with gastric acid hypersecretion it can be helpful to administer H_2 blocking agents or proton pump inhibitors with the extracts in order to prevent their inactivation by gastric acid. Steatorrhea develops in about 50–60% of patients with advanced chronic pancreatitis.

In advanced stages of chronic pancreatitis, usually after 7 or 8 years from clinical onset, diabetes can develop as a result of the destruction of islet cells by pancreatic fibrosis. It usually starts in a mild form that is treatable with oral antidiabetic agents or low doses of insulin but often progresses to a more severe form with higher insulin requirements. The complications of diabetes due to chronic pancreatitis are similar to those of primary diabetes. In particular, we studied the frequency of diabetic retinopathy in chronic pancreatitis and found that it is similar to that of patients with type I diabetes. Diabetes develops in about 50–60% of patients with advanced chronic pancreatitis.

Another task for the physician responsible for patients with chronic pancreatitis is to educate them regarding their diet. Prior to onset of the disease these patients are often hearty eaters and drinkers. In the early stages of the disease, when steatorrhea and diabetes are not yet present, there is no need for particular dietetic measures; it is important, however, that the diet be well balanced and that it meets the nutritional needs of the individual. It is generally advised to reduce fat intake, although there is no clear evidence that this is useful. Obviously, if there is decreased glucose tolerance, carbohydrate and sugar intake should be reduced. In more advanced stages of the disease, when steatorrhea may be present, the diet should be hypercaloric but, other than a reduction of fat intake, the patient should not be subjected to other restrictions unless diabetes is also present.

Regarding restrictions on activity, none should be imposed except in the case of patients who have severe steatorrhea or advanced diabetes; if their job entails heavy labor, they should be advised to seek less strenuous employment.

Complications

Of the various complications that can develop in the course of chronic pancreatitis, pseudocysts and stenosis (generally mild) of the retropancreatic portion of the common bile duct are the most frequent. Several less common ones can also be encountered (Table 32.2).

Pancreatic pseudocysts

Pseudocysts most commonly develop during the initial stages of chronic pancreatitis; their reported frequency varies from study to study, but they are fairly frequent, occurring in about 25–30% of cases. In surgical series their frequency is higher (about 50–60%). Most often pseudocysts present as a single lesion, but sometimes two or more can be seen; their size is variable, they are often symptomatic (persistent pain being the most frequent symptom), and they are occasionally complicated by rupture or infection. In our experience, in the great majority of cases the pseudocysts derive from

Table 32.2 Complications, associated diseases, and mortality in chronic pancreatitis.

Pancreatic pseudocysts	25–30%
Stenosis (usually mild) of the retropancreatic common bile duct	40–50%
Pancreatic cancer	1–3%
Extrapancreatic cancer	10–15%
Splenic vein thrombosis	2–5%
Pseudoaneurysm	2–3%
Duodenal obstruction	4–5%
Pancreatic fistula	2–3%
Pancreatic abscess	2–3%
Alcoholic liver diseases	25–40%
Cardiovascular diseases	20–30%
Mortality	20–35%

dilated ducts, and thus are true cysts; as they dilate, the epithelial lining can be lost, at which point they no longer appear to be true cysts. Among our patients with chronic pancreatitis, postnecrotic pseudocysts are rare, the main reason being that we see few patients (about 10%) who have had an acute necrotic attack.

As far as treatment is concerned, if the pseudocysts are asymptomatic and without complications they can be left untreated, but repeat ultrasound is recommended every 6–12 months to control their size. If they become painful or develop a complication, treatment becomes obligatory. Years ago the only treatment available was surgery; more recently this has been abandoned in favor of endoscopic intervention.

Another possibility in the treatment of painful pseudocysts in chronic pancreatitis is the administration of octreotide, a synthetic analog of somatostatin, which causes the cysts to shrink and eventually disappear. We have shown that this treatment (100 μg every 8 hours) is effective mainly when the cysts do not communicate with the Wirsung duct and if the drug is administered when their size is increasing. When these criteria are met, the pain disappears completely and definitively after 3–4 days of octreotide treatment, as the cysts begin to shrink in size; the cysts then disappear completely after 6–8 weeks of treatment.

We would like to point out that size alone is not an indication for treatment. Although it has been a guiding principle that cysts of greater than 5–6 cm in diameter should be treated, we feel that if the cysts are asymptomatic treatment is not necessary, regardless of their size. We have followed several patients whose cysts have been larger than 5 or 6 cm and stable in size for many years, during which they have also been pain-free; we believe that intervention is not necessary in these cases. Generally speaking, once cysts are treated they are no longer problematic.

Stenosis of the retropancreatic common bile duct

Stenosis of the distal portion of the common bile duct is a complication seen in both initial and advanced stages of chronic pancreatitis and can be observed in up to 40–50% of cases; it is generally mild and does not obstruct the flow of bile. The stenosis is caused by pancreatic fibrosis in the area of the duct. It can contribute to a generally mild and transient (lasting 3–10 days) form of jaundice that can occur during attacks of pain, when the already stenotic bile duct is compressed by pancreatic edema. This transient jaundice during attacks of abdominal pain occurs in about 30–40% of cases.

In about 5–10% of the patients with chronic pancreatitis the jaundice persists and requires treatment. It is due to complete obstruction of the retropancreatic common bile duct, most often by pancreatic fibrosis, although sometimes it is due to compression of the duct by a cyst of the pancreatic head or, more rarely, by cancers of the pancreatic head, which can complicate chronic pancreatitis. In these cases, it is necessary to perform a choledochojejunostomy. A stent is sometimes placed endoscopically, but these tend to become occluded, and the procedure is often complicated by the development of cholangitis; for this reason, it should only be used in carefully selected cases, such as in patients awaiting surgery or in those who present a high surgical risk.

Pancreatic cancer

Many studies have been published on the risk of pancreatic cancer in patients with chronic pancreatitis, but results have been conflicting: some have concluded that there is a risk, others that there is not or that it is very low. We believe that chronic pancreatitis is a risk factor for pancreatic cancer but that this risk is low, on the order of 1–3%. Lowenfels *et al.* reported a cumulative risk of pancreatic cancer in subjects with chronic pancreatitis who were followed for 10 and 20 years after the diagnosis of pancreatitis of 1.8 and 4% respectively.

The risk of pancreatic cancer has been reported to be very much higher in patients with hereditary chronic pancreatitis. Lowenfels *et al.* have shown that the estimated cumulative risk of pancreatic cancer to age 70 years in patients with this disease approaches 40%.

Extrapancreatic cancer

Patients with chronic pancreatitis have a high incidence (10–15%) of extrapancreatic cancer, the commonest sites being the upper and lower airways as well as the gastrointestinal tract. The reason for this increased incidence is not clear, but the abuse of tobacco and alcohol in these patients is thought to be responsible.

Splenic vein thrombosis

While splenic vein thrombosis is well known as a complication of chronic pancreatitis, its incidence is not. Bradley reported an incidence of 2% among his patients with this disease. In our experience, the incidence has been a little higher (about 5%). Thrombosis of the splenic vein is due to involvement of the vein by the chronic inflammatory process in the pancreas. It can result in the development of gastric or esophageal varices; although there are no precise data regarding the frequency with which these varices bleed, the percentage is generally low.

Pseudoaneurysm

This is a rare complication of chronic pancreatitis, seen in about 2–3% of cases. It usually occurs in association with pancreatic pseudocysts, the mechanism of formation being erosion of an expanding pseudocyst into a nearby artery. The vessels most commonly involved are the splenic, gastroduodenal, pancreaticoduodenal, and hepatic arteries. Pancreatic pseudoaneurysms cause bleeding that may be slow and intermittent or acute and massive. Treatment is necessary even if they are not actively bleeding because untreated pseudoaneurysms have a very high mortality rate. Bleeding can be successfully controlled by arteriographic transcatheter embolization or surgery.

Duodenal obstruction

This complication occurs in about 4–5% of patients with chronic pancreatitis. It is generally due to marked fibrosis of the head of the pancreas that involves the duodenum or to a pseudocyst; treatment consists of surgery for the former and endoscopic drainage or surgical treatment for the latter.

Pancreatic fistula

Pancreatic fistulas are a rare complication of chronic pancreatitis (2–3%). External fistulas generally develop after surgical procedures on the pancreas or after attacks of necrotic pancreatitis. Internal pancreatic fistulas are generally due to rupture of the main pancreatic duct or leakage from a pseudocyst. The main complications of internal fistulas are pancreatic ascites or pleural effusions.

Treatment consists of fasting, parenteral nutrition, octreotide (100 μg every 8 hours), or endoscopic stent placement; if the fistula persists surgery is indicated.

Pancreatic abscess

This is a rare complication that involves only about 2–3% of patients with chronic pancreatitis. The abscess often develops at the site of a previous pseudocyst. Treatment with antibiotics is generally unsuccessful, leaving surgery as the only viable alternative.

Alcoholic liver disease

Based on clinical studies, it was long believed that in patients with chronic alcoholic pancreatitis the damage from alcohol was limited to the pancreas and that liver involvement was rare. However, with histologic studies of the liver we and others have shown that a high percentage of these patients have alcoholic damage to the liver as well. In particular, in a study done on surgical biopsies of the liver taken from 50 patients with chronic alcoholic pancreatitis undergoing surgery for pancreatitis, we showed that 22 (44%) had associated alcoholic liver disease; of these 22, 13 had alcoholic hepatitis, 7 cirrhosis, and 2 steatosis. The percentage of alcoholic liver disease in this series of patients was similar to that found in the general alcoholic population.

We have seen that patients with chronic alcoholic pancreatitis who develop hepatic disease are most often those who drink larger quantities of alcohol (> 200 g of pure alcohol daily) and for a longer period of time (> 20 years). It is therefore important that patients with chronic alcoholic pancreatitis, especially those whose alcohol consumption is to the above-described extent, are periodically monitored with liver function and imaging tests for early recognition and timely treatment of any associated liver disease.

Cardiovascular lesions

Several investigators have reported an increased frequency of vascular lesions in patients with chronic pancreatitis, but while some have assumed that this was simply a coincidence, others have suggested that a causal relationship may exist. In a study of 54 patients with chronic pancreatitis (mean age 44 years, range 26–66), we found evidence of vascular involvement in 18 (33%) of the patients and in 5 (9%) of the controls. In particular, we found electrocardiographic signs of coronary artery disease in eight patients, as well as peripheral signs and symptoms of obliterative atherosclerotic disease in the lower extremities in 12 patients. No significant differences in the prevalence of the major vascular risk factors were noted between patients with vascular lesions and those without, or between the patients and the control subjects.

In another study, we showed that in 57 patients with chronic pancreatitis there was radiologic evidence of aortic calcification in 35 (41.4%), but only in 12 of 40 (30%) smoker controls. Interestingly, these patients had a mean age of 44 years (range 26–59), whereas in the general population aortic calcifications are rarely seen in persons under the age of 50–60 years. None of these patients with chronic pancreatitis had conditions associated with atherosclerosis, such as diabetes, arterial hypertension, obesity, or hyperlipidemia. It should be mentioned that aortic calcification is associated with a marked increase in risk of death by cardiovascular disease. These two studies indicate that, compared with the general population, patients with chronic pancreatitis have more frequent cardiovascular lesions and the lesions tend to develop at an earlier age; the reason for these findings is not clear.

Mortality

All the studies published on mortality in chronic pancreatitis have concluded that it is high. Ammann *et al.* in their study of 245 patients with chronic pancreatitis reported that 86 (35%) died; the mean age at death was 54 years in 54 patients with alcoholic pancreatitis and 66 years in 32 with nonalcoholic pancreatitis. In a study by Levy *et al.* of 240 patients with chronic pancreatitis, of whom 210 were drinkers, it was reported that after a mean of 20 years from the clinical onset of the disease, 57 patients (23.7%) were dead and that the average age at the time of death was 52 years.

The mortality rate for chronic alcoholic pancreatitis is higher than it is for idiopathic or other forms of chronic pancreatitis; as would be expected, among patients with alcoholic pancreatitis the mortality rate is higher for those who continue to drink. The main causes of death for these patients are cardiovascular disease, hepatic cirrhosis, extrapancreatic or pancreatic cancer, postoperative complications, complications of chronic pancreatitis or of diabetes, and alcoholism. In general, less than 20% of deaths are directly related to chronic pancreatitis.

Recommended reading

Ammann RW, Akovbiantz A, Largiader F, Schueler G. Course and outcome of chronic pancreatitis. Longitudinal study of a mixed medical–surgical series of 245 patients. *Gastroenterology* 1984;86:820–828.

Bender JS, Bouwman DL, Levison MA *et al.* Pseudocysts and pseudoaneurysms: surgical strategy. *Pancreas* 1995;10:143–145.

Bradley EL III. The natural history of splenic vein thrombosis due to chronic pancreatitis: indications for surgery. *Int J Pancreatol* 1987;2:87–92.

Gullo L, Barbara L. Treatment of pancreatic pseudocysts with octreotide. *Lancet* 1991;338:540–541.

Gullo L, Stella A, Labriola E *et al.* Cardiovascular lesions in chronic pancreatitis. A prospective study. *Dig Dis Sci* 1982;27:716–722.

Gullo L, Barbara L, Labò G. Effect of cessation of alcohol use on the course of pancreatic dysfunction in alcoholic pancreatitis. *Gastroenterology* 1988;95:1063–1068.

Gullo L, Parenti M, Monti L, Pezzilli R. Diabetic retinopathy in chronic pancreatitis. *Gastroenterology* 1990;98:1577–1581.

Gullo L, Casadei R, Campione O, Grigioni W, Marrano D. Alcoholic liver disease in alcoholic chronic pancreatitis: a prospective study. *Ital J Gastroenterol* 1995;27:69–72.

Gullo L, Tassoni U, Mazzoni G, Stefanini F. Increased prevalence of aortic calcification in chronic pancreatitis. *Am J Gastroenterol* 1996;91:759–761.

Gullo L, Ventrucci M, Tomassetti P, Migliori M, Pezzilli R. Fecal elastase 1 determination in chronic pancreatitis. *Dig Dis Sci* 1999;44:210–213.

Gullo L, Tomassetti P, Migliori M, Casadei R, Marrano D. Do early symptoms of pancreatic cancer exist that can allow an earlier diagnosis? *Pancreas* 2001;22:210–213.

Hansen TH, Laursen M, Christensen E *et al.* Chronic pancreatitis and extrapancreatic cancer. *Int J Pancreatol* 1995;18:235–240.

Hayakawa T, Kondo T, Shibata T, Sugimoto Y, Kitagawa M. Chronic alcoholism and evolution of pain and prognosis in chronic pancreatitis. *Dig Dis Sci* 1989;34:33–38.

Karlson BM, Ekbom A, Josefsson S *et al.* The risk of pancreatic cancer following pancreatitis: an association due to confounding? *Gastroenterology* 1997;113:587–592.

Lankisch PG, Lohr-Happe A, Otto J, Creutzfeldt W. Natural course in chronic pancreatitis. Pain, exocrine and endocrine pancreatic insufficiency and prognosis of the disease. *Digestion* 1993;54:148–155.

Layer P, Yamamoto H, Kalthoff L, Clain JE, Bakken LJ, DiMagno EP. The different courses of early and late onset idiopathic and alcoholic chronic pancreatitis. *Gastroenterology* 1994;107:1481–1487.

Levy P, Milan C, Pignon JP, Baetz A, Bernades P. Mortality factors associated with chronic pancreatitis. Unidimensional and multidimensional analysis of a medical–surgical series of 240 patients. *Gastroenterology* 1988;96:1165–1172.

Lowenfels AB, Maisonneuve P, Cavallini G *et al.* Pancreatitis and the risk of pancreatic cancer. *N Engl J Med* 1993;328:1433–1437.

Lowenfels AB, Maisonneuve P, DiMagno EP *et al.* Hereditary pancreatitis and the risk of pancreatic cancer. *J Natl Cancer Inst* 1997;89:442–446.

Miyake H, Harada H, Kunichik K, Ochi K, Kimura I. Clinical course and prognosis of chronic pancreatitis. *Pancreas* 1987;2:378–385.

Pradeep B, Sonnenberg A. Pancreatitis is a risk factor for pancreatic cancer. *Gastroenterology* 1995;109:247–251.

Saed ZA, Ramirez FC, Hepps KS. Endoscopic stent placement for internal and external pancreatic fistulas. *Gastroenterology* 1993;105:1213–1217.

Segal I, Parekh D, Lipschitz J *et al.* Treatment of pancreatic ascites and external pancreatic fistulas with a long-acting somatostatin analogue. *Digestion* 1993;54:53–58.

Woods MS, Traverso LW, Kozarek RA *et al.* Successful treatment of bleeding pseudoaneurysms of chronic pancreatitis. *Pancreas* 1995;10:22–26.

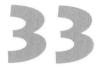

Conservative treatment of pain in chronic pancreatitis: guidelines for clinical routine

Pierluigi Di Sebastiano, Markus A. Weigand, Jörg Köninger, Fabio F. di Mola, Helmut Friess, and Markus W. Büchler

Introduction

Chronic pancreatitis is an inflammatory, often painful disease of the exocrine pancreas that leads to exocrine insufficiency. Its incidence is about 8.2 new cases per 100 000 inhabitants per year in western Europe. Complications encountered in chronic pancreatitis include biliary (10–30%) and duodenal (10–25%) obstruction and, as the disease progresses, maldigestion and diabetes mellitus.

However, the most disturbing complication of chronic pancreatitis is abdominal pain. Surgical management is often indicated in cases with medically intractable pain and this has also repercussions on the economic management of these patients. Three typical pain profiles that occur during the evolution of chronic pancreatitis have been described: (i) repeated episodes of acute pancreatitis (acinar necrosis) in early stages; (ii) spontaneous lasting pain relief in association with severe pancreatic dysfunction in the late stage of uncomplicated chronic pancreatitis; and (iii) persistent severe pain (or frequent recurrent episodes of pain) usually in association with local complications such as pseudocysts, ductal hypertension or extrapancreatic complications such as partial obstruction of the common bile duct, peptic ulcer, and opiate addiction. Clearly, the actual pathophysiology of abdominal pain remains elusive and several hypotheses have been postulated over the last few years.

At present, pancreatic and extrapancreatic mechanisms are implicated in the development of pain in chronic pancreatitis.

Pancreatic causes of pain

Acute inflammation of the pancreas

Acute inflammation is readily apparent when there is severe abdominal pain and tenderness, elevation of serum amylase and lipase, and evidence of acute pancreatic inflammation on computed tomography. The causes are likely to be the same as for inflammation associated with acute pancreatitis, involving activated enzymes and other injurious substances.

Increased pressure in the pancreatic ducts and tissue

Intrapancreatic ductal pressure might be related to pancreatic secretion itself and to the presence of an obstruction in the pancreatic duct. Therefore, many investigators have related the origin of pain to increased pressure in the pancreatic ducts and tissue. This ductal hypertension hypothesis as an explanation for pain in chronic pancreatitis is derived from observations that decompression of a dilated pancreatic duct or pseudocyst frequently relieves pain in patients with chronic pancreatitis. Pancreatic enzyme supplementation may also relieve pain in some patients with chronic pancreatitis. It is believed that the beneficial effect of pancreatic enzymes is explained by regulation involving cholecystokinin-mediated feedback between pancreatic exocrine secretion and the activity of proteases in the lumen of the small intestine. According to this hypothesis, administration of enzymes reduces hypercholecystokininemia in patients with chronic pancreatitis, thus resulting in less stimulation of the pancreas and subsequently lowered intraductal pressure and pain. Interestingly, different studies have shown that progressive pancreatic insufficiency, which appears several years after the first diagnosis, is often associated with a reduction in, and sometimes complete relief of, pain in patients with chronic pancreatitis, thus indicating that disease progression might "burn out" the pancreas itself, as mentioned before. In contrast, we have to consider that often pain in chronic pancreatitis is not related to the consumption of food, and even pain intensity, radiation, and duration are not constant. In addition, other studies have calculated that around 30% of the patients treated with decompressive surgery exhibit recurrent attacks of pain. On one hand, when patients are pain-free after surgery, this could often be due to the reduction of alcohol ingestion or to progressive pancreatic insufficiency. At present, the relationship between pancreatic parenchymal pressure and pain in chronic pancreatitis is still controversial.

Neurogenic inflammation

Recent concepts have focused on the possible involvement of the nervous system in chronic pain and the inflammatory process in chronic pancreatitis. Supporting this fascinating hypothesis, Keith *et al.* postulated that neural and perineural alteration might be important in the pathogenesis of pain in chronic pancreatitis. They demonstrated that pain severity correlated with the duration of alcohol consumption, pancreatic calcification and, more interestingly, with the percentage of eosinophil number in the perineural infiltrate, but not with duct dilatation.

A subsequent study demonstrated that there is an increase in both number and diameter of pancreatic nerve fibers in the course of chronic pancreatitis compared with normal pancreas. Also, there is an altered pattern of intrinsic and possibly extrinsic innervation of the pancreas in chronic pancreatitis, leading to upregulation of neuropeptides such as substance P and calcitonin gene-related peptide. Because both of these peptides are generally regarded as pain transmitters, these findings provided evidence that changes in pancreatic nerves themselves might be involved in the long-lasting pain syndrome in chronic pancreatitis.

Another interesting finding of these studies was the observation of close contacts between neuronal structures and immune cells in chronically inflamed pancreas, which led to the concept that neuroimmune mechanisms play a role in the pathogenesis of chronic pancreatitis and the accompanying abdominal pain. To confirm this interesting hypothesis, in a subsequent report the presence of growth-associated protein (GAP)-43, an established marker of neuronal plasticity, correlated with individual pain scores in patients with chronic pancreatitis.

Extrapancreatic causes of pain

Bile duct stenosis and duodenal stenosis due to extensive pancreatic fibrosis and inflammation are often considered putative extrapancreatic causes of pain. However, only a few authors are in accordance with this belief. Recently, Becker and Mischke described a pathologic condition named "groove pancreatitis" in 19.5% of 600 patients with chronic pancreatitis. This form of chronic pancreatitis is characterized by the formation of a scar plate between the head of the pancreas and the duodenum. Scars in the groove lead to complications also determined by the topography: disturbance in the motility of the duodenum, stenosis of the duodenum, and tubular stenosis of the common bile duct, which occasionally leads to obstructive jaundice. These alterations might be responsible for several symptoms present in chronic pancreatitis and also for postprandial pain, probably due to compression of several critical structures, such as nerves and ganglia, present between the pancreatic head and the duodenum.

Characteristics of pain in chronic pancreatitis

Pain is the leading symptom in chronic pancreatitis and should be treated to improve quality of life and to prevent excessive weight loss in these patients. Pain can be mild, moderate, or severe and increase or decrease over time. Multifactorial elements are involved and this may explain why all patients do not respond to the same treatment modality.

Pain in chronic pancreatitis is usually elicited by the activation of specific nociceptive receptors (nociceptors) and is thus referred to as *nociceptive pain*. However, it may also result from injury to sensory fibers or from damage to the central nervous system itself (*neuropathic pain*). Inflammation due to neural activity is called *neurogenic inflammation*. In healthy conditions, nociceptors in the pancreas are silent and are not activated by noxious stimulation. In chronic pancreatitis, however, inflammation, ischemia, elevated pressures, and release of substances such as prostaglandins, bradykinin, leukotrienes, and substance P sensitize nociceptors to the generation of action potentials and induce nociceptive pain. In addition, pain is also based on neuropathic changes such as proliferation of unmyelinated nerve fibers, destruction of the perineurium, neural edema, and damage to nerve fibers. Thus, nociceptive pain and neurogenic inflammation in chronic pancreatitis provide the rationale for medical, analgesic, and antiinflammatory treatment. In the beginning, patients should be examined for obvious abnormalities and extrapancreatic causes of pain. Surgical intervention should seriously be considered if long-term use of potent opioids is required for pain relief, before the development of narcotic addiction. In addition, surgery is recommended if pain no longer responds to analgesics or if complications in adjacent organs occur.

Conservative treatment of pain

Abstinence from alcohol

The first step in managing pain in chronic pancreatitis consists of the complete avoidance of alcohol. Alcohol abstinence can achieve pain relief in up to 50% of patients, but its effect seems to be restricted to patients with mild or moderate disease.

Analgesics

The treatment of pain in chronic pancreatitis is performed according to the three-step ladder of the World Health Organization for the relief of cancer pain (Fig. 33.1). The first step is for mild to moderate pain and consists of nonopioid analgesics. The second step is for moderate to severe pain and a nonopioid analgesic is combined with a mild opioid, which is titrated until pain relief is satisfactory. The third step is for severe pain and requires the use of a potent opioid such as morphine. Adjuvant drugs like tricyclic antidepressants may be used at each step on the ladder. However, as already mentioned above, when pain treatment in chronic pancreatitis requires the long-term use of potent opioids, surgical intervention should be considered.

Although the application of reasonable levels of analgesics is the first-line therapy for pain in chronic pancreatitis, there are no randomized studies comparing different drugs for pain therapy in chronic pancreatitis. Regular application of analgesic drugs should be preferred to drug intake on demand in order to provide consistent analgesia. Pain intensity should be regularly estimated by visual analog scale and the lowest drug dose for sufficient pain relief prescribed. Pain therapy should be coordinated and provided by one physician to avoid overprescription and to reduce the risk of abuse or addiction.

Acetaminophen (paracetamol) and metamizol
According to a consensus report from the German Society of Gastroenterology, acetaminophen or metamizol are the drugs of first choice for pain treatment in chronic pancreatitis. Acetaminophen is a drug with good analgesic and antipyretic properties and minimal adverse effects. In particular, no relevant gastrointestinal adverse effects of the drug in the recom-

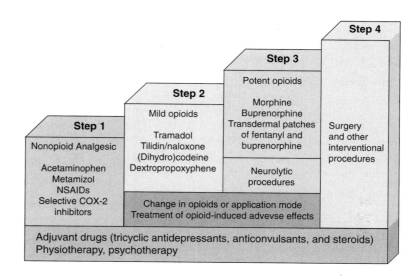

Figure 33.1 World Health Organization analgesic ladder for cancer pain adapted for pain management in chronic pancreatitis. COX, cyclooxygenase; NSAIDs, nonsteroidal antiinflammatory drugs.

mended dose is known. Acetaminophen may also have synergistic effects with other nonopioid analgesics.

Metamizol has potent analgesic and antipyretic effects and is the standard nonopioid analgesic in many countries. In addition to its analgesic properties, metamizol also has spasmolytic effects, which can be beneficial for pain treatment in chronic pancreatitis. A major adverse effect of metamizol is the risk of agranulocytosis. Because of this, metamizol is not approved in the USA and UK. When metamizol is used on a regular basis, a white blood cell count has to be performed regularly.

Unfortunately, acetaminophen and metamizol have only weak inhibitory activity against cyclooxygenase (COX) and therefore possess no antiinflammatory effects. Since inflammation is a major cause of the nociceptive and neuropathic pain during chronic pancreatitis, antiinflammatory analgesic agents may be beneficial under these conditions.

Nonsteroidal antiinflammatory drugs

Nonsteroidal antiinflammatory drugs (NSAIDs), with the exception of aspirin, inhibit COX-1 and COX-2 in a reversible manner and thus provide consistent analgesia and antiinflammatory action. In addition, they have antipyretic properties. NSAIDs are recommended as first-line drugs for the treatment of nociceptive pain (Table 33.1).

Although the inhibition of inflammation by NSAIDs is an attractive hypothesis because (neurogenic) inflammation is a key pathogenic factor in chronic pancreatitis, there are no studies confirming the superiority of antiinflammatory analgesics in chronic pancreatitis. Therefore, the potential adverse effects of NSAID treatment must be balanced with the potential benefits. The adverse effects of NSAIDs range from trivial, such as skin irritation or dyspepsia, to life-threatening, such as gastric ulceration and renal toxicity. In addition

Table 33.1 Drug overview for the management of pain in chronic pancreatitis.

Drug class	Generic name	Single dose (mg)	Dosing interval (hours)	Maximum dosage (mg)	COX-2 selectivity*
Nonacidic nonopioid analgesic	Acetaminophen	500–1000	6	4000 (6000)	
	Metamizol	500–1000	6	4000 (6000)	
Acidic nonopioid analgesic/NSAIDs	Diclofenac	50–100	8–12	150–200	4
	Ibuprofen	400–800	6–8	2400	0.4
	Naproxen	250–500	12	1000	0.3
Selective COX-2 inhibitors	Celecoxib	100–200–400	12	800	9
	Rofecoxib	12.5–25–50†	24	50	80
	Valdocoxib	20–40–80†	24	80	
Mild opioids	Tramadol/(retard)	50–100/(100)	6/(8–12)	400	
	Tilidin/(retard)	50–200/(50–100)	8/(12)	600	
Potent opioids	Morphine/(retard)	5–10/(10)	4/(8–12)	As required	
	Buprenorphine	0.2–0.4	6–8	4–5	Partial μ agonist
	Transdermal fentanyl	25–50 μg/hour	(48)–72		
	Transdermal buprenorphine	35–52.5 μg/hour	72		
Tricyclic antidepressants	Amitriptyline	25–50–100	24	In the evening	Sedating
	Clomipramine	20–50–100	24	In the morning	Mild stimulating
Anticonvulsants	Gabapentin	300–800	8	2400–(3600)	Start with low dosage
	Carbamazepine	200–400	6–8	1200–(1600)	Sedating

* The 80% inhibitory concentration ratios of COX-2 relative to COX-1 in human whole blood assays (Warner *et al.* 1999).
† Highest dosage only approved for treatment of acute pain.
COX, cyclooxygenase; NSAIDs, nonsteroidal antiinflammatory drugs.

to direct nephrotoxicity, patients with reduced glomerular filtration rate (especially when already taking diuretics), cirrhosis, and heart failure may be seriously affected by NSAIDs. Risk factors for gastrointestinal bleeding include old age, cirrhosis, and coagulation and platelet disorders. Thus, due to these adverse effects of NSAIDs, acetaminophen or metamizol may be the safer drugs for long-term use in chronic pancreatitis, at least in at-risk patients. If NSAIDs are used on a regular basis, proton pump inhibitors should be added.

COX-2 inhibitors

Recent data demonstrate that COX-2 is overexpressed in chronic pancreatitis and correlates with the stage of disease and diabetes mellitus. These data point to the treatment of pain in chronic pancreatitis with selective COX-2 inhibitors such as celecoxib, rofecoxib, and valdecoxib. However, the contribution of the constitutive COX-1 enzyme to pronociceptive pools of prostaglandins should not be discounted. Therefore, under certain conditions COX-2-selective drugs are suspected to be less analgesic than unselective COX inhibitors such as diclofenac. In addition, treatment with COX-2-selective analgesics turned out to be a double-edged sword. Although studies indicate a lower incidence of ulcer complications/symptomatic ulcers and a decreased rate of lower gastrointestinal clinical events with coxib treatment of rheumatoid arthritis compared with nonselective NSAIDs, the total incidence of non-gastrointestinal serious adverse events was increased. In particular, renal adverse events, blood pressure, annualized myocardial infarction rate, and mortality were higher with coxib use. Thus, the potential benefits of COX-2-selective inhibitors have to be weighed against potential harm. Because gastric ulcer complications are only reduced but not eliminated by selective COX-2 inhibitors, proton pump inhibitors cannot always be omitted when patients are treated with these drugs. At present, COX-2 inhibitors are not approved for pain treatment in chronic pancreatitis.

Opioids

If no sufficient pain relief is achieved by nonopioid analgesics, mild opioids should be added (Table 33.1). Treatment with opioids can be started with immediate-release formulations in order to titrate the opioid, and later can be continued with depot preparations to reduce the frequency of administration. Nausea and vomiting either settle with time or can be treated with standard antiemetics. In case of constipation laxatives may be prescribed.

Morphine is the standard potent opioid. However, injection of morphine increases constriction of the sphincter of Oddi, resulting in a 10–15 fold elevation in pressure in the common bile duct. This may worsen pain symptoms in chronic pancreatitis. In contrast, fentanyl is much less likely to cause this problem and buprenorphine has no undesireable effect on the biliary tract. Transdermal fentanyl and buprenorphine are effectively absorbed from a patch by the transdermal route, with a long duration of onset and offset suitable for providing stable blood levels over days.

Adjuvant drugs

Patients with chronic pancreatitis may often be depressed due to their pain syndrome. In addition, tricyclic antidepressants are classical drugs for treatment of neuropathic pain. Therefore, the addition of tricyclic antidepressants as adjuvant therapy is helpful in many cases. Depending on the patient's condition, either a sedating (amitriptyline) or a mild stimulating (clomipramine) tricyclic antidepressant has to be prescribed.

According to recent data for treatment of pain in diabetic neuropathy, anticonvulsants are now frequently recommended as drugs of first choice for neuropathic pain. In particular, gabapentin is now widely used for this indication. Gabapentin should be started in low doses such as 100 mg t.i.d. and daily increased to 300 mg t.i.d. or higher.

Secretory inhibition

Inhibition of gastric acid secretion by proton pump inhibitors such as omeprazole and pantoprazole leads to a higher duodenal pH and might therefore lessen stimulus-driven pancreatic secretion. In addition, patients with chronic pancreatitis show an enhanced risk of duodenal ulcer formation. Although no formal studies have demonstrated the effectiveness of proton pump inhibitors, they are used in many institutions especially when NSAIDs are used, because this approach is relatively easy and safe.

As mentioned above, application of high-dose pancreatic enzymes reduces hypercholecystokininemia in patients with chronic pancreatitis and thus may reduce pancreatic secretion and pain. Six studies and one metaanalysis investigating the effects of pancreatic enzyme therapy for pain in chronic pancreatitis have been performed, with controversial results. Only two studies using enzyme preparations in tablet form, which are believed to release pancreatic enzymes in the duodenum, showed a benefit. Thus, the role of pancreatic enzymes in reducing pain in chronic pancreatitis remains controversial. However, because high-dose pancreatic enzyme therapy carries only minor risks and may sometimes be helpful in pain management in chronic pancreatitis, a 6–8 week trial with preparations releasing enzymes in the duodenum seems to be worth trying.

Octreotide, a somatostatin analog, strongly inhibits pancreatic secretion. Although some patients may show some pain relief with high doses of octreotide, most patients do not. Since octreotide injections are painful and expensive and the effects very controversial, octreotide is not recommended for general use in chronic pancreatitis.

Other treatment options

The pancreas is innervated by sympathetic, parasympathetic, motor, and sensory fibers. The sensory fibers transmitting pain travel from the pancreas without synapsing in the splanchnic nerves to the dorsal root, transversing the celiac plexus and the sympathetic chain. Thus, blocking these nerve fibers anywhere along this path may theoretically provide pain relief in chronic pancreatitis.

Celiac plexus block is achieved with 25 mL of 50% alcohol on each side, which should be preceded by a positive diagnostic block with long-acting local anesthetics at least 1 day before. However, the results of this procedure have been disappointing. Leung *et al.* found that 12 of 23 patients with chronic pancreatitis had initially complete, and six patients partial, pain relief with celiac plexus block. However, the mean pain-free interval was only 2 months and repeated blocks were ineffective.

The role of transcutaneous electrical nerve stimulation, often used in other pain syndromes, is not yet determined for pain in chronic pancreatitis. In cases of severe pain in chronic pancreatitis which do not respond to medical or surgical therapy, celiac plexus block or transthoracic splanchniectomy or individual therapeutic options such as epidural local anesthetics or intrathecal administration of opioids via a subcutaneous infusion pump should be discussed. However, conservative treatment is not always successful in patients with chronic pancreatitis. Pain that significantly reduces the quality of life, especially if it requires morphine on a regular basis, may represent an indication for surgical treatment. Surgery for chronic pancreatitis is indicated in patients with pain refractory to medical measures. It can be performed with low mortality and morbidity and pain relief is achieved in the vast majority of patients.

Conclusions

For decades, physicians have been trying different approaches to the problem of pain in chronic pancreatitis. There is still disagreement about the mechanisms that contribute to the generation of pain and about the best method of managing pain in chronic pancreatitis.

Earlier pain hypotheses, for example those postulating increased intraductal and intraparenchymal pressure or postprandial pancreatic hyperstimulation by decreased enzyme secretion and insufficient functioning of the so-called negative feedback mechanism, are now seriously questioned as reliable explanations of abdominal pain in patients with chronic pancreatitis.

In the last 10 years we have learned about the role of altered nerve patterns in the inflamed pancreas and the overproduction of different neuromediators in the enlarged pancreatic nerves. In the light of these considerations, it is now clear that we must explore the pathophysiology of pain generation in order to develop new drugs to control pain in chronic pancreatitis. In addition, the lack of a good animal model of chronic pancreatitis remains a limiting factor in understanding the complete cascade of event that generate and sustain the long-lasting pain syndrome in the natural history of chronic pancreatitis.

Based on current knowledge there are no gold standards for the therapy of chronic pancreatic pain. A multidisciplinary approach based on individual pain history is recommended.

Recommended reading

AGA technical review: treatment of pain in chronic pancreatits. *Gastroenterology* 1998;15:765–776.

Andrén-Sandberg A, Hoem D, Gislason H. Pain management in chronic pancreatitis. *Eur J Gastroentereol Hepatol* 2002;14:957–970.

Beger HG, Krautzberger W, Bittner R, Büchler M. Duodenum-preserving resection of the head of the pancreas in patients with severe chronic pancreatitis. *Surgery* 1985;97:467–473.

Beger HG, Büchler M, Malfertheiner P (eds) *Standards in Pancreatic Surgery*. New York: Springer-Verlag, 1993: 41–46.

Bockman DE, Buchler M, Malfertheiner P, Beger HG. Analysis of nerves in chronic pancreatitis. *Gastroenterology* 1988;94:1459–1469.

Brown A, Hughes M, Tenner S, Banks PA. Does pancreatic enzyme supplementation reduce pain in patients with chronic pancreatitis: a meta-analysis. *Am J Gastroenterol* 1997;92:2032–2035.

Buchler M, Weihe E, Friess H *et al*. Changes in peptidergic innervation in chronic pancreatitis. *Pancreas* 1992;7: 183–192.

Büchler MW, Friess H, Müller M, Wheatley AM, Beger HG. Randomized trial of duodenum-preserving pancreatic head resection versus pylorus-preserving Whipple in chronic pancreatitis. *Am J Surg* 1995;169:65–69.

Di Sebastiano P, Fink T, Weihe E *et al*. Immune cell infiltration and growth-associated protein 43 expression correlate with pain in chronic pancreatitis. *Gastroenterology* 1997;112: 1648–1655.

Ditschuneit H. Treatment of pain in chronic pancreatitis by inhibition of pancreatic secretion with octreotide. *Gut* 1995;36:450–454.

Ebbehoj N, Borly L, Bulow J *et al*. Pancreatic tissue fluid pressure in chronic pancreatitis. Relation to pain, morphology, and function. *Scand J Gastroenterol* 1990;25: 1046–1051.

Hacker JF, Chobanian SJ. Pain of chronic pancreatitis: etiology, natural history, therapy. *Dig Dis* 1987;5:41–48.

Halgreen H, Pederson NT, Worning H. Symptomatic effect of pancreatic enzyme therapy in patients with chronic pancreatitis. *Scand J Gastroenterol* 1986;21:104–108.

Hiraoka T, Watanabe E, Katoh T *et al*. A new surgical approach for control of pain in chronic pancreatitis: complete denervation of the pancreas. *Am J Surg* 1986;152:549–551.

Ihse I, Borch K, Larsson J. Chronic pancreatitis: results of operations for relief of pain. *World J Surg* 1990;14:53–58.

Isaksson G, Ihse I. Pain reduction by an oral pancreatic enzyme preparation in chronic pancreatitis. *Dig Dis Sci* 1983;28:97–102.

Jansen JB. Pain in chronic pancreatitis. *Scand J Gastroenterol* 1995;212:117–125.

Kahl ST, Glasbrenner B, Schulz HU, Malfertheiner P. An integrated approach to the non-operative treatment of pain in chronic pancreatitis. In: MW Büchler, H Friess, W Uhl, P Malfertheiner (eds) *Chronic Pancreatitis:*

Novel Concepts in Biology and Therapy. Oxford, Berlin: Blackwell Publishing, 2002: 409–419.

Khalid A, Whitcomb DC. Conservative treatment of chronic pancreatitis. *Eur J Gastroentereol Hepatol* 2002;14:943–949.

Kloppel G. Pathology of chronic pancreatitis and pancreatic pain. *Acta Chir Scand* 1990;156:261–265.

Koliopanos A, Friess H, Roggo A, Zimmermann A, Büchler MW. Cyclooxygenase-2 expression in chronic pancreatitis: correlation with stage of the disease and diabetes mellitus. *Digestion* 2001;64:240–247.

Lankisch PG, Lohr-Happe A, Otto J, Creutzfeldt W. Natural course of chronic pancreatitis. Pain, exocrine and endocrine pancreatic insufficiency and prognosis of the disease. *Digestion* 1993;54:148–155.

Leung JW, Bowen-Wright M, Aveling W, Shorvon PJ, Cotton PB. Coeliac plexus block for pain in pancreatic cancer and chronic pancreatitis. *Br J Surg* 1983;70:730–732.

Malesci A, Gaia E, Fioretta A *et al*. No effect of long-term treatment with pancreatic extract on recurrent abdominal pain in patients with chronic pancreatitis. *Scand J Gastroenterol* 1995;30:392–398.

Malfertheiner P, Pieramico O, Buchler M, Ditschuneit H. Relationship between pancreatic function and pain in chronic pancreatitis. *Acta Chir Scand* 1990;156:267–271.

Manes G, Buchler M, Pieramico O, Di Sebastiano P, Malfertheiner P. Is increased pancreatic pressure related to pain in chronic pancreatitis? *Int J Pancreatol* 1994;15: 113–117.

Mössner J, Secknus R, Meyer J, Niederau C, Adler G. Treatment of pain with pancreatic extracts in chronic pancreatitis: results of a prospective placebo-controlled multicenter trial. *Digestion* 1992;53:54–66.

Mössner J, Keim V, Niederau C *et al*. Guidelines for therapy of chronic pancreatitis. Consensus Conference of the German Society of Digestive and Metabolic Diseases. *Z Gastroenterol* 1998;6:359–367.

Pitchumoni CS. Chronic pancreatitis: pathogenesis and management of pain. *J Clin Gastroenterol* 1998;27:101–107.

Prinz RA, Aranha GV, Greenlee HB, Kruss DM. Common duct obstruction in patients with intractable pain of chronic pancreatitis. *Am Surg* 1982;48:373–377.

Schlosser W, Schlosser S, Ramadani M, Gansauge F, Gansauge S, Beger HG. Cyclooxygenase-2 is overexpressed in chronic pancreatitis. *Pancreas* 2002;25:26–30.

Uhl W, Anghelacopoulos SE, Friess H, Büchler MW. The role of octreotide and somatostatin in acute and chronic pancreatitis. *Digestion* 1999;60(Suppl 2):23–31.

Warner TD, Guiliano F, Vojuovic I *et al*. Nonsteroid drug selectivities for cyclo-oxygenase-1 rather than cyclo-oxygenase-2 are associated with human gastrointestinal toxicity: a full in vitro analysis. *Proc Natl Acad Sci USA* 1999;96:7563–7568.

34 Endoscopic treatment of pain in chronic pancreatitis: really useful or only feasible?

Guido Costamagna and Andrea Tringali

Chronic pancreatitis is a progressive disease without a curative treatment. Therapeutic efforts have therefore centered on palliative treatment of pain, which is present in about 90% of cases. Abdominal pain is the predominant symptom of chronic pancreatitis that initially brings most of the patients to the physician's attention.

The typical epigastric pain radiating to the back is common, but any type of abdominal pain may occur. Pain is often worsened by eating or by the supine position. The pain presents a heterogeneous pattern, from relapsing episodes to persistent pain of varying intensity. The usual pattern is initial episodes of acute abdominal pain and recurrent episodes of acute "nonbiliary" pancreatitis; with progression of the disease the attacks become more frequent and severe, ultimately culminating in continuous pain requiring narcotic analgesic and frequent hospital admissions. In some patients the pain improves with time, particularly during the end stage of the disease, which often coincides with deterioration of pancreatic function. A small proportion of patients have painless disease or minimal pain throughout the course of their illness, and in these the clinical emphasis is usually on endocrine or exocrine insufficiency.

Pathogenesis of pain in chronic pancreatitis

The pathogenesis of pancreatic pain is often multifactorial and may vary at different stages of the disease, explaining why not all patients respond to the same treatment. These factors may include the following.

• Increased pancreatic parenchymal pressures (compartment syndrome) secondary to increased ductal pressure resulting from outflow obstruction caused by strictures, pancreatic stone, or compressing pseudocyst and to reduced parenchymal compliance caused by fibrosis.
• Inflammatory infiltration with fibrotic encasement of sensory nerves, and a neuropathy characterized by both increased number and size of intrapancreatic sensory nerves and by inflammatory injury to the nerve sheaths allowing exposure of the neural elements to toxic substances such as activated pancreatic enzymes, calcitonin gene-related peptide, and substance P.
• Pancreatic ischemia secondary to lack of compliance of the pancreatic gland that impairs blood flow leading to hypoxia and acidosis.
• Release of oxygen-derived free radicals associated with a round cell inflammatory response and tissue damage. Oxidative stress is responsible for mediating pain especially during acute exacerbations of chronic pancreatitis.
• Complications such as pseudocysts.

Endoscopic treatment of pain in chronic pancreatitis

The history of the endoscopic management of chronic pancreatitis begins in November 1976, when Cremer performed the first pancreatic sphincterotomy to treat an impacted pancreatic stone in the major papilla that was causing acute cholangitis. Subsequent historical steps in this field include pancreatic stenting in 1985 and extracorporeal shock-wave lithotripsy (ESWL) for pancreatic stones in 1987.

When major pain episodes due to chronic pancreatitis cannot be controlled by acceptable maintenance analgesics, intervals of narcotics, or reasonable and brief period of hospitalization, interventional therapy can be justified. Whether immediate treatment can change the natural history of progressive loss of exocrine and endocrine function is still not known, even though experimental and clinical evidence suggests that early ductal decompression may be beneficial in modulating the outcome of chronic pancreatitis.

Selection of candidates for endoscopic pancreatic duct drainage

In addition to standard laboratory tests and routine plain films of the pancreatic area for detection of pancreatic calcifications, magnetic resonance imaging (MRI) is currently the noninvasive modality of choice for selection of patients who might benefit from endoscopic treatment. Intravenous administration of secretin, which stimulates the secretion of fluid and bicarbonate, enhances visualization of the pancreatic ducts and acts as an endogenous contrast medium, a technique known as secretin-enhanced magnetic resonance cholangiopancreatography (S-MRCP). It gives appropriate information on the presence of downstream ductal obstruction or a cystic lesion and on pancreatic exocrine function by quantification of duodenal filling.

S-MRCP provides a diagnostic pancreatogram with which to identify those patients with a single obstruction in the head of the pancreas caused by an impacted ductal stone or a fibrotic stricture (or both). Those cases with Cremer type IV chronic pancreatitis are the best candidates for endotherapy.

Pancreatic sphincterotomy

Endoscopic pancreatic sphincterotomy is generally performed as the first step toward improving access to the pancreatic duct before pancreatic stone extraction or endoprosthesis insertion. Minor papilla sphincterotomy may be needed in up to 20% of patients in cases of dominant dorsal duct anatomy (complete or incomplete pancreas divisum or ansa pancreatica). In a subset of patients, pancreatic sphincterotomy by itself may be sufficient to resolve papillary stenosis causing upstream dilatation and/or to extract small nonobstructive pancreatic stones.

The early complication rate of pancreatic sphincterotomy seems to be lower in chronic pancreatitis than in other indications, perhaps because of the periductal fibrosis and limited amounts of nearby acinar tissue associated with chronic pancreatitis. Early complications occur in 4.1–16% of cases and include the exacerbation of mild pancreatitis (1.8–9%), bleeding (1.3–3.6%), cholangitis (0–4.3%) and, in rare cases, retroduodenal perforation (0.6%).

Endoscopic manometry using a variety of techniques has yielded conflicting results when sphincter of Oddi and main pancreatic duct pressures in patients with chronic pancreatitis were compared with controls. In patients with chronic pancreatitis, sphincter of Oddi function varied from normal to gross disturbances of basal and phasic contractions. Laugier and colleagues observed a significantly increased pressure response of the sphincter of Oddi and pancreatic duct to secretin stimulation in patients with early disease when compared with advanced disease associated with pancreatic duct dilatation. These changes may be construed as evidence of increased volume responses with early disease. The role of increased viscosity of pancreatic juice in chronic pancreatitis and the hypothesis that protein plugs may impact on the sphincter leading to obstruction and pain is yet to be confirmed.

The results of pancreatic sphincterotomy alone in the treatment of chronic pancreatitis was retrospectively assessed in 55 patients followed for a median time of 16 months (range 3–52): 34 patients (62%) reported significant improvement in their pain assessed using a numeric rating scale ($P < 0.01$).

Endoscopic treatment could be regarded as the initial management of choice for patients with early-onset (before the age of 35) idiopathic chronic pancreatitis. In our clinic, 11 patients with pain due to early-onset chronic pancreatitis were treated by endoscopic sphincterotomy (major and/or minor papilla) and stone extraction. One patient had a dominant pancreatic duct stricture on the head and underwent pancreatic stenting; the other cases were treated by pancreatic sphincterotomy (major and/or minor papilla) with or without stone extraction after ESWL. Seven patients (64%) remained free of pain relapses after a mean follow-up of 6.5 years (range 3–9.5). Causes of recurrent pain included stenosis of the pancreatic sphincterotomy, new pancreatic stricture formation, pancreatic stone migration, and pancreatic stent occlusion. All these complications were successfully retreated endoscopically. The frequency of hospitalization before and 1, 3, and 6 years after endoscopic treatment was significantly reduced.

In selected cases, such as early stage of chronic pancreatitis and early-onset idiopathic chronic pancreatitis, pancreatic sphincterotomy in the absence of pancreatic duct stricture and dilation can be proposed as a treatment for reducing the frequency of pain and recurrence of pancreatitis. Patients with an attack of "nonbiliary" pancreatitis are studied with S-MRCP and those who show signs of initial chronic pancreatitis (side-branch dilation, tortuous pancreatic duct) undergo clinical follow-up. In cases of a second attack of pancreatitis within 1–2 years pancreatic sphincterotomy can be proposed.

ESWL of pancreatic stones

Approximately one-third of patients with chronic pancreatitis have pancreatic stones and half of these will have the main portion of their stone burden within the main duct in the pancreatic head or body. Successful endoscopic stone extraction after pancreatic sphincterotomy depends on the size (< 10 mm), number (< 3), and pancreatic location (head or body) of the stones, and may not be possible if strictures are present or if the stones are impacted in the ductal wall. ESWL is necessary to fragment stones prior to endoscopic extraction in 36–44% of patients with chronic pancreatitis.

ESWL-related complications (organ damage or acute pancreatitis) are rare (0–12.5%) and mortality was absent in the largest published series and in our experience (300 pancreatic ESWL). Mild adverse effects of ESWL include petechiae on the skin in the area of shock-wave penetration, and in the gastric antrum.

The best fragmentation of pancreatic stones is obtained using a two-dimensional radiologic targeting system under conscious sedation or general anesthesia. In two series where ultrasound was used to localize the stones, the fragmentation rate was much lower. In cases where calcified pancreatic stones are present, radiologic targeting is easy and ESWL can be performed as a first procedure before therapeutic endoscopic retrograde cholangiopancreatography (ERCP). Results from the literature show that ESWL and endotherapy achieve stone fragmentation in 54–100% of cases, complete duct clearance in 44–74%, and complete or partial pain relief in 48–85% after a mean follow-up of 7–40 months; surgery is necessary due to persistence or recurrence of pain in 3–20% of patients (Table 34.1).

Table 34.1 Results of extracorporeal shock-wave lithotripsy (ESWL) and endotherapy for chronic calcific pancreatitis.

Study	Year	No. of patients	Fragmentation (%)	Complete clearance (%)	Complete or partial pain relief (%)	Need for surgery (%)	Mean follow-up (months)
ESWL and endotherapy							
Delhaye	1992	123	99	59	85	8	14
Schneider	1994	50	86	60	62	12	20
Johanns	1996	35	100	46	83	14	23
Costamagna *et al.*	1997	35	100	74	72	3	27
Adamek *et al.*	1999	80	54	ND	76	10	40
Brand *et al.*	2000	48	60	44	82	4	7
Farnbacher *et al.*	2002	125	85	64	48*	13	29
Kozarek *et al.*	2002	40	100	ND	80	20	30
ESWL alone							
Ohara	1996	32	100	75	86	3	44
Karasawa	2002	10	NA	NA	NA	NA	12

* Patients with complete pain relief during follow-up.
NA, not addressed.

Early outcome of pancreatic ESWL in combination with interventional endoscopy has been prospectively evaluated. After a mean follow-up of 7 months, there was a significant decrease in pancreatic duct diameter ($P < 0.001$) and pain score ($P < 0.0001$); weight gain occurred in 68% of patients and several quality-of-life scores improved significantly. Improvement in pain score was also correlated with weight gain, decrease in pancreatic duct diameter, and nonalcoholic etiology.

A large retrospective study analyzed 114 patients with pancreatic stones treated by ESWL and endotherapy. The authors assessed the criteria for success of treatment and univariate analysis showed that middle-aged patients, an early stage of chronic pancreatitis, and distal location of stones were significantly associated with a higher rate of treatment success and pain relief. Stones located in the pancreatic tail are usually less symptomatic because of frequent parenchymal atrophy. A statistically significant decrease in pain score ($P = 0.001$), yearly hospitalizations for pancreatitis ($P = 0.001$), and monthly use of narcotic medications was found after a mean follow-up of 2.4 years in another retrospective study focused on ESWL and endotherapy for chronic pancreatitis.

For patients with calcified stones but without a tight stricture and with residual exocrine function as shown on diagnostic S-MRCP, ESWL alone is a possible first-line treatment, endotherapy being considered in cases where this approach is not successful. The hypothesis is that after ESWL, pancreatic juice and fragments can pass spontaneously through the intact sphincter with relief of ductal obstruction. Two Japanese groups have examined the results of this approach, with preliminary results similar to those of ESWL in association with endotherapy.

Much of the available information on ESWL and endotherapy for the treatment of pain in chronic pancreatitis come from retrospective studies. New prospective trials are warranted to confirm the good results of pancreatic ESWL.

Pancreatic stenting

The main indication for endoscopic placement of a pancreatic stent in chronic pancreatitis is the presence of a dominant ductal stricture, defined as high grade of narrowing with one of the following characteristics:

- induction of pancreatic duct dilation (≥ 6 mm);
- prevention of contrast medium outflow alongside a 6 Fr nasopancreatic catheter;
- pain during perfusion of nasopancreatic catheter with saline.

Where there is persistence of pain after placement of a well-functioning pancreatic stent, ductal hypertension is not likely to be the cause of pancreatic pain and other causes must be investigated. Clinical results of pancreatic stenting are also a good predictive factor for the outcome of derivative surgery.

Early complications of pancreatic stenting in chronic pancreatitis include acute pancreatitis (3.9–39%) and bleeding (3.9%). Late complications include stent clogging (20%), stent migration (10%), pain recurrence or bouts of pancreatitis, and possibly infection. Technical success of pancreatic stenting in the course of ERCP is high (96–100%), with immediate pain relief in 82–94% of cases; this improvement lasts for 6 months in 74% of treated patients. Results are summarized in Table 34.2.

Mean pancreatic stent patency is 12 months (range 2–38) and symptomatic stent exchange is suggested instead of prophylactic therapy. In fact pancreatic stents, even when clogged, may function as a wick around which pancreatic juice can drain, sometimes for years. After stent removal, morphologic resolution of the pancreatic stricture is uncommon, but improvement of pain can be obtained even without stricture calibration. For example, after stent removal in 29/93 patients (53%) after a mean period of stenting of 15.7 months, 73% of these patients remained pain-free without a stent during a mean follow-up of 3.8 years.

As described for pancreatic sphincterotomy and ESWL, pancreatic stenting is also more effective in the treatment of pain in chronic pancreatitis especially in cases with a shorter history of symptomatic chronic pancreatitis. Thus early endoscopic ductal drainage in chronic pancreatitis is advisable. When endoscopic treatment of pain in chronic pancreatitis is not effective or the need for stent exchange becomes too frequent, surgery is the alternative treatment.

Recently, a prospective randomized trial compared the outcome of endotherapy and surgery in the treatment of chronic pancreatitis. Initial success rates were similar for both groups, but at 5-year follow-up complete absence of pain was more frequent after surgery (37% vs. 14%) while the rate of partial relief was similar (49% vs. 51%). Increase in body weight was greater by 20–25% in the surgical group, while new-onset dia-

Table 34.2 Results of stent therapy of main pancreatic duct strictures in chronic pancreatitis.

Study	Year	No. of patients	Stent diameter (Fr)	Early pain relief (%)	Mean stent patency (months)	Stricture resolution (%)	Need for surgery (%)	Mean follow-up (months)
Cremer et al.	1991	75	10	94	12	9	15	37
Binmoeller et al.	1995	93	5–7–10	74	6	NA	26	58
Ponchon et al.	1995	23	10	74	NA*	48	15	14
Smits et al.	1995	49	10	82	NA†	NA	6	34

* Planned stent exchange every 2 months.
† Elective stent removal after a median time of 6 months.
NA, not addressed.

betes developed with similar frequency in both groups. According to these data, surgery is superior to endotherapy for long-term pain reduction in patients with painful chronic pancreatitis. Because of its low degree of invasiveness, endotherapy can be offered as a first-line treatment, with surgery being performed in cases of failure or recurrence.

New technique: EUS-guided pancreaticogastrostomy

In cases of obstruction or rupture of the main pancreatic duct or when surgical reconstruction precludes access to the duodenal papillae, a new technique has been described for draining the pancreatic duct through an endoscopically created fistula to the digestive tract, under echographic and fluoroscopic guidance. The endoscopically created pancreaticogastrostomy is enlarged by balloon dilatation or a diathermic sheath, and kept open by a 6–10 Fr stent. Three of four patients with chronic pancreatitis treated by endoscopic ultrasound (EUS)-guided pancreaticogastrostomy had satisfactory relief of pain at a median follow-up of 1 year. Results of this technique are preliminary but promising. Future wider experience in tertiary centers specialized in biliopancreatic therapeutic endoscopy are expected.

Endoscopic drainage of pancreatic pseudocyst

In the setting of chronic pancreatitis, symptomatic

pseudocysts are commonly seen in association with stones or strictures and these also need to be addressed. Pancreatic pseudocysts may complicate the course of chronic pancreatitis in 20–40% of cases, and less than 10% will resolve spontaneously.

Pseudocysts communicating with the main pancreatic duct are amenable to transpapillary drainage. In the absence of a communication with the pancreatic duct, transmural drainage (cystgastrostomy or cystduodenostomy) can be performed under endoscopic control where there is visible bulging of the pseudocyst into the wall of the stomach or duodenum. With the advent of large-channel linear echoendoscopes, transmural drainage is feasible even in the absence of pseudocyst bulging when the gut lumen is more than 1 cm away from the pseudocyst.

The indications for pseudocyst drainage are the presence of pain, cyst enlargement, or complications (gastrointestinal and biliary obstruction, vascular occlusion, spontaneous infection, fistula formation with pleural cavity or adjacent viscera). Complex pseudocysts that are multiseptated, associated with necrosis, or associated with a totally disrupted main pancreatic duct are less amenable to endoscopic management. Asymptomatic pseudocysts can be safely observed with careful follow-up using computed tomography (CT) or MRI.

Pain related to pseudocysts can be relieved after endoscopic drainage with satisfactory results: clinical resolution of the cyst was observed in 86% of patients after transmural drainage and 84% of patients treated with transpapillary drainage. Complications of pseudocyst drainage are present in 10% of patients. Endoscopic cystenterostomy is associated with a higher complication rate than transpapillary drainage. The major complications reported are bleeding, retroperitoneal leakage, and infection.

Endoscopic drainage of the pancreatic duct in chronic calcifiyng pancreatitis

Figures 34.1–34.5 show the stages in endoscopic drainage of the pancreatic duct to alleviate chronic calcifying pancreatitis.

EUS-guided celiac plexus block/neurolysis

Pancreatic pain is predominantly transmitted through

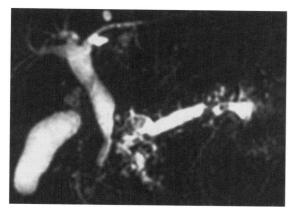

Figure 34.1 Magnetic resonance cholangiopancreatography shows marked dilation of the main pancreatic duct with obstructive stone in the head.

the celiac plexus and the splanchnic nerve. Celiac ganglion injection with alcohol or steroids has been performed percutaneously under CT guidance or sonographically (EUS) for patients still suffering after successful surgical or endoscopic drainage of the pancreatic duct, indicating that the mechanism of pain in these patients is not related to ductal obstruction. The role of EUS-guided celiac ganglion block is similar to percutaneous celiac block but it has the advantage of not having to traverse the aorta or the lumbar musculature with its associated risk (paraplegia) and discomfort. In addition, bacteria within the stomach may be translocated into the retroperitoneum during endoscopic transgastric blocks.

Injection of anesthetics and/or corticosteroids for temporary block is termed celiac plexus block (CPB) while injection of absolute ethanol that permanently destroys the plexus is called celiac plexus neurolysis (CPN). EUS-guided CPB /CPN was described in 1996; the procedure can be performed in 10 min under conscious sedation.

A prospective randomized comparison of EUS- and percutaneous CT-guided CPB for managing the pain of chronic pancreatitis showed that EUS-guided CPB provided more persistent pain relief than CT-guided block and was the preferred technique among the subjects studied. The effect of EUS-guided CPB with bupivacaine and triamcinolone has been prospectively assessed in 90 patients with chronic pancreatitis and pain unresponsive to current treatment options. Benefit was limited: significant pain relief was obtained in 55% of patients after 4 and 8 weeks of follow-up; persistent pain relief beyond 12 and 24 weeks was observed in 26% and 10% of patients, respectively. Three patients (3%) experienced diarrhea after EUS-guided CPB that resolved

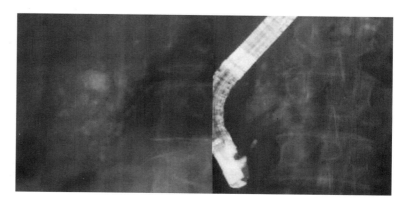

Figure 34.2 Radiograph shows pancreatic calcifications before (left) and after (right) extracorporeal shock-wave lithotripsy.

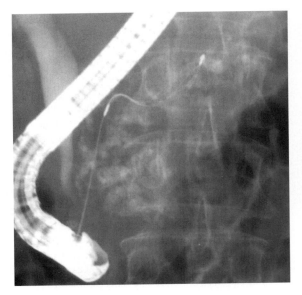

Figure 34.3 Stone extraction with a Dormia basket.

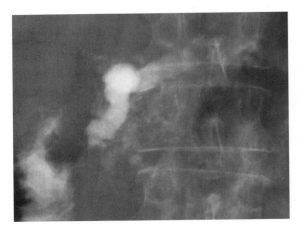

Figure 34.4 Pancreatic stricture in the head of the pancreas without outflow of contrast medium.

spontaneously within 7 days; one patient (1%) developed a peripancreatic abscess successfully treated with antibiotics. Procedure-related mortality was absent.

EUS-guided CPB and CPN provide transient pain relief in chronic pancreatitis and can be considered a therapy of last resort. Surgical videothoracoscopic splanchnicectomy in chronic pancreatitis is a new technique that provides long-lasting results compared with EUS-guided CPB. In a series of 44 patients who underwent videothoracoscopic splanchnicectomy,

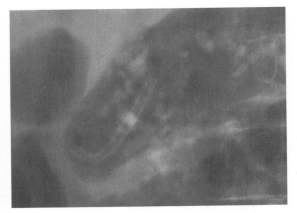

Figure 34.5 After placement of a 10 Fr pancreatic stent contrast medium is completely drained.

there was a 46% cumulative rate of pain relief 4 years after treatment.

Conclusions

During the natural history of chronic pancreatitis the duration of pain-free intervals is unpredictable and may last from weeks to many months, making it difficult to assess the value of different modalities of pain therapy. The management of pain in chronic pancreatitis is a team approach; the gastroenterologist, surgeon, endoscopist, radiologist, and psychiatrist are members of the team at various times.

Endoscopic management of chronic pancreatitis is safe, feasible, minimally invasive, often effective for years, and can be repeated. It should be applied as a first-line approach to improve the clinical condition of patients with this chronic disease. The best results are obtained when endoscopic treatment is performed early in the course of chronic pancreatitis. Proper patient selection, adequate expertise, and a supporting multidisciplinary infrastructure are essential.

A recent large multicenter study retrospectively assessed the long-term outcome in 1018 patients with chronic pancreatitis who had received endoscopic pancreatic ductal drainage in several large-volume centers. During a mean follow-up period of 5 years, 23% of the patients underwent surgery and 16% were still receiving endotherapy. After surgical drainage, 10% of the patients continued to receive endotherapy. Pancreatic exocrine and endocrine functions were not positively affected by endoscopic therapy. The long-term success of endotherapy was 86% in the entire group. Overall, on an intention-to-treat basis, 65% of the patients in this large series with painful chronic pancreatitis at initial presentation can be expected to be completely or nearly free of pain after 5 years, without needing surgery

Thus chronic pancreatitis has become a good candidate for endotherapy as an effective treatment for the relief of pain.

Recommended reading

Adamek HE, Jakobs R, Buttmann A et al. Long term follow-up of patients with chronic pancreatitis and pancreatic stones treated with extracorporeal shock wave lithotripsy. Gut 1999;45:402–405.

Beckingham IJ, Krige JEJ, Bornman PC et al. Endoscopic management of pancreatic pseudocysts. Br J Surg 1997;84: 1638–1645.

Binmoeller KF, Jue P, Seifert H et al. Endoscopic pancreatic stent drainage in chronic pancreatitis and a dominant stricture: long-term results. Endoscopy 1995;27:638–644.

Brand B, Kahl M, Sidhu S et al. Prospective evaluation of morphology, function, and quality of life after extracorporeal shock wave lithotripsy and endoscopic treatment of chronic calcific pancreatitis. Am J Gastroenterol 2000;95: 3428–3438.

Costamagna G, Gabbrielli A, Mutignani M et al. Extracorporeal shock wave lithotripsy of pancreatic stones in chronic pancreatitis: immediate and medium-term results. Gastrointest Endosc 1997;46:231–236.

Cremer M, Devière J, Delhaye M et al. Stenting in severe chronic pancreatitis: results of medium-term follow-up in seventy-six patients. Endoscopy 1991;23:171–176.

Delhaye M, Vandermeeren A, Baize M et al. Extracorporeal shock wave lithotripsy of pancreatic calculi. Gastroenterology 1992;102:610–620.

Delhaye M, Matos C, Devière J. Endoscopic management of chronic pancreatitis Gastrointest Endosc Clin North Am 2003;13:717–742.

Dite P, Ruzicka M, Zboril V. A prospective, randomized trial comparing endoscopic and surgical therapy for chronic pancreatitis. Endoscopy 2003;35:553–558.

Farnbacher MJ, Shoen C, Rabenstein T et al. Pancreatic duct stones in chronic pancreatitis: criteria for treatment intensity and successe. Gastrointest Endosc 2002;56:501–506.

Francois E, Kahaleh M, Giovannini M. EUS-guided pancreaticogastrostomy. Gastrointest Endosc 2002;56:128–133.

Gabbrielli A, Mutignani M, Pandolfi M et al. Endotherapy of early onset idiopathic chronic pancreatitis: results with long-term follow-up. Gastrointest Endosc 2002;55:488–493.

Gress F, Schmitt C, Sherman S et al. A prospective randomized comparison of endoscopic ultrasound and computed tomography-guided celiac plexus block for managing chronic pancreatitis. Am J Gastroenterol 1999;94:900–905.

Gress F, Schmitt C, Sherman S et al. Endoscopic ultrasound-guided celiac plexus block for managing abdominal pain associated with chronic pancreatitis: a prospective single center experience. Am J Gastroenterol 2001;96:409–416.

Jacobs R, Benz C, Leonhardt A. Pancreatic endoscopic sphincterotomy in patients with chronic pancreatitis. Endoscopy 2002;34:551–554.

Joahns W, Jakobeit C, Greiner L et al. Ultrasound-guided extracorporeal shock wave lithotripsy of pancreatic ductal stones: a six years experience. Can J Gastroenterol 1996; 10:471–475.

Karasawa Y, Kawa S, Aoki Y et al. Extracorporeal shock wave lithotripsy of pancreatic duct stones and patient factors related to stone disintegration. J Gastroenterol 2002;37: 369–375.

Kozarek RA, Bael TJ, Patterson DJ. Endoscopic pancreatic duct sphincterotomy: indications, technique and analysis of results. Gastroinest Endosc 1994;40:592–598.

Kozarek RA, Brandabur JJ, Ball JT et al. Clinical outcomes in patients who undergo extracorporeal shock wave lithotripsy for chronic calcific pancreatitis. Gastrointest Endosc 2002;56:496–500.

Ohara H, Hoshino M, Hayakawa T et al. Single application extracorporeal shock wave lithotripsy is the first choice for patients with pancreatic duct stones. Am J Gastroenterol 1996;91:1388–1394.

Okazaki K, Yamamoto Y, Ito K. Endoscopic measurement of papillary sphincter zone and pancreatic main ductal pressure in patients with chronic pancreatitis. Gastroenterology 1986;91:409–418.

Okolo PI, Pasricha PJ, Kalloo AN. What are the long-term results of endoscopic pancreatic sphincterotomy? Gastrointest Endosc 2000;52:15–19.

Ponchon T, Bory R, Hedelins F et al. Endoscopic stenting for pain relief in chronic pancreatitis: results of a standardized protocol. Gastrointest Endosc 1995;42:452–456.

Rosch T, Daniel S, Scholz M et al. Endoscopic treatment of chronic pancreatitis: a multicenter study of 1000 patients with long term follow-up. Endoscopy 2002;34:765–771.

Schneider HT, May A, Benninger J et al. Piezoelectric shock wave lithotripsy of pancreatic duct stones. Am J Gastroenterol 1994;89:2042–2048.

Smits ME, Badiga SM, Rauws EAJ et al. Long-term results of pancreatic stents in chronic pancreatitis. Gastrointest Endosc 1995;42:461–467.

Tarnasky PR, Hoffman P, Aabakken L et al. Sphincter of Oddi dysfunction is associated with chronic pancreatitis. Am J Gastroenterol 1997;92:1125–1129.

Wiersema MJ, Wiersema LM. Endosonography-guided celiac plexus neurolysis. Gastrointest Endosc 1996;44:656–662.

35 Management of maldigestion in chronic pancreatitis: a practical protocol

J. Enrique Domínguez-Muñoz

Exocrine pancreatic insufficiency with maldigestion is a major consequence of chronic pancreatitis. The probability of exocrine pancreatic insufficiency increases with time so that around 50% of patients with chronic pancreatitis develop exocrine pancreatic insufficiency at a median of 10–12 years from onset of the disease. By definition, exocrine pancreatic insufficiency is associated with maldigestion. Milder forms should be called "exocrine pancreatic dysfunction." Chronic diarrhea secondary to maldigestion is often the only symptom of chronic pancreatitis in the absence of pain. However, since exocrine pancreatic insufficiency develops slowly over time, patients tend to adapt their diet progressively, so that diarrhea is frequently not evident. Similarly weight loss is not marked with adequate nutritional support. Based on this, pancreatic function tests should always be carried out to detect or confirm maldigestion in patients with chronic pancreatitis.

The main clinical consequence of exocrine pancreatic insufficiency is fat maldigestion and steatorrhea. This is caused by the following.
- Studies on the fate of endogenously secreted pancreatic enzymes during gastrointestinal transit have demonstrated that lipase is the most unstable pancreatic enzyme. Most amylase activity and more than 20% of the protease activity produced by the pancreas and secreted into the duodenum is still present within the terminal ileum. Conversely, only 1% of lipase activity is still detectable at that intestinal level. This is because lipase is highly sensitive to proteolytic activity: it is hydrolyzed within the intestinal lumen by trypsin and, mainly, chymotrypsin.

- Lipase also suffers irreversible inactivation at acidic pH. This is frequently the pH found within the duodenum in patients with exocrine pancreatic insufficiency due to low pancreatic bicarbonate secretion.
- Compared with what occurs with amylase and proteases, the luminal digestive action of lipase is minimally compensated by nonpancreatic mechanisms (i.e., gastric lipase).
- The impairment of lipase secretion in the context of chronic pancreatitis occurs earlier than other enzymes.

Together with abdominal cramps and the typical characteristics of fatty stools associated with steatorrhea (loose, greasy, foul-smelling voluminous stools that are difficult to flush), which are not always evident because patients tend to limit fat ingestion, fat maldigestion causes several important clinical disturbances:
- fat maldigestion is the main cause of weight loss in patients with exocrine pancreatic insufficiency;
- circulating levels of micronutrients and vitamins are deficient in patients with fat maldigestion, among them magnesium, calcium, essential fatty acids, and vitamins A, D, E, and K;
- plasma levels of high-density lipoprotein C, apolipoprotein A-I, and lipoprotein A are also reduced, which has been related to an increased risk of cardiovascular events in patients with chronic pancreatitis.

The basis of the therapy of maldigestion in patients with chronic pancreatitis and exocrine pancreatic insufficiency consists of the oral administration of exogenous pancreatic enzymes. Together with this, diet has classically played an important role that nowadays should be reconsidered.

Which patients should be treated?

It is generally accepted that patients presenting with weight loss and those with symptoms associated with steatorrhea should be treated with dietary modifications and/or pancreatic enzyme supplements. The indication for treatment in patients with asymptomatic steatorrhea is strongly debated. Most authors maintain that dietary modifications and administration of exogenous pancreatic enzymes are unnecessary in asymptomatic patients. However, development of micronutrient and vitamin deficiency is independent of the presence of symptoms. In fact, circulating levels of fat-soluble vitamins are frequently low in asymptomatic patients with exocrine pancreatic insufficiency. Based on this and in order to prevent potentially relevant nutritional deficits, pancreatic enzyme substitution therapy should be prescribed in every patient with demonstrated exocrine pancreatic insufficiency and steatorrhea, independent of the presence or absence of associated symptoms.

Dietary modifications in the management of exocrine pancreatic insufficiency

Classically, the initial approach to patients with fat maldigestion was to restrict fat intake. The degree of restriction should be enough to abolish steatorrhea, and generally the intake of less than 20 g of fat daily was recommended. Medical therapy was limited to patients who continue to suffer from steatorrhea following dietary restrictions. This approach can no longer be supported.

Restriction of fat intake is linked to insufficient intake of fat-soluble vitamins, which are also malabsorbed as a consequence of fat maldigestion secondary to chronic pancreatitis. Because of exocrine pancreatic insufficiency, the potential vitamin deficiency is minimally compensated by oral vitamin supplements. Moreover, it has been demonstrated in an experimental model of exocrine pancreatic insufficiency in dogs that the coefficient of fat absorption, i.e., the proportion of ingested fat that is digested and absorbed, increases when oral enzyme supplements are added to a fat-enriched diet. However, the proportion of fat absorbed is lower when oral pancreatic enzymes are added to a low-fat diet.

As a consequence, dietary modifications are not recommended for the treatment of fat maldigestion. Only meals leading to abdominal pain or dyspeptic symptoms should be avoided. Cessation of alcohol intake is a general rule in patients with chronic pancreatitis. This has been associated with pain relief in a proportion of patients and, furthermore, some studies have suggested an increase in gastric lipase activity after alcohol abstinence. Whether this increase in gastric lipase activity is enough to prevent fat maldigestion and steatorrhea in some patients is questionable.

Medium-chain triglycerides, which are directly absorbed by the intestinal mucosa, can be useful for providing extra calories in patients with weight loss and a poor response to oral pancreatic enzymes. Furthermore, medium-chain triglycerides may be helpful in reducing steatorrhea in patients with an insufficient response to the medical therapy of exocrine pancreatic insufficiency.

Finally, patients with exocrine pancreatic insufficiency may require supplements of fat-soluble vitamins, among them retinol, calcidiol, α-tocopherol, and vitamin K.

Oral pancreatic enzyme supplements: how to obtain optimal therapeutic efficacy

The functional reserve of the exocrine pancreas is so important that fat maldigestion with steatorrhea does not occur until lipase secretion falls below 10% of normal. This means that 30 000 U of active lipase secreted postprandially within the duodenum are sufficient to guarantee fairly normal fat digestion and absorption. In terms of therapy, exogenous pancreatic supplements should be given orally in a dose and manner to ensure that at least 30 000 U of active lipase reach the duodenum together with meals. Several *in vitro* studies in the USA and Europe have shown that 1 U lipase equals 3 U of the US Pharmacopeia (USP) or European Pharmacopoeia (Eur.P) preparations, which are the units used in commercial pancreatic enzyme extracts. That means that 90 000 USP or Eur.P units of lipase should reach the duodenum in an active form to prevent steatorrhea in patients with exocrine pancreatic insufficiency.

Three main problems may prevent elimination of steatorrhea (Fig. 35.1).
• Pancreatic lipase is markedly acid sensitive and is

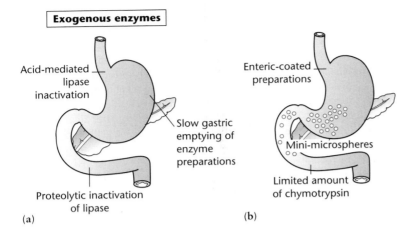

Exogenous enzymes

Acid-mediated lipase inactivation

Slow gastric emptying of enzyme preparations

Proteolytic inactivation of lipase

(a)

Enteric-coated preparations

Mini-microspheres

Limited amount of chymotrypsin

(b)

Figure 35.1 (a) Fate of exogenous pancreatic enzymes during gastrointestinal transit preventing elimination of steatorrhea. (b) Solutions for improving the efficacy of enzyme supplements in the management of exocrine pancreatic insufficiency.

irreversibly inactivated at pH 4.0 or lower. Therefore, orally administered lipase may be inactivated in the gastric cavity and be ineffective in preventing steatorrhea.

• Gastric emptying of pancreatic enzyme preparations should occur in parallel with gastric emptying of meals in order to ensure an optimal mixture within the duodenum. Pancreatic enzyme preparations frequently exhibit slow gastric emptying, leading to insufficient mixing with meals and low efficacy for the treatment of fat maldigestion.

• Pancreatic lipase suffers proteolytic inactivation in the intestinal lumen, mainly mediated by chymotrypsin. This, together with the effect of gastric acid, explains why only 8% of the lipase given orally reaches the duodenum in an active form and is able to exert its digestive activity. Therefore, a huge amount of lipase (around 1 million USP or Eur.P units) should be given orally together with meals in order to guarantee around 90 000 USP/Eur.P units in an active form within the duodenum.

Current commercially available enzyme preparations in the form of enteric-coated mini-microspheres avoid acid-mediated lipase inactivation and ensure gastric emptying of the enzymes in parallel with nutrients. In addition, these preparations include a very low amount of chymotrypsin in order to minimize proteolytic inactivation of lipase (Fig. 35.1). Based on this, there is nowadays no real place for nonenteric-coated enzymes in the management of exocrine pancreatic insufficiency secondary to chronic pancreatitis. However, nonenteric-coated enzyme preparations may be

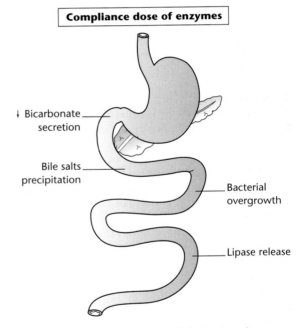

Compliance dose of enzymes

↓ Bicarbonate secretion

Bile salts precipitation

Bacterial overgrowth

Lipase release

Figure 35.2 Factors preventing total elimination of steatorrhea in patients with exocrine pancreatic insufficiency during therapy with enteric-coated pancreatic enzymes in the form of mini-microspheres.

useful in patients who are achlorhydric because of chronic atrophic gastritis or previous gastric surgery.

Despite the use of these modern commercial preparations, some factors may still prevent total elimination of steatorrhea (Fig. 35.2).

• Patient compliance is a key factor in the management of exocrine pancreatic insufficiency with oral pancreatic enzymes. Patients should understand the importance of the therapy and the correct administration schedule. In this sense, very recent clinical studies support the view that oral pancreatic enzymes should best be taken during a meal (one-quarter of the dose at the beginning of the meal, half of the dose during the meal, and the remaining quarter at the end of the meal).

• The prescribed dose of pancreatic enzymes should be high enough. Since some endogenous lipase secretion is usually preserved, a dose of 20 000–40 000 USP/Eur.P units of lipase in the form of enteric-coated mini-microspheres per meal is an adequate dose in a large proportion of patients. However, doses up to 80 000 U of lipase per meal are not infrequently needed.

• The abnormally low pancreatic secretion of bicarbonate that occurs in the context of advanced chronic pancreatitis with exocrine pancreatic insufficiency is associated with a limited buffer effect in the duodenal lumen. Because of this, a pH higher than 5.0, which is required for active lipase to be released from enteric-coated preparations, is not reached in distal segments of the small intestine.

• An acidic intestinal pH also leads to bile salt precipitation, which contributes to fat malabsorption.

• Up to 40% of patients with chronic pancreatitis have concomitant intestinal bacterial overgrowth. This is probably due to the known asynchrony between interdigestive gastrointestinal motility and pancreatic secretion that frequently occurs in patients with chronic pancreatitis. Bacterial overgrowth may contribute to maldigestion and malabsorption in patients with exocrine pancreatic insufficiency.

The first step to guarantee optimal efficacy of oral pancreatic enzymes in the management of exocrine pancreatic insufficiency is to confirm that patients take enzymes properly. Secondly, the dose of enzymes may be increased up to 80 000 USP/Eur.P units of lipase per meal. In cases in which this high dosage does not prevent steatorrhea, inhibition of gastric acid secretion may be of help. Finally, bacterial overgrowth should be considered in nonresponders (see Fig. 35.3).

Therapeutic role of the inhibition of gastric acid secretion

As mentioned above, gastric acid secretion may prevent

Oral pancreatic enzyme supplements in the form of enteric-coated mini-microspheres (20 000–40 000 USP/Eur.P units of lipase/meal)

Check compliance
Increase enzyme dose up to 80 000 USp/Eur.P units of lipase/meal

Inhibition of gastric acid secretion (standard dose of a proton pump inhibitor once a day or t.i.d.)

Test for bacterial overgrowth and treat if positive

Replace dietary fat by medium-chain triglycerides

Figure 35.3 A practical guide for treating exocrine pancreatic insufficiency secondary to chronic pancreatitis.

release of active lipase from enteric-coated granules within proximal segments of the small intestine. Moreover, an intraduodenal acidic pH, which is present up to 2 hours postprandially in patients with exocrine pancreatic insufficiency, leads to bile salt precipitation. Both effects may prevent total elimination of steatorrhea in patients treated with adequate doses of exogenous pancreatic enzymes in the form of enteric-coated mini-microspheres.

Several clinical trials have demonstrated that inhibition of gastric acid secretion with H_2-receptor antagonists and proton pump inhibitors (PPIs) improves the efficacy of oral pancreatic enzyme substitution therapy. Other authors have not confirmed this finding. Some important aspects should be taken into account in order to obtain a positive effect on fat maldigestion by inhibiting gastric acid secretion in patients treated with enteric-coated pancreatic enzymes.

291

- A maintained pH of 5.0 or higher is required to release lipase, as well as to avoid acid-mediated lipase inactivation and to ensure optimal lipolytic activity and amount of bile acids in micellar phase mixed with meals. This pH can be obtained in most patients by the administration of standard doses of a PPI once daily, at least 30 min before breakfast. In a proportion of patients, this single dose does not maintain its efficacy at the evening meal. In these cases, a double-dose PPI (before breakfast and dinner) may be required.

- Despite the use of an appropriate dose of PPI, an adequate amount of exogenous lipase is mandatory. It should be remembered that a dose of 90 000 USP/Eur.P units of lipase is required to correct fat malabsorption. This dose may to some extent be lower in patients with some pancreatic secretion.

Figure 35.3 summarizes the aspects mentioned above in a guide for treating exocrine pancreatic insufficiency in chronic pancreatitis in clinical practice.

How to control the efficacy of oral pancreatic enzyme substitution therapy

The efficacy of therapy of exocrine pancreatic insufficiency is usually evaluated by means of the clinical response, in terms of improvement of diarrhea, weight gain, or absence of further weight loss. However, we have recently demonstrated that most patients with adequate clinical control of exocrine pancreatic insufficiency with oral enzyme substitution therapy have abnormally low circulating levels of nutritional parameters, mainly fat-soluble vitamins. In addition, around one-third of patients have an abnormally low body mass index.

Fecal fat quantification during therapy is the gold standard for evaluating the effect of oral pancreatic enzymes in patients with fat maldigestion. However, this method requires patients to consume a diet containing around 100 g of fat daily for 5 days and to collect the total amount of feces produced over the last 3 days, which is not easy for most patients. In addition, feces should be processed in the laboratory, which is cumbersome and unpleasant.

As an alternative, our group has recently developed a breath test using ^{13}C-mixed triglyceride as substrate and an optimized solid test meal. The orally administered ^{13}C-labeled substrate is digested by endoge-

nous and exogenous pancreatic lipase, absorbed, and metabolized in the liver. As a consequence, $^{13}CO_2$ is released and exhaled in the breath, where it can be measured by mass spectrometry. The amount of $^{13}CO_2$ exhaled is directly related to the amount of fat digested and absorbed. This simple and noninvasive test, which can be easily applied to clinical routine, has shown high accuracy for the evaluation of the efficacy of oral pancreatic enzyme substitution therapy in patients with fat maldigestion secondary to chronic pancreatitis.

Recommended reading

Bruno MJ, Rauws EA, Hoek FJ, Tytgat GN. Comparative effects of adjuvant cimetidine and omeprazole during pancreatic enzyme replacement therapy. *Dig Dis Sci* 1994;39: 988–992.

Casellas F, Guarner L, Vaquero E, Antolin M, de Gracia X, Malagelada JR. Hydrogen breath test with glucose in exocrine pancreatic insufficiency. *Pancreas* 1998;16:481–486.

DiMagno EP. Gastric acid suppression and treatment of severe exocrine pancreatic insufficiency. *Best Pract Res Clin Gastroenterol* 2001;15:477–486.

DiMagno EP, Go VLW, Summerskill WHJ. Relations between pancreatic enzyme outputs and malabsorption in severe pancreatic insufficiency. *N Engl J Med* 1973;288:813–815.

Dutta SK, Bustin MP, Russell RM, Costa BS. Deficiency of fat-soluble vitamins in treated patients with pancreatic insufficiency. *Ann Intern Med* 1982;97:549–552.

Egberts JH, DiMagno EP. What is the dose of lipolytic activity that corrects human pancreatic steatorrhea? *Gastroenterology* 2000;118:A420.

Heijerman HG, Lamers CB, Bakker W. Omeprazole enhances the efficacy of pancreatin (pancrease) in cystic fibrosis. *Ann Intern Med* 1991;114:200–201.

Iglesias-García J, Iglesias-Rey M, Vilariño-Insua M, Domínguez-Muñoz JE. How to evaluate the efficacy of oral pancreatic enzyme substitution therapy in patients with exocrine pancreatic insufficiency? *Pancreatology* 2004;4: 190.

Layer P, Go VL, DiMagno EP. Fate of pancreatic enzymes during small intestinal aboral transit in humans. *Am J Physiol* 1986;251:G475–G480.

Montalto G, Soresi M, Carroccio A *et al.* Lipoproteins and chronic pancreatitis. *Pancreas* 1994;9:137–138.

Pieramico O, Domínguez-Muñoz JE, Nelson DK, Bock W, Büchler M, Malfertheiner P. Interdigestive cycling in chronic pancreatitis: altered coordination among pancreatic secretion, motility and hormones. *Gastroenterology* 1995;109:224–230.

Suzuki A, Mizumoto A, Sarr MG, DiMagno EP. Bacterial lipase and high-fat diets in canine exocrine pancreatic insufficiency: a new therapy of steatorrhea? *Gastroenterology* 1997;112:2048–2055.

Tran TMD, Van der Neucker A, Hendricks JE *et al*. Effects of a proton-pump inhibitor in cystic fibrosis. *Acta Paediatr* 1998;87:553–558.

36 Management of maldigestion in cystic fibrosis: tricks for an adequate outcome

Luisa Guarner

Introduction

Cystic fibrosis (CF) is one of the most common genetic illnesses in Caucasians. In 1989 the location of the mutated gene responsible for this disease was found to be on chromosome 7. The gene responsible for CF encodes a cell transmembrane conductance regulator present in the exocrine glands and is known as the cystic fibrosis transmembrane regulator (*CFTR*) gene. This gene is organized in 27 exons and more than 1000 mutations causing different forms of the disease are currently known. CF is a hereditary autosomic recessive disease with an incidence of approximately one case per 2500 live births in Caucasians. Recent data reported in Spain have estimated the incidence of CF to be 1 per 5300 live births.

Classical cystic fibrosis

The criteria defining classical CF were published by the Cystic Fibrosis Consensus Panel in 1998 and include the presence of one or more characteristic phenotypic features (chronic sinopulmonary disease, gastrointestinal and nutritional abnormalities, salt-loss syndrome, and obstructive azoospermia due to congenital bilateral absence of vas deferens), a history of CF in a sibling, or a positive newborn screening test result plus laboratory evidence of a *CFTR* abnormality (elevated sweat chloride concentration, identification of mutations in each *CFTR* gene known to cause CF, or abnormal nasal epithelial potential difference).

The atypical forms of the disease are generally due to the presence of a slight mutation and the clinical mani-festation is that of isolated azoospermia due to congential bilateral absence of vas deferens, several pulmonary diseases (disseminated bronchiectasis, diffuse panbronchiolitis, aspergillosis), and other digestive manifestations such as sclerosing cholangitis and chronic pancreatitis. Several studies have reported *CFTR* mutations in 30–37% of patients with chronic idiopathic pancreatitis and in 0–10% of patients with chronic alcoholic pancreatitis. The estimated risk of developing pancreatitis in patients with two *CFTR* mutations is much higher than that in the general population and increases extraordinarily when also associated with a mutation in the serine protease inhibitor Kazal type 1 (*SPINK1*) gene.

Malnutrition

The increase in life expectancy of patients with classical CF over the last two decades is spectacular. This has been due particularly to the advances in the treatment of respiratory complications and malnutrition. Respiratory function has been improved as a consequence of the strategy used in the antibiotic treatment of infections, especially in patients presenting with colonization by *Staphylococcus aureus*, *Haemophilus influenzae*, or *Pseudomonas aeruginosa* in whom early antibiotic treatment is currently recommended.

Malnutrition is directly related to worse prognosis for the disease. Good nutrition is known to reduce the incidence of respiratory infections and improves the quality of life. The cause of malnutrition is multifactorial, although pancreatic insufficiency is considered to be a fundamental factor. In patients with CF there is an imbalance between energy needs and calorie intake. On the one hand, it is known that energetic needs are increased mainly due to respiratory disease. On the other, calorie intake is reduced mainly because of malabsorption and maldigestion produced by pancreatic insufficiency and lower intestinal permeability to nutrients but also because of the restrictive diets indicated by physicians, anorexia, gastroesophageal reflux, and the liver involvement presented by some patients.

Nutritional deficiency may vary, with patients presenting with a range of symptoms, from depletion of fat deposits to severe protein malnutrition. The nutritional objective in these patients is to establish a positive energetic balance, minimizing losses and improving energy intake.

Pancreatic insufficiency

There is a good correlation between the genotype–phenotype and pancreatic involvement. Thus, the presence of two severe mutations produces pancreatic insufficiency in most patients, whereas a genotype with one or two slight mutations leads to preserved pancreatic function in most cases.

In recent years the prevalence of CF has shown an important rise in adult patients and this is due to not only to the greater life expectancy of the patients diagnosed during childhood but also to the diagnosis of adult patients because of better knowledge of the disease. Between 80 and 90% of the patients diagnosed with CF during childhood present with pancreatic insufficiency. However, this percentage falls to 16% when the diagnosis of the disease is made during adulthood. During childhood, improvement of the nutritional state favors adequate growth and development, decreases respiratory infections and, in general, increases the life expectancy of these patients. This is why treatment of pancreatic insufficiency in children is of particular importance.

Treatment of pancreatic insufficiency is based on the administration of pancreatic enzymes as oral supplements during meals. Deficits of amylase and trypsin are partially compensated by the patient's own metabolism; moreover, these enzymes are also stable in the commercial preparations used, which are obtained from the pancreas of the pig. Lipase, however, is more difficult to substitute. The production of salivary and gastric lipase is scarce and pig lipase is irreversibly inactivated by the action of gastric and duodenal acid,

similar to what occurs with human lipase. It has also been demonstrated that pig lipase is hydrolyzed in the small intestine by the action of trypsin and chemotrypsin.

In patients with CF the production of bicarbonate is particulary decreased. The CFTR protein is expressed in the apical membrane of proximal duct epithelial cells and mainly regulates the chloride channel, although some evidence has shown that alteration of CFTR also modifies the function of other channels such as that of bicarbonate. In fact, all patients with CF exhibit a reduction in the pancreatic secretion of bicarbonate regardless of pancreatic function.

At present, some enzymatic preparations are in the form of mini-microspheres (< 1.2 mm) that facilitate gastric emptying together with food. These microcapsules have an enteric coating that allows release of the enzymes only when the pH of the medium is greater than 5.5. These modifications facilitate enzyme function but, as previously mentioned, the duodenal pH of many patients with CF continues to be acid because of the lack of bicarbonate and this explains the subsequent lack of release of the enzymes in the duodenum and areas proximal to the jejunum, which is where absorption takes place. Thus, the delay in enzyme release may contribute to intraluminal maldigestion.

It is because of these limitations that, on occasions when levels of fecal fat are very high, treatment with pancreatic enzymes is able to reduce but not abolish steatorrhea. In this situation it is not difficult to understand why, in an attempt to provide better nutrition to patients, particularly children with CF, the dose of enzymes administered at each meal was increased; that is, until 1994, when the first cases of fibrosing colonopathy were diagnosed.

Fibrosing colonopathy

Fibrosing colonpathy has been recognized as a iatrogenic complication in CF. Since 1994, more than 80 cases have been described around the world, mainly limited to childhood cases, although several adult patients have recently been reported.

This complication of CF has been clinically characterized by persistent abdominal pain accompanied by intestinal subocclusion and, less frequently, bloody stools or chylous ascites. Radiologic study of the colon shows the presence of short or long stenosis which, on

Table 36.1 Characteristics of fibrosing colonopathy.

Clinical picture: persistent abdominal pain
Radiology: short or long colon stenosis
Pathologic anatomy:
    Severe submucosal fibrosis
    Loss of muscularis mucosa
    Infiltration by chronic inflammatory cells in the lamina
      propria
Treatment: surgery

---

occasions, may involve all the colon and even the end of the small intestine. Anatomopathologic study of surgical specimens has demonstrated that the external diameter of the colon is normal but the lumen is stenosed due to an extensive band of fibrosis in the lamina propria and the submucosa, with loss of muscularis mucosa and infiltration by chronic inflammatory cells (occasionally eosinophils) in the lamina propria (Table 36.1). Neither granulomas nor fistulas or transmural fissures, such as those observed in Crohn's disease, are found.

Initially, many predisposing factors were considered, such as a history of meconium ileus, previous surgery, corticoid treatment, treatment of pancreatic insufficiency with capsules of high enzymatic content, or a direct toxic action of the enteric coating of these capsules.

In a case–control study from 1990 to 1994, FitzSimmons and colleagues collected data from 114 centers of CF in the USA; 29 patients had been diagnosed with fibrosing colonopathy (all with surgical intervention) and 105 patients with CF and pancreatic insufficiency but without symptoms of colonopathy were used as controls. The study demonstrated that the mean dose of lipase used in treatment of the patients with fibrosing colonopathy was 2.6-fold greater than that used in the controls. Over the 12 months prior to diagnosis the mean lipase dose given to the fibrosing colonopathy patients was 50 046 U/kg body weight per day (corresponding to 12 512 U/kg per meal) whereas the mean lipase dose given to the controls was 18 985 U/kg per day (corresponding to 4746 U/kg per meal), and a very close relationship was found beween high dose of lipase and fibrosing colonopathy. These data have been confirmed in all the patients diagnosed in other countries.

Treatment of pancreatic insufficiency

Enzyme dosage should be individualized for each patient, although initially it is advisable to follow the recommendations of the US Cystic Fibrosis Foundation suggested in a consensus conference in 1995. Overall, these recommendations are based on the restriction of lipase, with the recommended lipase doses being 2000–4000 U per 120 mL of formula or breast milk in infants, 1000 U/kg per meal in children under the age of 4 years, and 500 U/kg per meal in children over 4 years of age. Half the dose recommended for meals should be used for snacks. In adults the approximate dose is that recommended for children over the age of 4 years, taking into account the greater body weight of adults and the fact that the diet of adults usually includes a lower fat content than that of children. In addition, it is very important to remember never to surpass the maximum lipase dose of 2500 U/kg per meal in order to avoid the development of fibrosing colonopathy.

With respect to the dose of lipase required, Stevens and colleagues reported that all the children they studied who were given a lipase dose of more than 6000 U/kg per meal were systematically administered a reduced dose of 2000 U. The clinical evolution and the nutritional status of these patients were followed over 1 year. Reduction in the dose of lipase produced no changes in either height or weight, demonstrating that high doses of lipase are not necessary for adequate nutrition and development.

Another important point to take into account is that no study has demonstrated any beneficial effect of pancreatic enzyme treatment in patients with CF without pancreatic insufficiency and thus their administration is not justified.

Follow-up

The dosage of enzymes is adjusted according to clinical and biochemical response, with an increase in dosage (up to the limits mentioned) if necessary. The disappearance of discomfort and abdominal distension, reduction in the number of depositions, and increase in weight and height of children and adolescents are evaluated on follow-up. Biochemical control of treatment efficacy is based on the determination of nutritional parameters (such as albumin) and fecal fat excretion (performed to calculate the coefficient of fat absorption).

Table 36.2 Cause of lack of response to treatment.

| Poor treatment compliance |
| Low intraluminal pH |
| Concomitant diseases |
| Bacterial overgrowth |
| Parasite infection |
| Intestinal inflammatory disease |
| Celiac disease |

In cases of poor response to treatment, other causes should be ruled out (Table 36.2). The first point is to ensure treatment compliance, particularly when the patient is an adolescent and does not wish to gain weight. Occasionally, as mentioned above, there may be greater duodenal acidity that impedes correct release of the enzymatic preparation. These patients may benefit from concomitant treatment with a proton pump inhibitor. Lastly, other diseases may cause steatorrhea and these may be associated with CF such as, in order of importance, bacterial overgrowth, parasitic infection (*Giardia lamblia*), inflammatory bowel disease (especially Crohn's disease), or celiac disease. Suspicion of one of these diseases should be confirmed by, respectively, a glucose breath test, the study of parasites in stool, or colonoscopy with ileoscopy or jejunal biopsy.

To ensure good nutritional status in these patients adequate food intake should be indicated that covers 120–150% of their recommended daily requirements, with 30–40% of the calories being obtained from fats. Periodic controls should be carried out to assess serum levels of the liposoluble vitamins, mainly A and E, with the administration of vitamin supplements if necessary. In cases of severe malnutrition, nutritional support with supplements or the placement of enteral nutrition is recommended with the addition of pancreatic enzymes.

Recommended reading

Bansi DS, Price A, Rusell C, Sarner M. Fibrosing colonopathy in an adult owing to over use of pancreatic enzymes supplements. *Gut* 2000;46:283–285.

Borowitz DS, Grand RG, Durie PR. Use of pancreatic enzyme supplements for patients with cystic fibrosis in the context of fibrosing colonopathy. Consensus Committee. *J Pediatr* 1995;127:681–684.

Chacravarti A, Buchwald M, Tsui LC. Identification of the cystic fibrosis gene: genetic analysis. *Science* 1989;245:1073–1080.

Cohn JA, Friedman KJ, Noone PG, Knowles MR, Silverman LM, Jowell PS. Relation between mutations of the cystic fibrosis gene and idiophatic pancreatitis. *N Engl J Med* 1998;339:653–658.

FitzSimmons SC, Burkhart GA, Borovitz D et al. High-dose pancreatic enzyme supplements and fibrosing colonopathy in children with cystic fibrosis. *N Engl J Med* 1997;336:1283–1289.

Guarner L, Rodriguez R, Guarner F, Malagelada J-R. Fate of oral enzymes in pancreatic insufficiency. *Gut* 1993;34:708–712.

Jackson R, Pencharz PB. Cystic fibrosis. *Best Pract Res Clin Gastroenterol* 2003;17:213–235.

Kerem B, Rommens JM, Buchanan JA et al. Relation of thickening of colon wall to pancreatic-enzyme treatment in cystic fibrosis. *Lancet* 1995;345:752–756.

Malats N, Casals T, Porta M, Guarner L, Estivill X, Real FX for the PANKRAS II Study Group. Cystic fibrosis transmembrane regulator (CFTR) ΔF508 mutation and 5T allele in patients with chronic pancreatitis and exocrine pancreatic cancer. *Gut* 2000;48:70–74.

Modolell I, Alvarez A, Guarner L, De Gracia J, Malagelada J-R. Gastrointestinal, liver, and pancreatic involvement in adult patients with cystic fibrosis. *Pancreas* 2001;22:395–399.

Modolell I, Guarner L, Malagelada J-R. Digestive system involvement in cystic fibrosis. *Pancreatology* 2002;2:12–16.

Noone PG, Zhou Z, Silverman LM, Jowell PS, Knowles MR, Cohn JA. Cystic fibrosis gene mutations and pancreatitis risk: relation to epithelial ion transport and trypsin inhibitor gene mutations. *Gastroenterology* 2001;121:1310–1319.

Ockenga J, Stuhrmann M, Ballmann M et al. Mutations of the cystic fibrosis gene, but not cationic trypsinogen gene, are associated with recurrent or chronic idiopathic pancreatitis. *Am J Gastroenterol* 2000;95:2061–2067.

Powell CJ. Colonic toxicity from pancreatins: a contemporary safety issue. *Lancet* 1999;353:911–915.

Ratjen F, Döring G. Cystic fibrosis. *Lancet* 2003;361:681–689.

Rosenstein BJ, Cutting GR for the Cystic Fibrosis Foundation Consensus Panel. The diagnosis of cystic fibrosis: a consensus statement. *J Pediatr* 1998;132:589–595.

Sharer N, Schwarz M, Malone G et al. Mutations of the cystic fibrosis gene in patients with chronic pancreatitis. *N Engl J Med* 1998;339:645–652.

Smyth RL, Van Velzen D, Smyth AR, Lloyd DA, Heaf DP. Strictures of ascending colon in cystic fibrosis and high-strength pancreatic enzymes. *Lancet* 1994;343:85–86.

Smyth RL, Ashby D, O'Hea U *et al.* Fibrosing colonopathy in cystic fibrosis: results of a case control study. *Lancet* 1995;346:1247–1251.

Stevens JC, Maguiness KM, Hollingsworth J, Heilman DK, Chong SKF. Pancreatic enzyme supplementation in cystic fibrosis patients before and after fibrosing colonopathy. *J Pediatr Gastroenterol Nutr* 1998;26:80–84.

Suarez L, Maiz L, Escobar H. Fibrosis quística. Tratamiento y pronóstico. In: S Navarro, M Perez-Mateo, L Guarner (eds) *Tratado de Páncreas Exocrino.* Barcelona: J&C Ediciones Médicas, 2002: 476–483.

Thiruvengadam R, Di Magno EP. Inactivation of human lipase by proteases. *Am J Physiol* 1988;18:G476–G481.

37 Management of exocrine pancreatic insufficiency associated with other clinical conditions: gastrointestinal surgery, diabetes mellitus, AIDS

Julio Iglesias-García

Exocrine pancreatic function after gastrointestinal surgery

The most important role of the stomach, apart from initiating digestion through the action of pepsin and hydrochloric acid, is to provide the duodenum with nutrient particles small enough (< 2 mm) and at the optimum rate to facilitate the digestive action of biliopancreatic secretions and duodenal enzymes and the absorption of digestion products. Gastric emptying is controlled by fundic distension, antral contractility, and pyloric motor activity. Two main reflexes coordinate these functions: antro-fundic reflexes (fundic distension in response to the presence of nutrients in the antrum) and duodeno-gastric reflexes (fundic distension and inhibition of antral motility in response to the presence of nutrients in the duodenum). Only when nutrient particles become smaller than 2 mm are they able to pass through the pylorus and advance into the duodenum in a slow and progressive way, making possible the digestive action of pancreatic secretion. Pancreatic secretion is stimulated by fundic distension (vagal stimulus) and release of cholecystokinin (CCK) (hormonal stimulus). CCK is released in response to CCK-releasing peptide, which is produced by the duodenal mucosa in response to the presence of nutrients, basically lipids, in the lumen (Fig. 37.1).

Alteration of any of these mechanisms due to anatomic changes after gastric, duodenal, and/or pancreatic surgery involves alterations in the digestive process.

Changes in digestive physiology after total or partial gastrectomy

Total or partial gastric resection eliminates the control that the stomach exerts on the arrival of nutrients in the duodenum with regard to both emptying rate and particle size. Antral resection is succeeded by the following.

- Loss of the antro-fundic reflex hinders the accommodation of nutrients in the gastric cavity and eliminates vagally mediated pancreatic stimulation.
- Loss of food-grinding capacity results in nutrient particles of a size not easy to digest by pancreatic and biliary secretions.
- The absence of a pylorus allows large particles, which cannot be properly digested, to pass into the intestinal lumen.
- In the case of Billroth II anastomosis, the duodenum is excluded from the transit of nutrients, making adequate release of CCK impossible and therefore reducing postprandial hormonal pancreatic stimulation.
- In the case of Billroth II anastomosis, there is also a lack of coordination between the arrival of nutrients and biliopancreatic secretion into the jejunum, so that it is impossible to achieve a correct mixture of nutrients and digestive enzymes.

All this explains the existence of secondary exocrine pancreatic insufficiency in patients after total or partial gastrectomy. There is also a marked reduction in exogenously stimulated pancreatic secretion (by intravenous secretin and cerulein), with a decrease of 74–92% in en-

Table 37.1 Frequency of steatorrhea in patients after surgical procedures on the pancreatic gland as reported in the literature.

Surgical procedure	Frequency of steatorrhea before surgery (%)	Frequency of steatorrhea after surgery (%)
Duodenopancreatectomy (Whipple)	5	55
Pylorus-preserving duodenopancreatectomy	4	64
Distal resection (40–80%)	3	19
Distal resection (80–95%)	9	38
Pancreaticojejunostomy	19	33

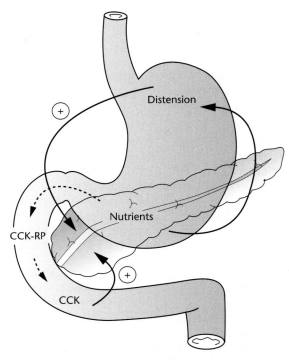

Figure 37.1 Control mechanism of postprandial exocrine pancreatic function. CCK, cholecystokinin; CCK-RP, cholecystokinin-releasing peptide.

Changes in digestive physiology after cephalic duodenopancreatectomy

In addition to the changes secondary to partial gastrectomy, duodenal resection hinders normal postprandial secretion of CCK, so that even though nutrients in the jejunum are able to stimulate pancreatic secretion, postprandial stimulation of this secretion is clearly decreased. Duodenectomy abolishes the fine control mechanism of gastric emptying, stimulation of biliopancreatic secretions, and the mixing of nutrient particles with digestive enzymes. This mixing is incomplete and occurs in distal segments of the gut, where the area for digestion and thus nutrient absorption are reduced.

Resection of the head of the pancreas induces an even more significant decrease in gland secretion. However, cephalic duodenopancreatectomy with preservation of the pylorus maintains the integrity of the antro-fundic reflex and therefore of exocrine pancreatic secretion mediated by the vagus. The antral function of grinding particles and the pyloric function of filtering large particles are also maintained. Even so, 64% of patients develop maldigestion with steatorrhea after this intervention (Table 37.1).

The development of bacterial overgrowth, due to the creation of an excluded upper jejunal loop and to reduction of gastric acid secretion, may contribute to the development of maldigestion after gastric and/or duodenopancreatic surgery.

Another important factor in the pathogenesis of maldigestion associated with gastrointestinal and pancreatic surgery is the negative feedback on pancreatic secretion mediated by the presence of nutrients in the ileum. As a consequence of all the aforementioned mechanisms, a significant quantity of nutrients reaches the ileal lumen, which activates contraregulatory mechanisms and inhibits pancreatic secretion, thereby aggravating maldigestion in such patients.

zyme and bicarbonate secretion with respect to levels prior to surgery. These facts define the existence of a primary postsurgical pancreatic insufficiency probably secondary to surgical denervation. All these alterations explain the presence of maldigestion in gastrectomized patients.

Changes in digestive physiology after distal pancreatic resection and after derivative surgery (lateral pancreatojejunostomy)

Resection of the distal pancreas does not affect gastroduodenal control of gastric emptying, biliopancreatic secretion, and nutrient mixing with digestive enzymes. However, loss of pancreatic parenchyma induces a diminution in the secretory capacity of the gland which, logically, depends on the extent of the resection: gland resections of less than 80% induce steatorrhea in only 20% of cases, whereas resections greater than 80% induce steatorrhea in around 40% of cases (Table 37.1).

Lateral pancreatojejunostomy constitutes a model of pancreatic–digestive asynchrony without gland or gastrointestinal resection. In these cases, even though the procedure does not alter gastroduodenal physiology or achieve pancreatic resection, the fact that pancreatic secretions drain directly into the jejunal loop produces maldigestion, with steatorrhea in one-third of these patients.

Evaluation of pancreatic function after pancreatic and gastrointestinal surgery

In operated patients it is essential to adopt a global approach to the digestive process, in order to determine the necessity for enzyme substitution treatment and to control its efficacy. In this sense, the optimized pancreolauryl test is probably too sensitive: almost every patient with partial or total gastrectomy and all patients with cephalic duodenopancreatectomy have an altered result in this test. In this group of operated patients, performing a direct test such as the secretin–cerulein test entails important methodologic problems, basically because of the difficulty of placing the probe correctly and the absence of method standardization. This is why fecal elastase quantification may be the best option in these patients. Fecal fat quantification, measured by the van de Kamer standard method or the newer near-infrared analysis, seems to be satisfactory in this setting. Our group has recently developed an optimized breath test with mixed triglyceride labeled with ^{13}C for the diagnosis of exocrine pancreatic insufficiency in chronic pancreatitis and in patients after gastrointestinal surgery, which shows great sensitivity and specificity compared with the classic fecal fat quantification. It is therefore a good alternative and easier to perform in clinical practice.

Treatment of maldigestion after gastrointestinal and/or pancreatic surgery

Every operated patient with fecal fat excretion greater than 15 g/day should be treated with oral pancreatic enzymes. There is also no discussion about the necessity of treating patients with a smaller degree of steatorrhea but with associated symptoms (weight loss, diarrhea, or dyspeptic symptoms). However, the necessity of treating patients with asymptomatic steatorrhea (< 15 g/day) is not clear. In our experience, substitution treatment is recommended because of the harmlessness of pancreatic enzymes and the high risk of developing nutritional deficits (liposoluble vitamins, trace elements) even if patients remain asymptomatic. Therefore, the majority of patients with partial or total gastrectomy, or with derivative or resective pancreatic surgery, should receive enzyme substitution treatment.

There are few studies comparing different enzyme preparations in patients after gastrointestinal and/or pancreatic surgical procedures. Enteric-coated pancreatic enzymes have proved to be effective in reducing steatorrhea in patients who undergo classic cephalic duodenopancreatectomy (Whipple's procedure) but less so in cases of preservation of pylorus or duodenum. In cases of stomach integrity, association with a proton pump inhibitor may be useful in increasing treatment efficacy. Patients suspected of having rapid intestinal transit, but who continue to exhibit steatorrhea despite correct substitution treatment, may benefit from drugs such as loperamide, which decreases intestinal transit time. The doses of enzymes required to treat fat maldigestion in surgical patients are similar to those employed in chronic pancreatitis. An important point is the optimization of substitution treatment by selecting the optimal dose of oral pancreatic enzymes. The classic method is by means of fecal fat quantification, using the same diagnostic methods described above (van de Kamer test, near-infrared analysis). Another alternative is the optimized breath test with mixed triglyceride, which is easier to apply in clinical routine. Figure 37.2 summarizes a protocol for the treatment of these patients.

Exocrine pancreatic function in diabetes mellitus

Endocrine and exocrine pancreatic tissues are closely related, both physiologically and anatomically. Patho-

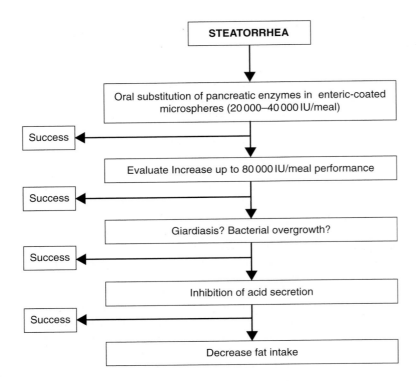

Figure 37.2 Algorithm for the treatment of steatorrhea in patients after gastric resection and/or duodenopancreatectomy.

logic conditions in exocrine tissue can induce alterations in endocrine function and vice versa. In diabetic patients, the pancreas is usually smaller, mainly related to involution of the exocrine pancreas. In patients suffering from juvenile diabetes, the pancreas is usually atrophic and fibrotic, with fatty infiltration and loss of acinar cells. Changes in exocrine tissue seem to be more pronounced in insulin-dependent diabetes mellitus (IDDM). In fact, nearly 50% of diabetic patients have pancreatic fibrosis and pathologic findings are more than twice as frequent as in controls.

Functional changes in exocrine pancreas in diabetes mellitus

There are several studies demonstrating impairment of pancreatic function in diabetic patients. Early reports in patients with diabetes mellitus suggested that exocrine pancreatic insufficiency occurred in both IDDM and noninsulin-dependent diabetes mellitus (NIDDM) (Table 37.2). Impairment of exocrine secretion diag-

nosed by secretin–cerulein test has been reported in 40–80% of cases.

The availability of an easily manageable pancreatic function test, such as the fecal elastase-1 test, promoted further research. These studies revealed that a significant number of patients with both types of diabetes have reduced fecal elastase-1. One study of over 400 diabetic patients showed impairment of exocrine pancreatic function (measured by fecal elastase) in 59% of NIDDM patients and also in 59% of IDDM patients. The largest study, including 536 patients with matched controls, showed that 11.8% of NIDDM patients had fecal elastase-1 levels below 100 µg/g compared with 3.8% of controls. Even though this test has poor sensitivity for mild exocrine pancreatic insufficiency, about 10% of patients had reduced fecal elastase levels characteristic of severe exocrine pancreatic insufficiency. In cases of NIDDM, exocrine pancreatic dysfunction seems to be less frequent than in IDDM, but is still much more frequent than in controls.

Table 37.2 Impairment of exocrine pancreatic function in diabetes mellitus.

Study	No. of patients	Patients with pancreatic dysfunction (%)	Test used
IDDM			
Frier (1976)	20	80	Secretin–CCK
Lankisch *et al.* (1982)	53	43	Secretin–CCK
Hardt (2000)	114*	57	Fecal elastase
Rathmann (2001)	112	26	Fecal elastase
NIDDM			
Hardt (2000)	114*	35	Fecal elastase
Icks (2001)	544	12	Fecal elastase

CCK, cholecystokinin; IDDM, insulin-dependent diabetes mellitus; NIDDM, noninsulin-dependent diabetes mellitus.
* Includes total (both IDDM and NIDDM).

Pathophysiologic concepts for exocrine dysfunction in diabetes mellitus

There are several hypotheses to explain these findings, the most important being the following:
• a deficit of insulin, which can induce atrophy of the gland;
• islet hormones have regulatory functions for exocrine tissue, and this may be impaired in patients suffering from diabetes mellitus;
• autonomic neuropathy may lead to impaired enteropathic reflexes, inducing pancreatic dysfunction;
• diabetic microangiopathy produces ischemic lesions, leading to pancreatic fibrosis and exocrine atrophy.
Even so, all these alterations do not satisfactorily explain the changes found in the pancreas of diabetic patients.

Other pathogenic concepts involve an autoimmune process (presence of autoantibodies against exocrine tissue) or viral infection leading to pancreatic gland destruction. All these hypotheses are under discussion as it is impossible at present to establish the exact mechanism that explains the pathogenesis of exocrine dysfunction and diabetes mellitus.

Management of exocrine pancreatic insufficiency in diabetic patients

The clinical spectrum seen in patients presenting with exocrine pancreatic insufficiency and diabetes mellitus is highly variable. It is frequent to find patients with some difficulties controlling glucose levels, with high levels of glycosylated hemoglobin, and requiring continuous modifications of insulin treatment, due to abnormal and variable absorption of different nutrients. Severe diabetic ketoacidosis or hypoglycemic coma has been described in relation to exocrine pancreatic insufficiency. However, in other cases it is possible to find the characteristic clinical picture of steatorrhea with diarrhea and noxious fatty stools, weight loss, and several other clinical manifestations related to malnutrition.

The methods used to study and evaluate pancreatic function in diabetic patients do not differ from those used in chronic pancreatitis or in cases of gastrointestinal and pancreatic surgery. It is possible to evaluate pancreatic function by studying pancreatic enzymes in feces, mainly pancreatic elastase, which is highly stable in the intestinal lumen, with concentrations in stool up to five times higher than in pancreatic secretions. Enzyme concentration is measured by enzme-linked immunosorbent assay (ELISA), without the problems related to potential inactivation of the enzyme during intestinal transit. The accuracy of this test in diagnosing pancreatic insufficiency is higher than the fecal chymotrypsin test. Because of its high efficacy and noninvasiveness, this test should be considered as the best option for detecting exocrine pancreatic insufficiency in this group of diabetic patients. Nevertheless, it must be taken into account that the fecal elastase test has not been validated for diabetic patients. Fecal fat quantification for diagnosing steatorrhea is also very important, because it enables precise control of substitution treatment with oral pancreatic enzymes. The optimized breath test with ^{13}C-labeled mixed triglycerides, mentioned above, is another alternative, permitting the evaluation of exocrine pancreatic function in a rapid noninvasive way with high accuracy, enabling its use in controlling substitution treatment.

The oral pancreatic enzymes used in this group of patients do not differ from the ones used in the treatment of pancreatic insufficiency secondary to chronic pancreatitis.

Based on all the aforementioned aspects, treatment with oral pancreatic enzymes in diabetic patients with proven exocrine pancreatic insufficiency should lead to an increase in body weight and normalization of nutritional status, with better management of glycemic homeostasis. In young patients, normalization of general development could also be attained. However, there are no data supporting enzyme supplementation in all diabetic patients regardless of their exocrine pancreatic function. It is very important that in diabetic patients suspected of suffering from exocrine pancreatic insufficiency, a minimal diagnostic work-up be employed to detect other causes of diarrhea.

Exocrine pancreatic function in AIDS

Intestinal malabsorption of nutrients has been reported in symptomatic human immunodeficiency virus (HIV) infection, in both adults and children. In these patients the intestinal mucosa is damaged, frequently showing villous atrophy and crypt hypertrophy. Although these findings may partially explain the malabsorption syndrome, morphologic changes in small intestinal mucosa often appear insufficient to explain severe malabsorption in HIV-infected patients. Another important point in this context may be an exocrine pancreatic insufficiency related, somehow, to pancreatic involvement. An autopsy study in HIV-infected children showed pancreatic abnormality in about 85% of cases, without any clear clinical manifestation of pancreatic disease, suggesting primary pancreatic involvement in HIV syndrome. Functional studies have demonstrated a high incidence of abnormalities in HIV-infected patients. Few papers have been published evaluating pancreatic function and fat absorption in HIV-infected patients. Some of these studies used the

tyrosil-p-aminobenzoic acid (PABA) test, showing a low percentage (10%) of patients with mild exocrine pancreatic insufficiency. More recently, newer studies have evaluated pancreatic function by applying more sensitive tests, such as fecal elastase concentration. One of these, which included 35 patients, showed that at least half of HIV-infected patients had some degree of pancreatic dysfunction. Overall, steatorrhea has been found in up to 26% of HIV-infected children and in up to 71% of adults. Generally, not less than 30% of patients have steatorrhea because of pancreatic dysfunction. However, the pathogenesis of steatorrhea in HIV-infected patients is probably multifactorial; in fact, intestinal malabsorption constitutes a determining factor of steatorrhea. Consequently, some patients had fat malabsorption due mainly to intestinal problems; however, these patients may have had a concomitant pancreatic insufficiency that worsened maldigestion.

It is difficult to establish the best test to evaluate exocrine pancreatic insufficiency in HIV-infected patients, mainly due to the unknown pathogenesis of malabsorption syndrome in these patients. In fact, there are only a few published data about the routine use of functional tests in these patients, using the PABA and fecal elastase tests. It would be useful to evaluate the alternatives of fecal fat quantification and breath test with mixed triglycerides, the only problem being that they can be altered by damaged intestinal mucosa.

The oral pancreatic enzymes used for treatment in HIV-infected patients do not differ much from the ones used in other cases of exocrine pancreatic insufficiency. Supplementation therapy with oral pancreatic enzymes has shown to reduce, or even abolish, fat malabsorption in HIV-infected patients. One published study demonstrated that during treatment, steatocrit values decrease significantly. It has recently been demonstrated that the severity of steatorrhea and improvement in fat absorption with substitution treatment are related to the severity of HIV disease. Thus, the more severe the clinical condition, the more severe the steatorrhea and the greater the improvement in fat absorption on pancreatic enzyme treatment. The efficacy of substitution treatment was not limited to patients with pancreatic dysfunction, so that oral pancreatic enzymes probably also modify the intestinal environment producing, for instance, a direct effect against bacterial overgrowth, with a positive effect on intestinal absorption.

In relation to symptoms derived from maldigestion,

pancreatic enzyme supplementation therapy may reduce stool fat loss, but only cures diarrhea in a minority of cases. Thus, pancreatic supplementation therapy may be useful in reducing stool fat loss, but only cures diarrhea in a minority of cases.

Finally, it must be remembered that the introduction of the new highly active antiretroviral therapy, which has been shown to significantly improve intestinal function in HIV-infected patients, may change the management of these patients, and the effectiveness of pancreatic enzyme treatment would then have to be reevaluated.

Recommended reading

Bruno MJ, Borm JJJ, Hoek FJ et al. Comparative effects of enteric-coated pancreatin microsphere therapy after conventional and pylorus-preserving pancreatoduodenectomy. Br J Surg 1997;84:952–956.

Büchler M, Malfertheiner P, Glasbrenner B, Friess H, Beger H. Secondary pancreatic insufficiency following partial and total gastrectomy. Nutrition 1988;4:314–316.

Caroccio A, Di Prima L, Di Grigoli C et al. Exocrine pancreatic function and fat malabsorption in human immunodeficiency virus-infected patients. Scand J Gastroenterol 1999;34:729–734.

Caroccio A, Guarino A, Zuin G et al. Efficacy of oral pancreatic enzyme therapy for the treatment of fat malabsorption in HIV-infected patients. Aliment Pharmacol Ther 2001;15:1619–1625.

Frier BM, Saunders JHB, Wormsley KG, Bouchier IAD. Exocrine pancreatic function in juvenile-onset diabetes mellitus. Gut 1976;17:685–691.

Friess H, Böhm J, Müller MW et al. Maldigestion after total gastrectomy is associated with pancreatic insufficiency. Am J Gastroenterol 1996;91:341–347.

Gröger G, Layer P. Exocrine pancreatic function in diabetes mellitus. Eur J Gastroenterol Hepatol 1995;7: 740–746.

Hardt PD, Krauss A, Bretz L et al. Pancreatic exocrine function in patients with type 1 and type 2 diabetes mellitus. Acta Diabetol 2000;37:105–110.

Icks A, Haastert B, Giani G, Rathmann W. Low fecal elastase-1 in type 1 diabetes mellitus. Z Gastroenterol 2001;39:823–830.

Lankisch PG, Manthey G, Otto J, Taulicar M, Willms B, Creutzfeldt W. Exocrine pancreatic function in insulin-dependent diabetes mellitus. Digestion 1982;25:210–216.

Rathmann W, Haastert B, Icks A et al. Low fecal elastase 1 concentrations in type 2 diabetes mellitus. Scand J Gastroenterol 2001;36:1056–1061.

38 Indications and timing of surgery in chronic pancreatitis

Werner Hartwig, Jens Werner, Markus W. Büchler, and Waldemar Uhl

Chronic pancreatitis is a benign inflammatory process of the pancreas characterized by progressive destruction of the gland with increasing fibrosis and disturbance of exocrine and endocrine function as a result of chronic inflammation. Chronic pancreatitis is associated with a mortality rate that approaches 50% within 20–25 years. Approximately 15–20% of patients die of complications associated with the disease, and most of the remaining deaths are due to factors such as trauma, malnutrition, infection, or tobacco abuse, which are frequently present among chronic alcoholics.

Chronic pancreatitis is not primarily a surgical disease. Nevertheless, surgeons will find themselves confronted by patients referred to them in the hope that there is surgical help for the agonizing symptoms of this disease. The predominant symptom of chronic pancreatitis is intractable upper abdominal pain, which affects over 85% of patients. Refractory to analgesics, pain persists in 85% and 55% of conservatively managed patients 5 and 10 years after diagnosis respectively. Other symptoms of chronic pancreatitis are those associated with exocrine and endocrine insufficiency. Exocrine pancreatic insufficiency occurs 10–20 years after onset of the disease and causes steatorrhea, malabsorption, weight loss, and subsequently cachexia. Manifestation of endocrine insufficiency with non-insulin- or insulin-dependent diabetes mellitus occurs later since the endocrine pancreas is more resistant to damage. Furthermore, chronic pancreatitis is frequently associated with disease-related complications of the organs neighboring the pancreas. These complications arise from either pseudocysts or an inflammatory pancreatic mass, which is often localized in the head of the pancreas. Such a mass may lead to compression of the portal or splenic vein, obstruction of the duodenum, stenosis of the common bile duct, and obstruction of the main pancreatic duct.

The adequate treatment of patients with chronic pancreatitis mandates an interdisciplinary approach of general physicians, gastroenterologists, and surgeons. The aim of this chapter is to clarify when and why in the course of chronic pancreatitis the general physician or the gastroenterologist should refer their patient to a surgeon to optimize therapy. The surgical procedures available for the treatment of this disease are outlined accordingly.

Indications for surgery

The treatment of chronic pancreatitis is primarily the field of general physicians and gastroenterologists, with severe abdominal pain as the domain of conservative measures. However, it is well known that as many as 50% of all patients with chronic pancreatitis will ultimately require surgical treatment, because conservative medical treatment cannot halt the progression of pain, exocrine and endocrine insufficiency, or pancreatitis-associated complications. It is when medical treatment fails that many patients are finally referred to the surgeon. At this time, patients are often addicted to narcotics, with their general and nutritional condition widely deteriorated. There are reports that surgery can have a positive influence on the progression of the disease, postponing the final "burn-out" of the pancreas which is characterized by exocrine and endocrine insufficiency. The concept of waiting for the final "burn-out," which in some cases may be associated with a

Table 38.1 Indications for surgery in chronic pancreatitis.

Intractable pain
Complications of fibrosis/pancreatic mass on neighboring
  structures
  Pancreatic duct stenosis
  Biliary obstruction
  Duodenal obstruction
  Splenic and/or portal vein obstruction
  Colonic obstruction
Complications of pseudocysts
  Persistent or symptomatic pseudocysts
  Pancreatic ascites and/or pleural effusion
  Pancreatic fistula
Suspicion of pancreatic carcinoma

decrease of pain, should no longer be a desirable treatment modality, since the morbidity and mortality of pancreatic surgery have decreased substantially in the last decades. Therefore, treatment of chronic pancreatitis should include an interdisciplinary approach to ensure optimized conservative treatment, endoscopic and interventional procedures, and surgery.

Surgery in chronic pancreatitis has to be directed at the following main objectives:

- to ameliorate pain;
- to treat local complications;
- to preserve or improve exocrine and endocrine function.

The indications for surgery in chronic pancreatitis are listed in Table 38.1 and are discussed in detail in the following section. The surgical interventions and, most importantly in the evaluation of treatment strategies, their long-term results, are outlined accordingly.

Pain

Severe abdominal pain is the dominant clinical symptom of chronic pancreatitis and the single most important indication for treatment of patients with this condition. Pain significantly affects quality of life, leads to drug addiction, and results in malnutrition because the patient is afraid to eat. The exact pathogenesis of pain in chronic pancreatitis is still not known, although various hypotheses based on pathomorphologic findings have been established. Two in particular are compelling. First, the duct pressure–pain hypothesis proposes that increased intraductal and intraparenchymal pressure due to distal compression or stenosis of the pancreatic duct causes pain. The second, which incorporates the increasing evidence from molecular biological and genetic research in recent years, proposes the concept of alterations in pancreatic nerves due to a persistent inflammatory process. Based on these mechanisms, two types of surgical intervention have been established: drainage and resection procedures. Recently, newer surgical approaches in chronic pancreatitis have been designed that combine the principles of these two techniques.

Patients with intractable pain not responding to medical treatment who are referred to a surgeon should first be considered for a drainage procedure in an attempt to preserve exocrine and endocrine pancreatic function. Pancreatic ducts identified as larger than 7 mm in diameter by endoscopic retrograde cholangiopancreatography (ERCP) or magnetic resonance cholangiopancreatography (MRCP) are amendable to successful decompression by an internal drainage operation. This approach is based on the assumption that pain relief is obtained by drainage of the dilated main pancreatic duct, thereby decreasing intrapancreatic ductal and parenchymal pressure. Lateral pancreaticojejunostomy, described by Puestow and Gillesby and subsequently modified by Partington and Rochelle, became the first surgical treatment widely considered to be effective for pain in chronic pancreatitis. This technique is associated with very low operative morbidity and mortality, and preserves endocrine and exocrine function. Unfortunately, while short-term pain relief is achieved in 80–90%, only 50–60% of patients remain pain-free at 5 years after operation. Therefore, lateral pancreaticojejunostomy should only be applied when a concomitant inflammatory mass in the pancreatic head cannot be detected. Otherwise, this mass, which is frequently associated with neuropathic changes and with alterations in organs neighboring the pancreas, may compromise adequate drainage of the main pancreatic duct in the long term and may result in the failure of the drainage procedure.

Patients with pain whose ducts are not dilated are not considered good candidates for drainage procedures. In these patients, resection procedures were started in the 1960s, assuming that pain is caused by the inflammatory process in the pancreas. Initially, distal pancreatectomies were performed with poor results regarding pain relief. Later, distal subtotal resections (95% of the

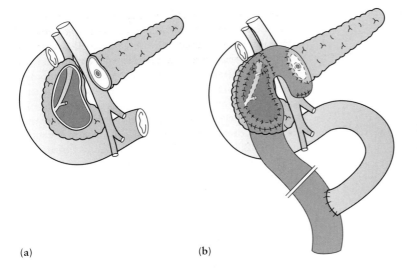

(a) (b)

Figure 38.1 Duodenum-preserving pancreatic head resection according to the Beger technique. (a) After resection of the chronically inflamed pancreatic head. (b) After reconstruction with a jejunal Roux-Y-loop with two anastomoses: (i) end-to-side pancreaticojejunal anastomosis, and (ii) side-to-side pancreaticojejunal anastomosis.

pancreas) were more effective for pain but rendered most patients diabetic. Today, the presence of a large pseudocyst in the tail, or the presence of a predominant inflammatory mass in the left pancreas, are the only indications for pancreatic left resection with good outcomes.

In patients with pancreatic head complications, the classical Whipple resection (pancreaticoduodenectomy), successfully performed first by Walter Kausch in 1909 and later reintroduced and further developed by Allen Oldfather Whipple, then became the standard operation in chronic pancreatitis for many years. Although the Whipple resection provides pain relief in up to 85% of patients, long-term results, especially with regard to quality of life, are poor. Postoperative digestive dysfunction, including gastric dumping, diarrhea, peptic ulcer, and dyspeptic complaints, may originate in the extended resection of organs not affected by the inflammatory process (lesser part of the stomach, duodenum and upper part of jejunum, and extrahepatic bile duct). Preserving the stomach, pylorus, and first part of the duodenum, the pylorus-preserving pancreaticoduodenectomy protects against gastric dumping, bile reflux, and marginal ulceration, and has provided better postoperative quality of life in some studies. Unfortunately, this technique is associated with postoperative delayed gastric emptying in 30–50% of patient. Keeping in mind that both the classical Whipple operation and the pylorus-preserving pancreaticoduo-

denectomy were originally designed to treat malignant disease, surgical approaches better suited for the treatment of chronic pancreatitis have been introduced in recent years.

Taking note of the drawbacks of existing surgical techniques for chronic pancreatitis, the duodenum-preserving pancreatic head resection was introduced by Beger *et al.* in 1972 (Fig. 38.1). By subtotal resection of the pancreatic head and by preserving the body and tail of the pancreas, pylorus, duodenum, and extrahepatic bile ducts, this operation preserves the normal anatomy of the upper gut and the normal passage of food through the stomach and the duodenum. The intention of the operation is to treat only the enlarged pancreatic head and to preserve the duodenum, with its crucial role in the regulation of digestion and glucose metabolism. This operation is indicated in patients suffering from intractable pain in combination with an inflammatory mass in the head of the pancreas, common bile duct obstruction, pancreatic duct obstruction, and/or obstruction of the retropancreatic vessels. In the hands of an experienced surgeon, this procedure is characterized by low morbidity and mortality (perioperative mortality almost nil), effective long-term pain relief in more than 80% of patients after a median of 5 years' follow-up, and low incidence rate of endocrine insufficiency.

Combining the two surgical principles of drainage and organ-preserving resection, Frey and Smith intro-

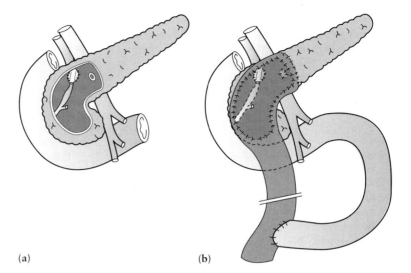

Figure 38.2 Duodenum-preserving pancreatic head resection according to the Bern technique. (a) After resection of the chronically inflamed pancreatic head, without cutting the gland in the isthmus. (b) After reconstruction with a jejunal Roux-Y-loop with side-to-side pancreaticojejunal anastomosis, including the bile duct.

(a)   (b)

duced a modification of the duodenum-preserving pancreatic head resection: longitudinal pancreaticojejunostomy with a local pancreatic head resection. This procedure seems comparable to the Beger operation. A randomized trial demonstrated comparable results concerning pain relief, control of complications in adjacent organs, postoperative quality of life, and preservation of exocrine and endocrine pancreatic function. The only difference found was a significantly lower postoperative morbidity with the Frey procedure. Therefore, both procedures are similarly effective and safe in the treatment of chronic pancreatitis.

By trying to combine the advantages of the Beger and the Frey procedures, Büchler and coworkers described a modified technique that allows resection of the pancreatic head without transection of the gland over the superior mesenteric vein (Fig. 38.2). Leaving behind only a thin bridge of pancreatic tissue in the dorsal aspect of the gland, the risk of bleeding complications can be minimized (advantageous in patients with portal hypertension), whereas radical excision of the pancreatic head with opening of the common bile duct (if necessary) can still be performed. In cases of multiple stenosis in the left-sided main pancreatic duct, a longitudinal incision of the duct with reconstruction by a longitudinal pancreaticojejunostomy can be added. Future prospective trials have to evaluate the long-term results of this modified technique.

Pancreatic duct stenosis

With respect to pancreatic duct morphology, ERCP or MRCP identifies two groups of chronic pancreatitis: normal/small-duct disease (2–5 mm) and large-duct disease (> 7 mm). The various forms of drainage procedures for large-duct pancreatitis have been described above. In small-duct disease, drainage procedures are not applicable, since the whole pancreas is infested by fibrosis and scarring. These patients are candidates for pancreatic resection. In most patients, the disease is most severe in the head of the pancreas. Surgical options include the Whipple procedure with or without preservation of the pylorus or the various techniques of duodenum-preserving pancreatic head resection. Izbicki and coworkers have recently described a technique combining drainage and local resection to treat the small-duct form of chronic pancreatitis. A longitudinal V-shaped excision of the ventral pancreas followed by drainage of the secondary and tertiary branches using longitudinal pancreaticojejunostomy has shown promising results in a small patient group. However, long-term results are not available yet.

Patients with pancreatic duct obstruction caused by an ampullary stenosis, strictures, or duct stones are often subjected to endoscopic transpapillary stenting. There are numerous reports suggesting that stents within the pancreatic duct relieve pain associated with chronic pancreatitis in the majority of patients. Others have shown limited benefit, with the need for additional surgery after stenting in 24% of patients or no benefit. However, since studies were not prospective, randomized, or blinded, valid data are missing. Therefore, prolonged stenting of the pancreatic duct in chronic pancreatitis should only be performed in specialized centers and in the setting of a clinical trial.

Biliary obstruction

Biliary obstruction in association with pain is the second most common indication for surgery, occurring in more than one-third of patients with advanced chronic pancreatitis. Unlike the abrupt cutoff as in malignant disease, common bile duct obstruction in chronic pancreatitis is characterized by a long tapered stricture, and almost always involves its intrapancreatic portion. Obstruction is usually due to fibrotic changes in the head of the pancreas extending into the wall of the duct, rather than to pressure by a pseudocyst. The earliest biochemical manifestation is the elevation of alkaline phosphatase and later the presence of jaundice. In the later course of the disease, jaundice is fixed and does not fluctuate or disappear. Such patients are at risk of cholangitis and, in the long term, of secondary biliary cirrhosis.

Endoscopic transpapillary drainage by means of a plastic stent may often be applied as the primary treatment of common bile duct stenosis associated with jaundice, although common bile duct stenting is successful in less than 30% of patients. In the long run, surgical procedures are necessary in those patients with persisting stenosis after stent removal. Repeated stent changes in the prolonged course of this benign disease are associated with numerous hospital admissions and encounter substantial morbidity.

Surgical therapy in patients with biliary obstruction has to address both the obstructed duct and the inflammatory process in the head of the pancreas. Overlooking a fibrotic stenosis of the bile duct is a pitfall when decompression or resection of a pancreatic pseudocyst or an inflammatory mass that has been blamed for the biliary compression is performed without a concurrent drainage procedure for the common bile duct. In patients with biliary obstruction, the duodenum-preserving pancreatic head resection, as described by Beger and adapted by Büchler, is perfectly suited to deal with the morphologic changes including the bile duct and the head of the pancreas. Procedures encouraging a bilioenteric bypass (e.g., hepaticojejunostomy utilizing a Roux-en-Y loop) will not suffice to achieve long-lasting pain relief, since resection of the underlying pain-inducing inflammatory process is not performed.

Duodenal obstruction

Symptomatic duodenal or biliary obstruction develops in 5–10% of patients with chronic pancreatitis. As published in a series of 58 patients by Warshaw, duodenal obstruction occurs almost exclusively in patients with large-duct disease and not in the small-duct form of chronic pancreatitis. Again, obstruction may be caused by a pseudocyst in the head of the pancreas or by direct spread of the fibroinflammatory process. Fibrotic and possibly ischemic changes in the duodenal wall, resulting in irreversible stenosis, are relatively rare. Importantly, other entities of duodenal stenosis, as caused by peptic ulcer disease for example, have to be excluded by endoscopy. Treatment of the duodenal stenosis can be directed at relieving the obstruction either by decompression of the pseudocyst or, most simply, by the creation of a gastrojejunostomy. However, since duodenal obstruction is rarely an isolated complication in chronic pancreatitis, a resection procedure including the mass or pseudocyst in the pancreatic head appears to provide the optimal solution in many cases.

Splenic and/or portal vein obstruction

In about 7–10% of patients with chronic pancreatitis, the portal or splenic vein is involved in the morphologic changes of the pancreas. As a result of inflammation, pseudocyst growth, or pancreatic mass formation, the compression or complete occlusion of the portal vein will result in thrombosis, portal hypertension, cavernous transformation of peripancreatic veins, and esophageal varices that may bleed. Whereas mild to moderate degrees of portal venous obstruction may be an indication for decompression (usually as part of an operation directed against other mechanical complications), such an operation is prohibitively hemorrhagic if there is complete thrombosis of the vein. For this reason, portal or superior mesenteric vein thrombosis with portal hypertension and cavernous transformation of the peripancreatic veins creates irremediable difficulties for pancreatic surgery, thus making complete resection of the pancreatic head dangerous and almost impossible. Some surgeons consider portal hypertension to be a contraindication to any procedure on the pancreas itself. However, performing a pancreatic head resection as described by Büchler with preservation of the dorsal aspect of pancreas, the risk of bleeding from the enlarged retropancreatic vessels is minimized.

In contrast, thrombosis confined to the splenic vein is no contraindication for surgery, since this is associated with a form of "segmental portal hypertension" that just creates gastric or esophageal varices. Splenectomy in these patients is effective in eliminating the risk of bleeding from these varices.

Colonic obstruction

Colonic obstruction by a pancreatic mass or pseudocyst is a rare complication of chronic pancreatitis. The obstruction may mimic colonic carcinoma but this can readily be excluded by colonoscopy. Bradley has published a series of 34 patients with strictures of the transverse colon and the splenic flexure, and concluded that when fibrosis and ischemia have caused irreversible mural changes and chronic ileus, this can only be relieved by segmental resection of the affected colon with end-to-end anastomosis. In cases of obstruction caused by pseudocysts, drainage procedures will result in relief of the narrowed colonic passage.

Persistent or symptomatic pseudocysts

Pancreatic pseudocysts are collections of pancreatic secretions surrounded by a nonepithelial-lined fibrous wall of granulation tissue. They develop in approximately 10–20% of patients with chronic pancreatitis. Pseudocysts may be asymptomatic and may resolve spontaneously. Enlarging pseudocysts, pseudocysts larger than 4–6 cm, or symptomatic pseudocysts inherit an increased risk of hemorrhage, rupture, infection, or compression of neighboring structures if left untreated. Rupture of pseudocysts or intracystic hemorrhage has been estimated to occur in 5–7% of patients, and can cause peritonitis or major intraabdominal or gastrointestinal bleeding, respectively. Massive hemorrhage into a pseudocyst, often from a branch of a splenic artery, requires emergency angiography and therapeutic embolization, followed by semielective operation with either resection or suture ligation of the bleeding point. Associated morbidity and mortality (bleeding accounts for 40–80% of deaths from chronic pseudocysts) exceeds by far the risks of elective surgery.

Therefore, elective surgery is generally the therapy of choice for patients with symptomatic pseudocysts or pseudocysts larger than 4–6 cm in diameter.

Surgical treatment options include internal drainage, external drainage, or resection procedures. The type of internal drainage depends on the location of the pseudocyst. Options include cystogastrostomy, cystoduodenostomy, and Roux-en-Y cystojejunostomy. For cysts located in the tail of the pancreas, distal pancreatectomy is often the best solution as long as functional pancreatic tissue can be spared. However, simple cyst drainage or cyst resection may not remove the underlying morphologic changes in the chronic inflamed pancreas. Thus, the remaining pancreatic duct obstruction or persisting pain may require additional drainage procedures or even resection.

Internal or external drainage may also be achieved endoscopically or in some form of interventional drainage. A transpapillary stent or the creation of a transgastric or transduodenal fistula by means of a plastic stent may be an alternative to surgical procedures. These interventional procedures are often performed repeatedly, even before the patient is seen by a surgeon. Recurrence of pseudocysts in these patients is high, and endoscopic procedures are not without risk. Most importantly, transendoscopic drainage assumes adherence between pseudocyst and the adjacent segment of intestine, which is present in only about 40% of cases. In the absence of such inflammatory adherence, separation of pseudocyst and enteric stoma may result in a high-risk, activated pancreaticoenteric fistula. Using external drainage by means of an indwelling catheter placed into the pseudocyst, resolution has been described for as many as 70% of cases when drainage exceeded 1 week. However, external drainage of pseudocysts may result in repeated infections or pancreatic fistula. Taking into account the increasing numbers of cystic neoplasms of the pancreas in recent reports, these interventional procedures carry the risk of draining a semimalignant or malignant cystic tumor that would otherwise have very good long-term survival rates when treated by radical resection. Using internal or external drainage techniques, it is imperative to ensure that the cystic structure to be drained is truly a pseudocyst and not a cystic neoplasm.

Pancreatic ascites and pleural effusion

Pancreatic juice can leak into the peritoneum from a

ruptured duct or pseudocyst, resulting in pancreatic ascites, or it can track into the pleural space, causing a pancreaticopleural fistula with pancreatic hydrothorax. Either one is a rare but significant complication in chronic pancreatitis, and both carry a mortality rate of around 20% if not treated adequately. The diagnosis is made by ultrasonography, paracentesis or thoracentesis (showing raised amylase and protein levels), and ERCP for the localization of the leak. Nonoperative methods, including repeated aspiration, parenteral nutrition, and the administration of octreotide to minimize pancreatic secretion, should be given a chance for about 2 weeks to cure patients. If pancreatic ascites persists, endoscopic or surgical intervention is indicated. Endoscopic stenting may offer a good alternative to surgery when the leak can accurately be localized by ERCP. However, most of these patients are treated surgically by anastomosis of a defunctionalized Roux-en-Y jejunal loop to the site of the fistula or by segmental pancreatic resection or left resection.

Pancreatic fistula

External pancreatic fistula most commonly occurs after pancreatic surgery or percutaneous external drainage of a pseudocyst, but is an unusual complication in the natural course of chronic pancreatitis. Pancreatic fistula must be suspected when clear fluid containing high concentrations of amylase drains from a cutaneous orifice after pancreatic intervention. Fistulas may drain up to 1 L of fluid per day. Most fistulas close spontaneously, providing that the general guidelines for the management of external gastrointestinal fistulas are followed. Octreotide can be used to decrease the volume of fistula drainage. However, there is no substantial proof that octreotide hastens the spontaneous closure of pancreatic fistulas. In cases where there is ductal obstruction between the site of the leak and the duodenum, surgery may be required to achieve fistula healing. This is most easily accomplished by a Roux-en-Y anastomosis with the jejunum over the opening where the leakage originates, a segmental pancreatic resection with both-sided anastomosis, or left resection if indicated.

Suspicion of malignancy

Confirming previous studies, recent reports indicate that pancreatic cancer develops in 2–3% of patients within 10 years and in roughly 4% within 20 years of diagnosis of chronic pancreatitis. The dilemma in chronic pancreatitis is the inability to exclude carcinoma preoperatively, even when modern imaging techniques like computed tomography, magnetic resonance imaging (MRI), or endoscopic ultrasound are applied. ERCP, in combination with toothbrush cytology, may be of value in some cases, with a sensitivity and specificity of toothbrush cytology of 20–25% and nearly 100% respectively. However, a stricture of the pancreatic duct of more than 10 mm, in the absence of ectatic side branches, should always suggest the presence of a malignant process. Also, fine-needle biopsy of a pancreatic process may add only limited information due to false-negative results, particularly when there is the problem of distinguishing a chronic inflammatory process associated with a pseudocyst from a cystic neoplasm of the pancreas. Furthermore, fine-needle aspiration is controversial because of possible tumor spread. Reflecting this problem, in many prospective series published on chronic pancreatitis, approximately 5–15% of patients were operated on because of the suspicion of carcinoma or inability to exclude a malignant origin of morphologic changes in the pancreas. To date, in about 95% of cases with chronic pancreatitis the diagnosis should be clear as a result of a careful work-up (including an all-in-one MRI), with a remaining risk of concomitant cancer in only 5% of patients. However, a surgeon's level of suspicion must always remain high as a pseudocyst or an inflammatory mass can masquerade as pancreatic carcinoma.

Timing of surgery

Almost no controversy exists about the timing of surgery in patients who present with local complications associated with chronic pancreatitis. Apart from complications due to pseudocysts, which may be observed for a few weeks in the hope of spontaneous resolution, surgery should be performed when complications are arising or are symptomatic. Endoscopic or interventional techniques may be of some help in the preoperative phase necessary to schedule the operation, for example in patients who present with severe jaundice and cholangitis due to biliary obstruction or in patients with bleeding from varices due to (segmental) portal hypertension. Surgery should not be delayed unnecessarily if there is the suspicion of malignancy in the chronic inflamed pancreas. In most other patients with chronic pancreatitis, however, the timing of surgery remains controversial.

The optimal timing of surgery in patients suffering severe pain is unclear. Pain may subside in the later course of chronic pancreatitis when the gland is globally insufficient ("burn-out" pancreas). Ammann *et al.* suggested that this may occur after a median time of 4.5 years from onset of symptoms. However, this expectation does not apply to the 50% of patients with persistently severe pain. Also Lankisch *et al.* confirmed a significant reduction of pain over time but found that more than 50% of patients still had significant pain after 10 years of observation. Despite exocrine insufficiency requiring enzyme replacement, 54% of alcoholics and 73% of nonalcoholics still experienced attacks of pain, and there was no reduction in pain with the development of endocrine insufficiency. In contrast, substantial long-term pain relief has been achieved by surgical intervention directed against an inflammatory mass or an enlarged pancreatic duct system. In a recent prospective long-term study (postoperative follow-up of 12.7 years), pain was definitely relieved by a single (drainage) procedure in approximately two-thirds of patients. Since these techniques are associated with low perioperative morbidity and mortality rates, surgical intervention should not only be regarded as the last opportunity to relieve intractable pain.

Recent studies suggest that the frequency of acute exacerbations in chronic pancreatitis can also be significantly reduced by surgery. In a study by Nealon *et al.* the mean rate of acute exacerbations was around six to seven events per year before surgery compared with one to two events per year after surgery. A similar finding was demonstrated in one of the largest single-center experiences ever published that included 504 patients with chronic pancreatitis who underwent duodenum-preserving pancreatic head resection. The frequency of hospital admissions for acute episodes decreased from 5.4 per patient before surgery to 2.7 after surgery. These results suggest that by changing the natural course of the disease, early surgical intervention is advantageous in the treatment of recurrent pain in chronic pancreatitis.

There is some evidence that surgery may also retard the progression of exocrine and endocrine insufficiency in chronic pancreatitis. In a series of 143 patients with chronic pancreatitis, deterioration of pancreatic function was slower in patients with dilated ducts treated by pancreatic duct drainage than in those with small-duct

disease treated nonoperatively. However, since this effect may also be due to differences in the patient population, this aspect is controversial. Based on recent publications, an interdisciplinary approach is recommended to define an individual treatment concept in patients with chronic pancreatitis. With regard to pancreatitis-associated complications, these may occur early or late in the disease progression. The optimal timing of surgery has to be defined accordingly.

Recommended reading

Ammann RW, Muellhaupt B. The natural history of pain in alcoholic chronic pancreatitis. *Gastroenterology* 1999; 116:1132–1140.

Bauer A, Uhl W, Tcholakov O, Wagner M, Friess H, Büchler MW. Pancreatic left resection in chronic pancreatitis: indications and limitations. In: MW Büchler, H Friess, W Uhl, P Malfertheiner (eds) *Chronic Pancreatitis: Novel Concepts in Biology and Therapy*. Oxford: Blackwell Science, 2002: 529–539.

Beger HG, Büchler M, Bittner RR, Oettinger W, Roscher R. Duodenum-preserving resection of the head of the pancreas in severe chronic pancreatitis. Early and late results. *Ann Surg* 1989;209:273–278.

Beger HG, Schlosser W, Friess HM, Büchler MW. Duodenum-preserving head resection in chronic pancreatitis changes the natural course of the disease: a single-center 26-year experience. *Ann Surg* 1999;230:512–519.

Bittner R, Butters M, Büchler M, Nagele S, Roscher R, Beger HG. Glucose homeostasis and endocrine pancreatic function in patients with chronic pancreatitis before and after surgical therapy. *Pancreas* 1994;9:47–53.

Bockman DE, Büchler M, Malfertheiner P, Beger HG. Analysis of nerves in chronic pancreatitis. *Gastroenterology* 1988;94:1459–1469.

Büchler M, Weihe E, Friess H *et al.* Changes in peptidergic innervation in chronic pancreatitis. *Pancreas* 1992;7: 183–192.

Ebbehoj N, Borly L, Bulow J *et al.* Pancreatic tissue fluid pressure in chronic pancreatitis. Relation to pain, morphology, and function. *Scand J Gastroenterol* 1990;25:1046–1051.

Frey CF, Smith GJ. Description and rationale of a new operation for chronic pancreatitis. *Pancreas* 1987;2:701–707.

Gloor B, Friess H, Uhl W, Büchler MW. A modified technique of the Beger and Frey procedure in patients with chronic pancreatitis. *Dig Surg* 2001;18:21–25.

Greenlee HB, Prinz RA, Aranha GV. Long-term results of side-to-side pancreaticojejunostomy. *World J Surg* 1990; 14:70–76.

Izbicki JR, Bloechle C, Knoefel WT *et al.* Drainage versus resection in surgical therapy of chronic pancreatitis of the head of the pancreas: a randomized study. *Chirurg* 1997;68: 369–377.

Izbicki JR, Bloechle C, Broering DC, Kuechler T, Broelsch CE. Longitudinal V-shaped excision of the ventral pancreas for small duct disease in severe chronic pancreatitis: prospective evaluation of a new surgical procedure. *Ann Surg* 1998;227:213–219.

Jalleh RP, Aslam M, Williamson RC. Pancreatic tissue and ductal pressures in chronic pancreatitis. *Br J Surg* 1991; 78:1235–1237.

Kahl S, Zimmermann S, Genz I *et al*. Risk factors for failure of endoscopic stenting of biliary strictures in chronic pancreatitis: a prospective follow-up study. *Am J Gastroenterol* 2003;98:2448–2453.

Lowenfels AB, Maisonneuve P, Cavallini G *et al*. Pancreatitis and the risk of pancreatic cancer. International Pancreatitis Study Group. *N Engl J Med* 1993;328:1433–1437.

Martin RF, Rossi RL, Leslie KA. Long-term results of pyloruspreserving pancreatoduodenectomy for chronic pancreatitis. *Arch Surg* 1996;131:247–252.

Nealon WH, Matin S. Analysis of surgical success in preventing recurrent acute exacerbations in chronic pancreatitis. *Ann Surg* 2001;233:793–800.

Nealon WH, Thompson JC. Progressive loss of pancreatic function in chronic pancreatitis is delayed by main pancreatic duct decompression. A longitudinal prospective analysis of the modified Puestow procedure. *Ann Surg* 1993;217:458–466.

Nealon WH, Townsend CMJ, Thompson JC. Operative drainage of the pancreatic duct delays functional impairment in patients with chronic pancreatitis. A prospective analysis. *Ann Surg* 1988;208:321–329.

Rattner DW, Fernandez-Del CC, Warshaw AL. Pitfalls of distal pancreatectomy for relief of pain in chronic pancreatitis. *Am J Surg* 1996;171:142–145.

Rosch T, Daniel S, Scholz M *et al*. Endoscopic treatment of chronic pancreatitis: a multicenter study of 1000 patients with long-term follow-up. *Endoscopy* 2002;34:765–771.

Sakorafas GH, Sarr MG, Farley DR, Farnell MB. The significance of sinistral portal hypertension complicating chronic pancreatitis. *Am J Surg* 2000;179:129–133.

Strasberg SM, Drebin JA, Soper NJ. Evolution and current status of the Whipple procedure: an update for gastroenterologists. *Gastroenterology* 1997;113:983–994.

Trede M, Carter DC. Preoperative assessment and indications for operation in chronic pancreatitis. In: M Trede, DC Carter (eds) *Surgery of the Pancreas*. Edinburgh: Churchill Livingstone, 1997: 313–328.

39 Surgical approaches to chronic pancreatitis: technical implications and outcome

Hans G. Beger, Bernd Mühling, Naoki Hiki, Zhengfei Zhou, Zhanbing Liu, and Bertram Poch

Chronic pancreatitis is an irreversible patchy inflammation of the pancreatic tissue that progresses to fibrosis due to duct changes subsequent to the necrotic–inflammatory processes in the pancreas. In industrialized countries, chronic alcoholic pancreatitis is the most frequent etiology; in Asian countries, the nutritional tropical pancreatitis prevails (Table 39.1). From a pathomorphologic point of view, patients with an inflammatory mass in the head of the pancreas frequently show focal necrotic lesions, small pseudocystic cavities, calcifications of the pancreatic parenchyma, and duct stones in the head area. Considering the head of the pancreas as the pacemaker, but not the cause, of chronic pancreatitis, the inflammatory mass in the head of the gland is the result of a variety of factors deriving from the anatomy (Table 39.2). In epidemiologic terms, chronic pancreatitis is a risk factor for the development of ductal pancreatic cancer. In the subset of patients suffering from chronic pancreatitis with an inflammatory mass, ductal pancreatic cancer was found in the pancreatic head in 6% of patients undergoing pancreatic head resection for long-lasting chronic pancreatitis (see Fig. 39.1).

In addition to the main abdominal symptoms of chronic pancreatitis, such as exocrine insufficiency and, in 20–40% of patients, endocrine insufficiency, pain is the decisive symptom, causing discomfort and limitations in daily life. Pain is considered to be a multifactorial process in chronic pancreatitis. Ductal and tissue hypertension, as well as chronic pancreatitis-associated neuritis with perineural inflammation and increased sensory neurotransmitters in the tissue–nerve environment, are the main factors (see Fig. 39.2).

Indications for surgery

The most important clinically relevant local complication in patients with chronic pancreatitis is stenosis of the main pancreatic duct, frequently caused by pancreatic duct stones. On the basis of investigations with endoscopic retrograde cholangiopancreatography (ERCP), common bile duct stenosis in the intrapancreatic segment of the duct is observed in about every second patient. One-third of these patients suffer some degree of cholestasis and around 15% develop clinical jaundice. Pseudocystic lesions are frequent in chronic pancreatitis; however, the indication for surgical drainage is mandatory in persistent large pseudocystic lesions not responding to interventional or endoscopic drainage. Severe duodenal stenosis has been documented in about 5–10%; portal vein compression, sometimes with the consequence of portal vein and/or splenic vein thrombosis, is observed in 12–20% of patients (Table 39.3). A difficult indication for surgery is inflammatory mass in the head of the pancreas which is not discriminable from a malignant process. Patients who suffer daily pain with the need for analgesic treatment should have surgical treatment (Table 39.4; see also Fig. 39.3).

There are three surgical principles for treatment: duct drainage, local excision of the pancreatic head using duodenum-preserving pancreatic head resection, and the major surgical procedure pylorus-preserving head resection. Only a minority of patients benefit from total pancreatectomy, in cases where exocrine and endocrine insufficiency are found in combination with a severe pain syndrome without an inflammatory mass in the head of the pancreas. The Whipple procedure, a

315

Table 39.1 Etiology of chronic pancreatitis.

Alcoholic (60–90%)
Idiopathic (20%)
Hereditary (< 10%)
Tropical
Associated with hyperparathyroidism
Pancreas divisum (< 1%)

Table 39.2 Head of the pancreas is the pacemaker of chronic pancreatitis: factors likely to be involved in causing inflammatory mass of the pancreatic head (IMH).

Anatomy of the pancreatic head: 40–50% of the pancreatic tissue
Embryologically two parts: dorsal and ventral pancreas
Two ductal systems with different drainage capacities: duct of Santorini, duct of Wirsung
Pancreas divisum
Development of IMH has been observed combined with a marked alteration of the ducts up to the confluence ("knee") of the ducts
Papilla–duct connections
Pancreaticobiliary maljunctions

Table 39.3 Chronic pancreatitis: frequency of local complications.

	Results in the literature	Authors' experience*
Common bile duct stenosis	23% (Frey 1990)	43%
Main pancreatic duct stones	< 90% (Nagai 1989)	20%
Pseudocysts	40–60% (Grace 1993)	32%
Necroses	49% (Amman 1996)	9%
Obstruction of duodenum	0.8% (Frey 1990)	23%
Portal vein and superior mesenteric vein, splenic vein obstruction/ thrombosis	10–20% (Warshaw 1997)	16%

* Department of General Surgery, University of Ulm, Germany, 1972–1998.

Table 39.4 Surgical options in chronic pancreatitis.

Duct drainage
Partington–Rochelle procedure
Coring-out modification of Frey
Gastrointestinal drainage of pseudocysts

Local resection
Duodenum-preserving pancreatic head resection
Spleen-preserving left resection

Major resection
Pylorus-preserving head resection
Total pancreatectomy

Historical
Whipple resection
Bypass procedure
Sphincteroplasty
Resection of splanchnic nerves

bypass operation, or sphincteroplasty are historical. A Whipple resection of the pancreatic head is an overtreatment of this benign disease and results in long-lasting disadvantages regarding maintenance of endocrine function and late morbidity. In case of a suspected malignancy, a pylorus-preserving head resection is indicated. The most frequently used duct drainage procedure is pancreatic duct drainage according to Partington–Rochelle, with a duct opening from the prepapillary area of both papillas up to the tail of the pancreas. The coring-out technique, described by Frey as a modification of the Partington–Rochelle/Frey procedure, removes a minor part of the ventral pancreas, but is different from duodenum-preserving pancreatic head resection, which results in subtotal resection of the pancreatic head.

The aims of surgical treatment for chronic pancreatitis are (i) pain relief, (ii) control of pancreatitis-associated complications of adjacent tissue, (iii) preservation of exocrine and endocrine pancreatic function, (iv) social and occupational rehabilitation, and (v) improvement of quality of life. The frequency of the surgical techniques currently used in the first author's institution are given in Table 39.5.

Table 39.5 Surgery in chronic pancreatitis: Ulm experience (905 patients).

Duct drainage: 121 patients (13%)
Left resection: 83 patients (9%)
Duodenal-preserving pancreatic head resection*: 548 patients (61%)
Pylorus-preserving head resection: 78 patients (9%)
Kausch–Whipple: 12 patients (1%)
Others: 63 patients (7%)

* Department of General Surgery, Free University of Berlin, November 1972 to April 1982, and Department of General Surgery, University of Ulm, May 1982 to September 2000.

Table 39.6 Pain relief after pancreatic duct drainage by pancreaticojejunostomy: results after more than 5 years of follow-up of 582 patients.*

Complete pain relief in 55%
Pain, but improved in 25%
Failure of pain control in 20%
Unsatisfactory long-term results in 25 + 20 = 45%

* *Sources*: Leger (1974), White (1979), Prinz (1981), Morrow (1984), Bradley (1987), Drake (1999), Greenie (1990), Wilson (1992), Adams (1994), Kestens (1996), Gonzales (1997), Shama (1998), Sidhu (2001).

Drainage procedure

Pancreatic duct drainage using the Partington–Rochelle modification of the Puestow technique results in a ventral incision of the dilated main pancreatic duct. A drainage procedure is most beneficial in patients with chronic pancreatitis who have a dilated main pancreatic duct without multiple stenosis of the side branches and who lack an inflammatory mass in the head of the pancreas. A critical point of the Partington–Rochelle modification is the excision of the ventral pancreatic tissue in the head of the pancreas at the level of the prepapillary ducts. The Frey modification of coring-out is similar to the Partington–Rochelle drainage procedure. The excised tissue has a wet weight of about 5 g. The Izbicki–Frey modification of the coring-out technique is equivalent to a duodenum-preserving subtotal head resection if the coring-out results in subtotal excision of the pancreatic head tissue. Long-lasting pain relief after pancreatic duct drainage using the Partington–Rochelle procedure (i.e., pancreaticojejunostomy) is achieved in only about 50% of patients. The figures given in Table 39.6 show that in patients undergoing a duct drainage procedure, 20% failed to gain relief from pain while 25% suffered further pain but a little less than preoperatively. Failure to control pain with the use of a duct drainage procedure is caused by tissue changes outside the duct system, mostly in patients with chronic pancreatitis and an inflammatory process in the head of the pancreas. Duct drainage into the jejunum is an inadequate treatment in these cases. It has been demonstrated that reappearance of pain after a duct drainage procedure is caused by an inflammatory mass; resection of this mass leads to a long-lasting pain-free status and improvement of the quality of life if the head of the pancreas is resected in a second surgical procedure. Furthermore, lateral duct-to-jejunum anastomosis is ineffective in chronic pancreatitis with side-duct stenosis through the pancreas.

Duodenum-preserving pancreatic head resection

The rationale for duodenum-preserving pancreatic head resection in chronic pancreatitis is removal of the main inflammatory process, considered to be the pacemaker of the disease, while preserving the upper gastrointestinal tract. The surgical procedure preserves the stomach, duodenum, and biliary tree. Preservation of the duodenum is superior to Whipple-type resection, which includes duodenectomy. Preservation of the duodenum has been shown to be very important because the duodenum is essential for the regulation of glucose metabolism and gastric emptying.

The duodenum-preserving head resection is based on two principal steps: (i) subtotal resection of the pancreatic head with removal of the inflammatory mass, while preserving the duodenum, extrahepatic common bile duct, gallbladder, and stomach, as well as the pancreatic parenchyma to a large extent; and (ii) restoration of the flow of pancreatic juice from the left pancreas, including neck, body, and tail, to the upper gastrointestinal tract by the use of a Roux-en-Y excluded upper jejunal loop. There are three technical steps in the procedure, starting with exposure of the head of the pancreas (Fig. 39.1). After tunneling of the pancreatic neck ventrally to the portal vein along the portal groove,

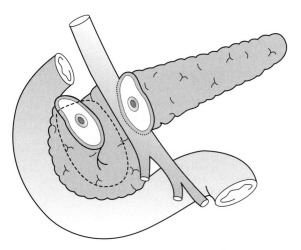

Figure 39.1 Duodenum-preserving pancreatic head resection: the first step is transection of the neck of the pancreas; resection line is along the mass of the pancreatic head.

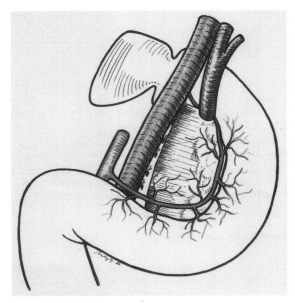

Figure 39.2 Duodenum-preserving pancreatic head resection: dorsal view of the pancreas. The dorsal capsule of the head of the pancreas is preserved. The dorsal pancreaticoduodenal arcades are intact.

transection of the pancreas along the duodenal border of the portal vein is performed. After transection of the pancreas, the pancreatic head and the duodenum are rotated by 90° to a ventral–dorsal position (Fig. 39.2). Subtotal resection of the pancreatic head along the intrapancreatic segment of the common bile duct leads in most cases to decompression of the narrowed common bile duct without opening the duct. The wet weight of an operative specimen after subtotal head resection with duodenum-preserving head resection is between 25 and 45 g; in 54 patients, the median was 28 g. After completion of the subtotal resection, a shell-like rest of the pancreatic head along the duodenal C-line is preserved. The dorsal pancreaticoduodenal arteries are preserved, whereas in most cases the ventral branch of the gastroduodenal artery has to be ligated. To restore flow of pancreatic juice into the upper intestine, a jejunal loop is separated and interposed (Fig. 39.3). Two pancreatic anastomoses have to be performed. In cases with stenosis of the common bile duct, due to inflammation of the duct wall, an additional internal biliary anastomosis between the bile duct and jejunal loop has to be carried out (Fig. 39.4). In cases with a biliary anastomosis, three connections to the jejunal loop are established: two pancreatic and one biliary anastomoses. In patients with multiple stenosis and dilatation of the main pancreatic duct in the body and tail, a side-to-side

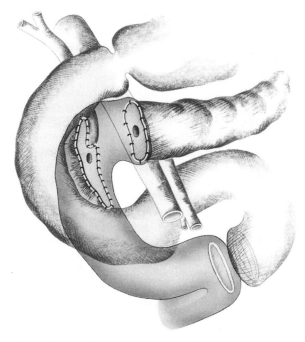

Figure 39.3 Duodenum-preserving head resection: reconstruction with a jejunal loop.

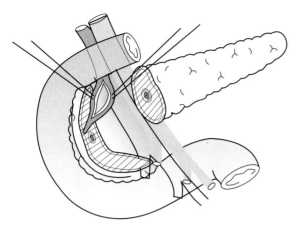

Figure 39.4 Duodenum-preserving pancreatic head resection with intrapancreatic stenosis of the common bile duct: additional biliary drainage into the jejunal loop has to be performed.

Table 39.7 Duodenum-preserving pancreatic head resection in chronic pancreatitis: early postoperative results (504 patients).*

Hospitalization (postoperative): 14.5 (7–87) days
Relaparotomy: 28 patients (5.6%)
Hospital mortality: 4 patients (0.8%)

* Department of General Surgery, Free University of Berlin, November 1972 to April 1982, and Department of General Surgery, University of Ulm, May 1982 to December 1998.

anastomosis has to be performed additionally (Fig. 39.5). Early postoperative results after duodenum-preserving head resection in chronic pancreatitis are given in Table 39.7.

Using the duodenum-preserving head resection, control of pain is achieved in about 90% of patients in the late follow-up (Table 39.8). With regard to endocrine function, the duodenum-preserving head resection results in improvement of glucose metabolism in 8–15% of patients. In the long-term follow-up, however, an

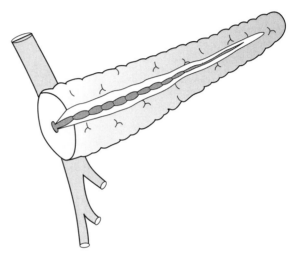

Figure 39.5 Multiple stenosis of the main pancreatic duct in the body and tail: duodenum-preserving pancreatic head resection is combined with a pancreaticojejunostomoses lateral-lateral.

Table 39.8 Late postoperative pain after duodenum-preserving pancreatic head resection in chronic pancreatitis (Beger 1999).

	Late postoperative follow-up		
	1984 2.0 years* 57 patients	1988 3.6 years* 109 patients	1997 5.7 years* 303 patients
Pain-free	92.8%	89%	91.3%
Continuing abdominal pain	7.2%	11%	8.7%
Abdominal complaints	—	12%	12%
Hospitalization due to attacks of pancreatitis	14%	11%	9%

* Median years of follow-up.

Table 39.9 Duodenum-preserving pancreatic head resection changes the natural course of chronic pancreatitis.

	1972–83 58 patients*	1972–87 128 patients†	1972–94 298 patients‡	1982–96 368 patients§
Follow-up	2.8 years (median) 57 patients	3.6 years 109 patients	6.0 years 258 patients	5.7 years (median) 303 patients
Follow-up rate	100%	96%	87%	94%
Pain-free	93%	89%	88%	91%
Continuing abdominal pain	7%	11%	12%	9%
Hospitalization for acute episode	14%	11%	10%	9%
Late death rate	3.6%	4.7%	8.9%	13%
Endocrine functions improved	15.8%	5.5%		11%
Professional rehabilitation	89%	67%	63%	69%
Quality of life/Karnorfsky 80–100				82%

* November 1972 to October 1983.
† November 1972 to December 1987.
‡ November 1972 to December 1994.
§ May 1982 to October 1996.

Table 39.10 Duodenum-preserving pancreatic head resection (DPPHR) versus Whipple resection in chronic pancreatitis: results of randomized trials.

Study	Procedures compared	Results
Buechler *et al.* (1995)	DPPHR vs. pylorus-preserving Whipple resection	DPPHR much superior with regard to postoperative morbidity, glucose metabolism, gastric emptying, and rehospitalization
Klempa *et al.* (1995)	DPPHR vs. Whipple resection	DPPHR superior with regard to postoperative morbidity, glucose metabolism, and rehospitalization
Izbicki *et al.* (1995)	DPPHR vs. Beger–Frey DPPHR*	Both methods equal with regard to pain control, glucose metabolism, postoperative morbidity, and quality of life
Izbicki *et al.* (1998)	Frey DPPHR* vs. pylorus-preserving Whipple resection	DPPHR superior with regard to postoperative morbidity, gastric emptying, and quality of life
Witzigmann *et al.* (2003)	DPPHR vs. Whipple resection	DPPHR superior with regard to postoperative morbidity, maintenance of endocrine function, rehospitalization, and quality of life

* Frey, modified by Izbicki.

increase in insulin-dependent diabetes occurs; after a median follow-up of 5.7 years, about 50% of patients are diabetic (Table 39.9). Table 39.10 shows the results of randomized clinical trials that compared duodenum-preserving pancreatic head resection with pylorus-preserving (Kausch–Whipple) resection and with the Izbicki–Frey modification. Duodenum-preserving head resection is superior or equal to the other procedures with regard to postoperative morbidity, postoperative maintenance of glucose metabolism, delay of gastric emptying, and low level of rehospitalization, as well as restoration of quality of life. In the long-term outcome after surgical treatment, it has been convincingly demonstrated that in a small group of patients the Partington–Rochelle procedure (i.e., duct drainage procedure) using the modification of Izbicki–Frey delays deterioration of function (Table 39.10). Duodenum-preserving pancreatic head resection is the surgical technique of choice in patients suffering chronic pancreatitis with an inflammatory mass in the head.

Pylorus-preserving pancreatic head resection in chronic pancreatitis

A complete pancreatic head resection is mandatory in chronic pancreatitis suspected to be associated with pancreatic cancer. In patients suffering long-lasting chronic pancreatitis, a malignant lesion is observed in 4–6%. The cancer risk in chronic pancreatitis is predicted to be increased 16-fold after 20 years.

The criteria for malignancy inlude the double-duct sign and continuously increasing CA-19-9 and/or CEA in the peripheral blood after biliary stenting of jaundiced patients. Most suggestive of cancer is positive cancer cell staining of biopsy material or of intraoperatively obtained frozen sections. Infiltration of the portal or superior mesenteric vein wall develops rarely in chronic pancreatitis but is more frequent in cancer. Increased mutations of K-*ras*, p53, p16, and DPC4 can be used as markers of carcinogenic process in the pancreas.

Conclusion

In chronic pancreatitis complicated by medically intractable pain, common bile duct stenosis, main pancreatic duct stenosis, portal vein compression, and duodenal stenosis, and in pancreas divisum, the application of duodenum-preserving pancreatic head resection with or without lateral duct drainage offers the benefits of low postoperative morbidity, pain-free status in 90% of patients, reduction in pancreatitis-related hospitalization to less than 5%, postoperative maintenance of endocrine status, professional rehabilitation in more than 60% of patients, and significant improvement in quality of life. In patients with main pancreatic duct dilatation without multiple main- and side-duct stenoses and without an inflammatory mass in the head, a Partington–Rochelle procedure or a Frey modification is the first choice for surgical treatment. In patients with a mass in the head of the pancreas, suspected to be an association of chronic pancreatitis with pancreatic cancer, a pylorus-preserving resection has to be performed once the diagnosis is confirmed by positive frozen section.

Recommended reading

Barton CM, Hall PA, Hughes CM, Gullick WJ, Lemoine NR. Transforming growth factor alpha and epidermal growth factor in human pancreatic cancer. *J Pathol* 1991;163: 111–116.

Beger HG, Büchler M. Duodenum-preserving resection of the head of the pancreas in chronic pancreatitis with inflammatory mass in the head. *World J Surg* 1990;14:83–87.

Beger HG, Büchler M, Bittner R, Oettinger W, Röscher R. Duodenum-preserving resection of the head of the pancreas in severe chronic pancreatitis: early and late results. *Ann Surg* 1989;209:273–278.

Birk D, Schoenberg MH, Gansauge F, Formentini A, Fortnagel G, Beger HG. Carcinoma of the head of the pancreas arising from the uncinate process: what makes the difference? *Br J Surg* 1998;85:498–501.

Bockman DE, Buchler M, Malfertheiner P, Beger HG. Analysis of nerves in chronic pancreatitis. *Gastroenterology* 1988;94:1459–1469.

Bordalo O, Bapista A, Dreiling D, Noronha M. Early pathomorphological pancreatic changes in chronic alcoholism. In: KE Gyr, MV Singer, H Sarles (eds) *Pancreatitis: Concepts and Classification.* Amsterdam: Elsevier/North-Holland, 1984: 642.

Büchler M, Malfertheiner P, Friess H, Senn T, Beger HG. Chronic pancreatitis with inflammatory mass in the head of the pancreas: a special entity? In: HG Beger, M Büchler, H Ditschuneit, P Malfertheiner (eds) *Chronic Pancreatitis.* Berlin: Springer-Verlag, 1990: 41–46.

Caldas C, Hahn SA, da Costa LT *et al.* Frequent somatic mutations and homozygous deletions of the p16 (MTS1) gene in pancreatic adenocarcinoma. *Nat Genet* 1994;8:27–32.

D'Ardenne AJ, Kirkpatric P, Sykes BC. Distribution of laminin, fibronectin, and interstitial collagen type III in soft tissue tumours. *J Clin Pathol* 1984;37:895–904.

Ebbehoj N. Pancreatic tissue fluid pressure and pain in chronic pancreatitis. Dan Med Bull 1992:39:128–133.

Friess H, Yamanaka Y, Büchler M *et al.* Increased expression of acidic and basic fibroblast growth factors in chronic pancreatitis. *Am J Pathol* 1994;144:117–128.

Friess H, Yamanaka Y, Büchler M, Kobrin MS, Tahara E, Köre M. Cripto, a member of the epidermal growth factor family, is overexpressed in human pancreatic cancer and chronic pancreatitis. *Int J Cancer* 1994;56:668–674.

Friess H, Yamanka A, Büchler M *et al.* A subgroup of patients with chronic pancreatitis overexpress the c-erbB-2 protooncogene. *Ann Surg* 1994;220:183–192.

Gansauge S, Gansauge F, Beger HG. Molecular oncology in pancreatic cancer. *J Mol Med* 1996;74:313–320.

Gansauge S, Schmid RM, Gansauge F *et al*. Genetic alterations in chronic pancreatitis: evidence for early occurrence of p53 but not K-ras mutations. *Br J Surg* 1998;85:337–340.

Gress TM, Müller-Pillasch F, Lerch MM *et al*. Balance of expression of genes coding for extracellular matrix proteins and extracellular matrix degrading proteases in chronic pancreatitis. *Z Gastroenterol* 1994;32:221–225.

Klöppel G, Maillet B. Pseudocysts in chronic pancreatitis: a morphological analysis of 57 resection specimens and 91 autopsy pancreata. *Pancreas* 1991;6:266–274.

Korc M, Friess H, Yamanaka Y, Kobrin MS, Büchler M, Beger HG. Chronic pancreatitis is associated with increased concentrations of epidermal growth factor receptor, transforming growth factor α, and phospholipase C-gamma. *Gut* 1994;35:1468–1473.

Lowenfels AB, Maisonneuve P, Cavallini G *et al*. Pancreatitis and the risk of pancreatic cancer: International Pancreatitis Study Group. *N Engl J Med* 1993;328:1433–1437.

Matsubara T, Sakurai Y, Funabiki T *et al*. K-ras point mutations in cancerous and noncancerous biliary epithelium in patients with pancreaticobiliary maljunction. *Cancer* 1996;77:1752–1757.

Oertel JE, Heffess CS, Oertel YC. Pancreas. In: SS Sternberg (ed.) *Diagnostic Surgical Pathology*. New York: Raven Press, 1989: 1057–1093.

Sarles H, Dagorn JC, Giorgi D, Bernard JP. Remaining pancreatic stone protein as "lithostatin." *Gastroenterology* 1990;99:900–905.

Schlosser W, Schoenberg MH, Siech M, Gansauge F, Beger HG. Development of pancreatic cancer in chronic pancreatitis. *Z Gastroenterol* 1996;34:3–8.

Shimoyama S, Gansauge F, Gansauge S, Oohara T, Beger HG. Altered expression of extracellular matrix molecules and their receptors in chronic pancreatitis and adenocarcinoma of the pancreas in comparison to normal pancreas. *Int J Pancreatol* 1995;18:227–234.

van Laethem JL, Deviere J, Resibois A *et al*. Localization of transforming growth factor beta l and its latent binding protein in human chronic pancreatitis. *Gastroenterology* 1995;108:1873–1881.

Warshaw AL. Pancreas divisum: a case for surgical treatment. *Adv Surg* 1988;21:93–109.

Watanabe M, Tanaka J, Masauji N *et al*. Detection of point mutation of K-ras gene codon 12 in biliary tract and ampullary carcinoma by modified two-step polymerase chain reaction. *Nippon Shokakibyo Gakkai Zasshi* 1993;90:789–794.

Weihe E, Nohr D, Müller S, Büchler M, Friess H, Zentel HJ. The tachykinin neuroimmune connection in inflammatory pain. *Ann NY Acad Sci* 1991;632:283–295.

Widmaier U, Schmidt A, Schlosser W, Beger HG. Die duodenumerhaltende Pankreaskopfresektion in der Therapie des Pancreas divisum. *Chirurg* 1997;68:180–186.

40 Management of chronic pancreatic pseudocyst: when to observe, when and how to drain

William R. Brugge

Introduction

Pancreatic pseudocysts are chronic inflammatory fluid collections associated with pancreatitis. Pseudocysts are the most common complication of acute and chronic pancreatitis and nearly one-third of patients with pancreatitis will develop a pseudocyst. Because the fluid cavities are not lined with an epithelium, they are not true cysts. The cavities are instead lined with a reactive granulation tissue that surrounds a collection of enzyme-rich fluid, debris, and necrotic tissue.

The treatment of pancreatic pseudocysts is highly variable, ranging from observation to surgical drainage. Drainage procedures via radiologic or endoscopic approaches are also an important option. An understanding of the pathogenesis of pseudocysts associated with chronic pancreatitis will aid the clinician in the selection of proper treatment.

Pathophysiology of pancreatic fluid collections and pseudocysts

Pseudocysts associated with chronic pancreatitis

Pseudocysts are chronic fluid collections that consist of pancreatic secretions and inflammatory debris and contain large concentrations of active proteolytic enzymes. The fluid collections may develop after an episode of acute pancreatitis or insidiously in the setting of chronic pancreatitis. Small pancreatic pseudocysts are usually intrapancreatic and have a thin wall. Large pseudocysts may be so large that they occupy areas remote from the pancreas. The histologic features of pseudocyst walls are similar in all types of pseudocysts, consisting of fibrosis and inflammatory tissue. Most pancreatic pseudocysts originate from large or small leaks from the ductal system and this feature can be demonstrated with endoscopic retrograde cholangiopancreatography (ERCP).

Focal fluid collections arising in the setting of acute pancreatitis

Acute peripancreatic fluid collections commonly arise during episodes of acute pancreatitis. The fluid collections may accumulate as a result of ductal disruptions or the liquefaction of necrotic pancreatic tissue. Simple fluid collections as a result of ductal leaks are usually unilocular and filled with pancreatic secretions that contain high concentrations of enzymes. Early in the formation of these fluid collections, the fluid is not well contained in the peripancreatic space and may spread throughout the peritoneal and retroperitoneal spaces. Early fluid collections located adjacent to organs such as the stomach, colon, liver, and mesentery are the source of older mature pseudocysts. Chronic fluid collections are contained by thick walls of fibrotic inflammatory tissue that often include the serosa of adjacent organs.

Complex fluid collections often originate from pancreatic tissue necrosis during acute pancreatitis. These focal fluid collections or phlegmons contain semisolid debris, inflammatory fluid, and high concentrations of pancreatic enzymes and can be divided into loculations by fibrotic septations. Complex fluid collections are particularly prone to infection and often require sampling and drainage.

Focal fluid collections arising from a duct leak

Leakage and accumulation of fluid from a disrupted pancreatic duct may occur without evidence of pancreatitis or tissue necrosis. Most commonly, simple leaks take place in the postoperative setting when an incomplete anastomosis breaks down and allows the escape of fluid from a duct. Nonsurgical injuries such as abdominal trauma and endoscopic instrumentation may also be responsible for ductal defects. These fluid collections are often unilocular and respond readily to closure of ductal defects.

Clinical manifestations

Most pancreatic pseudocysts cause mild symptoms. The most common symptom is early satiety and distension; these symptoms occur in 76–94% of patients. In general, the size of the pseudocyst and the duration of the clinical course are the most important predictors of symptoms. With large pseudocysts, there may be a palpable fullness or mass that is sensed by the patient or an examining physician. However, small pseudocysts and pseudocysts located behind the stomach or in the retroperitoneum are rarely detected by physical examination. Related to gastric compression, weight loss is observed in 20% of patients and is a result of poor intake as well as maldigestion. Jaundice, as manifest by icterus, dark urine, pruritus, and acholic stools, may be noted in 10% of patients. The onset of jaundice is usually slow, as a result of bile duct compression by the pseudocyst or the inflamed pancreas itself. Fever is unusual in chronic uncomplicated pseudocysts and its presence should raise the suspicion of an occult infection of a pseudocyst.

Pain from distension and compression

Gastric compression and poor emptying is commonly observed in large pseudocysts located in the head of the pancreas. Patients often complain of early satiety, nausea, and vomiting, particularly after meals. Duodenal obstruction may arise from the presence of the pancreatic pseudocyst or the fibrotic process in the pancreas. Large pseudocysts in the body and tail of the pancreas may also compress the stomach and cause early satiety. After attempted drainage, pseudocysts may dissect into the gastric wall and cause an intramural inflammatory process.

Bleeding

Acute or chronic gastrointestinal bleeding from a variety of sources is seen in 10–20% of patients with chronic pseudocysts. The most serious potential source of bleeding is from gastric varices that arise from splenic vein thrombosis. However, bleeding from varices that arise from splenic vein obstruction is unusual. A common associated lesion is portal hypertensive gastropathy, which may cause chronic gastrointestinal bleeding from the stomach.

Occasionally, bleeding may originate from within the pseudocyst cavity or necrotic pancreatic tissue. Since bleeding in a pseudocyst cavity usually originates from an arterial source, the bleeding may result in sudden and massive distension of the pseudocyst. Bleeding from pseudoaneurysms is the most common cause of significant bleeding and may be responsible for bleeding within pancreatic tissue as well as within the pseudocyst cavity. Spontaneous bleeding into a pseudocyst and communication with the main pancreatic duct results in hemosuccus pancreaticus, a rare form of upper gastrointestinal bleeding associated with pseudocysts. Blood-filled pseudocysts may also rupture into the stomach and cause bleeding within the lumen of the stomach. There are reports of hemobilia as a result of bleeding from a pseudocyst and subsequent erosion into the bile duct. Lower gastrointestinal bleeding may result from spontaneous erosion of a pseudocyst into the colon.

Infection

Infection of pseudocysts usually takes place within the protein-rich fluid of the pseudocyst cavity. Infections may be mild and transient, but more commonly are severe and result in a sepsis syndrome. Spontaneous infections are caused by proliferation of enteric organisms in the protein-rich fluid of the pseudocyst. Instrumentation combined with inadequate drainage may result in infection of a pseudocyst, particularly if there is necrotic tissue present within the pseudocyst cavity. Patients with an infected pseudocyst will present with abdominal pain, fever, or sepsis. Computed tomography (CT) may reveal the presence of air in the pseudocyst cavity, a highly specific sign of infection.

Similar findings have been reported with transabdominal ultrasound. Percutaneous CT- or ultrasound-guided aspirations are used to sample fluid for culture and Gram staining. False-positive diagnostic fluid aspirations with Gram stains are rare. In selected patients with signs of infection, aspiration studies reveal evidence of infection in more than 30% of patients. Despite the use of CT-guided aspiration for the diagnosis of early pancreatic pseudocyst abscess, the long-term mortality rate of treated pancreatic abscesses remains significant at 17%. Severe systemic infections occur when infected fluid communicates with the peritoneal cavity or the bloodstream, often in the setting of pancreatic necrosis. Long-term percutaneous drainage of infected pseudocysts is successful in 60–70% of patients but is less successful if the infection is associated with areas of tissue necrosis and complex infected fluid collections. Drainage of multiple infected fluid collections requires prolonged hospitalization and a combination of surgery and percutaneous drainage. The initial treatment of infected pseudocysts and fluid collections is percutaneous drainage, followed by surgery in patients with a poor response to drainage. Long-term use of external catheters for drainage is often complicated by the development of a cutaneous–pancreatic fistula. Endoscopic drainage of infected pseudocysts using ERCP avoids the complications of fistula formation but may contribute to the introduction of bacteria into a pseudocyst cavity. Internal drainage of infected pseudocysts has also been performed using endoscopic ultrasound (EUS) guidance and the approach avoids the risk of fistula formation. EUS-guided drainage of infected pseudocysts may be improved by prolonged drainage using nasocystic drains placed across the gastric wall. Surgical drainage of infected pseudocysts should be performed in patients not responding to endoscopic or radiologic drainage therapy. Despite these aggressive therapeutic approaches, the mortality rate of treated infected pseudocysts remains quite high (~10%).

Vascular injury associated with pseudocysts

Splenic vein thrombosis, the common vascular injury associated with pseudocysts, occurs in about 13% of patients with pseudocysts, particularly when the pseudocyst is located in the body or tail of the pancreas and is associated with chronic pancreatitis. The thrombosis presumably occurs in the lumen of the splenic vein compressed by the pancreas and/or the pseudocyst. Splenic vein thrombosis will also result in dilation of the short gastric veins, splenomegaly, and the formation of gastric varices. There are few symptoms related to this complication, except for the occasional bleeding from gastric varices and portal hypertensive gastropathy. At times, the patient with a pseudocyst may present solely with splenomegaly found on physical examination or hypersplenism. On rare occasions, splenic vein thrombosis may be complicated by extension of the thrombus into the portal vein.

Thrombocytopenia and leukopenia may arise from "hypersplenism," but it is rare for the patient to present with any symptoms relating to sequestration of platelets and white blood cells. The treatment of splenic vein thrombosis, splenectomy, is indicated in those patients with complications such as bleeding. The long-term results of splenectomy for the treatment of recurrent gastric variceal bleeding is excellent and is the treatment of choice.

Pseudoaneurysms are potentially the most lethal complication of chronic pancreatitis and pseudocysts. These focal inflammatory weaknesses of an arterial wall most commonly occur in the splenic and gastroduodenal arteries. The low-attenuation lesions are readily seen on cross-sectional imaging studies as dilated fluid-filled structures and may be confused with pancreatic fluid collections. The average size of pseudoaneurysms that require intervention is quite large, nearly 14 cm. However, the use of Doppler ultrasound and EUS can readily differentiate between fluid collections and pseudoaneurysms. EUS with color Doppler may also diagnose ruptured pseudoaneurysms. Prospective studies have demonstrated that 10% of patients with pancreatic pseudocysts have pseudoaneurysms as demonstrated by angiography. Pseudoaneurysms are the most common source of bleeding in pancreatic pseudocyst cavities. The treatment of bleeding from pseudoaneurysms includes surgical resection and angiographic techniques. Surgical techniques for the control of acute bleeding from pseudoaneurysms consist of arterial ligation and surgical resection. The reported surgical mortality rate for the control of bleeding from a pseudoaneurysm is high (> 10%). The angiographic control of bleeding from pseudoaneurysms consists of arterial embolization and is successful in 40–50% of patients with acute bleeding. Percutaneous arterial embolization may be used prophylactically to prevent bleeding from pseudoaneurysms.

Pancreatic biliary duct obstruction

Obstruction of the pancreatic biliary ducts is relatively common, particularly when the pseudocyst is located within the head of the pancreas. Local compression is the most common cause of ductal obstruction, although direct fibrotic involvement of the ducts is occasionally seen. Obstruction of the distal bile duct with resulting obstructive jaundice is the most common scenario. Although the degree of obstruction of the bile duct may be impressive, it is rare for the patient's symptoms to be related to biliary obstruction. Drainage of a pseudocyst associated with bile duct compression resolves the obstruction of the duct, particularly the bile duct. With long-term obstruction of the pancreatic biliary ducts, stones, sludge, and debris will commonly accumulate and may be responsible for episodes of cholangitis.

Diagnostic testing

Ultrasound/CT

Pseudocysts are readily seen with CT and appear as low-attenuation lesions within or adjacent to the pancreas (Fig. 40.1). Chronic pseudocysts are most

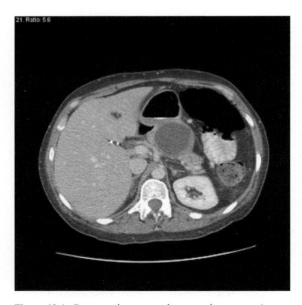

Figure 40.1 Computed tomography scan of a pancreatic pseudocyst in the body of the pancreas.

commonly round in shape and surrounded by a thick dense wall. Large pseudocysts may appear in the mediastinum or pelvis, or involve the mesentery. Prominent vessels, as depicted with color Doppler, adjacent to the pseudocyst wall are common and may represent paragastric varices and thrombosis of the splenic vein. Although pseudocysts are most commonly unilocular, fibrotic strands within the cavity may cause multiple septations, commonly encountered in patients with postpancreatitis, complex fluid collections. The pseudocyst cavity may also contain debris, blood, or infections that appear as high-attenuation areas within the fluid-filled cavity. It may be difficult to distinguish between pseudocysts and true pancreatic mucinous cysts associated with malignancy without the use of aspiration fluid analysis. Choledochocysts, as they appear on CT, may also be confused with pancreatic pseudocysts.

ERCP

Pancreatography in the setting of a pseudocyst often reveals a diffusely abnormal duct with changes of chronic pancreatitis evident. The main pancreatic duct may be partially or completely obstructed by compression of the pseudocyst. In more than half of patients, the pseudocyst will fill with contrast during retrograde pancreatography. Pancreatic ductal leaks are common and may originate from the pancreatic duct or may be small and originate from a secondary radicle. A normal pancreatogram should suggest the possibility of a cystic neoplasm rather than a pseudocyst. Retrograde injection of contrast into a pseudocyst may result in infection of the pseudocyst. Contamination of a pseudocyst cavity may be prevented by the use of antibiotics and minimizing the amount of contrast injected.

EUS

Using EUS, pseudocysts appear as anechoic fluid-filled structures adjacent to the upper gastrointestinal tract and pancreas (Fig. 40.2). Fluid collections associated with acute pancreatitis will not be surrounded with a wall, whereas pseudocysts are often surrounded by a thick hyperechoic rim. Calcifications in a cyst wall are highly suggestive of a mucinous cystadenoma rather than a pseudocyst. Within the pseudocyst cavity, EUS will readily demonstrate the presence of fluid. Debris in the dependent portion of the cavity is common and may

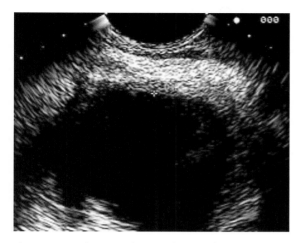

Figure 40.2 Endoscopic ultrasound image of a thick-walled pancreatic pseudocyst.

represent blood, infection, or necrotic material. Color Doppler of the wall often reveals multiple prominent vessels, including paragastric varices. EUS-directed fine-needle aspiration (FNA) with cyst fluid analysis will differentiate between pseudocysts and neoplastic cysts in more than 90% of patients.

Cyst aspiration

FNA of pseudocysts is performed for diagnostic or therapeutic purposes using CT/ultrasound or EUS for guidance. Since pseudocysts may be confused with true cysts of the pancreas in nearly 20% of patients, aspiration is performed to differentiate between pseudocysts and a wide variety of benign and malignant cystic neoplasms of the pancreas. If infection of a pseudocyst is suspected, the cyst should be aspirated for culture.

FNA of pseudocysts can be performed with a variety of techniques. The most common approach is to use CT/ultrasound guidance. A needle is placed through the abdominal wall and into the cystic cavity; small amounts of fluid are aspirated for cytology and tumor markers such as carcinoembryonic antigen (CEA). EUS can also be used to guide aspiration through the gastric or duodenal wall and is ideal for small cystic lesions. The aspirated fluid from a cystic lesion is examined cytologically for evidence of inflammatory cells. The presence of pigmented histiocytes is diagnostic of a pseudocyst, but this finding may be absent in a significant number of patients with a pseudocyst. If there is cytologic evidence of epithelial cells with the cyst fluid, this should raise the suspicion of a cystic neoplasm rather than a pseudocyst. The presence of granulocytes in the aspirated fluid is suggestive of an acute infection. A high concentration of amylase in aspirated fluid is predictive of a connection with the main pancreatic duct and helps confirm the diagnosis of a pseudocyst.

The cytologic analysis of a cystic lesion may not provide diagnostic material because of the low cellularity of cyst fluid. Cyst fluid tumor markers are often used to assist in differentiating between pseudocysts and cystic neoplasms. CEA is the most commonly used marker because mucinous cystic neoplasms secrete CEA into cystic fluid, whereas pseudocysts should have relatively low levels of CEA.

If there is any concern about an infected pseudocyst, the aspirated fluid should be sent for culture and sensitivity. Although Gram-negative enteric organisms are the most common organism, occasionally Gram-positive bacteria may infect a pseudocyst. Viral and mycobacterial infections of pseudocysts are very rare but *Candida* species may infect secondarily.

Treatment

Natural history

Small pseudocysts of less than 4 cm in diameter often resolve spontaneously and are rarely associated with clinical symptoms. In long-term observation studies, 9% of patients experience a complication of a pseudocyst. Spontaneous resolution of pseudocysts takes place through drainage into the gastrointestinal tract or the pancreatic duct. Of pseudocysts less than 6 cm, 40% will require drainage because of complications or persistence. Small pseudocysts located in the tail of the pancreas and arising from acute biliary pancreatitis have a very high rate of spontaneous drainage. In a large series, the overall mortality of pseudocyst drainage by any method was 9–14%. Prior to drainage, it is critical to confirm the diagnosis of a pseudocyst using fluid analysis and cytology. Mistakenly diagnosed pseudocysts that are drained with percutaneous drainage often do not resolve and may harbor occult malignancy.

Drainage

Pancreatic pseudocysts may be drained using a variety of approaches. Simple, one-time aspiration of pseudocysts rarely provides lasting resolution because of communication with the pancreatic ductal system. External drainage using CT/ultrasound guidance is the most common approach and should include the use of Doppler or contrast injection to order to differentiate between pockets of fluid and vascular structures. With CT/ultrasound guidance, a single pigtail drainage catheter is placed percutaneously into the fluid cavity and fluid is drained into an external collection system carried by the patient (Fig. 40.3). The short-term success rate for this relatively simple technique is very high (> 90%). Patients with communicating pseudocysts, as evidenced by high concentration of amylase in cyst fluid, and pancreatic duct strictures should not have percutaneous drainage because of the high risk of prolonged drained and fistula formation. Acutely ill patients with evidence of infection in the pseudocyst should be urgently aspirated and drained under ultrasound guidance at the bedside. Long-term success rates of external drainage are much lower than immediate success rates and a significant percentage of patients with external drainage will require surgical drainage. However, the placement of an external drain will not interfere with surgical drainage or excision if external drainage is not successful. The placement of the catheter across the stomach reduces the risk of subsequent external fistula formation and allows for subsequent transgastric stenting. Peripancreatic fluid collections complicated by infection are also easily drained with CT-guided catheters and external drainage. Pseudocyst fluid drained externally is collected over an average of 3 weeks into an external collection bag. When the drainage output becomes minimal, the catheter is removed. Contrast injection into the cyst cavity will demonstrate the size of the cavity and this finding can be used to monitor the progress of the chronic drainage. This technique is highly successful at resolving pseudocysts, but is plagued by infections and the need for an external bag. The average duration of external drainage is 24 days.

Surgical drainage of pseudocysts is performed by providing a large anastomosis between the pseudocyst wall and the stomach or small bowel. The anastomosis should be placed in the most dependent portion of the cystic cavity in order to maximize the chances of complete drainage. The cyst-gastrostomy or -enterostomy usually remains patent and functional for several months. ERCP is often performed prior to surgical drainage in order to evaluate the main pancreatic duct for evidence of strictures, fistula, and leaks. Surgical drainage is probably the best approach when the pseudocyst is complicated by areas of necrosis or infection, or involves adjacent organs such as the spleen. However, maturation of a pseudocyst wall over 4–6 weeks allows the formation of a thick wall that will provide a more secure anastomosis. Cyst-gastrostomy is the easiest approach and requires less operating time than cyst-jejunostomy. However, the risk of bleeding is greater with cyst-gastrostomy. A jejunal anastomosis is indicated in giant pseudocysts because drainage with a cyst-gastrostomy is often inadequate and the recurrence rate is quite high. An alternative to a cyst anastomosis is a longitudinal pancreaticojejunostomy, which has been reported to provide high rates of successful drainage and with fewer complications such as anastomotic bleeding. Pancreaticojejunostomy can be performed if there is an associated pancreatic duct diameter of more than 7 mm and is more likely to be successful if there is communication between the pseudocyst cavity and the main pancreatic duct. When the pseudocyst has resolved, the low output of fluid allows spontaneous closing of the anastomosis. Old reports of surgical drainage suggested high mortality and complication rates. More recent series report overall success rates for surgical drainage of 90%, with major complication rates of 9% and recurrence rates of 3%.

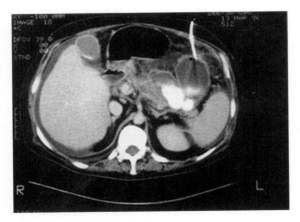

Figure 40.3 Percutaneous drainage of a pancreatic pseudocyst.

Laparoscopic techniques are being developed that will enable the surgeon to provide internal drainage and resection of necrotic tissue. However, these techniques are also associated with similar complications as reported with endoscopic drainage, i.e., cyst wall bleeding and postoperative cyst infection. If areas of pancreatic necrosis are encountered during the laparoscopic procedure, laparoscopy may enable surgeons to noninvasively remove areas of necrotic tissue.

Endoscopic drainage is the newest approach for the eradication of pseudocysts. It is used most commonly for uncomplicated unilocular pseudocysts. Drainage is accomplished either with a transpapillary approach with ERCP or with direct endoscopic drainage across the stomach or duodenal wall. A transpapillary approach with drainage is used when the pseudocyst communicates with the main pancreatic duct, usually in the head of the pancreas. The transpapillary approach has also proven successful in the drainage of infected pseudocysts or pseudocysts associated with strictures or leaks of the main pancreatic duct. The transgastric or duodenal approach is used when the pseudocyst is directly adjacent to the gastroduodenal wall. EUS is used to determine the size, location, and thickness of the pseudocyst wall (Fig. 40.2). A wall thickness of more than 1 cm or the presence of large intervening vessels or varices on EUS precludes the possibility of endoscopic drainage. Endoscopic-guided drainage may be performed using direct endoscopic or EUS imaging. With the presence of a visible bulge in the wall of the stomach or the duodenum, endoscopic drainage is successful by the placement of transmural catheters or stents (Fig. 40.4). EUS guidance is required if a bulge is not evident during the endoscopic evaluation prior to drainage. One-step EUS-directed drainage is now possible with pseudocyst drainage catheters that can be used in therapeutic echoendoscopes. This approach has proven highly successful and may be feasible for infected pseudocysts. Recently, endoscopic drainage of necrotic pancreatic tissue through an endoscopic cyst-gastrostomy has been reported in three patients. The success rate within 3 months of endoscopic drainage is reported to be more than 80%, with lower rates reported with alcoholic pancreatic disease. The improvement in endoscopic skills necessary for the successful performance of pseudocyst drainage takes place over about 20 cases and results in significant decreases in complications and the length of hospital stay. Overall, the complication rate of elective endoscopic drainage is

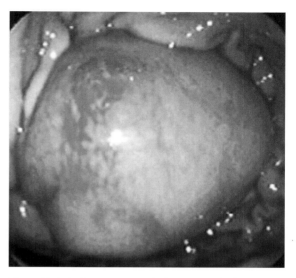

Figure 40.4 Endoscopic gastric bulge as a result of a pancreatic pseudocyst.

about 13%, with success rates of more than 90% and recurrence rates of 10–20%.

Conclusions

Small asymptomatic pseudocysts associated with chronic pancreatitis should be monitored. If there is any question about the diagnosis or the presence of an infection, cyst aspiration should be performed. Simple, chronic, uninfected, unilocular pseudocysts should be drained endoscopically when the expertise is available; otherwise this type of pseudocyst should be drained radiologically with an external drainage catheter. Complex, postnecrotic, multilocular pseudocysts should be managed with surgical drainage and/or resection.

Recommended reading

Andersson R, Cwikiel W. Percutaneous cystogastrostomy in patients with pancreatic pseudocysts. *Eur J Surg* 2002; 168:345–348.

Baril NB, Ralls PW, Wren SM *et al*. Does an infected peripancreatic fluid collection or abscess mandate operation? *Ann Surg* 2000;231:361–367.

Beckingham IJ, Krige JE, Bornman PC, Terblanche J. Long term outcome of endoscopic drainage of pancreatic pseudocysts. *Am J Gastroenterol* 1999;94:71–74.

Bender JS, Bouwman DL, Levison MA, Weaver DW. Pseudocysts and pseudoaneurysms: surgical strategy. *Pancreas* 1995;10:143–147.

Bhattacharya D, Ammori BJ. Minimally invasive approaches to the management of pancreatic pseudocysts: review of the literature. *Surg Laparosc Endosc Percutan Tech* 2003; 13:141–148.

Boerma D, van Gulik TM, Obertop H, Gouma DJ. Endoscopic stent placement for pancreaticocutaneous fistula after surgical drainage of the pancreas. *Br J Surg* 2000; 87:1506–1509.

Boggi U, Di Candio G, Campatelli A, Pietrabissa A, Mosca F. Nonoperative management of pancreatic pseudocysts. Problems in differential diagnosis. *Int J Pancreatol* 1999; 25:123–133.

Brugge WR. EUS-guided pancreatic fine needle aspiration: instrumentation, results, and complications. *Tech Gastrointest Endosc* 2000;2:149–154.

Byrne MF, Mitchell RM, Baillie J. Pancreatic pseudocysts. *Curr Treat Options Gastroenterol* 2002;5:331–338.

Carr JA, Cho JS, Shepard AD, Nypaver TJ, Reddy DJ. Visceral pseudoaneurysms due to pancreatic pseudocysts: rare but lethal complications of pancreatitis. *J Vasc Surg* 2000;32:722–730.

Cohen-Scali F, Vilgrain V, Brancatelli G *et al*. Discrimination of unilocular macrocystic serous cystadenoma from pancreatic pseudocyst and mucinous cystadenoma with CT: initial observations. *Radiology* 2003;228:727–733.

Deviere J, Bueso H, Baize M *et al*. Complete disruption of the main pancreatic duct: endoscopic management. *Gastrointest Endosc* 1995;42:445–451.

Fockens P, Johnson TG, van Dullemen HM, Huibregtse K, Tytgat GN. Endosonographic imaging of pancreatic pseudocysts before endoscopic transmural drainage. *Gastrointest Endosc* 1997;46:412–416.

Frossard JL, Amouyal P, Amouyal G *et al*. Performance of endosonography-guided fine needle aspiration and biopsy in the diagnosis of pancreatic cystic lesions. *Am J Gastroenterol* 2003;98:1516–1524.

Giovannini M, Pesenti C, Rolland AL, Moutardier V, Delpero JR. Endoscopic ultrasound-guided drainage of pancreatic pseudocysts or pancreatic abscesses using a therapeutic echo endoscope. *Endoscopy* 2001;33:473–477.

Hammel P. Diagnostic value of cyst fluid analysis in cystic lesions of the pancreas: current data, limitations, and perspectives. *J Radiol* 2000;81:487–490.

Harewood GC, Wright CA, Baron TH. Impact on patient outcomes of experience in the performance of endoscopic pancreatic fluid collection drainage. *Gastrointest Endosc* 2003;58:230–235.

Heider R, Behrns KE. Pancreatic pseudocysts complicated by splenic parenchymal involvement: results of operative and percutaneous management. *Pancreas* 2001;23:20–25.

Heider R, Meyer AA, Galanko JA, Behrns KE. Percutaneous drainage of pancreatic pseudocysts is associated with a higher failure rate than surgical treatment in unselected patients. *Ann Surg* 1999;229:781–787; discussion 787–789.

Mori T, Abe N, Sugiyama M, Atomi Y. Laparoscopic pancreatic cystgastrostomy. *J Hepatobiliary Pancreat Surg* 2002; 9:548–554.

Nealon WH, Walser E. Duct drainage alone is sufficient in the operative management of pancreatic pseudocyst in patients with chronic pancreatitis. *Ann Surg* 2003;237:614–620; discussion 620–622.

Parks RW, Tzovaras G, Diamond T, Rowlands BJ. Management of pancreatic pseudocysts. *Ann R Coll Surg Engl* 2000;82:383–387.

Seifert H, Dietrich C, Schmitt T, Caspary W, Wehrmann T. Endoscopic ultrasound-guided one-step transmural drainage of cystic abdominal lesions with a large-channel echo endoscope. *Endoscopy* 2000;32:255–259.

Sharma SS, Bhargawa N, Govil A. Endoscopic management of pancreatic pseudocyst: a long-term follow-up. *Endoscopy* 2002;34:203–207.

Usatoff V, Brancatisano R, Williamson RC. Operative treatment of pseudocysts in patients with chronic pancreatitis. *Br J Surg* 2000;87:1494–1499.

Yeo CJ, Bastidas JA, Lynch-Nyhan A, Fishman EK, Zinner MJ, Cameron JL. The natural history of pancreatic pseudocysts documented by computed tomography. *Surg Gynecol Obstet* 1990;170:411–417.

41 What is the epidemiologic impact of pancreatic cancer?

Joachim Mössner

Introduction

Pancreatic adenocarcinoma is the fourth leading cause of tumor deaths in men and the fifth leading cause in women, with 95% of all pancreatic malignancies being ductal adenocarcinomas. The 5-year survival rate of only 1–5% is one of the worst for any tumor. Thus it is of utmost importance to identify risk groups since only early diagnosis allows the chance of a curative resection. Among the potential risk factors, only nicotine has been clearly identified. A diet high in fat and calories seems to add some risk. According to a case–control study from northern Italy, attributable risks were 14% for tobacco smoking, 14% for high consumption of meat, and 12% for low consumption of fruit. The authors speculate that almost one-fourth of all cases of pancreatic carcinoma could be prevented by a healthy lifestyle. It is likely that a combination of factors, most of them associated with relatively small risk enhancements, may be responsible for the pathogenesis.

Furthermore, chronic inflammation of the pancreas (i.e., chronic pancreatitis) has been identified as a risk factor. This has been especially documented in chronic hereditary pancreatitis, a disease with early onset of inflammation; 5–10% of all cases of pancreatic cancer may be inherited. It will be a major challenge to identify these genetic alterations. In a population-based case–control study based on direct interviews with 526 incident cases and 2153 population controls, the following risk factors were identified: elevated body mass index (BMI) when combined with elevated caloric intake; diabetes mellitus (hyperinsulinemia); first-degree relatives; family history of colon, endometrial, ovary, and breast cancer; smoking; possibly heavy alcohol use in blacks.

I discuss the significance of various risk factors that have been proposed to play a role in the pathogenesis of pancreatic carcinoma.

Incidence

The incidence rate in industrialized Western countries is about 8–12/100 000 inhabitants and still increasing in some countries. In Europe the incidence is higher in northern and central Europe compared with southern Europe. In the USA, there is a geographic cluster of pancreatic cancers in areas of Louisiana and Mississippi. However, the factors responsible for clustering have not been identified. The rate for pancreatic cancers in the USA seems to be higher in urban areas and in counties with many residents of Scandinavian and East European descent. In all countries incidence almost equals mortality. The incidence rate between the ages of 40 and 44 is 19/100 000 and between the ages of 75 to 79 is 43/100 000 per year. Thus, the increase in incidence may be due to an increased lifespan. In the USA, the incidence and mortality of pancreatic cancer increased for several decades earlier in this century but have tended to level off in the last 25 years.

Rates seem to be higher in blacks than in whites and higher in men than in women. However, smoking may be a confounding factor. In the district of Malmö in Sweden, the incidence is higher for men than for women in all age groups above 44 years. No change in incidence over time was observed for men. In older and

331

middle-aged women there was a significant increase observed.

Risk factors

Chronic pancreatitis

Any type of chronic pancreatitis (i.e., alcohol-induced, tropical, hereditary) confers an increased risk of developing pancreatic carcinoma (Table 41.1). The duration of exposure to inflammation seems to be the major factor involved in the transition from a benign to malignant condition. According to case–control studies, the relative risk of developing pancreatic carcinoma in chronic pancreatitis varies from 2.3 to 18.5. In a prospective single-center cohort of almost 440 consecutive patients and a median follow-up of 9.2 years, four cases (1.1%) of pancreatic adenocarcinoma were observed in 3437 patient-years. The expected number of cases was 0.15% (standardized incidence ratio (SIR) 26.7). In most cases of pancreatic cancer in alcohol-induced chronic pancreatitis, smoking has to be considered as an important confounding factor.

The early diagnosis of pancreatic carcinoma in patients with chronic pancreatitis remains an unsolved problem. Despite the fact that K-*ras* mutations play a crucial role in the pathogenesis of pancreatic cancer, sequential determinations of this oncogene in pancreatic juice of patients with chronic pancreatitis does not allow a definite diagnosis. Some patients with chronic pancreatitis carry K-*ras* mutations yet do not develop carcinoma.

Diabetes mellitus

There is an association between diabetes and an elevated risk of pancreatic cancer (Table 41.1). Diabetes may be due to pancreatic damage caused by the cancer or to insulin resistance. However, preexisting long-term type II diabetes also seems to increase the risk of pancreatic carcinoma. One interpretation of these findings is that insulin might act as a promoter for pancreatic carcinogenesis. Human pancreatic adenocarcinomas express insulin receptors that can stimulate mitosis. Furthermore, high insulin levels could indirectly promote pancreatic carcinogenesis via insulin-like growth factor (IGF)-I released from the liver.

Dietary effects on pathogenesis might be partly mediated via insulin. However, in some studies the risk of developing pancreatic cancer declined with time after primary diagnosis of diabetes mellitus. One might speculate that this decrease is due to the loss of hyperinsulinemia in early type II diabetes. Another explanation is that in most cases diabetes is an early symptom of cancer or preneoplastic lesions. In a well-conducted case–control study from Italy, diabetes did not increase the risk of pancreatic cancer. Thus, in many cases of diabetes and pancreatic cancer, cancer might be the cause of diabetes and not vice versa. Especially in cases of atypical diabetes, i.e., lack of family history of diabetes, absence of obesity, and rapid progression to insulin dependence, one should consider pancreatic cancer. Further epidemiologic studies should differentiate between type I (insulin-dependent) and type II diabetes when evaluating the risk of pancreatic cancer.

Physical activity and body weight

Obesity, height, and physical activity might be related to the risk of pancreatic cancer. In 32 687 subjects, physical activity and BMI were not associated with pancreatic cancer mortality. The authors had reported similar findings some years earlier. However, insulin resistance is associated with anthropometric factors and physical activity. In a population-based case–control study from Canada, men with a BMI greater than 28.3 kg/m^2 were at increased risk of pancreatic cancer (adjusted odds ratio (OR) 1.90; 95% confidence interval (CI) 1.08–3.359). Decrease of weight in women and moderate and strenuous physical activity in men might reduce the risk. Thus, insulin resistance could be an etiologic factor in the pathogenesis of pancreatic cancer. In two US cohort studies conducted by mailed questionnaire with 10–20 years of follow-up, individuals with a BMI of at least 30 kg/m^2 had an elevated risk of pancreatic cancer compared with those with a BMI of less than 23 kg/m^2. An inverse relation was reported for moderate activity. According to these two studies, obesity significantly increased the risk of pancreatic cancer and physical activity appears to decrease the risk in those who are overweight. Obesity seems to contribute to the higher risk of this disease among blacks than among whites in the USA, particularly among women.

Table 41.1 Preexisting illnesses and the risk of pancreatic cancer.

Study	Study design	Risk
Asthma		
Stolzenberg-Solomon et al. (2002)	Cohort analysis of 172 subjects who developed pancreatic cancer 1985–97. Median 10.2 years follow-up among 29 048 male smokers, 50–69 years old	Increased
Diabetes		
Stolzenberg-Solomon et al. (2002)	Cohort analysis of 172 subjects who developed pancreatic cancer 1985–97. Median 10.2 years follow-up among 29 048 male smokers, 50–69 years old	Increased
Fischer (2001)	Metaanalysis, English literature, 1970–99	Diabetes of at least 5 years: increased risk
Silverman et al. (1999)	Population-based case–control study: 484 cases vs. 2099 controls, interview	Significant positive trend in risk with increasing years prior to diagnosis of cancer
Wideroff et al. (1997)	Discharge records of 109 581 individuals hospitalized with diagnosis of diabetes 1977–89 linked with national cancer registry records through 1993	Increased risk: SIR 2.1 (CI 1.9–2.4) with a follow-up time of 1–4 years. SIR declined to 1.3 (CI 1.1–1.6) after 5–9 years of follow-up
Lee et al. (1996)	Retrospective study: 282 inpatients with pancreatic cancer vs. 282 controls	Increased risk: OR 2.84
Everhart & Wright (1995)	Metaanalysis: published studies between 1975 and 1994; 20 of 30 case control and cohort studies met inclusion criteria, i.e., diabetes at least 1 year prior to cancer, RR calculation possible	Elevated risk: RR of pancreatic cancer for diabetics relative to nondiabetics 2.1 (CI 1.6–2.8)
La Vecchia et al. (1994)	Case–control study, northern Italy, 1983–92: 9991 patients below age 75 with incident, histologically confirmed neoplasms including 362 of the pancreas vs. 7834 subjects in hospital for acute, nonneoplastic, nonmetabolic disorders	Risk increased: RR 2.1 (CI 1.5–2.9). RR for pancreatic cancer declined from 3.2 in the first 5 years after diagnosis of diabetes to 2.3 at 5–9 years after diagnosis and to 1.3 (CI 0.7–2.3) at 10 or more years after diagnosis
Gullo et al. (1994)	720 patients with pancreatic cancer vs. controls from 14 Italian centers	Diabetes in 22.8% of pancreatic cancer patients vs. 8.3% of controls; 56.1% diabetes diagnosed either concomitantly with the cancer (40.2%) or within 2 years before the diagnosis of cancer (15.9%)
Noninsulin-dependent diabetes mellitus		
Balkau et al. (1993)	6988 working men aged 44–55 years. Follow-up 17 years. 312 diabetic subjects	After exclusion of deaths during the first 5 years of follow-up, RR in diabetic vs. normoglycemic men 4.9 (CI 1.3–18) after adjustment for age and tobacco consumption
Jain et al. (1991)	Case–control study, Toronto: 249 cancers vs. 505 controls	Increased risk: history of diabetes within 5 years

Continued

Table 41.1 *Continued*

Study	Study design	Risk
Gallstones		
Post cholecystectomy		
Schernhammer *et al.* (2002)	Prospective study: 104 856 women, 48 928 men. 16 years of follow-up.	No increased risk
Silverman *et al.* (1999)	Population-based case–control study: 484 cases, 2099 controls, interview	Cholecystectomy at least 20 years ago: 70% increased risk
Chow *et al.* (1999)	Population-based cohort study in Denmark. Discharge diagnosis of gallstones 1977–89. 60 176 patients, follow-up until death or 1993	Gallstones: no risk. Cholecystectomy: risks at 5 or more years of follow-up elevated for cancers of ampulla of Vater (SIR 2.0, CI 1.0–3.7) and pancreas (SIR 1.3, CI 1.1–1.6)
Schattner *et al.* (1997)	Retrospective case–control study. Abdominal ultrasound of 100 consecutive cases of pancreatic cancer and that of 140 age- and gender-matched controls	37 patients with pancreatic cancer had cholelithiasis (37%) compared with 23 (16%) of the control group ($P < 0.001$)
Ekbom *et al.* (1996)	Population-based cohort: 62 615 patients with cholecystectomy. Follow-up for pancreatic and periampullary cancer up to 23 years	261 pancreatic cancers vs. 216.8 expected, SIR 1.20 (CI 1.06–1.37)
Post papillotomy		
Karlson *et al.* (1997)	992 patients followed by linkage to the Swedish Death Registry and the Swedish Cancer Registry	No increased risk
Post gastrectomy		
Tascilar *et al.* (2002)	Multivariate and person-year analysis: cohort of 2633 patients	Increased risk of 1.8 (CI 1.3–2.6) 5–59 years postoperatively
Heberg *et al.* (1997)	Necropsy-based case–control study	No relation
Mack *et al.* (1986)	Case–control study, Los Angeles: 490 cases, working age vs. 420 controls. Home interviews: occupation, smoking, food, beverage consumption, medical history	Strong association between pancreas cancer and history of subtotal gastrectomy at any past time
Helicobacter pylori		
Stolzenberg-Solomon *et al.* (2001)	Nested case–control study: 29 133 male Finnish smokers, age 50–69 years	Seroprevalence of *H. pylori* 82% vs. 73% in controls. OR 1.87 (CI 1.05–3.34)
Malignancies		
Neugut *et al.* (1995)	Data from Surveillance, Epidemiology, and End results for the period from 1 January 1973 to 31 December 1990. Observed number of cases divided by the expected number	Risk of second primary cancer was elevated after: (a) lung cancer for men (RR 1.3) and women (RR 2.5) (b) head and neck cancer in women (RR 1.8) (c) bladder cancer in women (RR 1.5), related to smoking? (d) prostate cancer (RR 1.2)

Table 41.1 *Continued*

Study	Study design	Risk
Melanoma (without family history)		
Schenk *et al.* (1998)	Patients identified from Surveillance, Epidemiology, and End Results program of the National Cancer Institute: 43 781 patients with melanoma	Nearly twofold increased risk of subsequent carcinoma of the pancreas in patients diagnosed with malignant melanoma before age 50 years, SIR 1.76 (CI 0.80–3.34). Greatest risk occurred in young white females, SIR 2.27 (CI 0.73–5.30)
Chronic pancreatitis *Any type*		
Talamini *et al.* (1999)	715 cases of chronic pancreatitis with a median follow-up of 10 years	Significant increase in incidence of both extrapancreatic cancer (SIR 1.5, CI 1.1–2.0; $P < 0.003$) and pancreatic cancer (SIR 18.5, CI 10–30; $P < 0.0001$). Smoking contributes to increased risk
Karlson *et al.* (1997)	Swedish Inpatient Register with diagnosis of pancreatitis 1965–83. Recurrent pancreatitis, $n = 7328$; chronic pancreatitis, $n = 4546$. Follow-up through record linkage to nationwide Swedish Cancer Register, Death Register, and Migration Register	Excess risks for pancreatic cancer in all subcohorts. Risk declined with time! Persistent excess risk after 10 years restricted to patients with associated alcohol abuse (SIR 3.8, CI 1.5–7.9)
Fernandez *et al.* (1995)	Hospital-based case–control study, northern Italy, 1983–92, 362 cancer cases, 1408 controls, structured interview	Risk of pancreatic cancer higher (RR 6.9) 5 or more years after diagnosis of pancreatitis than in the first 4 years (RR 2.1). Tobacco and alcohol may be confounding factors
Ekbom *et al.* (1994)	Data collected from all inpatient medical institutions in Sweden 1965–83. Population-based cohort of 7956 patients with at least one discharge diagnosis of pancreatitis. Follow-up to 19 years	SIR 2.2 (CI 1.6–2.9). Absence of an increased risk 10 years or more after first discharge for pancreatitis argues against a causal relationship. Smoking is a confounding factor
Lowenfels *et al.* (1993)	Multicenter historical cohort study, 2015 subjects with chronic pancreatitis, recruited from clinical centers in six countries. 56 cancers during mean follow-up of 7.4 years. Expected cases adjusted for age and sex: 2.13	SIR 26.3 (CI 19.9–34.2). Cumulative risk of pancreatic cancer in subjects followed for at least 2 years increased steadily, and 10 and 20 years after diagnosis of pancreatitis it was 1.8%
Hereditary pancreatitis Lowenfels *et al.* (1997)	Longitudinal study. Initial criteria: early age (≤ 30 years) at onset of symptoms, positive family history, absence of other causes	Compared with expected number of 0.15, 8 pancreatic adenocarcinomas developed during 8531 person-years of follow-up. SIR 53 (CI 23–105)
Tropical pancreatitis Chari *et al.* (1994)	185 patients from the Diabetes Research Center in Madras, India. Follow-up for an average of 4.5 years	Six deaths (25%) from cancer of the pancreas. Average age at onset of pancreatic cancer 45.6 ± 7.3 years, considerably younger than for Western populations

CI, 95% confidence interval; OR, odds ratio; RR, relative risk; SIR, standardized incidence ratio.

Smoking

It has been known for many years that smoking confers an important risk factor for pancreatic cancer. Many well-defined case–control studies confirm that smoking increases the risk of pancreatic cancer (Table 41.2). According to a study using a computer model, the numbers of new pancreatic cancer patients in the EU up to 2015 could be reduced by 15% if all smokers discontinued the habit immediately. Since one-fourth of all cases seem to be attributable to smoking, prevention of up to 25% of all pancreatic cancers by cessation of smoking is discussed. However, in one study a decrease of risk was only observed more than 10 years after quitting.

Diet

According to case–control studies, meat and cholesterol are thought to slightly elevate the risk of pancreatic carcinoma. Heterocyclic amines and polycyclic aromatic hydrocarbons produced during the cooking of meat seem to be the responsible pathogenetic factors. In an Italian case–control study, pancreatic cancer risk was directly associated with consumption of meat (OR 1.43), liver (OR 1.43), and ham and sausages (OR 1.64), and inversely associated with consumption of fresh fruit (OR 0.59), fish (OR 0.65), and olive oil (OR 0.58). However, there are methodologic limitations of many descriptive and case–control studies. Thus, definite statements regarding the risk or benefit of any diet are not possible (Table 41.3).

Coffee

It is amazing how many epidemiologic studies have investigated the potential association between coffee and pancreatic cancer (Table 41.3). Obviously, the scientific community, as a major coffee consumer, was shocked by an early study published in a leading scientific journal that confirmed the risk association. However, this association could not be verified by most of the subsequent studies, except for an eventual risk of drinking more than three cups of coffee per day (Table 41.3).

Alcohol

Most studies have not detected an association between alcohol consumption and the risk of pancreatic cancer (Table 41.3). In a retrospective cohort based on the Swedish Inpatient Register, alcoholics had only a modest 40% excess risk of pancreatic cancer. The excess risk for pancreatic cancer among alcoholics is small and is influenced by the confounding factor of smoking.

Occupational and environmental risk factors

For all occupational risk factors studied, especially chlorinated hydrocarbons, there may be only a weak association with pancreatic cancer (Table 41.4). Interactions between environmental and occupational agents, lifestyle factors, and genetic susceptibility always remain a possibility. Thus, there is no convincing evidence to support specific environmental causes in most cases of pancreatic cancer.

Genes

The genetic alterations that develop during pancreatic carcinogenesis are increasingly understood. Acquired mutations have been identified in the oncogenes K-*ras* and *HER2/neu*, and in the tumor-suppressor genes *p16*, *p53*, *SMAD4*, and *BRCA2*. Several familial syndromes with known genetic defects have been implicated, but the majority of familial cases result from as yet undefined genes. Thus, the inherited genetic defects in familial pancreatic carcinoma are still not known. The pattern of inheritance is mostly autosomal dominant. In about 35% of families, additional tumor types such as melanoma and breast and prostate cancer can occur. There seems to be evidence for involvement of a major gene in the etiology of pancreatic cancer that influences "age at onset" of pancreatic cancer more than "susceptibility." According to a segregation analysis of 287 families that used an "age-at-onset" model, approximately 7% of the population appears to be at high risk of pancreatic cancer.

Pancreatic cancer is associated with several genetic syndromes, including hereditary breast cancer (*BRCA2*), familial atypical multiple mole melanoma syndrome (CDKN2A (*p16*) germline mutation), Peutz–Jeghers syndrome, von Hippel–Lindau disease, and hereditary nonpolyposis colorectal cancer. For example, according to a cohort study of 11 847 individuals from 699 families segregating a *BRCA1* mutation, mutation carriers were at a statistically significantly

Table 41.2 Smoking and the risk of pancreatic cancer.

Study	Study design	Risk
Cigarettes		
Lin *et al.* (2002)	Prospective cohort study, 110 792 inhabitants	RR for current smokers: 1.6 (CI 0.95–2.6) in males; 1.7 (CI 0.84–3.3) in females
Stolzenberg-Solomon *et al.* (2001)	Prospective study, 27 111 male smokers aged 50–69 years	Increased risk (highest compared with lowest quintile, cigarettes per day: HR 1.82; CI 1.10, 3.03; *P*-trend 0.05)
Ciu *et al.* (2001)	Population-based case–control study	Increased risk. Males: OR 1.8 (CI 1.2–2.8). Females: OR 2.1 (CI 1.4–3.1)
Nilsen *et al.* (2000)	Health screening survey in a county in Norway: 31 000 men, 32 374 women initially free from cancer. 12 years of follow-up	Twofold increased risk among current smokers. Dose–response association: number of cigarettes (*P* for trend, 0.02) and number of pack-years (*P* for trend, 0.02 for men and 0.01 for women)
Villeneuve *et al.* (2000)	Direct questionnaire data 76% of the cases: 583 pancreatic cancers vs. 4813 controls	Increased risk. Males with 35 or more cigarette pack-years: OR 1.46 (CI 1.00–2.14). Women reporting at least 23 cigarette pack-years of smoking: OR 1.84 (CI 1.25–2.69)
Harnack *et al.* (1997)	Prospective cohort study of 33 976 postmenopausal Iowa women	Elevated risk: < 20 pack-years and > 20 or more pack-years of smoking exposure: 1.14 (CI 0.53–2.45) and 1.92 (CI 1.12–2.30) times more likely to develop pancreatic cancer than nonsmokers
Partanen *et al.* (1997)	Population-based case–control study	Increased risk
Fuchs *et al.* (1996)	118 339 women aged 30–55 years, 49 428 men aged 40–75 years without cancer, 2 116 229 person-years of follow-up, pancreatic cancer diagnosed in 186 participants	Multivariate RR for current smokers: 2.5 (CI 1.7–3.6). Proportion of cancers attributable to smoking: 25%
Lee *et al.* (1996)	Retrospective study 282 inpatients with pancreatic cancer vs. 282 age- and sex-matched controls	OR increased with level of smoking
Ji *et al.* (1995)	Case–control study: 451 vs. 1552 controls. Interview	Increased risk: men OR 1.6 (CI 1.1–2.2); women OR 1.4 (CI 0.9–2.4). ORs increased with number of cigarettes smoked per day and with duration of smoking
Silverman *et al.* (1994)	Population-based case–control study 1986–89 in Atlanta, Detroit, and 10 counties in New Jersey. Direct interviews. 526 case patients vs. 2153 controls, aged 30–79 years	70% increased risk, positive trend in risk with increasing duration of smoking
Friedman & van den Eeden (1993)	Exploratory case–control study. People with multiphasic health check-ups in San Francisco Bay Area: 452 developed pancreatic cancer vs. 2687 controls	Increased risk: cigarette smoking, diabetes mellitus, higher levels of serum iron, iron saturation, body weight

Continued

Table 41.2 *Continued*

Study	Study design	Risk
Ghadirian *et al.* (1991)	Population-based case–control study, Quebec: 179 cancers vs. 239 controls	Smoking: OR 3.76 (CI 1.80–7.83). Smokers in the highest quintile of number of cigarettes: OR 5.15 vs. 3.99 for exsmokers
Howe *et al.* (1991)	Population-based case–control study, Toronto: 249 cancers vs. 505 controls. Lifetime history of smoking	Risk increased. Dose–response relationship with RR of 1.88, 4.61, 6.52 for tertiles of consumption for current cigarette smokers. Rapid decrease after quitting
Bueno de Mesquita *et al.* (1991)	Population-based case–control study, Netherlands: 176 cases vs. 487 controls. Interviewer-administered questionnaire: 58% interviewed directly	Positive dose–response effect of lifetime number of total cigarettes, i.e., nonfilter and filter, OR 1.00, 1.35, 1.40
Farrow *et al.* (1990)	Population-based case–control study, New Mexico: 148 cases vs. 188 controls. Interview cases or wives	Current smokers: OR 3.2 (CI 1.8–5.7)
Olsen *et al.* (1990)	Case–control study, Minneapolis-St Paul area: 212 cases vs. 220 controls. Family members interviewed about the subject's use of cigarettes, alcohol, coffee, and other dietary factors in the 2 years prior to death	OR for two packs or more of cigarettes per day: 3.92. OR for four or more drinks per day: 2.69. Coffee: no risk factor. Positive trend for beef and pork consumption. Negative trend for cruciferous vegetables
Falk *et al.* (1988)	Hospital-based case–control study, Louisiana: 363 cases vs. 1234 controls	Current smokers: twofold risk associated with moderate (16–25 cigarettes per day) and heavy ($\geq$ 26 cigarettes per day) smoking. Ex-smokers: no risk
Wynder *et al.* (1986)	Hospital-based case–control study of individuals aged 20–80 years in 18 hospitals, USA. Males: 127 cases vs. 371 controls. Females: 111 vs. 325	Cigarette smoking: increased risk in both sexes
Mack *et al.* (1986)	Case–control study, Los Angeles: 490 cases, working age vs. 420 controls. Home interviews: occupation, smoking, food, beverage consumption of tea, carbonated	Risk increased. Effect disappeared after a decade of nonsmoking. No association with past consumption, medical history beverages, beer, spirits, coffee
Heuch *et al.* (1983)	Prospective study, Norway: 16 713 individuals, 63 cases occurred	Positive association: chewing of tobacco, use of snuff. Weaker association: cigarette smoking. No association: pipe smoking or coffee drinking
MacMahon *et al.* (1981)	Case–control study: 369 patients with histologically proved cancer vs. 644 control patients. Interview about use of tobacco, alcohol, tea, coffee	Weak positive association: cigarette smoking No association: cigars, pipe tobacco, alcoholic beverages, tea. Strong association: smoking and weight

Table 41.2 *Continued*

Study	Study design	Risk
Ogren *et al.* (1996)	35 000 men and women below 55 years of age participated in a general health examination, 1974–92. Record linkage with the Cause of Death Register and the National Cancer Register	Weight gain > 10 kg since the age of 30: OR 1.8 (CI 0.9–3.6)
Weiss & Benarde (1983)		Temporal trends between pancreatic cancer prevalence related to temporal trend in cigarette smoking in USA 1920–78
Moolgavkar & Stevens (1981)		Difference in male and female rates in pancreatic cancer attributable to differences in smoking habits. Observed increase in mortality due to dramatic increase among smokers. Mortality rate among nonsmokers increased only slowly
Cigars		
Shapiro *et al.* (2000)	Prospective cohort of 137 243 US men; 12 years follow-up	No increased risk if smoke is not inhaled
Farrow *et al.* (1990)	Population-based case–control study, New Mexico: 148 cases vs. 188 controls. Interview cases or wives	No risk: pipe tobacco, cigars, chewing tobacco
Cessation of smoking		
Mulder *et al.* (2002)	Computer simulation model, Markov multistate type	Reduced
Cessation of smoking for more than 5 years		
Nilsen *et al.* (2000)	Health screening survey in a county in Norway: 31 000 men, 32 374 women initially free from cancer; 12 years of follow-up	No increased risk
Fuchs *et al.* (1996)		Less than 10 years, risk equals that of nonsmokers
Silverman *et al.* (1994)	Population-based case–control study 1986–89 in Atlanta, Detroit, and 10 counties in New Jersey, direct interviews, 526 case patients vs. 2153 controls, aged 30–79 years	Stopped smoking for more than 10 years: 30% reduction in risk. Quitters of 10 years or less: no risk reduction
Bueno de Mesquita *et al.* (1991)	Population-based case–control study, Netherlands: 176 cases vs. 487 controls. Interviewer-administered questionnaire: 58% interviewed directly	Risk after quitting 15 years or more examined in the low-smoking group only: no different from nonsmokers

CI, 95% confidence interval; HR, hazard ratio; OR, odds ratio; RR, relative risk.

Table 41.3 Dietary risk factors and pancreatic cancer.

Study	Study design	Risk
Alcohol		
Lin *et al.* (2002)	Prospective cohort study, 110 792 subjects	No effect
Michaud *et al.* (2001)	Semiquantitative food-frequency questionnaires (1986 Health Professionals Follow-Up Study and 1980 Nurses' Health Study), follow-up questionnaires	No effect
Villeneuve *et al.* (2000)	Direct questionnaire data 76% of the cases: 583 pancreatic cancers, 4813 controls	No effect
Kato *et al.* (1992)	Prospective study of 6701 American men of Japanese ancestry living in Hawaii	Risk of upper digestive tract cancers was increased even among heavy alcohol drinkers who were nonsmokers, RR 8.6 (CI 2.1–36.0)
Bueno de Mesquita *et al.* (1992)	Population-based case–control study, 1984–88, Netherlands: 176 pancreatic cancers vs. 487 controls	No increased risk: alcohol, coffee, tea
Ghadirian *et al.* (1991)	Population-based case–control study, Quebec: 179 cancers vs. 239 controls	Alcohol: lower risk
Heuch *et al.* (1983)	Prospective study, Norway, 16 713 individuals, 63 cases occurred	Strongest positive association: alcohol (RR 5.4)
Beer vs. wine vs. spirits		
Bouchardy *et al.* (1990)	Pooled analysis of three case–control studies, Italy, France, Switzerland: 494 cases vs. 1704 controls	No increased risk
Blacks vs. whites		
Silverman *et al.* (1995)	Population-based case–control study, direct interviews with 307 white, 179 black incident cases, 1164 white, 945 black controls	Increased risk: > 57 drinks/week Blacks: OR 2.2 (CI 0.9–5.6) Whites: OR 1.4 (CI 0.6–3.2) Compared with whites, blacks had higher ORs associated with heavy alcohol drinking
Coffee		
Lin *et al.* (2002)	Prospective cohort study, 110 792 subjects	No effect
Michaud *et al.* (2001)	Semiquantitative food-frequency questionnaires (1986 Health Professionals Follow-Up Study and 1980 Nurses' Health Study), follow-up questionnaires	No effect
Villeneuve *et al.* (2000)	Direct questionnaire data 76% of the cases: 583 pancreatic cancers, 4813 controls	No effect
Porta *et al.* (1999)	Case–case study	Ki-*ras* mutations in tumors: 77.7%. Mutations more common among regular coffee drinkers: 82.0% vs. 55.6%, $P = 0.018$. Dose relation between Ki-*ras* mutation and number of cups of coffee per week
Soler *et al.* (1998)	Case–control study 1983–92 in northern Italy on 362 patients with histologically confirmed, incident cancers of the pancreas, and 1552 controls	No effect
Harnack *et al.* (1997)	Prospective cohort study of 33 976 postmenopausal Iowa women	Elevated risk for those who drank > 17.5 cups of coffee per week compared with those who consumed < 7 cups per week

Table 41.3 *Continued*

Study	Study design	Risk
Gullo *et al.* (1995)	Case–control study: 570 pancreatic cancers vs. 570 controls; 14 centers in Italy	Increased risk for those who drank > 3 cups of coffee per day: OR 2.53 (CI 1.53–4.18)
Partanen *et al.* (1995)	Data on coffee consumption 20 years prior to diagnosis of cancer obtained from the next of kin of 662 cases of pancreas cancer and 1770 reference (stomach, colon, and rectum) cancers	No association
Stensvold *et al.* (1994)	10-year complete follow-up of 21 735 men and 21 238 women aged 35–54 years in Norway	No association
Lyon *et al.* (1992)	Population-based case–control study: 149 from proxy respondents	Increased risk: coffee drinkers (OR pancreatic cancers vs. 363 controls. Information 2.38), cigarette smokers (OR 2.27). Risk higher for users of decaffeinated coffee than users of regular coffee
Jain *et al.* (1991)	Case–control study, Toronto: 249 cancers vs. 505 controls	No association for coffee and alcohol
Ghadirian *et al.* (1991)	Population-based case–control study, Quebec: 179 cancers vs. 239 controls	Coffee: lower risk when consumed with meals, not on empty stomach
Clavel *et al.* (1989)	Hospital-based case–control study, France: 161 cases vs. 268 controls	No association between tobacco or alcohol consumption. Coffee consumption associated with increased risk with two or more cups per day vs. less: RR 2.27 (CI 1.11–4.64) and RR 1.45 (CI 0.82–2.55) among females and males respectively
La Vecchia *et al.* (1987)	Hospital-based case–control study, northern Italy: 150 cancers vs. 605 controls	No association with duration of consumption of coffee, decaffeinated coffee or tea
Nomura *et al.* (1986)	Prospective cohort study: 7355 men clinically examined, 1965–68; 21 pancreas cancers developed	No increased risk
Binstock *et al.* (1983)	Relationship of per-capita coffee imports, total dietary fat, saturated fat, cholesterol, tobacco, cigarettes, national income, 1957–65 to age-adjusted pancreatic cancer death rates of men and women from 22 countries, 1971–74	Bivariate partial correlation coefficients of coffee with pancreatic cancer mortality: significant (one-tailed) in 11 of 12 analyses, borderline significant in two-way ANOVA (two-tailed)
Wynder *et al.* (1983)	Case–control study, USA: 275 cases vs. 7994 controls. Interview	No association
Benarde & Weiss (1982)		Per-capita consumption of coffee and pancreatic cancer mortality in USA since 1950: temporal association, 10-year lag. Cigarette smoking: confounding factor
MacMahon *et al.* (1981)	Case–control study: 369 patients with histologically proved cancer vs. 644 control patients. Interview about use of tobacco, alcohol, tea, coffee	Coffee consumption in both sexes. Dose–response relation. RR after adjustment for cigarette smoking: up to two cups of coffee per day, 1.8 (CI 1.0–3.0); three or more cups per day, 2.7 (CI 1.6–4.7)
Decaffeinated coffee		
Wynder *et al.* (1986)	Hospital-based case–control study of individuals aged 20–80 years in 18 hospitals, USA. Males: 127 cases vs. 371 controls. Females: 111 vs. 325	No increased risk

Continued

341

Table 41.3 *Continued*

Study	Study design	Risk
Fat		
Saturated fat		
Stolzenberg-Solomon et al. (2002)	Prospective study, 27 111 male smokers aged 50–69 years	Elevation: HR 1.60; CI 0.96, 2.64; P trend 0.02
Binstock et al. (1983)	Relationship of per-capita coffee imports, total dietary fat, saturated fat, cholesterol, tobacco, cigarettes, national income, 1957–65 to age-adjusted pancreatic cancer death rates of men and women from 22 countries, 1971–74	Significantly related in univariate analyses, and in 11 of 12 bivariate partial correlation analyses; in ANOVA, significance borderline in 10 of 12 analyses
Butter, margarine		
La Vecchia et al. (1997)	Case–control study: 362 pancreatic cancer cases and 1502 controls	No effect
Fat from all sources		
Lyon et al. (1993)	Case–control study: 149 cases vs. 363 controls, Utah	Increased risk: in men OR 3.41 (CI 1.59–7.29); in women, fat from nonmeat and nondairy sources increased OR for upper tertile, 3.44 (CI 1.35–8.78). High levels of intake of red meat, chicken, fish, and dairy foods did not increase risk
Meat		
Saturated fat		
Michaud et al. (2003)	Prospective, 18 years, mailed questionnaire	No effect
Grilled red meat, method of meat preparation		
Anderson et al. (2002)	Case–control study	OR increased: 2.19
Ohba et al. (1996)	Community-based case–control study: 141 cases, 282 controls	Meat and animal viscera increased risk
Smoked meat		
Ghadirian et al. (1995)	Population-based case–control study of pancreatic cancer and nutrition among the Francophone population of Montreal: 179 cases, 239 controls	Smoked meat: RR 4.68 (CI 2.05–10.69)
Protein		
Farrow et al. (1990)	Population-based case–control study, New Mexico: 148 cases vs. 188 controls	Risk increased with increasing protein intake. No association between pancreatic cancer risk and intake of total fat, saturated fat, cholesterol, ω-3 fatty acids, or vitamins A, C
Salt		
Ghadirian et al. (1995)	Population-based case–control study of pancreatic cancer and nutrition among the Francophone population of Montreal: 179 cases, 239 controls	High consumption of salt: RR 4.28 (CI 2.20–8.36)
Various		
Ghadirian et al. (1995)	Population-based case–control study of pancreatic cancer and nutrition among the Francophone population of Montreal: 179 cases, 239 controls	Dehydrated food: RR 3.10 (CI 1.55–6.22). Fried food: RR 3.84 (CI 1.74–8.48) Refined sugar: RR 2.81 (CI 0.94–8.45)

Table 41.3 *Continued*

Study	Study design	Risk
Ji *et al.* (1995)	Case–control study in Shanghai: 451 vs 1552	No association: preserved animal foods, fresh red meat, organ meat, poultry Risk increased: preserved vegetables, deep fried, grilled, cured, or smoked foods
Baghurst *et al.* (1991)	Case–control study, South Australia: 104 cancers vs. 253 controls. Quantitative food-frequency questionnaire, 179 items, about diet 1 year prior to diagnosis	Food items consumed more by cases than controls: boiled eggs, omelettes, sweet, fatty items. RR for the highest quartile of cholesterol 3.19 (CI 1.58–6.47)
Bueno de Mesquita *et al.* (1991)	Case–control study, Netherlands: 164 cancers vs. 480 controls. Semi-quantitative food-frequency questionnaire about diet 1 year prior to diagnosis. Half the cases directly interviewed	Increased risk: high consumption of eggs, fish, low consumption of vegetables
Zatonski *et al.* (1991)	Case–control study, south-west Poland: 110 cancers vs. 190 controls. Diet history	Increased risk: cholesterol, RR 1.90, 3.77, 4.31 for the 3 upper quartiles compared with the lowest
Howe *et al.* (1990)	Case–control study, Toronto: 249 cases vs. 505 controls	Positive association with total caloric intake, RR 2.39 (CI 1.18–4.83) (highest vs. lowest quartile). Inverse associations with fiber from fruit, vegetable, cereal sources
Mills *et al.* (1988)	Prospective study among 34 000 California Seventh-day Adventists, 1976–83; 40 deaths from pancreas cancer occurred	Compared with all US whites, Adventists have decreased risk of pancreas cancer, SMR 72 for men, 90 for women, not statistically significant
Norell *et al.* (1986)	Population-based case–control study, Sweden: 99 cases vs. 138 population controls vs. 163 hospital controls	Risk increased: higher consumption of fried, grilled meat, RR 1.7 (CI 1.1–2.7) for weekly intake; RR 13.4 (CI 2.4–74.7) for associations found with other fried or grilled foods, not with meat other than fried or grilled Risk increased with the intake of margarine, RR 9.7 (CI 3.1–30.2) No excess risk associated with high intake of butter Low risk associated with frequent consumption of fruits, vegetables, particularly carrots, RR 0.3 (CI 0.2–0.7) citrus fruits, RR 0.5 (CI 0.3–0.9) No associations: coffee, artificial sweeteners, alcohol consumption Threefold increase in risk: smoking at least one pack of cigarettes daily
Gold *et al.* (1985)	Case–control study, Baltimore: 201 cancers vs. 201 hospital and nonhospital controls	Increased risk: white bread Decreased risk: raw fruits, vegetables, diet soda, white wine No association: coffee
Durbec *et al.* (1983)	Retrospective study: 69 cancer patients vs. 199 normal subjects interviewed	RR increases with fat and alcohol intake. No association with protein intake. Decreased risk: carbohydrate intake and duration of alcohol consumption

ANOVA, analysis of variance; CI, 95% confidence interval; HR, hazard ratio; OR, odds ratio; RR, relative risk; SMR, standardized mortality ratio.

Table 41.4 Occupational, medical, and environmental risk factors for pancreatic cancer.

Study	Study design	Risk
Acrylamide Marsh *et al.* (1999)	Cohort of 8508 workers with potential exposure to acrylamide	Significant 2.26-fold risk (CI 1.03–4.29) with cumulative exposure to acrylamide > 0.3 mg/m^3.years. No exposure–response relation
Aluminum polycyclic aromatic hydrocarbons Romundstad *et al.* (2000) Ronneberg *et al.* (1999)	Cancer incidence 1953–96 among 11 103 men employed for more than 3 years	Higher incidence, no dose correlation
Cadmium Schwartz *et al.* (2000)	Metaanalysis	SMR 166; CI 98–280; $P = 0.059$
Chlorinated hydrocarbon solvents Ojajarvi *et al.* (2001)	Metaanalysis, 1969–98	Weak excesses: trichloroethylene, MRR 1.24; polychlorinated biphenyls, MRR 1.37; methylene chloride, MRR 1.42; vinyl chloride, MRR 1.17; carbon tetrachloroethylene, MRR 3.08; chlorohydrin, MRR 4.92 No risk: tetrachloride
Organochlorine pesticides Clary & Ritz (2003)	Pesticide reporting system for residents of high-use areas: pancreatic cancer vs. random controls	Elevated for long-term residents in areas with highest dose
Hoppin *et al.* (2000)	Serum from 108 pancreatic cancer cases and 82 controls aged 32–85 years	Polychlorinated biphenyls (PCBs) and transnonachlor: significantly greater among cases than controls. Subjects in the highest tertile of PCBs ($\geq$ 360 ng/g lipid): OR 4.2
Pesticides, fungicides, and herbicides Ji *et al.* (2001)	Case–control study	Increased risk: ORs of 1.3 and 1.4 for low and moderate/high exposure to pesticides Fungicides: OR 1.5 Herbicides: OR 1.6
Alguacil *et al.* (2000)	Direct interview with patient; 164 pancreatic cancer cases	For each type of pesticide group: moderately increased ORs in the high-intensity category. Highest for arsenical pesticides (OR 3.4, CI 0.9–12.0). ORs for aniline derivatives, dyes, and organic pigments: higher for high-intensity exposure
Chromium: medium/high level of exposure Weiderpass *et al.* (2003)	Cohort including all female workers born 1906–45	RR of exposure 1.8 (CI 1.0–3.1)
DDT (Ethylan and DDD) Garabrant *et al.* (1992)	Cohort mortality study among 5886 chemical manufacturing workers. Nested case–control study: 28 cancer cases vs. 112 matched controls. Next of kin interview	Increased risk: RR for ever exposed compared with never exposed 4.8 (CI 1.3–17.6) DDT risk: heavy and prolonged exposure
Education Ferraroni *et al.* (1989)	Case–control study, Italy: 214 cases vs. 1944 controls	No association

Table 41.4 *Continued*

Study	Study design	Risk
Formaldehyde		
Collins *et al.* (2001)	Metaanalysis: 14 studies	Small increase of risk in the studies overall (MRR 1.1, CI 1.0–1.3) limited to embalmers (MRR 1.3, CI 1.0–1.6), pathologists, anatomists (MRR 1.3, CI 1.0–1.7). Other factors responsible?
Kernan *et al.* (1999)	63 097 persons who died from pancreatic cancer in the period 1984–93; 252 386 persons who died from causes other than cancer	Occupational exposure associated with a moderately increased risk: ORs 1.2, 1.2, 1.4 for subjects with low, medium, and high probabilities of exposure
Latitude		
Kato *et al.*		Internationally and within Japan, strong positive association between latitude and pancreatic cancer mortality, strong negative association with the average temperature: "factors related to latitude or average temperature other than diet involved?"
Lead		
McDonald & Potter (1996)	Lead poisoning in 454 children, 1923–66	Two pancreatic cancers many years later
Leather		
Mikoczy *et al.* (1996)	Case–control study cohort of 2487 workers employed for at least 6 months during the period 1900–89 in Swedish leather tanneries: 68 cancer cases (lung, stomach, bladder, kidney, nasal, pancreatic cancers, soft-tissue sarcomas) vs. 178 controls	Association of exposure to leather dust and pancreatic cancer: OR 7.19 (CI 1.44 to 35–89) Data tentative due to small numbers
Costantini *et al.* (1989)	2926 male workers at tanneries compared with national mortality	Slight increase of risk: SMR 146 (CI 39–373)
Resin: vinyl resins and polyethylene		
Selenskas *et al.* (1995)	Case–control study: 28 cancers vs. 140 controls	Increased risk in men with more than 16 years of exposure: RR 7.15 (CI 1.28–40.1)
Styrene		
Kolstad *et al.* (1995)	36 610 workers of 386 plastics companies and 14 293 workers not exposed to styrene. Follow-up from 1970 to 1990	IRR 2.2, 17 cases, CI 1.1–4.5
Sulfite pulp		
Rix *et al.* (1997)	2238 workers employed 1955–90, historic cohort, followed until 1993	Risk of pancreatic cancer almost doubled (7 observed, SIR 1.88, CI 0.75–3.88)
Thorotrast		
Nyberg *et al.* (2002)	Computerized linkage of a cohort with the Swedish Cancer Register	SIR significantly increased for cancers at all sites (3.0), largest for primary liver and gallbladder cancer (SIR 39.2)
Polednak *et al.* (1983)	Cohort of 3039 men employed 1940–73 at a company involved in the production of thorium	SMRs high: 2.01 (CI 0.92–3.82). Smoking a confounding factor
Undefined biological research		
Rachet *et al.* (2000)	Metaanalysis: 45 studies	Low overall risk: RR ranging from 0.5 to 6.3. Confounding factors?

Continued

Table 41.4 *Continued*

Study	Study design	Risk
Various occupational exposures		
Ojajarvi *et al.* (2000)	Metaanalysis: 1969–98	Chlorinated hydrocarbon solvents, MRR 1.4; nickel, MRR 1.9; chromium, MRR 1.4; polycyclic aromatic hydrocarbons, MRR 1.5; organochlorine insecticides, MRR 1.5; silica dust, MRR 1.4; aliphatic and alicyclic hydrocarbon solvents, MRR 1.3. Weak or nonpositive: acrylonitrile, arsenic, asbestos, diesel engine exhaust, electromagnetic fields, formaldehyde, flour dust, cadmium, gasoline, herbicides, iron, lead, synthetic vitreous fibers, oil mist, wood dust. Occupational etiologic fraction of pancreatic cancer estimated at 12%
Kauppinen *et al.* (1995)	Case–control study in Finland: exposure histories for 595 incident cases of pancreatic cancer vs. 1622 controls	Elevated risk: ionizing radiation, OR 4.3 (CI 1.6–11.4); nonchlorinated solvents, OR 1.6–1.8; pesticides, OR 1.7 (CI 0.8–3.4); inorganic dust containing crystalline silica, OR 2.0 (CI 1.2–3.5); heat stress, OR 2.2 (CI 0.8–6.6); rubber chemicals including acrylonitrile, OR 2.1 (CI 0.9–4.7) No association: asbestos, chromates, cleaning agents, waxes, polishes
Ji *et al.* (1999)	451 pancreatic cancer patients newly diagnosed in 1990–93 and 1552 controls randomly selected from Shanghai residents. Information on lifetime job history and other factors obtained by direct interview	Increased risk of pancreatic cancer in men: electrician, OR 7.5 (CI 2.6–21.8); metal workers, OR 2.1 (CI 1.0–4.8); toolmakers, OR 3.4 (CI 14–7.1); plumbers and welders, OR 3.0 (CI 1.2–7.5); glass manufacturers, potters, painters, and construction workers, OR 2.6 (CI 1.1–6.3)
Partanen *et al.* (1994)	Job history information from next of kin of 625 incident cases of pancreatic cancers vs. 1700 cancers of stomach, colon, rectum	Increases in risk suggested: stone mining, OR 3.7; cement and building materials, OR 11.1; pharmacists and sales associates in pharmacies, OR 12.9; male wood machinists, OR 4.1; male gardeners, OR 6.7; female textile workers, OR 5.4; male transport inspectors and supervisors, OR 9.4
Pietri *et al.* (1990)	Case–control study, France: 171 cases vs. 317 controls	Increased risk for workers in: food industry, OR 1.86; leather industry, OR 1.63; textile industry, OR 2.30; printing, OR 1.54; building materials, OR 2.16
Falk *et al.* (1990)	Hospital-based case–control study in high-risk area of Louisiana, 1979–83: 198 cases vs. 209 controls	Elevations in risk: white-collar occupations
Waste		
Schwartz *et al.* (1998)	Florida's population-based cancer registry. Whites with median household income, per county. Prevalence of cigarette smoking. Measures of per-capita municipal solid waste collection	Incidence for pancreatic cancer from 0 to 8.1/100 000 per year. Correlation with income ($r = 0.35$), cigarette smoking ($r = 0.39$), and solid waste ($r = 0.47$), especially yard trash (due to herbicides, insecticides?)

CI, 95% confidence interval; IRR, individual relative risk; MRR, meta-relative risk; OR, odds ratio; RR, relative risk; SIR, standardized incidence ratio; SMR, standardized mortality ratio.

Table 41.5 Genetic risk factors of pancreatic cancer.

Study	Study design	Risk
Family history		
Fernandez *et al.* (1994)	Case–control study, northern Italy: 362 pancreatic cancers vs. 1408 controls	RR 3.0 (CI 1.4–6.6)
Smoking and number of family members having pancreatic carcinoma		
Rulyak *et al.* (2003)	Nested case–control study	Additional risk factor in familial pancreatic carcinoma: OR 3.7
Black vs. white		
Silverman *et al.* (2003)	Population-based case–control study	No difference. Increased risk in blacks due to different lifestyle
Young *et al.* (1975)		Increased risk in blacks
Familial atypical multiple mole melanoma (FAMMM)		
Vasen *et al.* (2000)	Dutch FAMMM families with a 19-bp deletion in exon 2 of the *p16* gene (*p16*-Leiden)	Cumulative risk at age 75: 17% Only in FAMMM carrying the *p16* mutation

CI, 95% confidence interval; OR, odds ratio; RR, relative risk.

increased risk for pancreatic cancer (relative risk 2.26, 95% CI 1.26–4.06, $P = 0.004$).

Family history of pancreatic cancer confers a 1.5–13-fold elevated risk of developing pancreatic cancer (Table 41.5). In a nested case–control study, one-third of families demonstrated genetic anticipation. The mean age of onset decreased by two decades between generations. Furthermore, smoking seems to be a very strong risk factor in familial pancreatic cancer kindreds. In families with multiple affected first-degree relatives the risk is further increased. However, familial clustering of pancreatic cancer could also be due to chance, exposure to environmental factors such as cigarette smoking, and/or polygenetic or mendelian inherited factors. In a study from the Swedish Family-Cancer Database of 10.2 million individuals and 21 000 pancreatic cancers, the SIR for pancreatic adenocarcinoma was increased (1.73, 95% CI 1.13–2.54) when a parent presented with pancreatic cancer. Pancreatic cancer showed an association with parental lung, rectal, or endometrial cancer and with melanoma. The SIR for pancreatic cancer was about 10 among offspring who were diagnosed before the age of 50 years. The population-attributable proportion of familial pancreatic cancer in this study was only 1.1%, lower than the data in the literature. In another study

from Canada, the lifetime risk of pancreatic cancer was 4.7% for first-degree relatives of pancreatic cancer cases. The risk increased up to 7.2% for relatives of cases diagnosed before age 60, and was 12.3% for relatives of patients with multiple primary cancers. In another study, the risk of pancreatic cancer in the sporadic pancreatic cancer kindreds was not significantly greater than expected. However, there was a significantly increased 18-fold risk of pancreatic cancer when more than one family member was affected. In a subset of familial pancreatic cancer kindreds with three or more affected family members at the time of enrolment, there was even a 57-fold increased risk. When stratified by age, the risk was mainly confined to relatives over the age of 60.

For many decades, the incidence of pancreatic cancer has been 50–90% higher among blacks than among whites in the USA. Established risk factors such as cigarette smoking, long-term diabetes mellitus, and family history of pancreatic cancer account for 46% of the disease in black men and for 37% in whites. This might explain all but 6% of the excess risk among blacks. Among women, the authors report that other factors may contribute to the racial disparity, i.e., moderate to heavy alcohol consumption and elevated BMI. According to this study, in the absence of these risk factors,

Table 41.6 Factors reducing risk of pancreatic cancer.

Study	Study design	Risk
Aspirin		
Menezes *et al.* (2002)	Hospital-based case–control study	Not reduced
Energy-adjusted carbohydrate intake		
Stolzenberg-Solomon *et al.* (2002)	Prospective study, 27 111 male smokers aged 50–69 years: Alpha-Tocopherol, Beta-Carotene Cancer Prevention Study cohort	HR 0.62; CI 0.37, 1.03; P-trend 0.02
Dietary folate		
Stolzenberg-Solomon *et al.* (2001)	Prospective study, 27 111 male smokers aged 50–69 years	Slight decreased risk: adjusted HR comparing the highest with the lowest quintile of dietary folate intake: 0.52 (CI 0.31, 0.87); P-trend 0.05
Various nonsteroidal antiinflammatory drugs		
Anderson *et al.* (2002)	Prospective study	RR reduction with any current use of aspirin vs. no use: 0.57
Olive oil		
La Vecchia *et al.* (1997)	Case–control study: 362 pancreatic cancer cases and 1502 controls	Reduced risk: multivariate OR 0.76 for intermediate and 0.60 for highest score of intake
Various fruits, vegetables, etc.		
Ohba *et al.* (1996)	Community-based case–control study: 141 cases, 282 controls	Vegetables, traditional Japanese foods, e.g., tofu, deep-fried tofu, raw fish, and tempura: reduced risk
Ji *et al.* (1995)	Case–control study in Shanghai: 451 vs. 1552	Risks inversely associated: vegetables, fruits, dietary fiber, eggs
Kalapothaki *et al.* (1993)	Hospital-based case–control study: 181 patients vs. 181 controls. Semiquantitative food-frequency questionnaire	No associations for total energy, total protein, fat, saturated fat, monounsaturated fat, dietary cholesterol, total carbohydrates, sucrose, vitamin C, vitamin A, riboflavin, or calcium
Lyon *et al.* (1993)	Case–control study: 149 cases vs. 363 controls, Utah	No protective effect among men who consumed large amounts of fruits, vegetables, or high-fiber foods. Protective effect in women for these foods: OR for upper tertile of fruit consumption, 0.37 (CI 0.18–0.81); OR for upper tertile of vegetable consumption, 0.32 (CI 0.13–0.74); OR for upper tertile of fiber consumption, 0.28 (CI 0.12–0.67)
Olsen *et al.* (1991)	Case–control study, Minnesota: 212 cases vs. 220 controls. Family interviews about diet 2 years prior to death	Negative trends observed for polyunsaturated fat, linoleic acid, vitamin C, i.e., vegetables, citrus fruits

Table 41.6 *Continued*

Study	Study design	Risk
Baghurst *et al.* (1991)	Case–control study, South Australia: 104 cancers vs. 253 controls. Quantitative food-frequency questionnaire, 179 items, about diet 1 year prior to diagnosis.	Food items consumed less: vegetables, fruits
Zatonski *et al.* (1991)	Case–control study, south-west Poland: 110 cancers vs. 190 controls. Diet history	Decreased risk: vitamin C, RR 1.10, 0.30, 0.37
La Vecchia *et al.* (1990)	Hospital-based case–control study, northern Italy: 247 cancers vs. 1089 controls	Some tendency for risk reduction with more frequent fruit consumption
Mills *et al.* (1988)	Prospective study among 34 000 California Seventh-day Adventists, 1976–83; 40 deaths from pancreas cancer occurred	Decreased risk: increasing consumption of vegetarian protein products, beans, lentils, peas, dried fruit
Vitamins: α-tocopherol, β-carotene		
Rautalahti *et al.* (1999)	29 133 participants in the Alpha-Tocopherol, Beta-Carotene Cancer Prevention Study. Male smokers	No efffect

CI, 95% confidence interval; HR, hazard ratio; OR, odds ratio; RR, relative risk.

Table 41.7 Role of Aspirin.

Study	Study design	Risk
Menezes *et al.* (2002) Schernhammer *et al.* (2004)	Hospital-based case–control study 88.378 women, Nurses Health Study, interview every two years	Not reduced. Aspirin intake at least 650 mg/week >20 years: increased risk 58%. RR 1.43; CI 1.05–1.95. Potential confounding factors: selection bias, overweight, diabetes, smoking. Discarding patients who developed cancer within the first two yrs of aspirin intake: no increased risk, RR 1,15; CI 0.83–1.59. Potential explanation: aspirin intake due to pain in unknown pancreatic cancer (confounding by indication)

pancreatic cancer incidence rates among blacks would probably not exceed those among whites of either sex.

Table 41.6 outlines the factors that have been found to reduce the risk of pancreatic cancer, and Table 41.7 reports important new work on the role of aspirin.

Recommended reading

Furuya N, Kawa S, Akamatsu T, Furihata K. Long-term follow-up of patients with chronic pancreatitis and K-ras gene mutation detected in pancreatic juice. *Gastroenterology* 1997;113:593–598.

Ghadirian P, Liu G, Gallinger S et al. Risk of pancreatic cancer among individuals with a family history of cancer of the pancreas. *Int J Cancer* 2002;97:807–810.

Gullo L, Pezzilli R, Morselli-Labate AM. Diabetes and the risk of pancreatic cancer. Italian Pancreatic Cancer Study Group. *N Engl J Med* 1994;331:81–84.

Gullo L, Pezzilli R, Morselli-Labate AM. Coffee and cancer of the pancreas: an Italian multicenter study. The Italian

Pancreatic Cancer Study Group. *Pancreas* 1995;11:223–229.

Hanley AJ, Johnson KC, Villeneuve PJ, Mao Y, Canadian Cancer Registries Epidemiology Research Group. Physical activity, anthropometric factors and risk of pancreatic cancer: results from the Canadian enhanced cancer surveillance system. *Int J Cancer* 2001;94:140–147.

Hemminki K, Li X. Familial and second primary pancreatic cancers: a nationwide epidemiologic study from Sweden. *Int J Cancer* 2003;103:525–530.

Lowenfels AB, Maisonneuve P, Cavallini G *et al*. Pancreatitis and the risk of pancreatic cancer. International Pancreatitis Study Group. *N Engl J Med* 1993;328:1433–1437.

Lowenfels AB, Maisonneuve P, DiMagno EP *et al*. Hereditary pancreatitis and the risk of pancreatic cancer. International Hereditary Pancreatitis Study Group. *J Natl Cancer Inst* 1997;89:442–446.

Lynch HT, Brand RE, Deters CA, Shaw TG, Lynch JF. Hereditary pancreatic cancer. *Pancreatology* 2001;1:466–471.

McCarty MF. Insulin secretion as a determinant of pancreatic cancer risk. *Med Hypotheses* 2001;57:146–150.

MacMahon B, Yen S, Trichopoulos D, Warren K, Nardi G. Coffee and cancer of the pancreas. *N Engl J Med* 1981;304:630–633.

Maisonneuve P, Lowenfels AB. Chronic pancreatitis and pancreatic cancer. *Dig Dis* 2002;20:32–37.

Malka D, Hammel P, Maire F *et al*. Risk of pancreatic adenocarcinoma in chronic pancreatitis. *Gut* 2002;51:849–852.

Michaud DS, Giovannucci E, Willett WC, Colditz GA, Stampfer MJ, Fuchs CS. Physical activity, obesity, height, and the risk of pancreatic cancer. *JAMA* 2001;286:921–929.

Michaud DS, Giovannucci E, Willett WC, Colditz GA, Fuchs CS. Dietary meat, dairy products, fat, and cholesterol and pancreatic cancer risk in a prospective study. *Am J Epidemiol* 2003;157:1115–1125.

Ogawa Y, Tanaka M, Inoue K *et al*. A prospective pancreatographic study of the prevalence of pancreatic carcinoma in patients with diabetes mellitus. *Cancer* 2002;94:2344–2349.

Rulyak SJ, Lowenfels AB, Maisonneuve P, Brentnall TA. Risk factors for the development of pancreatic cancer in familial pancreatic cancer kindreds. *Gastroenterology* 2003;124:1292–1299.

Silverman DT. Risk factors for pancreatic cancer: a case–control study based on direct interviews. *Teratogenesis Carcinog Mutagen* 2001;21:7–25.

Silverman DT, Hoover RN, Brown LM *et al*. Why do Black Americans have a higher risk of pancreatic cancer than White Americans? *Epidemiology* 2003;14:45–54.

Soler M, Chatenoud L, La Vecchia C, Franceschi S, Negri E. Diet, alcohol, coffee and pancreatic cancer: final results from an Italian study. *Eur J Cancer Prev* 1998;7:455–460.

Thompson D, Easton DF, Breast Cancer Linkage Consortium. Cancer incidence in BRCA1 mutation carriers. *J Natl Cancer Inst* 2002;94:1358–1365.

Ye W, Lagergren J, Weiderpass E, Nyren O, Adami HO, Ekbom A. Alcohol abuse and the risk of pancreatic cancer. *Gut* 2002;51:236–239.

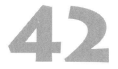

42 Molecular basis of pancreatic carcinogenesis: which concepts may be clinically relevant?

Martin Wirtz, Joanne Nyarangi, Jörg Köninger, and Helmut Friess

The pancreas consists of acinar, ductal, and endocrine cells and is a mitotically quiescent tissue that is highly differentiated. In the past decades, there has been a significant increase in our knowledge of the biology and pathophysiology of pancreatic cancer, but a great number of the mechanisms involved are yet to be fully comprehended.

In normal eukaryotic cells, cell growth, cell differentiation, and cell death are controlled and regulated through various signals that are well coordinated to enable the maintenance of cell homeostasis. In malignant cells, such as in pancreatic cancer, increased dysregulation of important signaling pathways has been observed and many such neoplastic cells need neither mitogenic signaling to develop and further proliferate, nor do they react to inhibitory signals. This is thought to be the result of molecular changes that have been mainly observed in protooncogenes and oncogenes, tumor-suppressor genes, DNA repair genes, and longevity genes that control apoptosis (programmed cell death). Hanahan and Weinberg have described the typical characteristics of tumor cell growth (Table 42.1).

In pancreatic cancer, some genes and gene products have been reported to be mutated, amplified, decreased, or overexpressed. These include growth factors and their receptors (Table 42.2) and important intracellular signal transducers like protein-serine/threonine kinases (e.g., AKT2) and guanine nucleotide-binding proteins (e.g., K-*ras*) and nuclear transcription factors (e.g., c-*myc*, c-*fos*).

In the next sections some of the most important factors involved in the molecular biology and pathophysiology of pancreatic adenocarcinomas are outlined in

more detail, including some growth factors and their receptors and different therapeutic approaches in regard to these.

Epidermal growth factor receptor family and its ligands

Members of the epidermal growth factor (EGF) receptor family consist of four homologous transmembrane proteins that bind various growth actors, thereby resulting in signal transduction. The EGF receptor (EGFR) family consists of the following members:

- human EGFR type 1 (HER1/EGFR/c-erbB1);
- human EGFR type 2 (HER2/c-erbB2/Neu);
- human EGFR type 3 (HER3/c-erbB3);
- human EGFR type 4 (HER4/c-erbB4).

EGFR-1 belongs to one of the most extensively researched growth factor receptors in oncology and it has been found to be significantly overexpressed in human pancreatic cancer. EGFR-1 is a 170-kDa glycosylated phosphoprotein that exerts a profound effect on cell differentiation. Furthermore, it is a potent mitogenic factor for a variety of cultured cells of both ectodermal and mesodermal origin. The molecular structure of EGFR consists of an extracellular ligand-binding domain, a transmembrane domain, and an intracellular domain with tyrosine kinase activity.

EGF and transforming growth factor (TGF)-α are prototype growth factors and can bind to EGFR, resulting in its activation. Early studies in pancreatic cancer showed that the overexpression of EGFR is associated with increased production of EGF and TGF-α, thereby promoting autocrine and paracrine

351

Table 42.1 Basic characteristics of tumor cells and the role of growth factors and their receptors in pancreatic cancer. (After Hanahan & Weinberg 2000.)

Characteristics of malignant growth	Pancreatic cancer*
Autonomous growth control	Increased expression of EGF, FGF, PDGF, IGF, and their receptors
Resistance to growth inhibition	Increased expression of TGF-β and its receptors; *Smad4* mutation *Smad6/7* overexpression
Resistance to apoptosis	Increased expression of EGF, IGF, and their receptors
Angiogenesis	Increased expression of VEGF, FGF-2, and their receptors
Invasiveness and metastasis	Increased expression of HGF, TGF-β, NGF, uPA, and their receptors; decreased expression of KAI-1

* See text and Table 42.2 for definition of abbreviations.

Table 42.2 Important families of growth factors and their receptors that play a major role in pancreatic cancer.

	Growth factor	Receptor
Epidermal growth factor (EGF) family	EGF	EGFR (HER1)
	TGF-α	HER2
	Cripto	HER3
	Amphiregulin	HER4
	Betacellulin	
	HB-EGF	
	Epiregulin	
Fibroblast growth factor (FGF) family	FGF-1	FGFR-1
	FGF-2	FGFR-2
	KGF	FGFR-3
		FGFR-4
Insulin-like growth factor (IGF) family	IGF-I	IRS-1
	IGF-II	IRS-2
Hepatocyte growth factor (HGF) family	HGF	c-met
Platelet-derived growth factor (PDGF) family	PDGF	PDGFR-α
		PDGFR-β
Vascular endothelial growth factor (VEGF) family	VEGF	Flk-1/KDR
	VEGF-C	Flt-1
	PD-ECGF	
Nerve growth factor (NGF) family	NGF	TrkA
Transforming growth factor (TGF)-β family	TGF-β1	TβRI
	TGF-β2	TβRII
	TGF-β3	TβRIII
	Activin-βA	actRI/Ib
	Activin-βB	actRII
	Inhibin-α	BMPR-IA
	BMP-2	BMPR-II
Urokinase plasminogen activator	uPA	uPAR

BMP-2, bone morphogenic protein-2; HB-EGF, heparin-binding EGF-like growth factor; KGF, kartilague growth factor.

loops that boost cell proliferation and malignant transformation. In addition to EGF and TGF-α, EGFR is further activated by different peptide ligands, e.g., heparin-binding EGF-like growth factor (HB-EGF), amphiregulin, betacellulin, neuregulin, and epiregulin among others, that bind to its extracellular fragment with high affinity and trigger a signaling cascade that results in cell proliferation and other cell functions. All these growth factors share high homology with EGF.

In accordance with early results obtained from human pancreatic cancer tissue, cultivated human pancreatic cancer cell lines show overexpression of betacellulin. EGF and HB-EGF promote the expression of betacellulin mRNA and it is assumed that betacellulin expression in pancreatic cancer cells is additionally regulated by other ligands of the EGF family. These observations suggest that upregulation of a growth factor may induce enhanced expression of other growth-promoting factors, thereby multiplying its own mitogenic activity tremendously.

A further member of the EGF family is amphiregulin. Immunohistochemical analysis has revealed that one-third of pancreatic cancer tissues exhibit cytoplasmic amphiregulin expression. It was also found that this expression was frequently associated with coexpression of EGFR. Survival analysis of tumor-resected patients revealed shorter survival for the patients with increased coexpression of both factors compared with those without simultaneously increased expression.

In contrast, neither HB-EGF nor the coexpression of HB-EGF and EGFR is associated with poorer patient prognosis, indicating that overexpression of growth factors is not definitely accompanied by a poor survival prognosis. Recent studies have shown that epiregulin, which is expressed in pancreatic carcinoma, also possesses the potential to stimulate pancreatic cancer cell growth *in vitro*.

The significance of the HER1 signaling pathway on the pathogenesis and growth behavior of pancreatic cancer is also underlined by correlation of the molecular findings with clinical outcome. Simultaneously high levels of HER1, TGF-α, and/or EGF are related to reduced patient survival postoperatively, indicating that this signaling cascade plays a significant role in the growth and malignant transformation of pancreatic cells and blockage of the EGF signalling pathway seems to be a clinically relevant target.

The c-*erb2* gene (HER2) encodes a receptor not capable of directly binding a ligand. This receptor acts as a coreceptor for other EGFRs. *In vitro* studies indicate that HER2 leads to malignant cell transformation, as previously shown for other EGFRs. Interestingly, high HER2 expression levels are associated with better tumor differentiation and not with shorter survival and poorer prognosis.

In accordance with the findings for the HER1 receptor, the expression of HER3 is significantly overexpressed in pancreatic adenocarcinomas. Correlation analysis revealed an association of HER3 overexpression with poor prognosis and shorter postoperative survival in pancreatic cancer.

HER4 serves as receptor for different ligands, such as betacellulin, HB-EGF, epiregulin, as well as the neuregulins. Recently, it was reported that lack of HER4 expression might increase the metastatic capacity of pancreatic cancer cells. However, since HER4 levels in UICC stages I and II are increased but are comparable to those in normal pancreatic tissue in stages III and IV, the role of HER4 in pancreatic cancer is still not clearly understood and deserves further investigation.

Since the EGF family and its receptors are involved in tumor progression and mediate growth effects in pancreatic cancer, they serve as targets for new treatment concepts. It is the aim of these concepts to interrupt EGFR signal transduction and thereby inhibit tumor growth (Table 42.3). *In vitro* studies have revealed the antitumoral effects of amphiregulin antisense oligonucleotides in pancreatic cancer cell lines. These antisense oligonucleotides are constructed to bind amphiregulin mRNA and to inhibit translation of amphiregulin mRNA to the functional protein. This concept is still experimental and not yet validated for anticancer treat-

Table 42.3 Examples of tested therapeutic approaches in anticancer treatment by inhibition of EGF-family peptides and their receptors.

Therapeutic approach	Target molecule
Tyrosine kinase inhibitor (e.g., PKI116, ZD 1839)	HER1
Antibody (e.g., CD225, Astra HER1-Antibody, Herceptin)	HER1, HER2
Dominant-negative receptors	HER1
Riboenzymes	HER2
Antisense oligonucleotides	Amphiregulin

ment in humans. Another approach for interrupting EGFR signal transduction is to create a dominant-negative EGFR. In this approach, the ligand binds to the receptor but without causing signal transduction. Recent *in vitro* studies using this technique revealed promising results with regard to growth inhibition of pancreatic cancer cells. Furthermore, tyrosine kinase inhibitors (e.g., PKI116 and ZD1839) have been used to block EGFR signal transduction and led to growth inhibition of cancer cell lines and of pancreatic cancer xenografts in nude mice.

The most promising therapeutic approach for disrupting growth factors and their signaling cascades involves the use of HER antibodies, e.g., Herceptin and C225. Recently, treatment of human pancreatic cancer cell lines and tumor xenografts in nude mice with a combination of an anti-EGFR antibody, gemcitabine, and radiation was examined. Treatment of cancer cells with a combination of Erbitux, gemcitabine, and radiation produced the highest induction of apoptosis and inhibition of proliferation *in vitro*. Moreover, combination treatment resulted in complete regression of xenograft tumors for more than 250 days.

Phase I trials with monoclonal HER antibodies showed antibody binding to tumor EGFRs and demonstrated saturation of the receptors. Phase Ib/IIa trials in advanced head and neck cancer revealed good clinical response in combination with radiochemotherapy. Over 500 patients have been treated with the monoclonal antibody C225 and have shown only little evidence of immunogenicity, with only 4% of patients developing antibodies against C225.

Transforming growth factor-β and its receptors

TGF-β belongs to an important family of cytokines that bind to specific cell-surface receptors. These cytokines influence cell division, cell death, structure of the extracellular matrix, and angiogenesis. Three TGF-β isoforms (TGF-β1, TGF-β2, and TGF-β3) and three types of TGF-β receptor (TβRI, TβRII, and TβRIII) have been characterized. All three TGF-β isoforms are overexpressed in pancreatic cancer *in vivo*. However, only TβRI and TβRII, but not TβRIII, are overexpressed in pancreatic cancer tissues. Since the TGF-β signaling pathway is upregulated in the extracellular compart-

ment, it was thought that it might support cell invasiveness, metastasizing potential, and angiogenesis. This hypothesis was supported by analysis of the survival time of pancreatic cancer patients and expression of TGF-β isoforms which showed that overexpression of these factors was associated with aggressive tumor growth and reduced postoperative survival.

Since TGF-β functions as a strong inhibitor of proliferation in cells of epithelial origin, it was not understood why pancreatic cancer cells remain resistant to the inhibitory signals of TGF-β. However, further molecular analysis of the TGF-β pathway revealed that the loss of growth inhibition in pancreatic cancer can be explained by mutations of the tumor-suppressor gene *Smad4/DPC4*, which is a crucial signaling molecule in the intracellular TGF-β pathway. Mutated *Smad4/DPC4* therefore represents one possibility by which TGF-β-induced growth inhibition is abolished. The mutation of this gene is identified in about 50% of pancreatic adenocarcinomas, which suggests that *Smad4/DPC4* may have a specific promoting role in pancreatic tumorigenesis.

Deletion or mutational inactivation of the *Smad4/DPC4* gene correlates with loss of responsiveness to TGF-β-induced growth inhibition and TGF-β-inducible p21[wafl] expression. Additionally, wild-type *Smad4/DPC4* transfection can reestablish TGF-β-inducible reporter gene activity in a *Smad4/DPC4*-null human pancreatic adenocarcinoma cell line, indicating the critical function of *Smad4* in pancreatic carcinogenesis.

The TGF-β signaling pathway inhibitors Smad6 and Smad7 are also markedly overexpressed in pancreatic cancers. Smad6 and Smad7 expression is localized in cancer cells within the tumor mass and also to a lesser extent in the endothelial cells and chronic pancreatitis-like areas adjacent to the tumor. Transfection experiments in human pancreatic carcinoma cells with Smad6 and Smad7 show complete abrogation of the growth-inhibitory effects of TGF-β. These *in vitro* and *in vivo* data suggest that pancreatic cancer cells have various barriers to their TGF-β signaling which may thus allow the cancer cells to escape TGF-β-induced growth inhibition while still allowing expression of metastasis-promoting genes. In addition, tumor cell-derived TGF-β may act in a paracrine manner to enhance angiogenesis and suppress cancer-directed immune mechanisms.

A study that investigated whether lack of TβRII expression and loss of TGF-β signaling play a role in radiation resistance of pancreatic cancer cells reported that the loss of function of TβRII may enhance resistance to radiation-induced apoptosis.

Fibroblast growth factor and its receptors

The fibroblast growth factor (FGF) gene family consists of a group of homologous growth-promoting polypeptides:
- FGF-1, also referred to as acidic fibroblast growth factor (aFGF);
- FGF-2, also referred to as basic fibroblast growth factor (bFGF);
- FGF-3 (also named int-2);
- FGF-4 (also named Kaposi FGF);
- FGF-5, FGF-6, FGF-7 (also named keratinocyte growth factor);
- FGF-8 (also named androgen-induced growth factor);
- FGF-9.

aFGF and bFGF are closely related prototypes of this family which are chemotactic toward fibroblasts, promote cellular differentiation, migration, and angiogenesis, and participate in tissue repair.

Analysis of aFGF and bFGF in pancreatic tissue has revealed their marked overexpression in pancreatic cancer. Correlation of immunhistochemical data with clinicopathologic parameters indicated that the presence of aFGF and bFGF is associated with advanced tumor stage. In addition, bFGF but not aFGF immunoreactivity in pancreatic cancer cells is associated with a shorter postoperative patient survival period.

Four high-affinity FGF receptors (FGFR-1, FGFR-2, FGFR-3, and FGFR-4) have been described to date. They are expressed in normal as well as in pancreatic cancer tissue. Overexpression of FGF-1 and FGF-3 is present in many pancreatic cancer tissues and the concomitant overexpression of aFGF, bFGF, and FGFR-1 in human pancreatic cancer indicates that paracrine and autocrine activation of this growth-promoting pathway may play a role in the induction and progression of this particular cancer.

Inhibition of tumor angiogenesis as a therapeutic approach

Hypoxia in solid malignant tumors

Healthy human organs exhibit Po_2 levels of 24–66 mmHg, whereas in solid tumors these values decrease to 10–30 mmHg due to increased oxygen consumption or ineffective and reduced oxygen supply. Measurement of Po_2 in pancreatic cancer tissues reveals even lower levels of up to 3 mmHg. Recent data indicate that tumor hypoxia plays a crucial role in local and systemic tumor progression, leading to a more aggressive clinical phenotype. Graeber *et al.* demonstrated increased growth of p53 mutated cells under low oxygenation conditions in tumor tissues, whereas wild-type *p53* clones underwent apoptosis under these conditions (Fig. 42.1).

Furthermore, clinical tumor treatment by means of chemotherapy and radiotherapy is based on cell cycle disruption, particularly in cells with high mitotic activity, which is normally a characteristic of tumor cells. Since proliferating cells consume more oxygen than dormant cells, sufficient oxygenation is required to achieve adequate response to radiotherapy and chemotherapy. Therefore, the poor response of pancreatic cancer to chemotherapy and radiotherapy is in part thought to be related to the low oxygenation in the tissue.

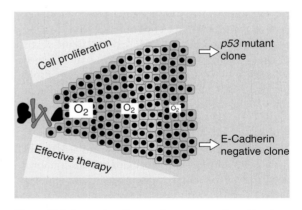

Figure 42.1 Increasing distance from tumor cells to blood vessels leads to hypoxia in the tumor. Hence, the doubling rate of the tumor decreases and therefore the efficacy of antitumor therapy. Hypoxia leads to the selection of malignant cell clones, such as those with *p53* mutation and those lacking E-cadherin expression.

Table 42.4 Characteristics of blood vessels in tumor tissue.

Heterogeneous irregular vessel structure
Decreased blood flow
Arteriovenous shunts
Blind-ending vessels
Missing innervation, no inner muscular layer
Fenestrated endothelial layer and basal layer

Interestingly, there is broad heterogeneity of oxygenation in solid tumors. Frequently they present with areas of extreme hypoxia adjacent to regions with normal oxygenation, i.e., conditions of high and low oxygenation alternate. Taking this into account, it is obvious that solid tumors such as pancreatic cancer have a heterogeneous response to anticancer treatment.

Blood vessels in tumor tissue exhibit numerous features that are different from those seen in normal blood vessels (Table 42.4). These vessels are mainly responsible for the tumor-specific "microenvironment." Within a tumor there are often totally avascular areas (> 1 mm), whereas large arterial but hypoxic tumor vessels (>20 μm diameter) with Po_2 values lower than 5 mmHg are found in the neighborhood. In addition, it is reported that the presence of hypoxic areas is influenced by neither the distance to and the diameter of surrounding vessels nor the arterial flow and oxygenation levels.

The important and prominent role of tumor angiogenesis was first described by Folkman, who postulated the phenomenon of "tumor dormancy" in the absence of neovascularization. It is recognized that angiogenesis is not only essential for tumor growth but is also implicated in the initial progression from premalignant tumor to invasive cancer, and in the growth of dormant micrometastases into clinically detectable metastatic lesions.

Angiogenesis is a complex process regulated through the production of several proangiogenic and antiangiogenic factors. Under physiologic conditions, inhibitory factors such as endostatin predominate, but various signals can tip the balance in favor of angiogenesis, the so-called "angiogenic switch." The main signaling molecules responsible for this phenomenon are vascular endothelial growth factor (VEGF) and bFGF. Further details are shown in Fig. 42.2.

Recent studies reveal evidence that antiangiogenic therapy may be a powerful tool for antitumor thera-

pies. Avascular tumors are only able to reach a diameter of 1 mm. Therefore, tumor cell survival is closely associated with tumor angiogenesis, which is mainly regulated by angiogenic cytokines. The most important angiogenic factor is VEGF and its receptors (VEGF-RI, VEGF-RIII). Endothelial cells express these receptors and respond to VEGF by migration and proliferation. This mechanism is not active under physiologic conditions. However, if Po_2 decreases, due to arteriosclerosis or uncontrolled tumor growth, VEGF is produced and secreted to induce new blood vessels. The detailed mechanisms by which the cells recognize low oxygenation levels and by which signaling pathways react to hypoxia are still not clearly understood. However, it is known that hypoxia activates specific transcription factors, such as hypoxia inducible factor (HIF)-1. HIF-1 itself regulates VEGF synthesis and thereby promotes angiogenesis and better oxygenation of the tumor cells.

At the annual meeting of the American Society of Oncologists in 2003, the promising results of a large clinical trial were presented showing that the antiangiogenic drug Avastin prolonged the lives of patients with advanced colon cancer. In contrast, no benefits of Avastin could be shown in an earlier breast cancer trial. Avastin is an antibody that blocks VEGF, thereby inhibiting angiogenesis. The reasons why the anti-VEGF antibody worked in the colon cancer trial but not in the breast cancer trial are not obvious. They are thought to lie in the differences in the two patient groups and in the different natures of their cancers. Currently, there are a number of clinical trials that are evaluating the impact of different antiangiogenic drugs in cancer therapy.

The impact of this new therapeutic approach on pancreatic cancer deserves to be investigated in randomized controlled clinical trials. Since Büchler et al. demonstrated that VEGF and its receptors regulate angiogenesis and local tumor growth in pancreatic cancer, it has been assumed that antiangiogenic therapy could also play a role in pancreatic cancer treatment.

Significance of present knowledge

Even if our knowledge of the biology and pathophysiology of pancreatic cancer is still fragmentary, a number of the above-mentioned studies show that certain molecular changes in pancreatic cancer are associated with enhanced tumor aggressiveness and shortened postoperative survival times. Although the specific

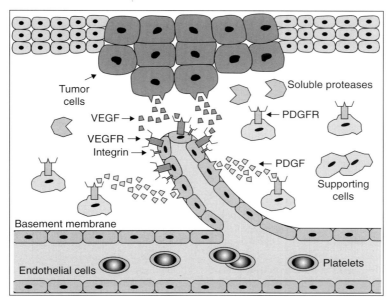

Figure 42.2 Simplified overview of key steps in angiogenesis. Proangiogenic factors, e.g. vascular endothelial growth factor (VEGF), are released by tumor cells and diffuse into the surrounding tissue. VEGF binds to the endothelial cells of preexisting blood vessels and activates these. This cross-link between the tumor cells and the endothelial cells results in the secretion and activation of various proteolytic enzymes, e.g., matrix metalloproteinases that degrade the basement membrane and the extracellular matrix. The stimulation of activated epithelial cells by growth factors results in the migration of epithelial cells toward the tumor. The development of new blood vessels is supported by integrin molecules, such as a$_v$b$_3$-integrin. To stabilize the new vessels, supporting cells are attracted by the endothelial cells depositing a new basement membrane and secreting growth factors, such as platelet-derived growth factor (PDGF). PDGFR, platelet-derived growth factor receptor; VEGFR, vascular endothelial growth factor receptor. (After Cristofanilli *et al.* 2002.)

mechanisms involved in these processes are yet to be entirely explained, the present knowledge could still find use, e.g., particular proteins as diagnostic and prognostic genetic markers. This could, in future, allow the selection of those cancer patients with a potentially poor prognosis, who would then be subjected to extended surgical and more aggressive adjuvant therapy that could improve their chances of survival. Some of the aforementioned growth factors and their ligands could not only be used in the development of genetic screening tests for early diagnosis of pancreatic cancer, but could also act as specific targets for specific pharmacotherapy.

A milestone in these explorations is the use of anti-EGF and anti-HER antibodies (Herceptin), which are already in clinical use for some cancers but have still not been tested for pancreatic cancer. Further studies will be addressed to evaluate these antitumoral strategies in pancreatic cancer.

This knowledge of the molecular biology and a better understanding of the pathophysiology of pancreatic cancer is therefore of extreme importance and deserves further research in order to develop better diagnostic and therapeutic concepts.

Recommended reading

Buchler P, Reber HA, Buchler MW, Friess H, Hines OJ. VEGF-RII influences the prognosis of pancreatic cancer. *Ann Surg* 2002;236:738–749.

Carraway KL III, Cantley LC. A neu acquaintance for erbB3 and erbB4: a role for receptor heterodimerization in growth signaling. *Cell* 1994;78:5–8.

Cristofanilli M, Charnsangavej C, Hortobagyi GN. Angiogenesis modulation in cancer research: novel clinical approaches. *Nat Rev Drug Discov* 2002;1:415–426.

Folkman J, Klagsbrun M. Angiogenic factors. *Science* 1987;235:442–447.

Friess H, Yamanaka Y, Kobrin MS, Do DA, Buchler MW, Korc M. Enhanced erbB-3 expression in human pancreatic cancer correlates with tumor progression. *Clin Cancer Res* 1995;1:1413–1420.

Hanahan D, Weinberg RA. The hallmarks of cancer. *Cell* 2000;100:57–70.

Kleeff J, Ishiwata T, Maruyama H *et al.* The TGF-beta signaling inhibitor Smad7 enhances tumorigenicity in pancreatic cancer. *Oncogene* 1999;18:5363–5372.

Kleeff J, Maruyama H, Friess H, Buchler MW, Falb D, Korc M. Smad6 suppresses TGF-beta-induced growth inhibition in COLO-357 pancreatic cancer cells and is overexpressed in pancreatic cancer. *Biochem Biophys Res Commun* 1999;255:268–273.

Kleeff J, Maruyama H, Ishiwata T *et al.* Bone morphogenetic protein 2 exerts diverse effects on cell growth in vitro and is expressed in human pancreatic cancer in vivo. *Gastroenterology* 1999;116:1202–1216.

Korc M, Chandrasekar B, Yamanaka Y, Friess H, Buchler M, Beger HG. Overexpression of the epidermal growth factor receptor in human pancreatic cancer is associated with concomitant increases in the levels of epidermal growth factor and transforming growth factor alpha. *J Clin Invest* 1992;90:1352–1360.

Longnecker DS. Molecular pathology of invasive carcinoma. *Ann NY Acad Sci* 1999;880:74–82.

Lu Z, Friess H, Graber HU *et al.* Presence of two signaling TGF-beta receptors in human pancreatic cancer correlates with advanced tumor stage. *Dig Dis Sci* 1997;42:2054–2063.

Massague J, Chen YG. Controlling TGF-beta signaling. *Genes Dev* 2000;14:627–644.

Skobe M, Rockwell P, Goldstein N, Vosseler S, Fusenig NE. Halting angiogenesis suppresses carcinoma cell invasion. *Nat Med* 1997;3:1222–1227.

Yamanaka Y, Friess H, Kobrin MS, Buchler M, Beger HG, Korc M. Coexpression of epidermal growth factor receptor and ligands in human pancreatic cancer is associated with enhanced tumor aggressiveness. *Anticancer Res* 1993;13:565–569.

43

Genetic basis of pancreatic carcinogenesis: which concepts may be clinically relevant?

Felix Lluis

In 1988, Perucho *et al.* reported that most human pancreatic carcinomas contain a mutant K-*ras* gene. Over the past 15 years, many studies have been conducted to elucidate the genetics involved in pancreatic carcinogenesis. Human pancreatic tissue, including pancreatic adenocarcinoma (Fig. 43.1), has been difficult to obtain for research purposes until a number of cell lines and models of the disease in experimental animals became available in laboratories worldwide. In addition, new insights have been gained with the introduction of molecular biology techniques. As a result, relevant advances have contributed to a change, at least partly, in the classical nihilistic approach so widely present among basic scientists and clinicians when facing a disease with such a dismal prognosis.

The present chapter begins with a brief update on the pivotal role played by certain oncogenes and tumor-suppressor genes in pancreatic carcinogenesis, followed by a concise description of their involvement in the cell-cycle alterations present in pancreatic adenocarcinoma. Although the occasional reader may find it somewhat difficult, the concepts are simple and essential for obtaining a general picture of what is known and relevant today in pancreatic carcinogenesis. The section ends with a summary of the frequency of fundamental genetic aberrations present in pancreatic adenocarcinoma.

The genetics of pancreatic carcinogenesis is a fast-evolving field. An update on what is known about the initial genetic events that occur in preneoplastic and early lesions is offered. In addition, a summary of recent developments in methodology that may further our understanding of the disease has been added under

a heading entitled New directions in research. The present chapter can only aim at enhancing the curiosity of readers by giving a simple brushstroke of the yet unfinished painting entitled "genetics of pancreatic carcinogenesis." This is why a short section on gene therapy has also been included.

Finally, two sections with some practical value from the clinical standpoint are included. The first, devoted to hereditary pancreatic adenocarcinoma, outlines the genetic syndromes related to the development of the disease. Unfortunately, discussion about recommendations for screening is far beyond the scope of the present chapter. The interested reader will find all the necessary information in the guidelines included in the Recommended reading section. To end the chapter, a summary of our group's work over the last 10 years on the detection of K-*ras* mutations in the diagnosis of pancreatic adenocarcinoma is included. The reader is advised that many other authors have made significant contributions in this field. My purpose is to portray a comprehensive picture of these clinically relevant matters without entering into a long discussion that, no doubt, can easily be found elsewhere.

In pancreatic carcinogenesis, the role played by genetic aberrations in the clinical setting is far from settled. As is the case with other pancreatic diseases, such as acute or chronic pancreatitis, many scientific societies advise that patients be treated in specialized multidisciplinary units comprising surgeons, gastroenterologists, pathologists, and radiologists. In pancreatic adenocarcinoma, the collaboration of molecular biologists and genetic counsellors with the more traditional faculty specialists mentioned above seems only appropriate. This is why at-risk patients requiring so-

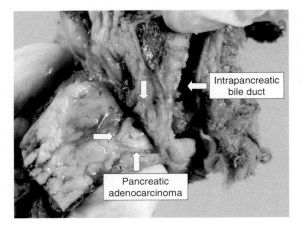

Figure 43.1 Specimen of a duodenopancreatectomy showing a small pancreatic adenocarcinoma in the vicinity of the intrapancreatic bile duct.

phisticated screening procedures should be referred to these specialized multidisciplinary units.

Basic genetic aberrations in human pancreatic adenocarcinoma

K-*ras*

Most pancreatic adenocarcinomas contain a mutation in codon 12 of the K-*ras* gene. Although its frequency varies depending on the geographic location of the population studied, K-*ras* mutation is an early and relevant event in human pancreatic carcinogenesis, also present in premalignant lesions. The aspartic acid substitution (GAT) accounts for 50% of mutations, the valine substitution (GTT) 30%, the arginine (CGT) 11%, and the cysteine (TGT) 6%. The spectrum of K-*ras* mutations in pancreatic adenocarcinoma may suggest geographic differences or might reflect the action of different carcinogens. In those patients with tumors not bearing the K-*ras* mutation, a distinct tumorigenic pattern must be considered. The K-*ras* gene codes for a 21-kDa protein that acts as mediator in the intracellular cascade of events elicited by growth factors leading to protein synthesis. K-*ras* plays a pivotal role in cell proliferation and differentiation. Mutated K-ras protein remains activated always, thereby its transforming potential.

p53

Most genetic aberrations in the *p53* tumor-suppressor gene found in pancreatic adenocarcinoma are missense mutations in the conserved domains of the protein. Frameshift mutations are also present. Correlations have been made between specific mutations and some genotoxic agents (i.e., ultraviolet light, aflatoxin-rich diets) in pancreatic adenocarcinoma. Mutations in the *p53* gene lead to loss of the normal inhibitory role of P53 protein in several cell-cycle regulatory mechanisms, and hence to the development of the malignant phenotype. P53 also plays a critical role favoring apoptosis in the presence of cellular damage. In all, *p53* has been considered the guardian of the genome. Its loss of function severely damages cell regulatory mechanisms.

p16

The cell cycle is regulated by the sequential activation and deactivation of cyclin-dependent kinases (CDKs). The P16 protein is a specific inhibitor of CDK4–6, which in turn phosphorylate the retinoblastoma protein. The *p16* gene is located in the *INK4a* locus of chromosome 9, near the *INK4b* locus responsible for the synthesis of P15, another inhibitory protein involved in the transforming growth factor (TGF)-β pathway. In many pancreatic adenocarcinomas, *p16* is inactivated by either mutation or homozygous deletion. In addition, germline *p16* mutations are present in patients with inherited predisposition to develop mole melanomas associated with pancreatic adenocarcinomas (see below).

DPC4/Smad4

Mutated in more than half of pancreatic adenocarcinoma, *DPC4/Smad4* plays a central role in the TGF-β inhibitory pathway. A recent study using preoperative assessment by immunohistochemistry of human pancreatic adenocarcinoma showed that loss of *DPC4/Smad4* expression improved resectability and survival after resection, whereas resection did not benefit those patients whose tumors expressed *DPC4/Smad4*.

Rb1

Mutations are present in a small proportion of pancreatic adenocarcinoma. The locus lies next to the *BRCA2*

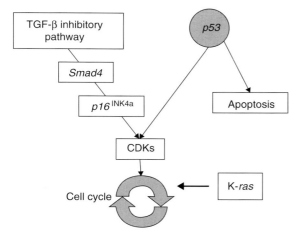

Figure 43.2 Cell cycle in pancreatic adenocarcinoma showing the specific gene aberrations most frequently encountered. CDKs, cyclin-dependent kinases; TGF, transforming growth factor. (Adapted from Mangray & King 1998.)

Table 43.1 Frequency of genetic aberrations in pancreatic adenocarcinoma.

K-*ras*	70–100%
p16^{INK4a}	30–95%
p53	45–75%
DPC4	50–55%
Rb1	0–10%

Microdissection techniques have allowed the detection of genetic alterations in premalignant lesions of the pancreas that are similar to those occurring in advanced pancreatic adenocarcinoma, albeit at a lower frequency. These findings were the basis for a proposed model of pancreatic carcinogenesis similar to the more established one in colorectal cancer. The sequential acquisition of aberrations in the K-*ras* oncogene, and in the tumor-suppressor genes *p53*, *DPC4*, and *p16*, leads to profound and irreversible changes in cell-cycle regulation that result in pancreatic cancer initiation and progression. Cancer cells that express an activated form of Ras must silence the expression of tumor suppressors such as *p53* and *p16*^{INK4A}. Such a mechanism may indeed facilitate human pancreatic cancer progression.

Depending on the target population and the molecular techniques available, the frequency of genetic aberrations in pancreatic adenocarcinoma varies widely (Table 43.1).

gene, responsible for hereditary breast cancer and involved in some hereditary forms of pancreatic adenocarcinoma.

Cell-cycle alterations in pancreatic adenocarcinoma

K-*ras* mutation could be the first step in pancreatic carcinogenesis, followed by disruption of the main mechanisms involved in cell-cycle regulation, primarily *p53* and *p16* mutations, but also aberrations occurring in CDKs and the various steps of the TGF-β inhibitory pathway (Fig. 43.2).

In addition to its effect as a tumor suppressor via the *Smad* pathway in a minority of tumors, pancreatic adenocarcinoma among them, TGF-β plays a role in promoting tumor metastasis. In fact, the growth-inhibitory effect of TGF-β is lost during multistep tumorigenesis; rather, an array of direct TGF-β and *ras*-mediated actions favoring tumorigenesis prevail (i.e., migration, invasiveness, transformation, angiogenesis). It has recently been shown that soluble TGF-β inhibitors are effective in reducing tumor metastasis when administered as circulating drugs in experimental models.

Epidemiology and risk factors

Tobacco smoking and diabetes mellitus preceding the diagnosis of cancer for more than 1 year are two well-established risk factors for pancreatic adenocarcinoma. Tobacco smoking may account for as much as one-quarter of all cases. In diabetic patients, a K-*ras* mutation-independent pathway with increased risk for pancreatic adenocarcinoma has been described recently.

Intraductal precursor lesions

There is a need to unravel the mechanisms involved in the initiation and progression of pancreatic cancer. Progress needs to be made in the elucidation of the

361

mechanisms by which normal cells become tumorigenic. Pancreatic cancer is derived from pancreatic ductal epithelial cells. In order for cancer cells to proliferate they must subvert both the machinery that controls the cell division cycle and the process of programmed cell death (apoptosis).

There is no screening test available for early pancreatic adenocarcinoma, and pancreatic tissue can only be obtained by means of invasive techniques. A number of morphologic studies have recognized intraductal proliferations with atypia as putative precursors of malignant invasive pancreatic adenocarcinoma. By means of modern molecular techniques, it is now clear that hyperplastic pancreatic duct lesions are the precursors of the malignant phenotype. Based on this, K-*ras* mutations may occur early in precursor lesions, yet it is not a necessary event in the progression to pancreatic adenocarcinoma since some invasive tumors do not harbor the mutation. Aberration of *p16* appears to develop later, also in a cumulative fashion as the degree of atypia increases; *p53* and *Smad4* inactivation are late events in the neoplastic progression of intraepithelial lesions (Fig. 43.3). Once the appropriate tools are developed, it may prove reasonable in the future to screen for early pancreatic cancer.

Preneoplastic intraductal lesions appear to be early events in pancreatic carcinogenesis. Previously, analysis of *p53* had been performed by immunohistochemistry. Using microsatellite analysis, alterations in at least one tumor-suppressor gene (*p16*, *p53*, *DPC4*) have been found in 60% of preneoplastic intraductal lesions. Loss of heterozygosity of *p53* occurred even

in morphologically normal-appearing ductal epithelium near the tumor. Allelic loss analysis of selected genes may be useful in characterizing the intermediate steps in the development of early pancreatic adenocarcinoma.

According to some authors, however, intraepithelial pancreatic lesions might be the actual precursors of invasive neoplasm or merely the seeding of an already existing malignant tumor. Moreover, it is unclear whether ductal epithelial cells are the sole origin of pancreatic adenocarcinoma; instead, pluripotential pancreatic cells, including islet cells, may be the common ancestor.

Experimental models

Orthotopic implantation of solid fragments of human pancreatic adenocarcinoma in the pancreatic area of nude mice has a high success rate, the xenograft reproducing the pattern of local growth and distal dissemination. In this model system, mutations in K-*ras*, *p53*, *p15*, and *Smad4* genes can be acquired in the more advanced stages of pancreatic tumor dissemination.

In order to determine the role of K-*ras* in the initiating events of pancreatic carcinogenesis, transgenic mice have been generated that target mutant Ki-*ras* and the cytokeratin 19 promoter to ductal cells. These mice develop an intense periductal lymphocytic infiltration and an increase in cell adhesion-related molecules such as N-cadherin. These findings are a reminder of the early events that take place in the development of a pancreatic malignant lesion of ductal origin.

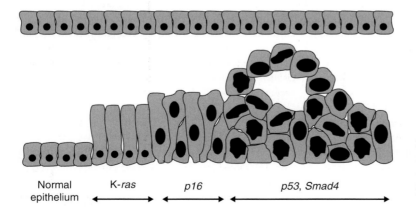

Figure 43.3 Pancreatic intraepithelial neoplasm. Tumor progression is accompanied by the accumulation of genetic aberrations. (Adapted from Wilentz *et al.* 2000.)

New directions in research

Microsatellite instability

Microsatellite instability is the result of mismatch repair defects occurring during DNA replication. DNA replication errors are more frequently found in tumors harboring the so-called mutator phenotype. There are tumors with widespread instability and tumors with low instability, the latter being indistinguishable both in genotype and phenotype from stable tumors. In a study of 100 patients, pancreatic adenocarcinomas with widespread instability (13%) were significantly associated with poor differentiation, and patients had a significantly longer survival time. In contrast, pancreatic adenocarcinomas with low microsatellite instability (13%) were associated with a higher frequency of K-*ras* and *p53* mutations, and patients had a shorter survival time. These results suggest that high microsatellite instability may represent a distinct and more benign tumorigenic pathway in patients with pancreatic adenocarcinoma.

Colony formation

A new improved laboratory method to detect, and possibly diagnose, cancer based on polymerase colony formation has been applied to the study of K-*ras2* and *p53* gene mutation analysis and loss of heterozygosity.

Tumor markers

CA-19-9 is the most widely used serum marker for pancreatic cancer detection and follow-up. Serum markers, also elevated in chronic pancreatitis and other neoplasms, derive from blood group-related antigens and glycoproteins contained in epithelial mucins. At present, several mucin genes have been characterized, and their role in the diagnosis of premalignant lesions and established tumors is being examined.

Telomerase

Human telomerase is a DNA-dependent RNA polymerase that maintains telomere length. It is found in tumor cells but not in normal tissues, other than germ cells and hematopoietic stem cells. The expression of telomerase exhibits a significant relationship with the clinical stage of pancreatic adenocarcinoma and may be a useful tool in diagnosis and prognosis.

Identifying candidate genes

Despite the significant progress that has taken place over the last 15 years or so, much needs to be known regarding genetic changes that occur during pancreatic carcinogenesis and tumor progression. With new methodologies, identifying new markers and genes involved in solid tumor development has become a promising area of research. We are now aware of hundreds of new genes that may be relevant in pancreatic cancer. Recently, a method that uses cDNA microarray technology allows an insight into the global expression patterns of thousands of genes that may be involved in cancer. Microdissection of tumor tissue samples and comparison of findings with those present in the surrounding fibrosis and in the normal pancreas can disclose new genetic aberrations that occur specifically in pancreatic cancer cells. Some overexpressed genes may bear a putative role in pancreatic carcinogenesis and become targets for therapy; for example, genes involved in cell-to-cell and matrix-to-cell interactions, cytoskeletal remodeling, proteolytic activity, and calcium homeostasis were found to be overexpressed in pancreatic cancer tissue.

Gene therapy

Pancreatic adenocarcinoma is an excellent candidate for therapy using the molecular oncology approach. Current treatment success is so limited that oncologists will welcome novel strategies. It is a deadly disease (>90% of patients die within 1 year of diagnosis, often a painful and debilitating process) and is relatively uniform in its molecular abnormalities. Despite this, multiple genes undergo either activation or inactivation during tumor development and progression.

Advances in understanding the genetic basis of pancreatic carcinogenesis have allowed the identification of targets for therapeutic intervention. Gene therapy involves the transfer of genetic constructs into the cancer cell by means of viral or physical vectors (i.e., liposomes). Induced alterations include restoration of tumor-suppressor genes or blockade of oncogenes, enhancement of the immunologic response against tumor cells, and induction of the bystander effect in the vicinity of treated cells. At present, with the exception of a few clinical trials, gene therapy for pancreatic cancer is limited to preclinical studies.

Tumor-suppressor gene therapy requires efficient

systems of gene delivery. Adenoviral vectors may have advantages over other viral and nonviral vectors in that they have been assayed *in vitro* and administered successfully *in vivo*. Using this approach, introduction of wild-type *p53* into mutant cells decreased proliferation and restored apoptosis, provided that no other genetic abnormality was present downstream in cancer cells.

Several studies have shown that inhibiting only K-*ras* is not sufficient to completely eradicate pancreatic adenocarcinoma cells. A recently identified melanoma differentiation-associated gene (*mda-7*) has proved useful for gene-based therapy of diverse human tumors. In contrast, pancreatic cancer was resistant to *mda-7*, a trait that could be linked to mutant K-*ras*. An approach that combined inhibition of mutated K-ras with expression of *mda-7* resulted in a striking synergistic growth-inhibitory and antisurvival effect on pancreatic cancer. These observations may provide evidence for a new and effective strategy for gene therapy in pancreatic cancer.

Hereditary pancreatic adenocarcinoma

Overall, 5–10% of cases of pancreatic adenocarcinoma are due to various hereditary factors. Screening in specialized units, using molecular and imaging techniques as well as genetic counseling, is advisable for family members with known cancer syndromes.

1 An increased risk for pancreatic adenocarcinoma has been shown in relatives of patients with pancreatic adenocarcinoma. Individuals at risk include those with two or more first-degree relatives with pancreatic adenocarcinoma, one first-degree relative younger than 50 years, or two or more second-degree relatives one of whom presents with pancreatic adenocarcinoma at a young age.

2 *BCRA2* germline mutations are associated with a high risk of developing pancreatic adenocarcinoma, with low penetrance. The sporadic mutation appears at a late stage in the development of pancreatic intraepithelial neoplasia.

3 The finding of multiple atypical nevi, familial clustering of cutaneous malignant melanoma, and increased incidence of extracutaneous cancers depicts the syndrome of familial atypical multiple mole melanoma (FAMMM), an autosomal dominantly inherited syndrome that exhibits germline *p16* and CDK4 mutations.

4 Patients with hereditary pancreatitis, who harbor a mutation in the cationic trypsinogen gene *PRSS1*, are at higher risk of developing pancreatic adenocarcinoma. Autoactivation of trypsin resulting in repeated attacks of pancreatitis can provide a mitogenic stimulus leading to pancreatic adenocarcinoma.

5 Germline mutation in one of the DNA mismatch repair genes (*hMSH2*, *hMLH1*, *hPMS1*, *hPMS2*), which causes microsatellite instability and hereditary nonpolyposis colorectal carcinoma, is also associated with some cases of pancreatic adenocarcinoma.

In the USA, the National Familial Pancreas Tumor Registry has been established at Johns Hopkins Hospital. As of July 2004, 1329 families had been enrolled, the largest reported collection of familial cases of pancreatic cancer. Patients with familial pancreatic cancer, inherited in an autosomal dominant fashion, are at higher risk of developing the disease. Detection of patients at high risk could benefit from early treatment. However, diagnosis of precancerous lesions such as pancreatic dysplasia may prove difficult. At this time, a single genetic test is not available for screening of family members of pancreatic cancer patients. A study of 20 affected family members provided evidence for a major locus for familial pancreatic cancer on the long arm of chromosome 4.

Role of detection of K-*ras* mutations in the clinical diagnosis of pancreatic adenocarcinoma

Over the past decade we have conducted a series of studies, mostly prospective, on the usefulness of K-*ras* mutation detection as an adjuvant in the clinical diagnosis of pancreatic adenocarcinoma. Samples were obtained from paraffin-embedded archival blocks, ultrasound- or computed tomography-guided fine-needle aspirates of pancreatic masses, fresh tumor tissue after pancreatic resection, pancreatic juice collected during endoscopic retrograde cholangiopancreatography, or plasma of patients with pancreatic masses or suspected pancreatic cancer, as well as from patients with chronic pancreatitis.

Using paraffin-embedded blocks, detection of K-*ras* mutations increased the sensitivity of cytology alone by more than 10% in the diagnosis of suspected pancreatic carcinoma. Analysis of K-*ras* mutations should be restricted to cell blocks containing suspicious cells, normal-appearing duct cells, or when there is insufficient material for the cytologic examination. Using fresh fine-needle aspirates of pancreatic masses and a polymerase chain reaction (PCR)-based technique (with a detection limit of one mutant allele in the presence of 10^3 wild-type alleles), even more cases could be classified correctly.

The mutant K-*ras* gene was also found in plasma DNA samples in 12 of 44 (27%) patients with pancreatic adenocarcinoma; this finding was significantly related to tumor stage, mainly in the presence of distant metastases. Finally, patients with pancreatic carcinoma with the mutant K-*ras* gene in plasma DNA exhibited a significantly shorter survival time than patients with the wild-type gene. In addition, K-*ras* mutations were detected in the plasma DNA of 2 of 37 (5%) patients with chronic pancreatitis. Moreover, *p53* and K-*ras* mutations can be detected in a minority of pancreatic juice samples from patients with chronic pancreatitis in the absence of malignancy. K-*ras* mutation analysis of pancreatic juice may complement cytologic evaluation in the diagnosis of pancreatic carcinoma, despite its limited contribution to clinical decision-making. The presence of K-*ras* mutations in chronic pancreatitis classifies a subgroup of patients at risk of pancreatic carcinoma, who should be evaluated carefully by long-term follow-up.

Recommended reading

Akhurst RJ. TGF-β antagonists: why suppress a tumor suppressor? *J Clin Invest* 2002;109:1533–1536.

Brentnall TA, Bronner MP, Byrd DR, Haggitt RC, Kimmey MB. Early diagnosis and treatment of pancreatic dysplasia in patients with a family history of pancreatic cancer. *Ann Intern Med* 1999;131:247–255.

Butz J, Wickstrom E, Edwards J. Characterization of mutations and loss of heterozygosity of p53 and K-ras2 in pancreatic cancer cell lines by immobilized polymerase chain reaction. *BMC Biotechnology* 2003;3:11. Available from http://www.biomedcentral.com/1472–6750/3/11

Capellá G, Villanueva A, Erill N, Lluís F. Molecular epidemiology of protooncogene and tumour-suppressor gene mutations. In: JP Neoptolemos, NR Lemoine (eds) *Pancreatic Cancer: Molecular and Clinical Advances*. Oxford: Blackwell Science, 1996: 169–180.

Cascalló M, Mercadé E, Capellà G et al. Genetic background determines the response to adenovirus-mediated wild-type p53 expression in pancreatic tumor cells. *Cancer Gene Ther* 1999;6:428–436.

Castells A, Puig P, Mora J et al. K-ras mutations in DNA extracted from the plasma of patients with pancreatic car-cinoma. Diagnostic utility and prognostic significance. *J Clin Oncol* 1999;17:578–584.

Eberle MA, Pfützer R, Pogue-Geile KL et al. A new susceptibility locus for autosomal dominant pancreatic cancer maps to chromosome 4q32–34. *Am J Hum Genet* 2002;70:1044–1048.

Iacobuzio-Donahue CA, Maitra A, Olsen M et al. Exploration of global gene expression patterns in pancreatic adenocarcinoma using cDNA microarrays. *Am J Pathol* 2003;162:1151–1162.

Löhr M, Muller P, Mora J et al. p53 and K-ras mutations in pancreatic juice samples from patients with chronic pancreatitis. *Gastrointest Endosc* 2001;53:734–743.

Lüttges J, Galehdari H, Bröcker V et al. Allelic loss is often the first hit in the biallelic inactivation of the p53 and PC4 genes during pancreatic carcinogenesis. *Am J Pathol* 2001;158:1677–1683.

Mangray S, King TC. Molecular pathology of pancreatic adenocarcinoma. *Front Biosci* 1998;3:1148–1160.

Mora J, Puig P, Boadas J et al. K-ras gene mutations in the diagnosis of fine-needle aspirates of pancreatic masses: prospective study using two techniques with different detection limits. *Clin Chem* 1998;44:2243–2248.

Pour PM, Pandey KK, Batra SK. What is the origin of pancreatic adenocarcinoma? *Mol Cancer* 2003;2:13. Available from http://www.molecular-cancer.com/content/2/1/13

Reyes G, Villanueva A, García C et al. Orthotopic xenografts of human pancreatic carcinomas acquire genetic aberrations during dissemination in nude mice. *Cancer Res* 1996;56:5713–5719.

Schneider G, Schmid M. Genetic alterations in pancreatic carcinoma. *Mol Cancer* 2003;2:15. Available from http://www.molecular-cancer.com/content/2/1/15

Slebos RJC, Hoppin JA, Tolbert PE et al. K-ras and p53 in pancreatic cancer: association with medical history, histopathology, and environmental exposures in a population-based study. *Cancer Epidemiol Biomark Prev* 2000;9:1223–1232.

Su Z, Lebedeva IV, Gopalkrishnan RV et al. A combinatorial approach for selectively inducing programmed cell death in human pancreatic cancer cells. *Proc Natl Acad Sci USA* 2001;98:10332–10337.

Ulrich CD for the Consensus Committees of the European Registry of Hereditary Pancreatic Diseases, the Midwest Multi-Center Pancreatic Study Group, and the International Association of Pancreatology. Pancreatic cancer in hereditary pancreatitis: consensus guidelines for prevention, screening and treatment. *Pancreatology* 2001;1:416–422.

Villanueva A, García C, Paules AB et al. Disruption of the antiproliferative TGF-β signaling pathways in human pancreatic cancer. *Oncogene* 1998;17:1969–1978.

Wilentz RE, Iacabuzio-Donahue CA, Argani P et al. Loss of expression of DPC4 in pancreatic intraepithelial neoplasia: evidence that DPC4 inactivation occurs late in neoplastic progression. *Cancer Res* 2000;60:2002–2006.

44 Clinical assessment of pancreatic cancer: is there a chance for early diagnosis?

Parviz M. Pour

Introduction

Despite advances made in the clinical and biological aspects of pancreatic cancer, the disease has retained its grave deadly course. It is still the fifth leading cause of cancer death in both men and women, accounting for more than 27 000 deaths annually in the USA. Its 5-year survival rate is still below 5%. Despite significant improvements in diagnostic tools, early detection is not possible and there are no efficient therapeutic modalities. The only effective therapy, surgery, is still limited to about 25% of patients and, even in these patients, cancer recurrence has remained unavoidable. These problems are based on our inability to understand the natural course and biology of the disease. The current molecular biological approach has not been helpful in gaining the necessary information. Numerous attempts to diagnose the disease at early curable stages by utilizing tumor-associated antigens, sophisticated imaging techniques, and molecular biology have proved disappointing.

The prevention of diseases requires adequate knowledge of the anatomy, physiology, pathophysiology, and biology of the tissue involved. Because of the complex structure of the pancreas, which is composed of different exocrine and endocrine cells, and the well-established interaction between the different cell types, knowledge of this tissue is fragmentary at best. Considering the findings of the past century and recent clinical achievements, it is obvious that interactions between the endocrine and exocrine tissues are much more intimate than generally believed. From our experience during the last 30 years, pancreatic islets have far more functions than merely providing digestive and growth hormones. Indeed, they seem to play the role of gatekeeper of the pancreas.

Starting in 1974, our research on pancreatic cancer has led us to conclude that alteration of glucose metabolism is, thus far, the only reliable marker for pancreatic cancer. The following data are evidence that islet cells play a crucial role in the normal as well as diseased pancreas and that alterations of islet-cell function and differentiation appear very early during pancreatic carcinogenesis. This alteration should be considered a signal for the development of pancreatic cancer.

Structural and biological consideration

The development of β cells only in the pancreas, but the formation of glucagon and somatostatin also in the gut epithelium, clearly points to specific environmental (pancreas) requirements for the genesis and neogenesis of these cells. At the same time it highlights the importance of β cells for the pancreas. Although many factors have been suggested to be important for islet-cell development, the issue is still far from clear. Besides transcriptional factors (IDX1, Neuro D, STF-1, etc.), glucagon-like peptide 1 and extendin-4, glucose-dependent insulinotropic polypeptide, mesenchyme, and defined culture medium seem to play a role in islet-cell differentiation *in vitro*. Although *in vivo* islet-cell regeneration can be induced by cellophane wrapping, islet neogenesis-associated proteins, partial pancreatectomy, or duct ligation, the *in vitro* production of β cells has remained a problem. However, recent studies of β-cell production *in vitro* are promising. The specific metabolic requirement for β cells is also highlighted by their response to toxic substances, such as streptozotocin, which selectively destroys β cells both *in vivo* and *in vitro*. However, recovery from streptozotocin-induced β-cell injury seems to depend on the age of the animals at the time the drug is administered, again highlighting the complexity of β-cell differentiation.

When we assemble the fragmented information on pancreatic anatomy and physiology, the importance of the islets for the whole pancreas becomes obvious. It was Henderson who wondered about the remarkable distribution of the islets within the pancreas. This unique distribution—unlike other endocrine tissues, which form a solid gland—is undeniable evidence for the importance of the islets in the function and integrity of the pancreas. This pattern of distribution of the islets and their almost constant size (ranging between 50 and 500 μm) is a reminder of the physical law that the total surface area of many small spheres (islets) is larger than the surface area of a single sphere (gland) of the same volume. This constant size appears to be "optimized" because in all mammals, regardless of body volume, the size and distribution of the islets is the same. In the Syrian hamster one islet is located in every 1.1 mm of the tissue. Yet, even in the same mammalian species, there are differences between the islets themselves. The cell population of islets in the pancreatic lobe derived from the ventral anlage (processus uncinatus) is different from that originating from the dorsal anlage (body and tail). In the latter tissue, compact spherical islets are predominantly found, whereas in the uncinate process the islets are rather ill-defined and diffuse. The most striking difference between the islets in these two anatomic regions is their cellular composition. Cells containing pancreatic polypeptide (PP) are the most abundant and cells containing glucagon the least common cell type in the uncinate process; the situation is reversed in the remainder of the pancreas. Another remarkable characteristic of the pancreas is that the endocrine cells are not confined to the islets. A single or small group of islet cells can be found randomly distributed within the exocrine tissue, primarily within the normal ductal epithelium. This pattern of islet-cell distribution, along with the irregular, almost diffuse arrangement of PP cells (Fig. 44.1), is an indication that islet cells are in total control of the function and growth of the exocrine pancreas.

The functional importance of the endocrine cells for the development and growth of exocrine tissue is also apparent during the embryonic period. The absolute

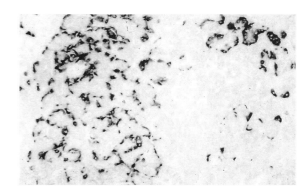

Figure 44.1 Distribution of pancreatic polypeptide (PP) cells in the normal pancreas. Note the irregular arrangement of the cells, many of which are incorporated into the ductal epithelium (upper right corner). Anti-PP antibody, ABC (avidin–biotin complex) method, × 70.

necessity for the presence of islet cells for pancreatic development is highlighted by the study showing that when one of the islet cell-specific transcriptional factors, PDX1, is removed from mice by targeted mutagenesis, the embryos fail to develop a pancreas. Also, there is accumulating evidence that islet cells are essential not only for pancreatic development and function but also for its diseases.

Pancreatic carcinogenesis

Based on the histology of most pancreatic cancers, which mimic ductal structure, it is a common belief that these carcinomas derive from ductal cells. Admittedly, looking at human pancreatic tumors, which are generally detected at later stages due to their late clinical symptoms, this assumption appears obvious. It became possible to examine the stepwise development of pancreatic tumors at all stages of carcinogenicity only after the hamster model was established. When treated with the pancreatic carcinogen *N*-nitrosobis(2-oxopropyl)amine (BOP), Syrian golden hamsters develop pancreatic adenocarcinomas that mimic the human disease morphologically, biologically, and molecular biologically. In this model, most tumors develop within islets, which appear to play a fundamental role in pancreatic carcinogenesis. The following observations support the unequivocal role of islets in the process of carcinogenesis.

1 Pretreatment of hamsters with streptozotocin, which causes the destruction of pancreatic b cells, inhibits pancreatic carcinogenicity of BOP.

2 Genetically diabetic hamsters with atrophic islets are resistant to the pancreatic carcinogenic effect of BOP, whereas the pancreas of a nondiabetic strain with intact islets is not.

3 Stimulation of islet cell proliferation (nesidioblastosis) enhances the pancreatic carcinogenicity of BOP.

4 Transplantation of homologous islets into the submandibular gland (nontarget tissue of BOP) of hamsters and subsequent treatment of the recipient hamsters with BOP results in the development of ductal-type adenocarcinomas in the transplanted islets.

5 Malignant transformation of hamster pancreatic islets by BOP *in vitro*. Although the treatment of cultured hamster pancreatic ductal cells also led to the formation of ductal adenocarcinomas, these tumors, contrary to those derived from islet cells, did not show mutation of the K-*ras* oncogene, the most common genetic abnormality in human pancreatic adenocarcinomas. Additionally, only the cultured islets cells treated with BOP showed inactivation of the $p16^{INK4a}$ gene (homozygous deletion), which is found in 90–100% of human pancreatic adenocarcinomas.

The cell of origin of pancreatic cancer

The most striking finding during the early stages of pancreatic carcinogenesis is the development of tiny, initially hard to detect, ductular structures that appear before any alterations in the ductal system. These ductular structures, which expand gradually to occupy the entire islet, form either patterns consistent with human serous cystadenoma or progress to hyperplasia and atypia and culminate in the formation of malignant glands that invade the surrounding tissue even when they are microscopic in size. In contrast, lesions in ducts develop much later and, as in human tumors, remain within the ductal boundary for a long time before they invade.

The mechanisms behind the development of intrainsular ductules are not yet completely understood. It has been assumed that islet cells derive from precursor cells that apparently reside within the ductal/ductular epithelium and which give rise to either ductal cells or islet cells. Using immunohistochemical procedures with antibodies against the islet hormones, a single or small

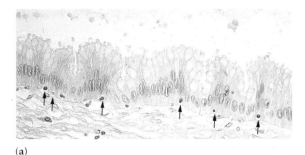

(a)

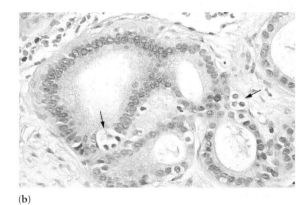

(b)

Figure 44.2 Clear cells in ductal epithelium. (a) Small cells with the round nuclei and clear cytoplasm (*Helle Zellen*) at the base of hyperplastic ductal epithelium (arrows) in an elderly person. (b) Several clear cells in hyperplastic ductal epithelium in an elderly person without clinical disease of the pancreas. Groups of the light cells are bulged out into the interstitium (arrows). A few light cells are within, and at the base of, the epithelium (mid field). H&E, × 120.

group of immunoreactive cells are detectable at the base of the ductal epithelium. In some instances, the number of these endocrine cells equals or even exceeds the number of ductal cells. In routinely prepared hematoxylin/eosin-stained tissues, there are cells with relatively small and round nuclei and a typical perinuclear halo (Fig. 44.2). These cells, first described by the Austrian pathologist Feyrter in 1953 as *Helle Zellen* (light cells), may or may not immunoreact with antibodies against islet cell hormones, although cytologically they are indistinguishable from each other. The nonimmunoreactive cells seem either to move toward the lumen to form ductal cells or show exophytic growth to become immunoreactive cells (Fig. 44.2b).

So if islet cells and ductal cells derive from these, apparently, precursor or stem cells, why should not these cells also reside within the islets to give rise to either islet cells or ductular cells? In fact, using specific techniques, the assumed stem cells, termed variably as "nesidioblasts," "clear cells," "muddy cells," "precursor cells," or "chromophobe cells," have been described in the islets of some mammals, including humans.

Studies using long-term culture of human and hamster islets showed that islet cells of both species have the potential to transdifferentiate to ductular, intermediary, and acinar cells. The transdifferentiated cells express α_1-antitrypsin, vimentin, nestin, cytokeratin 7, cytokeratin 19 or pancytokeratin, carbonic anhydrase II, CA-19-9, and/or DU-PAN-2. This transdifferentiation potency of islet cells has also been documented by several independent researchers. In the hamster pancreas, this process is not limited to ductal cell transdifferentiation and includes the formation of various pancreatic and extrapancreatic cell populations, such as hepatocytes, clear cells, and mucinous and oncocyte-like cells.

The transdifferentiation potency of islet cells is not restricted to the *in vitro* condition. We have found that in 70% of pancreatic cancer patients, who clinically have altered glucose tolerance, islet cells lose their reactivity to anti-insulin and express the same ductal cell markers as expressed in cancer cells, including CA-19-9, DU-PAN-2, and Tag-72, and develop intrainsular ductular structures (Figs 44.3 & 44.4) that express the same antigens. The occurrence of the same antigen in islet cells and intrainsular ductular cells within the same islet indicates a causal relationship between the altered islet cells and intrainsular ductular cells. In answer to the critique that such lesions have never been described by other investigators in the human pancreas, it must be argued that these minute early lesions are hard to find in the human pancreas because the developing malignant lesions replace the islets. Using conventional histologic techniques with limited number of samples, such lesions can escape recognition, although they can be observed occasionally during a vigorous search. In cancerous areas, the malignant intrainsular glands are hard to distinguish from invasive cancer. Islets are the favorite site for tumor invasion (the mechanism of which is discussed elsewhere), making it difficult to distinguish intrainsular malignant cells as primary or secondary. The lack of invasive patterns, such as destruction and compression, can help to make

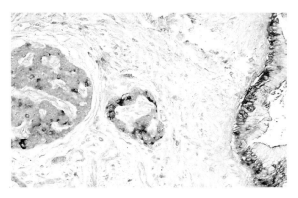

Figure 44.3 Expression of CA-19-9 in many islet cells (left) and in cancer cells (right). Most of the cells in the atrophic islet (middle) are also stained. Anti-CA-19-9, ABC (avidin–biotin complex) method, ×120.

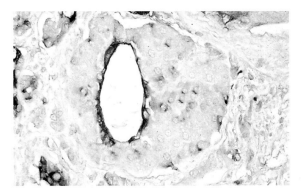

Figure 44.4 An islet in a patient with pancreatic cancer. Many islet cells and the ductal cells within the islet express DU-PAN-2, as do the surrounding cancer cells. Anti-DU-PAN-2 antibody, ABC (avidin–biotin complex) method, ×120.

a decision (Fig. 44.5). The involvement of islet cells in carcinogenesis is also highlighted by the presence of endocrine cells within the hyperplastic and malignant ductal epithelium, in both humans and hamsters. In some cases, the endocrine cells are present not only on the base of the epithelium, where they usually reside, but also within the multilayer epithelium and in papillary folding (Fig. 44.6), a finding that highlights their active participation in the proliferation and malignant process. The presence of these endocrine cells only in well-differentiated but not in poorly-differentiated or

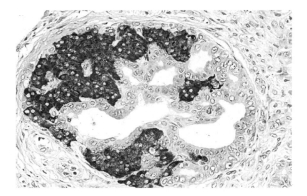

Figure 44.5 An enlarged islet in a patient with pancreatic cancer. Malignant glands have replaced most islet cells without any signs of islet cell destruction, including invasion of the islet cells and the surrounding tissue. In some areas intact islet cells are present within the malignant epithelium (e.g., lower right area). Anti-insulin antibody, ABC (avidin–biotin complex) method, × 120.

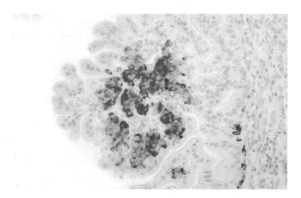

Figure 44.6 Papillary projection of a well-differentiated pancreatic adenocarcinoma. Numerous insulin-producing cells are seen at the base and within the papillary fold. Anti-insulin, ABC (avidin–biotin complex) method, × 120.

anaplastic cancers parallels the advanced loss of cellular differentiation in cultured islets, where the cells lose every known islet-cell marker.

Clinical studies supporting the role of islets in pancreatic carcinogenesis

Although it has been known for almost a century that nearly 80% of patients with pancreatic cancer have im-

paired glucose metabolism, either frank diabetes or impaired glucose tolerance (IGT), the reason has remained a mystery. Remarkably, the degree of IGT and diabetes in these patients has been known to vary. Some patients require insulin treatment whereas others do not. Fasting serum glucose levels may be in the normal range, but an oral glucose tolerance test may yield a diagnosis of IGT. On the other hand, a small subset of patients shows normal glucose metabolism. It is possible that differences in the patient population are the reason that morphologic and molecular biological approaches have not provided clues for understanding the biology of this dismal disease.

The association between diabetes and pancreatic cancer has remained a matter of controversy. According to recent studies, IGT or diabetes mellitus develops shortly before the clinical manifestations of the disease or is diagnosed at the first clinical admission. There are, however, a few who believe that diabetes is a predisposing factor, especially in cases where diabetes is present for more than 5 years before the diagnosis of cancer. Since the latency of pancreatic cancer is unclear, and the development of some cancers seems to take as long as 10 years, the role of diabetes as a predisposing factor remains questionable. Consequently, it appears that the development of pancreatic cancer is associated with the abnormality in islet cell function. Some suggested mechanisms include the primary alteration of islet cells by the carcinogen or secondary damage by cancer cells, either directly or via the production of substances that affect islet cell function.

Experimental studies in the hamster model described above and anecdotal observations indicate that islet cells may also play a role in pancreatic carcinogenesis in humans. This is highlighted by the development of altered glucose metabolism in small tumors that are located in the periphery of the pancreas but which do not cause chronic pancreatitis and in the very early stages of cancer development. The involvement of islet cells in pancreatic carcinogenesis explains at least some of the clinical observations.

Based on the published data and our experience, glucose intolerance is a pancreatic cancer-associated symptom as well as the result of the primary alteration of islet-cell function and differentiation in response to causative carcinogens. Experimental studies have shown that glucose intolerance coincides with the first appearance of microscopic pancreatic tumors. Studies have also shown that changes in islet hormones accompany the early development of pancreatic cancers. These hormone changes and insulin resistance resemble the metabolic changes in pancreatic cancer patients. In humans, IGT or diabetes has been noticed in small, localized, and early pancreatic cancer. In Japanese patients, IGT was the only abnormality in patients with small pancreatic cancer.

The overwhelming opinion that pancreatic cancer develops from ductal epithelium might be the reason why islet-cell alterations in pancreatic cancer patients have not been the focus of research. When we studied the pattern of islet cells immunohistochemically in 14 pancreatic cancer specimens, 14 chronic pancreatitis samples, and 10 normal pancreata as controls, we found that 10 of 14 cancer specimens showed a significant loss of islet β cells. Of the 10 cases, IGT was confirmed in four but no information was available about glucose metabolism in the remaining cases. The incidence of islet-cell alterations in our material (72%) correlates with the frequency of abnormal glucose metabolism in pancreatic cancer patients. Remarkably, most altered islet cells were in the vicinity of the cancer. In only one case was the abnormality also found in an area remote from the cancer. Since tumor-free pancreatic tissues were available in only five cases, the frequency of islet cell alteration in the teletumoral area could not be determined. Other noteworthy findings associated with this abnormality were the signs of altered islet cell differentiation, including the formation of intrainsular ductular structures and the expression of tumor-associated antigens CA-19-9, TAG-72, and/ or DU-PAN-2 in islet cells and intrainsular ductular cells (see Fig. 44.3). This finding indicates that in these patients islet cells have the ability to form an abnormal cell population.

Possible mechanism of altered glucose metabolism in pancreatic cancer

It has been proposed that amylin, a peptide with a molecular weight of 2030, or other yet unknown substances released from cancer cells are responsible for the development of IGT. Because we believe that most cancers arise from altered islet cells, the production of these substances from cancer cells is self-explanatory. Cancer cells are known to inherit some of the biological properties of the cells from which they are derived. Indeed, several studies show the expression of neuroen-

docrine markers in pancreatic cancer cells. From a pathophysiologic point of view, the production of diabetogenic material from islet cells appears more plausible, as it is well known that islet cells have the potential to produce many different pancreatic and extrapancreatic peptides simultaneously. They also have the ability to shift from synthesis of one hormone to synthesis of another. A good example is the coproduction and corelease of insulin and amylin, the synchrony of which is altered in pancreatic cancer. The improvement in IGT and diabetes after tumor resection (70% pancreatectomy or curative resection) by no means indicates that it was the tumor that produced the diabetogenic substances, because removal of cancer tissue also removes the altered islet cells that may actually have produced the diabetogenic material. Moreover, we must be aware that nearly all well-differentiated pancreatic cancers contain endocrine cells, sometimes in remarkably high numbers (Fig. 44.7), which could also be the source of altered hormone production and which are also removed with the cancer. For example, although tumor extracts from diabetic patients with pancreatic cancer showed a marked reduction of glycogen synthesis in skeletal muscles, examination of the tumor revealed that tumor tissue contained islet hormones. Although from a clinical standpoint the issue of whether the diabetogenic material is produced by cancer cells or altered islet cells is trivial, elucidation of the mechanism is

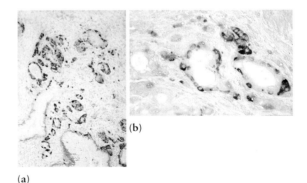

Figure 44.7 Presence of a large number of islet cells within the malignant epithelium. (a) Many β cells are incorporated within the glandular structures. Anti-insulin antibody, ABC method, ×25. (b) Malignant glandular structures containing more endocrine than cancer cells. Multilabeling technique, ×120.

crucial to understanding the biology of the disease and in planning future diagnostic and therapeutic modalities.

Differences in the clinical expression of pancreatic cancer

Although it appears that alteration of glucose metabolism can provide a diagnostic marker, some observations complicate the issue. According to clinical observations, only 60–70% of patients develop IGT or diabetes and the minority (30–40%) do not. Although IGT improves after surgery in many patients, in some it does not or it gets even worse. There are conflicting reports and inadequate information on the incidence of peripheral insulin resistance, IGT, and diabetes before and after surgery. According to one study, 59% of pancreatic cancer patients with either diabetes (45%) or IGT (14%) show improvement after curative surgery, whereas studies by Permert *et al.*, using a hyperglycemic clamp method, show normalization of IGT and improvement of diabetes in around 60% of patients. Consequently, it can be assumed that 10–40% of pancreatic cancer patients either do not show any improvement of the abnormality after surgery or IGT becomes worse. The latter figures could be even higher if one considers that postoperative improvement of IGT and diabetes could be due to the postoperative physical condition and dietary regimens of the patients rather than the consequence of tumor removal. It is unclear whether the observed improvement is just temporary or if the abnormality reappears at the time of tumor recurrence. Although many reasons could be responsible for the lack of postoperative improvement of glucose metabolism in the subset of patients, it is highly possible that altered islet cells producing diabetogenic substances exist in a teletumoral area not removed by surgery or some hidden (metastatic) tumors are left behind, for example in the liver.

Since in a follow-up study glucose homeostasis increasingly worsened in patients who did not have curative surgery, the extent of the tumor and/or altered islets seems to be responsible for glucose metabolism. There are, as yet, no studies examining the extent of islet cell alteration within, around, and remote from cancer. Also, there are limited follow-up studies of patients after surgery.

Possible etiologic factors for islet-cell alteration in pancreatic cancer

The results of our 30 years of experience in human and experimental pancreatic cancer has led us to believe that islet cells are the primary targets of carcinogens. In our view, all pancreatic tumors, endocrine or exocrine, are derived from islets. The structure of the carcinogen determines the phenotypic expression of the ensuing tumors. Streptozotocin, a nitrosamide, produces islet-cell tumors, whereas BOP, a nitrosamine, induces a ductal type of tumor. In hamsters and humans, cultured islet cells transdifferentiate into ductal cells. In hamsters, BOP treatment of isolated purified islets leads to tumor cells that grow *in vivo* as ductal adenocarcinoma. When we treat cultured human ductal and islet cells with BOP, only the treated islet cells are able to grow in a serum-free medium and show K-*ras* mutation, a marker for pancreatic cancer (unpublished results). In an ongoing study we are following the characteristics of these cells and expect their malignant transformation.

The most convincing support for our view is the finding that all drug-metabolizing enzymes, which are believed to be involved in the metabolism of environmental carcinogens, including tobacco-specific carcinogen, nitrosamines, polycyclic aromatic compounds, and aromatic amines, are primarily or exclusively expressed in the islet cells of humans and laboratory species. Considering the anatomy of the blood supply of the pancreas, where a major portion of the arterial blood goes to islets before nourishing the exocrine pancreas, the presence of drug-metabolizing enzymes in islet cells is understandable. Hence, islet cells seem to play the role of pancreatic filters. The availability of these enzymes makes islet cells the primary target of blood-borne carcinogens. Because most of these enzymes are present in a higher concentration or exclusively in islet cells in the head of the pancreas, the frequent occurrence of pancreatic cancer in the head may be explained. Carcinogen-induced alterations in the islets in teletumoral regions of the pancreas could be the reason for the altered production of hormones and, hence, the maintenance of IGT after tumor removal. This explanation, however, is not conclusive because not all pancreatic cancer patients develop a glucose metabolic abnormality. Is this related to the different biology of cancer, as has been suggested by a study where a correlation was found between the degree of IGT severity and the histologic type of cancer? Is this because tumors develop from islets in patients with IGT or diabetes and, in a minority of the patients, from other cells? Or could this be related to the severity and extent of islet-cell damage? Nevertheless, the data suggest that, with regard to the glucose metabolic alteration, there are at least three subsets of pancreatic cancer patients, possibly with tumors of different biology. The published data and our own experience suggest the following subsets (Fig. 44.4):

1 pancreatic cancer patients without IGT or diabetes (IGT–, about 20–30%);

2 pancreatic cancer patients with IGT or diabetes (IGT+, about 70–80%), whose glucose intolerance or diabetes improves postoperatively (IGT+/–);

3 patients in whom the abnormality does not or only slightly improves (IGT+/+) after tumor resection.

Possible mechanism of differing clinical presentation of pancreatic cancer

Reasons for the glucose metabolic abnormality in pancreatic cancer are not well understood. The suggestion that islet-cell destruction by cancer cells is the principal cause has been refuted, mainly because even small and localized tumors in the head of the pancreas are associated with abnormal glucose tolerance.

A few studies dealing with the alteration of islet hormones at the tissue level have found a reduction in the number of β cells in pancreatic cancer patients. No information is available on the frequency and extent of the process, and its specificity for pancreatic cancer. The question of specificity is important because about 45–75% of patients with chronic pancreatitis also develop abnormal glucose tolerance or frank diabetes mellitus. Consequently, it is reasonable to assume that damage to the islets by scar tissue and inflammation, which are also associated with pancreatic cancer, could be the underlying mechanism.

Clearly, disturbance of the subtle balance between exocrine and endocrine tissue by cancer, with associated inflammation and sclerosis, is expected to lead to deregulation of hormone secretion. However, because even localized and small tumors in the head of the pancreas not affecting islet-rich areas of the organ cause the glucose metabolic abnormality, it is likely that a factor or factors produced by cancer cells play a role. This view is supported by the finding that surgical removal of tumor by 85–90% pancreatectomy improves diabetes and normalizes glucose metabolism.

Several clinical studies have shown significant changes in the serum levels of islet hormones in pancreatic cancer patients, but little is known about the patterns of islets at the tissue level. In one study a reduction in β cells has been reported but the extent of the alterations and their specificity for pancreatic cancer have not been investigated. The latter issue deserves particular attention, because glucose-abnormality and diabetes also occurs in chronic pancreatitis. Therefore, we systematically examined the patterns of islets in pancreatic cancer in comparison with chronic pancreatitis and the normal pancreas. We selected archival pancreatic cancer specimens that had tumor-free areas close to and remote from the cancer because, as stated earlier, it is believed that factors released by cancer cells affect the islets directly via a paracrine pathway.

In 10 pancreatic cancer specimens, a significant reduction in β cells was found. Also, in eight of them, a significant increase in α cells was found as well. This result thus correlates with the incidence of pathologic serologic hormone levels in pancreatic cancer patients. Reasons for the lack of similar alterations in the four other patients are obscure. We could not find any correlation between islet alterations, sex, age, smoking habit, alcohol consumption, stage of the disease, and tumor morphology. We also did not find any significant changes in the islet-cell distribution in the chronic pancreatitis specimens, even within sclerotic and fibrotic tissue. Therefore, the suggestion that fibrosis or sclerosis associated with pancreatic cancer may have caused the β-cell loss by obstructing blood vessels could be excluded. Consequently, the described islet alteration appears to be specific for pancreatic cancer. Because pathologic islet hormone serum levels also occur in chronic pancreatitis patients, it seems that the mechanism of altered glucose metabolism in the two diseases differs. In chronic pancreatitis the abnormality seems to be due to altered insulin secretion, whereas in pancreatic cancer the defect appears to be in the machinery of insulin synthesis as evidenced by the reduced levels of insulin and C-peptide as well as of amylin, which is normally costored and cosecreted with insulin. Endocrine cells were found in the malignant epithelium in nine of our ten cases with β-cell alteration. Similar findings have been reported in up to 80% of cases. Also, the presence of nesidioblastosis in four of our ten cases with decreased β-cell number could reflect a compensatory process against β-cell loss. The question of why β cells in pancreatic cancer are exclusively affected remains to be investigated.

The increase in α cells, which was more pronounced in cancer tissue from diabetics than in tissue from diabetics without cancer, coincides with the serologic findings. The abnormality also differs from hormonal changes in chronic pancreatitis, where serum concentrations of glucagon have been found to be reduced or normal. Nevertheless, in our chronic pancreatitis samples we could not detect any alteration in the number of glucagon cells, possibly because it is the secretion of glucagon that is affected not the number of α cells. Also, contrary to clinical observations of increased somatostatin levels in pancreatic cancer patients, we could not find any significant changes in the number of somatostatin cells. Whether the source of increased serum somatostatin is derived from pancreatic or extrapancreatic somatostatin cells remains to be seen.

The greater alteration of islets within or immediately around cancer supports the hypothesis that factors released by cancer cells play a role in this process. Because alterations like hydropic swelling were also found in tissues remote from cancer, although in lesser degree, a humoral pathway also seems to exist. Examination of pancreatic tissue further away from the cancer would clarify this. If this is found to be the case, the identification of the causative factor(s) released from cancer cells could present an early pancreatic cancer marker, especially in view of the findings that an abnormality in glucose metabolism also occurs in small localized cancers.

One of the reasons for the differing results in the published data and pancreatic hormone levels in pancreatic cancer patients could be the inclusion of different subsets of patients with pancreatic cancer in these studies. It may be that the anatomic location of the tumor plays a role in these differences. Tumors in the head region obstructing the main pancreatic duct can cause severe (secondary) chronic pancreatitis and, hence, diabetes. However, there are differences in diabetes induced by chronic pancreatitis and pancreatic cancer. For example, diabetes improves after a 70% pancreatectomy in pancreatic cancer but not after surgical intervention in chronic pancreatitis. According to our recent studies, the size and cell constitution of islets are significantly different between primary pancreatitis and pancreatitis caused by cancer. Contrary to the islets in pancreatic cancer patients, which are of normal size or enlarged, about 95% of the islets in primary chronic pancreatitis measure less than 100 μm in diameter. Moreover, tumors developing in the upper and dorsal half of the head of the pancreas do not affect the pancreatic duct very much and hence are not accompanied by a significant chronic pancreatitis. Whether these tumors cause diabetes is unclear. Another argument against the role of secondary pancreatitis in the induction of diabetes derives from the experience that even patients with small tumors in the periphery of the pancreas not causing chronic pancreatitis show abnormal glucose tolerance.

Another major shortcoming of past studies is the lack of adequate control groups. There is not a single study that correlates the morphologic findings of both cancer and islet cells with plasma hormone levels of the patients. To our knowledge, there is only one limited study that compares the hormone levels in pancreatic cancer patients with that of healthy and noninsulin-requiring diabetic persons: a low level of plasma amylin was found in patients with type II diabetes and in those with pancreatic cancer and diabetes, and an increased level of amylin in pancreatic cancer patients without diabetes. Such correlative studies could provide important data for an understanding of the disease. For example, a low insulin level in a patient with IGT and altered islet cells could reflect impaired insulin release or synthesis in the altered islets. In fact, an inverse relationship has been found between the number of insulin cells in islets and the fasting plasma glucose level, suggesting that the alteration of islet cells is the primary cause of the glucose abnormality in these patients. Other studies also point to the primary alterations of islet cells, including reduced insulin and C-peptide response after glucose load and an increase in proinsulin secretion. The Σproinsulin/ΣC-peptide ratio, which has been found to be increased in pancreatic cancer with IGT but decreased after tumor removal, further substantiates the functional alteration of islet cells.

From a therapeutic point of view, the identification of a different subpopulation of pancreatic cancer patients is important because these patients could respond differently to therapeutic modalities. For example, does the genetic constitution of the tumors from the different pancreatic cancer subpopulations differ? Can the pattern of IGT help to better distinguish between sporadic and familial pancreatic cancer? If IGT is due to the substances released from islet cells or cancer cells, then is it expected that IGT+/− patients become IGT+/+ after tumor recurrence? If that is the case, the recurrence of the abnormality, and possibly its severity, could have predictive value. The existing results indicate that the occurrence of diabetes in pancreatic cancer cannot be explained by a single mechanism. The increase in peripheral insulin resistance, suppression of insulin secretion, impaired proinsulin conversion, altered fat and carbohydrate metabolism, presence of acute or chronic pancreatitis, medications for underlying disease, altered nutritional habits, weight loss, and many other factors seem to play important roles in the development and course of pancreatic cancer.

Conclusion

Past attempts to develop early diagnostic modalities have proven useless. The expression of tumor-associated antigens may have value in monitoring the disease but are unable to detect the cancer in early developmental stages. Despite the promising molecular biological approach, the method lacks specificity as the K-*ras* mutation is not specific for pancreatic cancer and can be found in patients with chronic pancreatitis as well as in individuals without pancreatic diseases. The most sophisticated imaging techniques are still unable to detect tumors less than 5 cm with accuracy. The frequent association between pancreatic cancer and IGT offers the most logical approach for detecting small tumors in most patients. This method could be applied readily in individuals prone to pancreatic cancer, including members of pancreatic cancer and hereditary chronic pancreatitis. Our studies pointing to the role of islets in pancreatic cancer and in the development of altered glucose metabolism should be further investigated. The development of a multidisciplinary program involving researchers in various fields of medicine, toxicology, nutrition, cellular and molecular biology, and epidemiology is a necessary step in revealing the true nature of this deadly disease.

Recommended reading

Ahren B, Andren-Sandberg A. Glucose tolerance and insulin secretion in experimental pancreatic cancer in the Syrian hamster. *Res Exp Med* 1993;193:21–26.

Bonner-Weir S, Baxter LA, Schuppin GT, Smith FE. A second pathway for regeneration of adult exocrine and endocrine pancreas. A possible recapitulation of embryonic development. *Diabetes* 1993;42:1715–1720.

Bouwens L. Transdifferentiation versus stem cell hypothesis for the regeneration of islet beta-cells in the pancreas. *Microsc Res Tech* 1998;43:332–336.

Bouwens L, Kloppel G. Islet cell neogenesis in the pancreas. *Virchows Arch* 1996;427:553–560.

Cersosimo E, Pisters PW, Pesola G, McDermott K, Bajorunas D, Brennan MF. Insulin secretion and action in patients with pancreatic cancer. *Cancer* 1991;67:486–493.

Gittes GK, Galante PE, Hanahan D, Rutter WJ, Debase HT. Lineage-specific morphogenesis in the developing pancreas: role of mesenchymal factors. *Development* 1996;122:439–447.

Gullo L, Ancona D, Pezzilli R, Casadei R, Campione O. Glucose tolerance and insulin secretion in pancreatic cancer. *Ital J Gastroenterol* 1993;25:487–489.

Jonsson J, Carlsson L, Edlund T, Edlund H. Insulin-promoter-factor 1 is required for pancreas development in mice. *Nature* 1994;371:606–609.

Kimura W, Morikane K, Esaki Y, Chan WC, Pour PM. Histological and biological patterns of microscopic ductal adenocarcinomas detected incidentally at autopsy. *Cancer* 1998;82:1839–1849.

Muscarella P, Knobloch TJ, Ulrich AB *et al.* Identification and sequencing of the Syrian golden hamster (*Mesocricetus auratus*) p16(INK4a) and p15(INK4b) cDNAs and their homozygous gene deletion in cheek pouch and pancreatic tumor cells. *Gene* 2001;278:235–243.

Ordonez NG, Balsaver AM, Mackay B. Mucinous islet cell (amphicrine) carcinoma of the pancreas associated with watery diarrhea and hypokalemia syndrome. *Hum Pathol* 1988;19:1458–1461.

Permert J, Ihse I, Jorfeldt L, von Schenck H, Arnquist HJ, Larsson J. Improved glucose metabolism after subtotal pancreatectomy for pancreatic cancer. *Br J Surg* 1993;80:1047–1050.

Permert J, Ihse I, Jorfeldt L, von Schenck H, Arnqvist HJ, Larsson J. Pancreatic cancer is associated with impaired glucose metabolism. *Eur J Surg* 1993;159:101–107.

Permert J, Larsson J, Westermark GT *et al.* Islet amyloid polypeptide in patients with pancreatic cancer and diabetes. *N Engl J Med* 1994;330:313–318.

Pour PM, Kazakoff K, Carlson K. Inhibition of streptozotocin-induced islet cell tumors and N-nitrosobis(2-oxopropyl)amine-induced pancreatic exocrine tumors in Syrian hamsters by exogenous insulin. *Cancer Res* 1990;50:1634–1639.

Pour PM, Weide L, Liu G *et al.* Experimental evidence for the origin of ductal-type adenocarcinoma from the islets of Langerhans. *Am J Pathol* 1997;150:2167–2180.

Pour PM, Schmied BM, Ulrich AB, Friess H, Andren-Sandberg A, Buchler MW. Abnormal differentiation of islet cells in pancreatic cancer. *Pancreatology* 2000;1:110–116.

Pour PM, Standop J, Batra SK. Are islet cells the gatekeepers of the pancreas? *Pancreatology* 2002;2:440–448.

Rosenberg L, Rafaeloff R, Clas D *et al*. Induction of islet cell differentiation and new islet formation in the hamster: further support for a ductular origin. *Pancreas* 1996;13:38–46.

Schmied B, Liu G, Moyer MP *et al*. Induction of adenocarcinoma from hamster pancreatic islet cells treated with *N*-nitrosobis(2-oxopropyl)amine in vitro. *Carcinogenesis* 1999;20:317–324.

Schmied BM, Liu G, Matsuzaki H *et al*. Differentiation of islet cells in long-term culture. *Pancreas* 2000;20:337–347.

Standop J, Schneider MB, Ulrich A *et al*. The pattern of xenobiotic-metabolising enzymes in the human pancreas. *J Toxicol Environ Health* 2002, in press.

Ulrich AB, Schmied BM, Matsuzaki H *et al*. Increased expression of glutathione *S*-transferase-pi in the islets of patients with primary chronic pancreatitis but not secondary chronic pancreatitis. *Pancreas* 2001;22:388–394.

Yuan S, Rosenberg L, Paraskevas S, Agapitos D, Duguid WP. Transdifferentiation of human islets to pancreatic ductal cells in collagen matrix culture. *Differentiation* 1996;61:67–75.

45 What can be expected from tumor markers in pancreatic cancer?

Thomas Seufferlein and Guido Adler

The dismal prognosis of pancreatic cancer is mostly due to the fact that this tumor is usually diagnosed at a late stage. There are no specific early symptoms and diagnostic imaging has limitations. As a result, the disease often eludes detection during its formative stages. Therefore, accurate tools for early diagnosis and screening are particularly important for this tumor. We also need markers that allow estimation of prognosis, disease progression, and treatment response and which help us to select the optimum therapeutic strategy for a patient.

Alterations in gene sequences, expression levels, and protein structure or function are used as tumor markers. This field is fast-moving and expanding, but also littered with numerous examples of might-have-beens. Very few markers have passed successfully from the bench to the bedside. In this chapter we highlight the present state of tumor markers in pancreatic cancer and point out developments that may lead to a diagnostic breakthrough in the near future. Because 80–90% of tumors of the exocrine pancreas are adenocarcinomas of ductal cell origin, we focus on markers for ductal pancreatic adenocarcinoma.

CA-19-9

CA-19-9 is the most frequently used serum-based marker for pancreatic cancer. The protein is a carbohydrate cell-surface antigen (sialylated lacto-*N*-fucopentose) related to the Lewis blood group substance. It was originally isolated in 1979 as a colorectal cancer-specific antigen and it is found in the normal epithelial cells of the gallbladder, biliary ducts, pancreas, and stomach. The elevation of CA-19-9 in pancreatic and other malignancies is thought to be due to increased production and secretion of the antigen from malignant cells. Multiple studies have shown that while elevations in serum CA-19-9 appear useful in the diagnosis of adenocarcinoma of the upper gastrointestinal tract and in the surveillance of colon cancer, its greatest sensitivity is in the detection of pancreatic adenocarcinoma. To date, CA-19-9 is considered one of the most useful tumor markers for pancreatic malignancies. However, up to 30% of patients with pancreatic cancer do not exhibit elevated serum CA-19-9 levels. The sensitivity of the CA-19-9 serum assay ranges between 69 and 93%, the specificity between 46 and 98%. The higher the level of CA-19-9, the greater the sensitivity and specificity of the assay. Elevations in CA-19-9 correlate with the degree of tumor differentiation and with the extent of disease. Consequently, CA-19-9 levels are lower in patients with localized disease and this marker is therefore of little use as a screening marker to detect early pancreatic cancers. It has been suggested that very high levels of CA-19-9 indicate unresectable tumors and that the pretreatment CA-19-9 level is a strong predictor of survival. There are conflicting results about whether the response of CA-19-9 to chemotherapy and/or radiotherapy is useful for predicting survival. In addition, CA-19-9 is a useful marker for detecting recurrent disease and can therefore be used for the surveillance of patients after surgery for pancreatic cancer.

A general clinical problem is to determine whether a pancreatic mass is due to malignancy or chronic pancreatitis. Furthermore, if chronic pancreatitis is established, it is important to know whether there is any sign of malignant transformation. CA-19-9 is of very limited value in solving this problem, since elevated CA-19-9 levels are also found in benign processes such as acute and chronic pancreatitis, chronic liver disease, and biliary tract disease. Consequently, in patients with suspected pancreatic cancer due to chronic pancreatitis, the sensitivity and specificity of serum CA-19-9 in the detection of pancreatic cancer were only 44% and 80% respectively. Marked elevations of CA-19-9 are essentially limited to cirrhosis and acute obstructive cholangitis. Biliary obstruction in the absence of cholangitis does not usually produce significant elevations of CA-19-9. The elevated CA-19-9 levels seen with obstructive cholangitis may be due to increased production from the inflamed epithelial cells, along with leakage into the serum due to elevated biliary tract pressure. In the setting of acute inflammatory processes, serum CA-19-9 values generally return to normal when biliary drainage is achieved and infection resolves. Thus, an elevated serum CA-19-9 as a marker for malignancy must be interpreted with caution when a pancreatic mass is associated with an inflammatory hepatobiliary process.

Genetic markers for the detection of pancreatic cancer in tissues

Because of a better understanding of the genetic progression of many common neoplasms, DNA mutations in oncogenes or tumor-suppressor genes are increasingly used as genetic markers. Studies in pancreatic cancers and preneoplastic lesions, the so-called pancreatic intraepithelial neoplasia (PanIn), led to the discovery of specific genetic modifications that occur at early stages of pancreatic carcinogenesis. For example, overexpression of $p21^{WAF/CIP1}$ is an early event in precursor lesions, whereas $p53$ alterations and the loss of $DPC4/Smad4$ are late events in PanIn development.

Ki-*ras* mutations

Activating Ki-*ras* mutations are the first genetic changes detected in the progression to pancreatic cancer. They occur in about 30% of lesions that show the earliest stages of histologic disturbance. Therefore, the analysis of Ki-*ras* mutations has been regarded as a milestone in the early detection of pancreatic cancer. Ki-*ras* point mutations at codon 12 are also detectable in 75–100% of pancreatic cancer tissues. However, ductal lesions in patients with chronic pancreatitis, and in the normal pancreas also, exhibit Ki-*ras* mutations without additional indications of neoplastic transformation such as severe dysplasia or mutated P53 protein. Furthermore, Ki-*ras* mutations are found in benign pancreatic tumors. Thus, Ki-*ras* as a single marker is not sufficient to establish the diagnosis of pancreatic cancer in a tissue sample.

p53

Alterations in $p53$ are late events in PanIn development. Overexpression of $p53$ is almost exclusively found in pancreatic cancers and not in benign pancreatic tumors. However, only about half of pancreatic cancers exhibit $p53$ mutations, which limits the value of $p53$ analysis for the diagnosis of pancreatic cancer.

Telomerase

Telomerase is a ribonucleoprotein that is involved in telomere maintenance. The enzyme is required for immortalization of cells and is expressed by almost every cancer. Telomerase activity has been found in up to 90% of malignant pancreatic tumors but is virtually absent from benign tumors, suggesting that telomerase is activated concomitantly with carcinogenesis. Telomerase activity could therefore be an interesting marker for pancreatic cancer. However, telomerase assays that determine the precise level of enzyme activity should be used, since low levels of telomerase can be detected in noncancerous tissues leading to false-positive results in less accurate assays.

KOC

The *KOC* (KH domain containing protein overexpressed in cancer) gene is highly overexpressed in pancreatic cancer. Recent data suggest that *KOC* is a highly specific and sensitive marker for pancreatic cancer in tissue samples.

Mucin family

Mucins are heavily glycosylated, high-molecular-weight glycoproteins that play a protective role for epithelial tissues and are possibly involved in the renewal and differentiation of the epithelium, cell adhesion, and cellular signaling. An aberrant expression pattern of mucins can be detected in various malignancies. Mucins may promote the invasive and metastatic potential of tumors by contributing to the cell-surface adhesion properties and through morphogenetic signal transduction. MUC-1 has been shown to be overexpressed in pancreatic adenocarcinomas and PanIns by immunohistochemistry. Other groups have reported that MUC-4 is the only mucin that is differentially expressed at the mRNA level in pancreatic cancers. Expression of MUC-4 is found in up to 89% of pancreatic cancers and in all PanIn grades, particularly PanIn 3 lesions. However, a few nonneoplastic lesions, including reactive ducts in chronic pancreatitis, are also MUC-4 positive in immunohistochemistry.

Pancreatic cancer markers in serum

A highly sensitive and specific marker that is detectable in the serum of patients at risk of developing pancreatic cancer would be ideal for screening. Apart from CA-19-9, only few such markers have been described. As described above, CA-19-9 is not suitable as an early marker and is not elevated in up to 30% of patients with pancreatic cancer.

Apart from proteins, DNA mutations can be detected in serum or plasma samples. The mechanism by which this DNA is released is poorly understood. Ki-*ras* mutations were found in the plasma of 27% of patients with pancreatic cancer, particularly when distant metastases were present. Such mutations are also detectable in about 5% of patients with chronic pancreatitis. Thus, Ki-*ras* mutation analysis in serum is specific but has low sensitivity.

The epidermal growth factor receptor (EGFR) is overexpressed in the majority of pancreatic cancers. EGFR mRNA is detectable in the peripheral blood of 18% of patients with pancreatic cancer and not in healthy controls. Thus, this marker may be very specific but is not sensitive enough for screening.

MUC-4 mRNA can also be detected in peripheral blood mononuclear cells of pancreatic cancer patients, but is undetectable in peripheral blood mononuclear cells of healthy volunteers or patients with chronic pancreatitis or other cancers. MUC-4 may indeed be useful in differentiating between chronic pancreatitis and pancreatic cancer in patients with a pancreatic mass.

Pancreatic juice: the best screening material for pancreatic cancer?

Because of the difficulties in obtaining biopsy specimens from patients with suspected pancreatic cancer and the low sensitivity of serum-based approaches, much hope has been placed in the analysis of pancreatic juice.

Unfortunately, Ki-*ras* polymerase chain reaction (PCR) of pancreatic juice or bile has a low sensitivity for diagnosing pancreatic cancer. In a prospective trial, codon 12 mutations of the Ki-*ras* gene were detected in pancreatic juice and bile of 38% of patients with pancreatic cancer, 8% of patients with chronic pancreatitis, 18.7% of patients with other malignancies, and 7.3% of patients with benign diseases or normal findings. In different studies, Ki-*ras* mutations were detected in pancreatic juice of up to 30% of noncancerous patients and in more than 60% of patients with benign mucous cell hyperplasia of pancreatic ductal epithelium with chronic inflammation. However, more sensitive and/or quantitative PCR tests may allow differentiation of pancreatic cancer from chronic pancreatitis. Using quantitative assays such as restriction fragment length polymorphism (RFLP) or hybridization protection assays, Ki-*ras* mutations can be detected in up to 84% and 65% of pancreatic cancers respectively.

Mutations of *p53* in pancreatic juice were detected in 42% of pancreatic cancers. However, no mutations were detectable in mucin-producing adenomas or in chronic pancreatitis or normal tissue, making *p53* a specific but not very sensitive marker. Combined analysis of Ki-*ras* and *p53* mutations may therefore enhance the genetic diagnosis of pancreatic cancer.

Assessing prognosis

The most relevant prognostic factors in pancreatic cancer to date are tumor grade, tumor size greater than 45 mm, resection margin involvement, and perineural invasion. Interestingly, in one study loss of *DPC4/Smad4* expression in pancreatic cancer correlated with resectability and was associated with improved survival after resection, whereas resection did not improve survival in patients whose tumor expressed *DPC4/Smad4*. Aberrant expression $p21^{WAF1}$, cyclin D1, *p53*, or *p16^{INK4a}* was not associated with a difference in survival.

Various other markers have been associated with poor prognosis in pancreatic cancer. The presence of anti-p53 antibodies in serum is likely to predict a poor prognosis for patients after surgery for pancreatic cancer. Similarly, the detection of plasma Ki-*ras* mutations correlates with shorter survival of patients with pancreatic cancer. Patients with pancreatic tumors that reexpress the pancreatic duodenal homeobox gene (*PDX1*), which is normally expressed in pancreatic duct cells during pancreatic development, have a significantly worse prognosis than those with *PDX1*-negative tumors. In addition, overexpression of the pancreatitis-associated protein correlates with short survival. The detection of disseminated tumor cells in the peritoneal cavity and bone marrow using antibodies against CA-19-9, 17-1A tumor-associated antigen, and cytokeratins correlates inversely with survival of patients after surgery for pancreatic cancer.

Gene expression analysis in pancreatic cancer

Microarray analysis is widely used to detect changes in gene expression in cancer. This technique allows rapid assessment of the expression of thousands of genes in one experiment and can be used to identify differences in gene expression pattern in different samples. One major aim of gene expression analysis in pancreatic cancer is the identification of novel genes that are differentially expressed in pancreatic cancer as compared with normal pancreas or pancreatitis tissue and may hence be classified as "candidate disease genes." Indeed, using this technique, multiple candidate disease genes for pancreatic cancer have been identified. Genes overexpressed in pancreatic cancer are associated with processes such as cell–cell and cell–matrix interactions, cytoskeletal remodeling, proteolytic activity, calcium homeostasis, cell proliferation, and host desmoplastic response. An alternative approach is the serial analysis of gene expression (SAGE), a comprehensive cloning and sequencing method that is used to identify and quantify gene expression, particularly of low-copy-number genes. Using a SAGE approach, mesothelin has been identified as a new marker for pancreatic cancer.

Microchip-based approaches have also been developed for high-throughput analysis, such as screening a large number of samples for mutations in oncogenes. For diagnostic purposes it is ultimately desirable to select a small number of candidate genes that can be spotted on a diagnostic chip in order to detect tumors in samples such as pancreatic juice or fine-needle aspirates with high sensitivity and specificity.

Expression profiling also furthers our understanding of the molecular pathology of pancreatic cancer. Various programs are underway to characterize the different PanIn stages at the level of gene expression. Using state of the art bioinformatics, the specific gene expression pattern of a tumor can be linked to prognosis or drug activity patterns. This will be used in future to select patients for treatment and to predict responsiveness of the patient's tumor to chemotherapeutic agents or targeted therapies.

The future of all markers: proteomic pattern analysis?

Until recently, the search for cancer-related proteins for early disease detection has been conducted on a case by case basis. Proteins have been identified that are overexpressed as a consequence of the disease process and are shed into body fluids. This approach, as shown above, is laborious and time-consuming. The emerging field of clinical proteomics is especially well suited to the discovery and implementation of novel biomarkers, including their posttranslational modifications. Recently, using mass spectrometry-driven proteomic analysis, a proteomic profile was derived from sera of patients with prostate and ovarian cancer as well as from sera of unaffected patients. Using this information the investigators established a unique discriminatory pattern of peptides in the serum of patients with prostate and ovarian cancer. This algorithm enabled them to correctly identify patients with prostate and ovarian cancer in a blinded set of samples. Surprisingly, even patients with Stage I ovarian disease were correctly identified. Similar data in pancreatic cancer are not yet available. However, proteomic pattern diagnosis might be a real step forward in the early diagnosis of pancreatic cancer in serum samples.

What can be expected from tumor markers in pancreatic cancer?

In the foreseeable future CA-19-9 will continue to be the most widely used marker for monitoring response or disease progression. The conclusion to be drawn from the multiple studies examining single markers is that there is no single marker that allows early detection of pancreatic cancer with high sensitivity and specificity in a compartment that is readily accessible such as serum. Given the complex genetic profile of pancreatic cancer, it is also predictable that such a marker is unlikely to be found. However, microarray analysis on diagnostic chips containing a set of distinctive candidate genes may in future enable us to differentiate between normal pancreas, chronic pancreatitis, and pancreatic cancer and to detect the formative stages of this disease in tissue samples or pancreatic juice. Ultimately, proteomic pattern analysis in serum samples could be the revolution in the early diagnosis of pancreatic cancer.

References

Andrianifahanana M, Moniaux N, Schmied BM et al. Mucin (MUC) gene expression in human pancreatic adenocarcinoma and chronic pancreatitis: a potential role of MUC4 as a tumor marker of diagnostic significance. *Clin Cancer Res* 2001;7:4033–4040.

Argani P, Iacobuzio-Donahue C, Ryu B et al. Mesothelin is overexpressed in the vast majority of ductal adenocarcinomas of the pancreas: identification of a new pancreatic cancer marker by serial analysis of gene expression (SAGE). *Clin Cancer Res* 2001;7:3862–3868.

Biankin AV, Morey AL, Lee CS et al. DPC4/Smad4 expression and outcome in pancreatic ductal adenocarcinoma. *J Clin Oncol* 2002;20:4531–4542.

Buchholz M, Boeck W, Fensterer H. Use of DNA arrays/microarrays in pancreatic research. *Pancreatology* 2001;1: 581–586.

Caldas C, Kern SE. Related K-ras mutation and pancreatic adenocarcinoma. *Int J Pancreatol* 1995;18:1–6.

Castells A, Puig P, Mora J et al. K-ras mutations in DNA extracted from the plasma of patients with pancreatic carcinoma: diagnostic utility and prognostic significance. *J Clin Oncol* 1999;17:578–584.

Eskelinen M, Haglund U. Developments in serologic detection of human pancreatic adenocarcinoma. *Scand J Gastroenterol* 1999;34:833–844.

Gress TM, Muller-Pillasch F, Geng M et al. A pancreatic can-

cer-specific expression profile. *Oncogene* 1996;13:1819–1830.

Halm U, Schumann T, Schiefke I et al. Decrease of CA 19–9 during chemotherapy with gemcitabine predicts survival time in patients with advanced pancreatic cancer. *Br J Cancer* 2000;82:1013–1016.

Iacobuzio-Donahue CA, Maitra A, Olsen M et al. Exploration of global gene expression patterns in pancreatic adenocarcinoma using cDNA microarrays. *Am J Pathol* 2003;162: 1151–1162.

Koizumi M, Doi R, Toyoda E et al. Increased PDX-1 expression is associated with outcome in patients with pancreatic cancer. *Surgery* 2003;134:260–266.

Logsdon CD, Simeone DM, Binkley C et al. Molecular profiling of pancreatic adenocarcinoma and chronic pancreatitis identifies multiple genes differentially regulated in pancreatic cancer. *Cancer Res* 2003;63:2649–2657.

Luttges J, Diederichs A, Menke MA et al. Ductal lesions in patients with chronic pancreatitis show K-ras mutations in a frequency similar to that in the normal pancreas and lack nuclear immunoreactivity for p53. *Cancer* 2000;88:2495–2504.

Maitra A, Adsay NV, Argani P et al. Multicomponent analysis of the pancreatic adenocarcinoma progression model using a pancreatic intraepithelial neoplasia tissue microarray. *Mod Pathol* 2003;16:902–912.

Micke O, Bruns F, Schafer U et al. CA 19–9 in the therapy monitoring and follow-up of locally advanced cancer of the exocrine pancreas treated with radiochemotherapy. *Anticancer Res* 2003;23:835–840.

Mu DQ, Wang GF, Peng SY. p53 protein expression and CA19.9 values in differential cytological diagnosis of pancreatic cancer complicated with chronic pancreatitis. *World J Gastroenterol* 2003;9:1815–1818.

Mueller F, Bommer M, Lacher U et al. KOC is a novel molecular indicator of malignancy. *Br J Cancer* 2003;8:699–701.

Ringel J, Faulmann FG, Brandt R et al. MUC4 mRNA in peripheral blood mononuclear cells (PBMC) as a potential tumor marker for pancreatic cancer. *Proc ASCO* 2001; 42:A616.

Saad ED, Machado MC, Wajsbrot D et al. Pretreatment CA 19–9 level as a prognostic factor in patients with advanced pancreatic cancer treated with gemcitabine. *Int J Gastrointest Cancer* 2002;32:35–41.

Schlieman, Ho HS, Bold RJ. Utility of tumor markers in determining resectability of pancreatic cancer. *Arch Surg* 2003;138:951–955.

Slesak B, Harlozinska-Szmyrka A, Knast W et al. Tissue polypeptide specific antigen (TPS), a marker for differentiation between pancreatic carcinoma and chronic pancreatitis. A comparative study with CA 19–9. *Cancer* 2000;89: 83–88.

Trumper L, Menges M, Daus H *et al.* Low sensitivity of the ki-ras polymerase chain reaction for diagnosing pancreatic cancer from pancreatic juice and bile: a multicenter prospective trial. *J Clin Oncol* 2002;20:4331–4337.

Uemura K, Hiyama E, Murakami Y *et al.* Comparative analysis of K-ras point mutation, telomerase activity, and p53 overexpression in pancreatic tumours. *Oncol Rep* 2003;10:277–283.

Xie MJ, Motoo Y, Iovanna JL *et al.* Overexpression of pancreatitis-associated protein (PAP) in human pancreatic ductal adenocarcinoma. *Dig Dis Sci* 2003;48:459–464.

Yamaguchi Y, Watanabe H, Yrdiran S. Detection of mutations of p53 tumor suppressor gene in pancreatic juice and its application to diagnosis of patients with pancreatic cancer: comparison with K-ras mutation. *Clin Cancer Res* 1999;5:1147–1153.

46 Stage classification of pancreatic cancer

Antonio Farré

Introduction

The long-term prognosis of patients with pancreatic cancer remains dismal. Surgical resection is the only potential curative therapy but this is frequently unfeasible due to locally advanced disease or to its extrapancreatic extension at diagnosis. Preoperative evaluation and staging of the disease must be carried out to assess tumor resectability, exclude the presence of extrapancreatic invasion, and prevent unnecessary operative exploration. If localized disease is confirmed, the anatomic relationship with peripancreatic major vessels must be evaluated. Encasement or invasion of the celiac axis or common hepatic or superior mesenteric arteries is an absolute contraindication to surgery. In the case of the venous system, if nonobstructive venous involvement is observed, surgical resection and reconstruction should be evaluated by an experienced team of surgeons who will determine when the tumor should be amenable to complete extirpation. In the presence of distant metastatic disease, palliative therapy only should be considered.

Stage classification

Stage classification of cancer is based on the observation that survival rates are higher when the disease is localized than when it has spread beyond the organ of origin. Staging of cancer is used to analyze and compare groups of patients. In order to create a global system of cancer staging and to ensure a common language is used, in 1987 the Union Internationale Contre le Cancer (UICC) and the American Joint Committee on Cancer (AJCC) agreed to simultaneously publish a classification based on the TNM system, an expression of the anatomic extent of the disease. New editions of the *TNM Classification of Malignant Tumors* (UICC) and the *Cancer Stage Manual* (AJCC) are developed periodically. Stage classification of exocrine pancreatic cancer is also included in this system.

In the stage classification of exocrine pancreatic cancer (Table 46.1), the TNM classification describes the anatomic extent of tumor at the primary site (T), the presence or absence of tumor in regional lymph nodes (N), and the presence or absence of metastasis (M). T is divided into four major categories (T1–T4), depending on the size or spread of the primary tumor. N and M are divided into two categories (0–1) depending on the absence or presence of regional lymph-node metastasis and the absence or presence of distant metastasis, respectively. Isolated tumor cells or small clusters of tumor cells less than 0.2 mm that can be detected by immunohistochemistry or molecular methods in lymph nodes or at distant sites should be classified as N0 or M0 respectively, as their significance from a biological point of view is not yet established.

The TNM system classifies the individual TNM elements separately and then groups them into stages. Stage grouping in the case of exocrine pancreatic cancer is basically distributed in five stages (0–IV).
Stage 0 corresponds to carcinoma *in situ*, N0, M0.
Stage I is subdivided into Stage IA, which includes only T1, and Stage IB, which includes only T2.
Stage II is differentiated into Stage IIA (T3, N0, M0) and Stage IIB (T1–3, N1, M0);
Stage III includes T4, any N and M0.
Stage IV includes any T, any N, and M1.

Table 46.1 TNM classification and stage grouping of exocrine pancreatic cancer. (From Greene *et al.* 2002.)

Primary tumor (T)

TX	Primary tumor cannot be assessed
T0	No evidence of primary tumor
Tis	Carcinoma *in situ*
T1	Tumor limited to the pancreas, 2 cm or less in greatest dimension
T2	Tumor limited to the pancreas, more than 2 cm in greatest dimension
T3	Tumor extends beyond the pancreas but without involvement of the celiac axis or the superior mesenteric artery
T4	Tumor involves the celiac axis or the superior mesenteric artery (unresectable primary tumor)

Regional lymph nodes (N)

NX	Regional lymph nodes cannot be assessed
N0	No regional lymph node metastasis
N1	Regional lymph node metastasis

Distant metastasis (M)

MX	Distant metastasis cannot be assessed
M0	No distant metastasis
M1	Distant metastasis

Stage grouping

Stage 0	Tis	N0	M0
Stage IA	T1	N0	M0
Stage IB	T2	N0	M0
Stage IIA	T3	N0	M0
Stage IIB	T1	N1	M0
	T2	N1	M0
	T3	N1	M0
Stage III	T4	Any N	M0
Stage IV	Any T	Any N	M1

Despite discrepancies between different surgical teams, most surgeons apply the following criteria of nonresectability: (i) celiac axis or hepatic artery origin invasion; (ii) superior mesenteric artery invasion; (iii) portal vein or superior mesenteric vein invasion (semicircular encasement or extension superior to 15 mm); and (iv) distant metastasis. Therefore, according to the UICC/AJCC stage classification, only certain T1 tumors, corresponding to Stage IA, are resectable and very few of the tumors classified as Stage IB and IIA (T2–3, N0, M0) are candidates for resection.

The pathologic classification (pTNM) and stage grouping is based on examination of a surgically resected specimen and can be used as a guide to the need for adjuvant therapy and prognosis. Since only a minority of patients with pancreatic cancer undergo surgical resection of the pancreas, a single TNM classification must apply to both clinical and pathologic staging.

In 1993, the Japanese Pancreatic Society (JPS) proposed a more complex stage classification, with more detailed evaluation of the degree of invasion. In contrast with the UICC/AJCC system, in the JPS TNM classification T refers only to tumor size and is recorded as T1 when tumor is 2.0 cm or less, T2 when 2.1–4.0 cm, T3 when 4.1–6.0 cm, and T4 when over 6.1 cm. Local extent of tumor is expressed as S, indicating serosal invasion (S 0, 1, 2, 3); RP, indicating retroperitoneal invasion (RP 0, 1, 2, 3); and PV, indicating portal vein invasion (PV 0, 1, 2, 3), where 0 is absence of invasion, 1 suspected invasion, 2 definite invasion, and 3 severe invasion. The N factor is divided into four grades: N0, no metastasis; N1, primary lymph-node group metastasis; N2, secondary lymph-node group metastasis; and N3, tertiary lymph-node group metastasis. The M factor, distant metastasis, is divided into M0, no distant metastasis, and M1, distant metastasis.

Major differences between the UICC/AJCC and JPS classifications concern local tumor spread and the extent of lymph-node involvement. The JPS classification is a more accurate reflection of disease prognosis but is complex and difficult to use. Taking into account all the pros and cons in the application of both systems (UICC/AJCC and JPS), a new pancreatic cancer TNM classification and stage grouping system has been proposed by Japanese authors based on a combination of the two systems, and draws on the merits of both.

The TNM system (UICC/AJCC and JPS) does not include other nonanatomic prognostic factors currently in use or under study, such as cytologic and histologic observations, serum measurements of tumor expression, and enzyme and genetic measurements, that may influence outcome predictions and treatment decisions. Once they are correctly identified and validated, such data might become candidates for future incorporation in the TNM staging system.

In this way, the extent of surgical resection, when possible, has recently promoted the increasing use of the R classification based on histopathologic analysis of the resected material, where R0 is complete resection with clear margins, R1 complete resection with positive resection margins, and R2 incomplete resection of macroscopic tumor. The R classification is not part of the TNM system but is prognostically of great significance.

Morphologic tumor staging

Early diagnosis of pancreatic cancer is extremely difficult. In Western countries, usually only 15–20% of patients with pancreatic cancer are candidates for resection compared with about 80% who will receive palliative treatment only. The late presentation of the disease is due to a combination of the silent behavior of the tumor in its early development and delay in diagnosis as a result of late presentation of the patient and lack of sufficiently sensitive diagnostic tools to identify localized disease. New multimodality treatment can be achieved with an improvement in preoperative staging and a better selection of patients for surgical therapy. As previously mentioned, the aim of staging is to detect those patients who have potentially resectable localized cancer from those with locally unresectable or metastatic disease.

Preoperative and perioperative staging can be based on the results obtained with currently available imaging techniques used in the diagnosis of pancreatic cancer. The diagnostic procedures generally used in the work-up of patients with suspected pancreatic cancer are highly sensitive and accurate in predicting those patients who will not be candidates for resection, thus avoiding unnecessary laparotomy. The prediction of unresectability may be as high as 90% when correlated with intraoperative findings. However, at present there are major difficulties in accurately predicting resectability, as almost 30% of patients considered to be eligible for resection are found to have either small hepatic or peritoneal metastasis or invasion of vascular structures.

Computed tomography

Helical computed tomography (CT) is now considered one of the most accurate methods in the diagnosis and staging of pancreatic cancer. Furthermore, CT-guided biopsy by fine-needle aspiration (FNA) can be performed at the initial scan to obtain histologic samples to confirm the diagnosis and/or the presence of metastasis. The accuracy of helical CT for staging unresectable carcinomas is virtually 100%. However, CT has proven far less reliable in predicting resectability, with an accuracy of 70–80%. Dual-phase helical CT, performed with contrast enhancement, provides information on tumor location and its resectability, affording excellent evaluation of its relationship to the celiac axis, superior mesenteric artery, and portal and superior mesenteric veins, as well as to the presence of enlarged lymph nodes, hepatic metastases, and/or ascites (Fig. 46.1). The presence of locally advanced tumor extension into the soft-tissue planes surrounding the celiac axis, mesenteric artery, superior mesenteric and portal veins, or retroperitoneum is assessed. The criteria of lymph-node involvement are often impossible to evaluate from size alone. Normal-size lymph nodes may contain tumor, and enlarged lymph nodes may be the result of inflammatory or reactive hyperplasia. Helical CT also appears to be limited in the detection of small hepatic and peritoneal metastasis. Despite the improved accuracy of CT, approximately 15–20% of patients may have unsuspected metastasis. Liver and peritoneal metastasis smaller than 1.0 cm are difficult to detect by CT.

Multislice CT has recently been introduced. It provides an improvement in anatomic volume coverage and also separates arterial from venous image acquisition phases. Reconstruction by three-dimensional imaging of peripancreatic vasculature in an attempt to determine vascular involvement by pancreatic cancer is controversial.

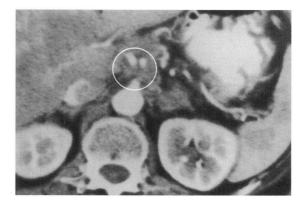

Figure 46.1 Unresectable pancreatic cancer: contrast-enhanced helical CT showing a 3-cm hypodense mass in the body of the pancreas (encircled area) that invades and occludes celiac axis.

Endoscopic ultrasonography

Endoscopic ultrasonography (EUS) is a reliable method for pancreatic tumor detection. The close proximity of the transducer to the pancreatic area ameliorates the resolution of this procedure in comparison with transcutaneous techniques. EUS can diagnose tumors as small as 5 mm in diameter and characterize their extension, assessing resectability by its capacity to determine vascular invasion and lymph-node enlargement. Incipient venous infiltration may be detected by EUS and may therefore be helpful in predicting resectability. The application of color Doppler ultrasound technology has enhanced the assessment of vascular involvement. EUS-guided FNA of suspicious tissues is safe and can provide reliable and useful information for the management of these patients. FNA performed during an EUS procedure also helps to establish a diagnosis of malignancy, with an accuracy of 90%. The inability to completely evaluate the liver for metastasis is a disadvantage of this technique.

Magnetic resonance imaging

Although the results from magnetic resonance imaging (MRI) rival those obtained by helical CT, this is not a standard procedure in the work-up of patients with pancreatic cancer and their preoperative staging. MRI is comparable to CT in detection of pancreatic cancer, enlarged lymph nodes, and hepatic metastasis. High-resolution and functional imaging have notoriously improved the arterial and venous definitions necessary for evaluation of resectability. Magnetic resonance cholangiopancreatography (MRCP) is excellent and provides information about the site and extent of hepatic biliary obstruction and periampullary strictures, often making endoscopic retrograde cholangiopancreatography unnecessary. The combination of MRCP with pancreatic MRI accurately predicts resectability. Altered renal function and allergies to iodine-based contrast agents that impede the use of CT are probably the main indications for the use of MRI in staging of pancreatic cancer.

Positron emission tomography

Positron emission tomography (PET) with ^{18}F-fluorodeoxyglucose (^{18}F-FDG) is a nonaggressive technique based on the greater incorporation of glucose and its analog ^{18}F-FDG in malignant cells compared with mostly healthy tissues. ^{18}F-FDG does not undergo further metabolism in tumor cells and remains trapped for a sufficient time to allow for imaging. It is not a first-line diagnostic method in pancreatic cancer and its utility in this tumor has not yet been well established. As the hypermetabolism of glucose is not restricted to malignancy but can also occur in certain inflammatory and infective conditions, PET images may be falsely positive in the presence of pancreatitis. Highly differentiated tumors and those with blood glucose levels above 130 mg/dL may not metabolize the PET marker and there may be difficulties in interpreting false-negative results. The main strength of PET lies in its ability to detect distant metastasis not imaged by CT. PET shows the best detection rate for the staging of lymphatic metastases. PET images can be fused with CT and/or MRI images, aiding accuracy in the detection of tumor spread.

Laparoscopy

Laparoscopy, the only nonimaging technique in the work-up, has been proposed for staging pancreatic cancer and thereby avoiding an unnecessary laparotomy. Superficial liver metastasis and peritoneal dissemination are frequently found in pancreatic cancer patients. These implants commonly measure no more than a few millimeters and can only be detected by direct visualization via laparoscopy or at laparotomy. Several series have demonstrated that the routine use of laparoscopy identifies occult metastatic disease in up to 40% of cases deemed resectable by other studies. In 10–20% of patients with apparently resectable tumor in the head of the pancreas according to CT, laparoscopy will reveal either distant metastasis or local invasion that contraindicates pancreaticoduodenectomy. In the case of carcinoma of the body or tail of the pancreas, this prevalence almost doubles. However, the role of routine preoperative staging laparoscopy is controversial, especially in tumors located in the head of the pancreas. It seems reasonable to perform laparoscopy, prior to laparotomy, in patients with a tumor considered potentially resectable, especially if it is located in the body or tail of the pancreas.

Conclusions

Data obtained during preoperative staging of pancreatic cancer allows classification of the tumor with regard to its potential resectability and thus ensures more appropriate treatment. Patients with a pancreatic cancer considered to be resectable have a long-term survival rate of 20% and a median survival of 15–20 months, whereas patients with locally advanced nonmetastatic disease have a median survival of 6–10 months. Patients with metastatic disease have the shortest median survival that varies between 3 and 6 months.

Contrast-enhanced multislice CT is the standard imaging procedure for classifying patients as having localized resectable, locally advanced, or metastatic pancreatic cancer. Additional procedures such as EUS, MRI, MRCP, and PET are best reserved for those cases in which CT yields equivocal findings or in patients who cannot undergo contrast-enhanced CT. Laparoscopy prior to laparotomy should be reserved for patients deemed resectable because of a 10–20% incidence of occult liver or peritoneal metastasis not detected by imaging methods.

Recommended reading

Alazraki N. Imaging of pancreatic cancer using fluorine-18 fluorodeoxyglucose positron emission tomography. *J Gastrointest Surg* 2002;6:136–138.

DiMagno EP, Reber HA, Tempero MA. AGA technical review on the epidemiology, diagnosis, and treatment of pancreatic ductal adenocarcinoma. American Gastroenterological Association. *Gastroenterology* 1999;117:1464–1484.

Greene FL, Page DL, Fleming ID *et al.* (eds) *AJCC Cancer Staging Manual*, 6th edn. Berlin: Springer-Verlag, 2002: 157–164.

Habr F, Akerman P. Role of endoscopic ultrasound in the diagnosis and staging of pancreatic cancer. *Front Biosci* 2000;5:30–35.

Horton KM. Multidetector CT and three-dimensional imaging of the pancreas: state of the art. *J Gastrointest Surg* 2002;6:126–128.

Japan Pancreas Society. *Classification of Pancreatic Carcinoma.* Tokyo: Kanehara & Co., 1996: 1–65.

Pisters PWT, Lee JE, Vauthey JN *et al.* Laparoscopy in the staging of pancreatic cancer. *Br J Surg* 2001;88:325–337.

Sheridan MB, Ward J, Guthrie JA *et al.* Dynamic contrast-enhanced MR imaging and dual-phase helical CT in the pre-operative assessment of suspected pancreatic cancer: a comparative study with receiver operating characteristic analysis. *Am J Roentgenol* 1999;173:583–590.

Sobin LH, Wittekind C (eds) *International Union Against Cancer (UICC), TNM Classification of Malignant Tumours*, 6th edn. New York: John Wiley & Sons, 2002: 93–96.

Tsunoda T, Eto T, Tsuchiya R. Staging of pancreatic cancer: a new Japanese stage classification based on TNM factors. In: H Beger, AL Warshaw, MW Büchler, DL Carr-Locke, JP Neoptolemos, C Russel, MG Sarr (eds) *The Pancreas.* Oxford: Blackwell Science, 1998: 943–949.

47 Imaging diagnosis and staging of pancreatic cancer: which methods are essential?

Marchelle J. Bean, Karen M. Horton, and Elliot K. Fishman

Introduction

The radiologic diagnosis and staging of pancreatic cancer depends predominantly on high-quality cross-sectional imaging. With advancements in computer and scanner technology, three-dimensional software programs, and the increasing availability of multidetector scanners, computed tomography (CT) emerges as the imaging modality of choice for the detection, staging, and follow-up of patients with pancreatic cancer. Although other imaging modalities, such as magnetic resonance imaging (MRI) and ultrasound perform an adjunctive role, CT is considered the primary imaging method for pancreatic imaging.

Evolution of CT scanning

The introduction of CT into clinical practice in the late 1970s finally made possible direct noninvasive imaging of the pancreas. Prior to this time, pancreatic imaging was limited to ultrasound, nuclear medicine, and barium studies. Such evaluations only inferred the presence of pancreatic disease by visualizing secondary signs such as displacement of bowel and widening of the duodenal C-loop. In fact, when these early examinations were positive, patients typically exhibited large tumors, which were not amenable to curative surgical intervention. Similarly, angiography was limited to the creation of vascular maps since this method is not able to visualize the pancreas directly. In contrast with these other imaging modalities, CT is able to directly and non-invasively visualize the pancreas and peripancreatic structures including the mesenteric and portal vessels. In addition, potential sites of metastases, including the liver and peripancreatic lymph nodes, can be imaged during a single examination.

Today, over 20 years later, CT remains the primary study for evaluating the pancreas. However, significant advancements in CT technology, along with the introduction of three-dimensional imaging techniques, have substantially improved pancreatic imaging. Understanding these changes is essential to fully appreciate the current role of CT in imaging pancreatic pathology. Advanced CT imaging of pancreatic cancer can improve patient outcome by correctly detecting tumor earlier as well as accurately evaluating the extent of disease in order to identify patients who could potentially benefit from aggressive surgical management.

Multidetector CT and three-dimensional imaging

CT plays an essential role in evaluation of pancreatic cancer. It has emerged as the gold standard in pancreatic imaging due to two major innovations: the development of multidetector CT (MDCT) scanners and improvements in three-dimensional imaging software and hardware.

The introduction of MDCT scanners in the late 1990s revolutionized CT scanning. MDCT offers the latest advances in CT technology by combining multiple rows of detectors and faster gantry rotation speeds. Early CT scanners acquired data in 10-mm slices at a rate of 1 slice per minute, producing limited visualization of small tumors and adjacent vasculature. The introduction of single detector spiral scanners in the late 1980s was definitely an improvement over conventional dynamic scanners, but these scanners still had limited speed and resolution. In contrast, the new 16-slice MDCT scanners allow pancreatic imaging with 0.75-mm slices, at a rate of 32 slices per second. In fact, the entire abdomen can be scanned in less than 10 s. This results in high-resolution datasets and has greatly improved three-dimensional imaging and CT angiography (CTA).

Three-dimensional CT imaging is essential when evaluating a patient with suspected pancreatic pathology. In the past, a CT examination was acquired and reviewed in the axial plane only, which is not adequate when evaluating complex anatomy. MDCT scanners still acquire the data in the axial plane, but instead of a series of slices the data are actually a volume. This volume can then be viewed with three-dimensional software to better display the anatomy and/or pathology. The three-dimensional CT dataset is manipulated using different orientations and cut planes in order to best demonstrate the pancreas and peripancreatic vasculature. Also, the radiologist is able to adjust the window level, center, brightness, and opacity in order to accentuate certain structures such as soft tissue or vessels. CTA information obtained from the same dataset can be reconstructed using volume rendering and maximum-intensity projection (MIP) techniques. This noninvasive method allows faster and more accurate visualization of vascular encasement/invasion of the celiac axis, superior mesenteric artery, superior mesenteric vein, and portal vein.

CT technique

Oral and intravenous contrast

For detection of pancreatic lesions, proper patient preparation and technique is essential. Patient preparation includes optimal contrast administration (oral and intravenous) as well as the acquisition of thin high-resolution slices. Oral contrast (1 L of water) is administered over 20 min to ensure adequate delineation and distension of small bowel. Water as an oral contrast agent also optimizes visualization of potential small periampullary masses and allows performance of CTA of the peripancreatic vessels, without complicated editing.

Fast bolus injection of 100–120 mL intravenous contrast at a rate of 3–5 mL/s through a 19–20 gauge catheter placed in an antecubital vein produces the parenchymal enhancement and vascular opacification

necessary for the visualization and staging of pancreatic lesions.

Scan protocol

For detailed imaging of the pancreas, we utilize our 16-slice MDCT (Siemens Sensation 16, Siemens, Malvern, PA) to obtain 0.75-mm slices through the liver and pancreas. These thin slices greatly improve the three-dimensional dataset.

With these faster scanning capabilities, dual-phase imaging of the pancreas is now possible, with the acquisition of both arterial- and venous-phase datasets using a single bolus injection of contrast. Arterial-phase images are acquired 25 s after the start of the injection, while portal venous-phase images are obtained at 60 s. Therefore high-resolution arterial and venous vascular maps can be created that are comparable to conventional angiography and serve as an essential anatomic map for staging and presurgical evaluation.

CT evaluation of pancreatic cancer

The overall 5-year survival rate for pancreatic adenocarcinoma is les than 5%, with the majority of patients presenting with advanced disease at the time of diagnosis (70–90%). The goal of CT is to detect the tumor and to determine which patients are candidates for surgical resection. The criteria for pancreatic cancer resectability include the absence of hepatic metastasis, peritoneal metastasis or lymph-node involvement, as well as the lack of vascular encasement.

Imaging features

Normal pancreas
The detection of pancreatic pathology relies upon an appreciation of the normal appearance of the pancreas. The pancreas is classically divided into head, neck, body, and tail. The pancreatic head lies within the duodenal sweep, anterior to the junction of the left renal vein and inferior vena. An extension of the left and caudal portion of the head is the uncinate process, which extends adjacent to the superior mesenteric vessels and has a tongue-like pointed contour. Immediately to the left of the head and resting ventrally to superior mesenteric vessels is the pancreatic neck. The pancreatic body rests behind the lesser sac and stomach with its dorsal

surface abutting the splenic vein. The pancreatic tail is often at the same level or cephalad to the pancreatic body and follows the splenic vessels into the splenic hilum.

The normal upper limit for width of the pancreatic head is 2.5–3 cm. The normal anterior–posterior width of the body of the pancreas varies, but 2.0 cm is generally accepted as the upper limit of normal. The maximum normal width for the pancreatic tail is approximately 1.5 cm. These are only rough guidelines for judging the size of the pancreas.

The normal pancreas demonstrates homogeneous enhancement on both the arterial- and venous-phase images. The pancreatic duct can be seen in normal patients, but should measure less than 2 mm in diameter. In addition the peripancreatic fat should be homogeneous and a good fat plane should be visible between the pancreas and adjacent structures.

Tumor detection

The majority of pancreatic cancers occur as a focal mass in the head/neck (65%), with only 20% located in the body and 10% in the tail (Fig. 47.1). However, approximately 5–10% of tumors will result in diffuse enlargement of the entire gland and can be a diagnostic challenge. The entire pancreas can be enlarged as a result of diffuse tumor infiltration of the gland or as a result of pancreatitis caused by a focal mass. It is sometimes difficult to distinguish the two on a single CT scan.

In the past, the CT diagnosis of pancreatic cancer relied heavily on the visualization of a discrete mass, a 3–6 cm mass being the classic description. This is still true, but today's CT technology also allows visualization of smaller masses as well as subtle density and textural differences as clues to an underlying malignancy.

On noncontrast examinations, a tumor may appear as a region of subtle hypodensity often due to edema and necrosis. However, most pancreatic tumors are difficult to visualize without intravenous contrast. With faster scanners, dual-phase (arterial and late phase) imaging is of paramount importance to ensure optimal gland enhancement, allowing detection of subtle and small tumors (< 2 cm) by alteration in density of the pancreas, as well as evaluation of vascular involvement. Arterial-phase imaging is superior for detection of some pancreatic tumors (islet cell), while venous-phase imaging is better in other instances when the tumor and gland have maximal differentiation of en-

hancement (adenocarcinoma). Therefore it is essential to always acquire images during both the arterial and venous phases.

In contrast-enhanced studies, most adenocarcinomas will enhance less than adjacent parenchyma, appearing as a low-density mass. However, small tumors, which do not distort the shape of the gland, may be detected only during arterial-phase scanning, appearing as a subtle region of low attenuation. On venous-phase imaging, these small tumors often appear isodense with normal pancreas and are therefore undetectable. Other small tumors may not be apparent on arterial images and are only detected on late-phase scanning.

Arterial-phase imaging is also key for less common vascular pancreatic tumors including islet-cell tumors, and hypervascular metastasis such as renal cell carcinoma or carcinoid. With arterial-phase imaging, hypervascular lesions enhance more than the normal pancreas, appearing hyperdense to normal pancreatic tissue. These lesions often wash out rapidly, becoming isodense with the pancreas on venous-phase sequences.

In some patients, it may not be possible to visualize small pancreatic masses directly. In these cases, the presence of secondary signs, including duct dilatation or gland atrophy, are clues to the presence of an underlying mass. For example, pancreatic and common bile duct dilation in the absence of a stone is very suspicious of a small pancreatic or periampullary mass, even if the actual tumor is not visible. Similarly, an abrupt transition in pancreatic duct caliber is highly suspicious for tumor at the transition point, even if no discrete mass is visible. Atrophy of the pancreas distal to a mass is also a common secondary finding.

Pancreatic cancer versus pancreatitis

Difficulty can occasionally arise when trying to distinguish pancreatic cancer from pancreatitis since the CT findings can overlap. Common CT features in patients with chronic pancreatitis include gland atrophy, dilatation of the pancreatic and bile ducts, pancreatic calcifications, and pseudocyst formation. However, focal pancreatic enlargement can occur that can simulate pancreatic tumor. An abrupt change in caliber of the pancreatic duct favors pancreatic cancer over pancreatitis even if no lesion is identified. In chronic pancreatitis, dilated ducts tend to be irregular, while dilation due to pancreatic mass is often smooth or beaded.

In pancreatitis and invasive pancreatic carcinoma, peripancreatic tissues may demonstrate an increase in

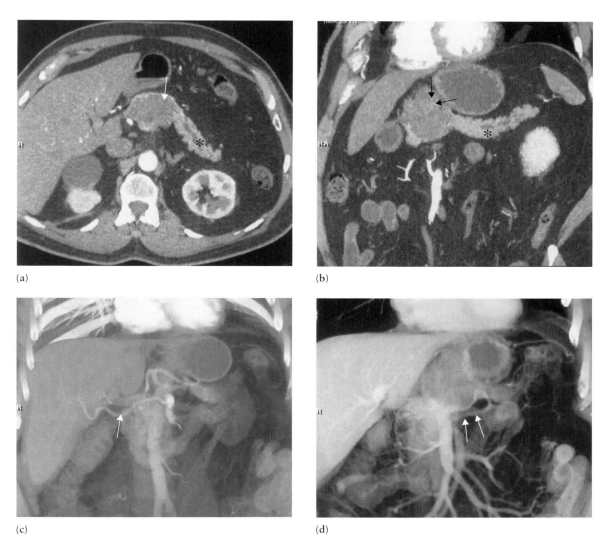

(a)

(b)

(c)

(d)

Figure 47.1 African-american male, 67 years old, with pancreatic adenocarcinoma arising from the neck and extending cephalad. (a) Axial and (b) off-axis oblique images demonstrating adenocarcinoma (arrow) producing focal pancreatic enlargement with decreased attenuation compared with the remainder of the pancreas resulting in obstruction and dilatation of the pancreatic duct (asterisk).

(c) Three-dimensional volume-rendering coronal of arterial anatomy showing patent arteries and a replaced right hepatic artery (arrow). (d) Three-dimensional volume-rendering coronal of venous anatomy demonstrating the mass producing narrowing and near-complete occlusion of the splenic vein rendering the tumor unresectable (arrows).

density of the peripancreatic fat. One finding that may help distinguish pancreatitis from a neoplastic process is preservation of a rim of normal fat around the superior mesenteric artery and superior mesenteric vein in pancreatitis.

As opposed to pancreatitis, pancreatic tumors are metabolically active, consuming increased amounts of glucose relative to the remaining pancreatic tissue. On this basis, ^{18}F-fluorodeoxyglucose (FDG) positron emission tomography (PET) may distinguish between cancer and pancreatitis. Pancreatic cancer demonstrates increased uptake of FDG, with accuracy reported to be 88–90%. This technique may also be useful for differentiating postoperative recurrence from surgical/radiation change. In addition, biopsy, endoscopic retrograde cholangiopancreatography (ERCP), and/or close serial follow-up with CT are often required to help differentiate focal pancreatitis from carcinoma.

Vascular involvement
The role of CT imaging includes not only the detection of a pancreatic mass but also accurate staging of the disease. Since the pancreas lacks a true capsule, invasion of adjacent soft tissue, fat, and vessels is common. Pancreatic carcinoma extension results in obliteration of normal peripancreatic fat. Tumor extension can involve duodenum, gastric antrum, posterior gastric wall, transverse colon, spleen, splenic flexure of the colon, porta hepatis, and blood vessels. When the fat plane is lost between a pancreatic mass and an adjacent organ, there is presumed to be direct extension of tumor. However, in some instances, fat plane obliteration may only indicate abutment by tumor, or may be caused by fibrous proliferation rather than tumor invasion itself. In addition, microscopic invasion of surrounding tissue may occur without gross obliteration of the fat plane. In the absence of metastatic disease, resectability depends on local tumor extensions and vascular involvement. In the majority of cases, vascular involvement with tumor renders a patient unresectable (Fig. 47.2).

Studies comparing helical CT to standard angiography for the detection of arterial involvement conclude that both methods are equivalent for diagnosing arterial invasion. For minor arteries, including anterior superior pancreaticoduodenal and posterior superior pancreaticoduodenal arteries, angiography was more

successful. However, encasement and invasion of these minor vessels is not a contraindication for pancreatic resection and such demonstration is not crucial for determining tumor resectability.

Tumor involvement of blood vessels appears as circumferential encasement and narrowing of the vessels, focal invasion, or complete occlusion. A CT grading system for vessel involvement (arterial and venous) by tumor was developed by Lu *et al*. Vessel invasion with tumor is prospectively graded, based on circumferential contiguity of tumor to vessel, on a scale from 0 to 4. Zero represented no soft tissue touching vessel; each number then corresponded to the percentage of vessel in contact with soft tissue in 25% increments, so that $1 = 25\%$ and $4 = 100\%$. This study found that patients with grade 3–4 involvement (> 50% circumference vessel abutted with tumor) were unresectable due to vascular involvement, with a sensitivity and specificity for unresectability of 84% and 98%. Nakayama *et al*. performed a similar study and found different grading criteria for arteries versus veins. Nakayama proposed that grade 3–4 criteria indicated unresectability for venous structures, but found arterial structures with this grade were sometimes surrounded by inflammatory/fibrous tissue rather than tumor, and therefore criteria were deemed less useful for peripancreatic arteries.

Other signs of tumor vessel involvement include change in vessel caliber or occlusion. Findings are often better visualized with three-dimensional volumetric reconstruction. Vessels run in numerous different planes and different angles. While some vessels may be best visualized on axial images, the majority of vessels, which run perpendicular to standard axial images, are better evaluated by CTA with three-dimensional, real-time, volumetric data manipulation. One study revealed that the negative predictive value of resectable tumor only on axial images was 70%. With the addition of CTA to the axial examination, negative predictive value improved to 96%.

The celiac artery and its branch vessels are commonly involved in patients with large pancreatic masses, especially tumors of the pancreatic body and tail. It is important to identify major branches off the celiac axis, including hepatic, splenic, and gastroduodenal arteries. Superior mesenteric artery is the vessel most commonly involved with pancreatic cancer because of its close approximation to the pancreatic head and neck. These vessels are best viewed using a coronal/

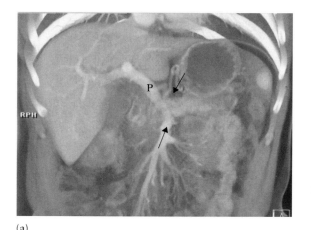

(a)

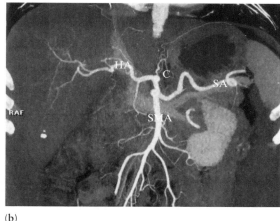

(b)

Figure 47.2 White male, 46 years old, with resectable moderately differentiated adenocarcinoma of the pancreatic head. (a) Coronal three-dimensional volume rendering revealing the pancreatic head adenocarcinoma abutting the portal vein/splenic vein confluence producing minimal compression of the portal vein (arrow; P, portal vein).

Common bile duct and pancreatic duct dilatation noted. (b) Coronal three-dimensional maximum-intensity projection showing normal arterial anatomy. HA, hepatic artery; C, celiac artery; SA, splenic artery; SMA, superior mesenteric artery.

anterior projection and sagittal views similar to conventional invasive angiograms (Fig. 47.3).

The portal vein runs perpendicular to axial images and is optimally visualized with three-dimensional reconstruction using a coronal oblique projection in order to demonstrate the complete extrahepatic portal vein and its junction with the mesenteric vessels and splenic vein. Splenic vein involvement occurs with tumors of pancreatic body and tail. Gastroepiploic collaterals appear when there is significant narrowing or occlusion of the splenic vein with tumor. Isolated splenic vein involvement is rare; however, patients may still be considered candidates for resection and splenectomy with limited, isolated splenic vein involvement. Superior mesenteric vein involvement renders patients unresectable. Since this vessel is intimately associated with uncinate process, head, and neck of pancreas, involvement occurs with tumors in these regions, also often narrowing the superior mesenteric vein and its confluence with the portal vein. Marked narrowing of superior mesenteric vein without adequate collaterals can induce small bowel loop ischemia (Fig. 47.4).

Biliary obstruction

Pancreatic cancer may cause biliary obstruction that results in a clinical presentation of painless jaundice, necessitating percutaneous biliary drainage to relieve symptoms and prevent sepsis/cholangitis. Biliary obstruction often results from tumors in the pancreatic head, uncinate process, or ampulla due to close association of pancreatic and common bile ducts. On axial CT, the classical appearance of obstruction is the double duct sign. This term arises from a lesion that produces occlusion of both pancreatic and common bile ducts, resulting in dilatation that appears as two large, easily visible ducts. While this sign is highly suspicious for pancreatic cancer, other conditions can produce a similar appearance, including ampullary carcinoma, cholangiocarcinoma, and chronic pancreatitis. The maximum normal dimension of the common bile duct is 6 mm. This can be slightly larger when patients are elderly or have undergone cholecystectomy. Normal pancreatic duct size is 1–2 mm.

Biliary dilatation can be seen by ultrasound as well as by MRI/magnetic resonance cholangiopancreatography

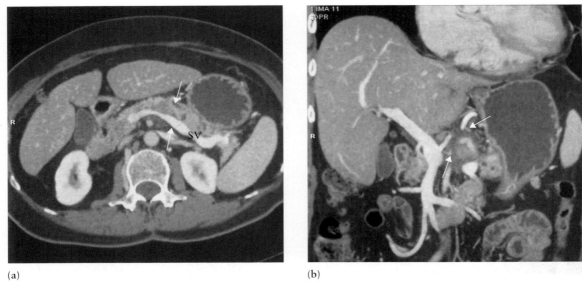

(a)   (b)

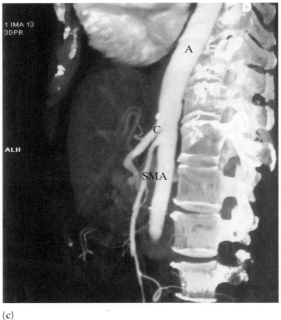

(c)

Figure 47.3 African-american female, 69 years old, with a pancreatic body adenocarcinoma. (a) Axial and (b) three-dimensional volume-rendering coronal images showing the pancreatic tumor encasing (arrows) the superior mesenteric artery and splenic vein (SV). These vessels are markedly narrowed but not occluded. (c) Lateral maximum-intensity projection showing narrowing of superior mesenteric artery (SMA); C, celiac artery; A, aorta.

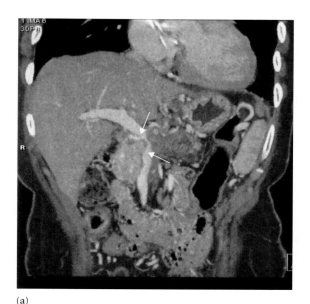

(a)

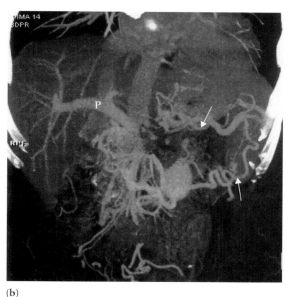

(b)

Figure 47.4 African-american female, 52 years old, with an infiltrating unresectable pancreatic neck/body adenocarcinoma. (a) Three-dimensional volume rendering demonstrating pancreatic adenocarcinoma occluding the portal vein/splenic vein confluence (arrow) and surrounding the celiac axis and superior mesenteric artery. (b) Coronal maximum-intensity projection again showing occlusion of the portal vein/splenic vein confluence with extensive collateralization of vessels (arrows); P, portal vein.

(MRCP). MRCP has an advantage over CT, as biliary fluid is inherently bright on T2-weighted sequences and therefore does not require addition of contrast for evaluation. However, the main disadvantage of MRCP remains rooted in the long acquisition time. Previously, CT cholangiography required oral or intravenous biliary contrast agents. Three-dimensional, volume-rendering, post-processing techniques have made these biliary contrast agents less necessary. With MDCT and three-dimensional processing, settings can be chosen to display biliary structures as high density, allowing better visualization and evaluation, a technique known as three-dimensional volume-rendered cholangiopancreatography (3D-VRCP). VRCP allows determination of length and level of obstruction. With this method of evaluation, pancreatic lesion, vasculature, metastasis, and biliary drainage planning can be performed with one study. VRCP is not only capable of detecting the level of obstruction, but may also reveal aberrant anatomy or multilevel obstruction/metastasis that could potentially alter biliary drainage. Another possible approach to CT imaging of the biliary tree is three-dimensional virtual CT cholangiopancreatoscopy. This technique allows endoscopic visualization of the biliary tree that correlates well with ERCP. Virtual methods and real-time evaluation allow manipulation of datasets so that all intrahepatic and extrahepatic ducts can be viewed in any orientation, contrary to percutaneous transhepatic cholangiography and routine ERCP. When a lesion is detected with VRCP, data settings can be altered to display adjacent pancreatic tissue, facilitating work-up and staging of tumor.

Extrapancreatic extension

Pancreatic metastases most commonly spread to liver, lymph nodes, peritoneum, and lung. Careful evaluation of the liver is crucial, as hepatic involvement precludes curative operative management. CT emerges as the primary, most accurate modality for detecting liver metastasis. Accuracy for detection of lesions larger than 1 cm has been reported at 91% for four-slice

MDCT. With thinner collimation and faster scanning capabilities of MDCT, smaller hepatic lesions are routinely detected, even when less than 5 mm. Lesions this small often cannot be accurately characterized by most imaging methods and therefore accuracy decreases in some studies to 75%. Hepatic surface metastases are also difficult to diagnose with imaging, and are more readily identified during surgical palpation of the hepatic capsule.

The majority of pancreatic liver metastases are hypovascular and are more readily visualized during venous-phase examination. Some pancreatic tumors, predominantly islet-cell tumors, produce hypervascular metastases necessitating arterial-phase imaging to aid detection. These hypervascular foci of hepatic spread enhance and wash out quickly, and therefore may be missed when only venous imaging is performed.

Pancreatic tumors commonly spread to celiac axis and superior mesenteric lymph nodes. Other nodal groups that may be involved include paraaortic, pericaval, retrocrural, and porta hepatis chains. Small normal lymph nodes in porta hepatis and peripancreatic regions are common. CT detection of tumor spread to lymph nodes primarily rests on size criteria. Lymph nodes larger than 1 cm are considered pathologic. However, smaller (1–2 mm) lymph nodes may also contain tumor, and are often undetectable by CT. A study by Zehman et al. used TNM staging for pancreatic cancer on CT and found nodal accuracy for pancreatic cancer to be only 58%.

Small peritoneal metastases may be seen with imaging, but frequently can be missed and only detected at surgery. Unexpected ascites strongly suggests peritoneal metastasis even though discrete lesions may not be visible.

Less common pancreatic neoplasms

Tumors of exocrine origin, including ductal adenocarcinoma, account for approximately 95% of pancreatic tumors. The remaining 5% result from rare tumors, including islet cell, lymphoma, and metastases to the gland. Mesenchymal tumors are extremely rare.

Neuroendocrine tumors/islet-cell neoplasms

Neuroendocrine tumors are an uncommon neoplasm of younger individuals, with an incidence of approximately five cases per million persons per year. These lesions have an increased incidence in patients with von Hippel–Lindau disease. Islet-cell tumors are considered functional when clinical symptoms present from excess hormone production. Approximately half of these rare neoplasms are hormonally active. Hormonally active tumors are diagnosed when smaller because of the development of clinical symptoms caused by active peptides secreted by tumor. These are almost always diagnosed with biochemical abnormalities. Nonfunctioning tumors present later, after reaching a larger size and causing symptoms from mass effect or metastasis. Reported sensitivity for CT detection of islet-cell tumors is 71–82%. Very small lesions in neck and body may be missed, and are sometimes confused for adjacent vascular structures. Three-dimensional reconstruction allows multiple views and easier detection of these small lesions, with separation from adjacent vessels.

Hormonally active islet-cell tumors are classified according to the hormones produced and include insulinomas, gastrinomas, glucagonomas, somatostatinomas, and tumors secreting vasoactive intestinal peptide. Insulinomas are the most common of the five islet-cell subtypes and are most commonly benign. This tumor induces marked elevation of serum insulin level, resulting in normal to intractably low glucose levels and symptoms of hypoglycemia. Insulinomas typically present at 2 cm or less in size. The second most common active tumor is gastrinoma, resulting in Zollinger–Ellison syndrome. Individuals with this neoplasm have severe peptic ulcer disease, abdominal pain, diarrhea, esophagitis, and weight loss from elevated levels of gastrin. Approximately 60% of gastrinomas are malignant. Both insulinomas and gastrinomas are associated with multiple endocrine neoplasia (MEN) type 1 syndrome. Remaining subclasses of functioning tumors account for less than 5% of all islet-cell tumors.

The rarity of this entity makes diagnosis and localization methods controversial. Invasive imaging modalities include selective celiac and mesenteric arteriography, venography, and venous sampling. Less invasive imaging tests include gadolinium-enhanced MRI, somatostatin receptor imaging, and endoscopic ultrasound. However, advancements and technologic improvements render dual-phase MDCT the gold standard. Both functioning and nonfunctioning islet-cell tumors are hypervascular. Identification of these tumors requires intravenous bolus injection of contrast with dual-phase imaging to visualize hypervascular enhancing mass. Islet-cell tumors demonstrate significant enhancement, best detected on arterial-phase studies. This tumor blush allows distinction of an islet-cell neoplasm from the more common low-density hypovascular adenocarcinoma. The small size of functioning islet-cell tumors often does not distort the gland at the time of clinical presentation. Metastases from islet-cell tumors to the liver are also hypervascular and best seen on arterial-phase images as hyperattenuating masses in the liver.

Only surgical resection offers a definitive cure for these tumors. When such cancers are malignant, they are often slow-growing and indolent, with a 5-year survival of 49–56%. Other tumors mimicking hypervascular pancreatic lesions are metastases from other organs, including renal cell carcinoma and melanoma.

Cystic pancreatic lesions

Cystic tumors of the pancreas are uncommon, accounting for only 1% of pancreatic tumors and 10% of all cystic lesions of the pancreas; 85% of cystic pancreatic lesions are pseudocysts, with true pancreatic cysts being uncommon.

Pancreatic pseudocysts lack an epithelial lining as opposed to true cystic neoplasms. Pseudocysts typically develop after an episode of pancreatitis, trauma, or alcoholism, resulting in the leakage of pancreatic secretions extravasated from a disrupted duct that form a fluid collection. Radiographic characteristics favoring a pseudocyst rather than a cystic neoplasm include a thin-walled cyst lacking septations, loculations, calcification, or solid enhancing components of tissue. Pseudocysts lack a blood supply and also demonstrate a communication between cyst and pancreatic duct, typically on ERCP.

Cystic pancreatic neoplasms tend to be slow-growing and are often large at diagnosis. Patients often present with a long history of intermittent abdominal/low back pain, nausea and vomiting, and potentially early satiety. Occasionally, a mass can be palpated in the left upper quadrant when the lesion has reached sufficient size.

Cystic tumors can be classified as mucinous cystic neoplasms (macrocystic adenomas/adenocarcinomas), serous cystadenomas (microcystic adenomas), and intraductal papillary mucinous tumors. Cystic tumors harboring malignant potential include mucinous cystic neoplasms, intraductal papillary mucinous tumors, papillary cystic neoplasms, and cystic islet-cell tumors.

Mucinous cystic tumors

Mucinous cystic neoplasms, the most common cystic tumor, are proliferative cysts developing from pancreatic duct epithelium and are potentially malignant. These tumors occur predominantly in middle-aged women during the fifth and sixth decades of life. More than 90% of these lesions develop in the pancreatic tail or body. This entity appears mass-like, typically with few, large (> 2 cm) cysts. Tumors may be well defined with thin-walled cysts; however, more often they are thick-walled with mural papillary projections into cyst cavities. There are areas of septations, septal thickening, calcification, and regions of enhancement on CT/MRI following contrast injection. Cystic spaces may comprise mucin, hemorrhagic fluid, or other debris. Ultrasound shows a multilocular fluid containing mass with good through transmission and acoustic enhancement. Ultrasound has advantages over CT/MRI, more clearly defining the extent of internal septations, mural nodules, and solid components of cyst and cyst wall. CT/MRI demonstrates a fluid-filled mass, often with calcifications. Following injection of contrast there is often enhancement of cyst wall, internal septations, mural nodules, and intracavitary projections. While all imaging modalities display the architecture of the lesion, none can differentiate benign versus malignant masses unless invasion or metastasis has occurred. The 5-year survival is greater than 95% for benign or borderline mucinous cystic neoplasm, with long-term survival rates of 50–75% for fully resected malignant tumors.

Serous cystic tumors

Serous cystadenomas are the second most common cystic tumor and tend to affect females older than 60 years or individuals with von Hippel–Lindau disease. Serous cystadenomas are almost always benign, although differentiation between this and the malignant form requires histopathologic correlation. Benign lesions usually present with vague abdominal pain or a palpable mass often growing to a large size before diagnosis. Serous cystic neoplasms can occur throughout the gland, but are most commonly located in the pancreatic head. Tumors comprise multiple small (1 mm to 2 cm) cysts, but can also appear solid. Of these tumors, 40% contain calcification and 13% demonstrate a central scar. A honeycomb enhancement pattern is common for this hypervascular lesion due to thin fibrous septae interspersed between innumerable tiny cysts. Some tumors may contain larger cysts mimicking mucinous cystic tumors. Although serous lesions have little to no malignant potential, resection is the only way to definitely differentiate this lesion from mucinous malignant tumors.

Intraductal papillary mucinous tumors

Intraductal papillary mucinous tumors (IPMTs), which account for 1–2% of pancreatic exocrine neoplasms and 12% of cystic pancreatic lesions, are slow-growing papillary tumors arising within the main pancreatic duct and/or branches. These tumors secrete thick mucin, leading to ductal dilatation and obstruction with cyst formation, potentially inducing chronic pancreatitis. They most commonly occur in men, with a mean age of 65 years, and are considered a premalignant lesion requiring surgical resection.

Dual-phase contrast-enhanced CT with thin slices demonstrates ductal abnormalities in approximately 97% of cases with IPMT. Diagnosis can be suggested on CT, with main pancreatic duct dilatation greater than 2 mm and obstruction as well as dysmorphic duct calcifications mimicking chronic pancreatitis. Of these tumors, 55–60% develop in head or uncinate process of pancreas. Main pancreatic duct involvement may be diffuse, with parenchymal atrophy, or segmental. Dilated branch pancreatic duct lesions appear as clusters of small cysts with a grape-like appearance or as a single cystic lesion with lobulated margins. Mural nodules, mass lesions, or ductal calcifications may be present, as well as a bulging papilla and communication between cystic lesions and duct. CT also evaluates IPMT extension, lymph nodes, vascular involvement, liver metastasis, or peritoneal dissemination. A patulous ampulla of Vater with extruding mucus is considered diagnostic on ERCP. Other ERCP/MRCP findings include polypoid or amorphous filling defects in addition to duct dilatation.

Overall, the majority of cystic pancreatic neoplasms have a better long-term prognosis than pancreatic adenocarcinoma, especially when diagnosed at an earlier stage. Other uncommon pancreatic tumors include lymphoma and metastases to pancreas, including those from breast, lung, and renal cancer and melanoma.

Postoperative examination

Of patients with pancreatic cancer, 10–15% have potentially resectable disease at the time of diagnosis. In these individuals, a pancreaticoduodenectomy (Whipple procedure) offers a chance for cure and increased longevity. Patients undergoing a Whipple procedure have a greater than 30% 5-year survival rate, whereas those with unresectable disease have a less than 2% survival rate at 3 years.

A Whipple procedure entails a duodenectomy, antrectomy, cholecystectomy, removal of common bile duct, and resection of pancreatic head. The resulting surgical anastomoses consist of a gastrojejunostomy, hepaticojejunostomy, and pancreaticojejunostomy. When possible, depending on the extent of disease, the Whipple procedure may be modified to spare the pylorus, creating a duodenojejunostomy instead of a gastrojejunostomy.

Following a Whipple procedure, spiral CT is the study of choice for evaluating postoperative complications, response to treatment, local recurrence, and metastatic disease. Postoperative appearance following a Whipple procedure is complex, with changes resulting from surgery, radiation, and chemotherapy. These postoperative and posttreatment complications may simulate residual/recurrent disease and make differentiation between a benign and malignant process difficult. Knowledge of the surgery performed, including modifications, date of surgery in relationship to imaging, and administration of radiation and chemotherapy, as well as comparison to old studies, is essential for accurate discrimination between recurrence and normal postoperative findings.

Normal postoperative findings

The typical routine follow-up CT is usually obtained at 3–6 months. The most common findings after a

Whipple procedure is pneumobilia. The hepaticojejunostomy can be identified by following the intrahepatic biliary air to the porta hepatis. Good bowel opacification is necessary to distinguish normal bowel from recurrent tumor. The jejunum is usually positioned to the right side of the remaining pancreas, resulting in a pancreaticojejunostomy. The gastrojejunostomy is typically to the right of the stomach and additional oral contrast should be administered immediately prior to scanning to insure optimal distension and visualization. Lymph nodes in the surgical bed measuring less than 1 cm are commonly reactive and should regress with time.

Soft-tissue stranding at the operative site and around major vessels is a common nonspecific postoperative finding. Similar stranding is present following radiation administration. Typically, these postoperative inflammatory changes should be stable or decrease over a 6-month period, and often resolve by 13 months. Radiation also tends to induce thickening of the gastric antrum and gastrojejunostomy, mesenteric fat stranding in the radiation port, fatty infiltration of the liver, and decreased function of those portions of the kidneys within the radiation port.

Postoperative complications

Patients are only imaged in the immediate postoperative period if there is suspicion for procedural complications. The most common indication for early imaging after surgery is to evaluate for surgical complications. When procedural-related problems are suspected, quick identification and diagnosis is essential as reoperation denotes a poor outcome and is a predictor of decreased long-term survival. Findings most often necessitating reoperation include hemorrhage, abscess, and fascial dehiscence.

Following surgery, 19–23% of patients develop delayed gastric emptying due to gastric outlet obstruction. CT may show a distended stomach with narrowing of the gastric outlet; however, upper gastrointestinal swallowing studies more accurately define the region of narrowing and obstruction.

After a Whipple procedure, 17% of patients develop pancreatic fistulas, especially when surgery is for excision of a periampullary mass. Diagnosis is predominantly clinical, with greater than 50 mL of amylase-laden fluid in surgical bed drainage on or after the tenth postoperative day. Treatment does not necessarily require surgery and CT is reserved for identifying loculated fluid collections.

Other postoperative complications include wound infection and dehiscence, abdominal abscess, and breakdown of surgical anastomosis causing peritonitis and pancreatitis. Vascular complications are uncommon but may include hepatic artery injury, portal vein thrombosis, and splenic infarction.

Recurrent and metastatic disease

After a Whipple procedure, follow-up imaging with CT is essential to detect recurrence. Several normal postoperative and postradiation findings may mimic recurrent disease. Distinction with imaging methods depends on stability or regression of findings over time. Though unusual, indeterminate cases can be biopsied. More commonly, follow-up imaging is performed to assess stability of findings. Individuals whose findings progress are highly suspicious. Additional clues to detection of persistent disease include a history of positive margins at time of surgery, an elevated CA-19-9, or an increase in size or new soft-tissue mass.

Pancreatic cancer may recur within the surgical bed (53%), especially in patients with known residual tumor or metastases to distant sites. Liver metastases are low-density lesions with minimal or delayed enhancement. Regional lymph nodes measuring less than 1 cm commonly appear immediately in the postoperative period but should decrease in size and number over time when free of tumor. Metastatic lung and peritoneal carcinomatosis occurs commonly, appearing as soft-tissue masses. Soft tissue encasing peripancreatic vessels may be due to tumor or postinflammatory/postoperative changes. Typical patterns of recurrence include tumor around the the superior mesenteric artery and superior mesenteric vein.

Radiation treatment is routine following a successful Whipple procedure. Not only does radiation induce difficulty in interpretation of postoperative examinations, mimicking tumor, but also potentially induces other complications, including thickening of stomach and small bowel within the therapy field. Inflammatory changes of peripancreatic tissues and within treatment bed consist of increased soft-tissue density and induration. Knowledge of these processes helps accurate determination of recurrence versus successful treatment.

Conclusion

Evaluation of pancreatic cancer, resectability, and postoperative course is a complex process requiring accurate knowledge of disease, appearance, and behavior in addition to proper radiographic examination technique. While many modalities may play a contributory role in evaluation of pancreatic cancer, CT remains the gold standard for a comprehensive detailed examination. Significant advances in CT technology, including MDCT, CTA, and three-dimensional techniques, optimizes pancreatic imaging, allowing more accurate detection and staging of pancreatic cancer.

Recommended reading

Balci NC, Semelkab RC. Radiologic diagnosis and staging of pancreatic ductal adenocarcinoma. *Eur J Radiol* 2001;38: 105–112.

Cieszanowski A, Chomicka D, Andrzejewska MG. Imaging techniques in patients with biliary obstruction. *Med Sci Monit* 2000;6:1197–1202.

Curry CA, Eng J, Horton KM. CT of primary cystic pancreatic neoplasms: can CT be used for patient triage and treatment? *Am J Roentgenol* 2000;175:99–103.

De Lima JE Jr, Javitt MC, Mathur SC. Mucinous cystic neoplasm of the pancreas. *Radiographics* 1999;19:807–811.

Fernandez-del Castillo C, Warshaw AL. Cystic tumors of the pancreas. *Surg Clin North Am* 1995;75:1001–1016.

Horton KM, Fishman EK. Multidetector CT angiography of pancreatic carcinoma. Part 1: evaluation of arterial involvement. *Am J Roentgenol* 2002;178:827–831.

Horton KM, Fishman EK. Multidetector CT angiography of pancreatic carcinoma. Part 2: evaluation of venous involvement. *Am J Roentgenol* 2002;178:833–836.

Ichikawa T, Peterson MS, Federle MP *et al.* Islet cell tumor of the pancreas: biphasic CT versus MR imaging in tumor detection. *Radiology* 2000;216:163–171.

Johnson PT, Heath DG, Hofmann LV *et al.* Multidetector-row computed tomography with three-dimensional volume rendering of pancreatic cancer: a complete preoperative staging tool using computed tomography angiography and volume-rendered cholangiopancreatography. *J Comput Assist Tomogr* 2003;27:347–353.

Kato T, Fukatsu H, Kengo I *et al.* Fluorodeoxyglucose positron emission tomography in pancreatic cancer: an unsolved problem. *Eur J Nucl Med* 1995;22:32–39.

Kuszyk BS, Blueratee DA, Urban BA *et al.* Portal-phase contrast-enhanced helical CT for the detection of malignant hepatic tumors: sensitivity based on comparison with intraoperative and pathogenic findings. *Am J Roentgenol* 1996; 166:91–95.

Lu DS, Reber HA, Krasny RM *et al.* Local staging of pancreatic cancer: criteria for unresectability of major vessels as revealed by pancreatic-phase, thin section helical CT. *Am J Roentgenol* 1997;168:1439–1443.

Nakayama Y, Yamashita Y, Kadota M *et al.* Vascular encasement by pancreatic cancer: correlation of CT findings with surgical and pathologic results. *J Comput Assist Tomogr* 2001;25:337–342.

Nino-Murcia M, Jeffrey RB Jr. Multidetector-row CT and volumetric imaging of pancreatic neoplasms. *Gastroenterol Clin* 2002;31(3).

Phan GQ, Yeo CJ, Hruban RH *et al.* Surgical experience with pancreatic and peripancreatic neuroendocrine tumors: review of 125 patients. *J Gastrointest Surg* 1998;2:472–482.

Prassopoulos P, Raptopoulos V, Chuttani R *et al.* Development of virtual CT cholangiopancreatoscopy. *Radiology* 1998;209:570–574.

Raptopoulos V, Steer ML, Sheiman RG *et al.* Use of helical CT and CT angiography to predict vascular involvement from pancreatic cancer: correlation with findings at surgery. *Am J Roentgenol* 1997;168:971–977.

Sachs JR, Deren JJ, Sohn M *et al.* Mucinous cystadenoma: pitfalls of differential diagnosis. *Am J Gastroenterol* 1989;84: 811–816.

Scatarige JC, Urban BA, Horton KM. Visual survey of cancer dissemination: classic patterns on helical CT. Abdomen and pelvis. 2001;25:••–••.

Scatarige JC, Horton KM, Sheth SS *et al.* Pancreatic parenchymal metastases: observations on helical CT. *Am J Roentgenol* 2001;176:695–699.

Sheth SS, Hruban RK, Fishman EK. Helical CT of islet cell tumors of the pancreas: typical and atypical manifestations. *Am J Roentgenol* 2002;179:725–730.

Taouli B, Vilgrain V, O'Toole D *et al.* Intraductal papillary mucinous tumors of the pancreas: features with multimodality imaging. *J Comput Assist Tomogr* 2002;26:223–231.

Thompson GB, van Heerden JA, Grant CS *et al.* Islet cell carcinomas of the pancreas: a twenty-year experience. *Surgery* 1988;104:1011–1017.

Tsuneo I, Kunihiro M, Hiroshi F *et al.* Radiologic diagnosis of pancreatic carcinoma. *Semin Surg Oncol* 1998;15:23–32.

Valls C, Andía E, Sanchez A. Dual-phase helical CT of pancreatic adenocarcinoma: assessment of resectability before surgery. *Am J Roentgenol* 2002;178:821–826.

Zeman RK, Cooper C, Zeiberg AS *et al.* TNM staging of pancreatic carcinoma using helical CT. *Am J Roentgenol* 1997;169:459–464.

48 The role of endoscopic ultrasound in the diagnosis and assessment of the resectability of pancreatic cancer

Marc Giovannini

Introduction

Endoscopic ultrasound (EUS) of the digestive tract is a relatively recent technique: the first publications date from the early 1980s. The history of EUS can be divided into two parts, the first in the 1980s and 1990s, when EUS was essentially descriptive. During this period, EUS allowed better definition of the degree of locoregional extension of cancers of the esophagus, stomach, pancreas, and rectum. It also enabled the diagnosis of common bile duct stones to be made in a less invasive manner than by endoscopic retrograde cholangiopancreatography (ERCP). However, it rapidly became apparent that the specificity of EUS images was low (around 50–60%), particularly for the diagnosis of neoplastic ganglions and pancreatic masses. The appearance in 1991 of sector-based linear probes enabled EUS-guided biopsies to be made of these lesions. This increased the specificity of EUS significantly, particularly for the diagnosis of cancerous lesions (now about 95%).

EUS and staging of pancreatic cancer

The role of EUS in malignant pathology of the pancreas is twofold.
1 EUS is the best technique for the diagnosis of small tumors (< 3 cm in diameter). Its sensitivity is greater than that of tomodensitometric (TDM) examination, percutaneous ultrasound, or magnetic resonance imaging (MRI) and equal to that of ERCP without sharing its invasive character. Nevertheless, the specificity of EUS for differentiating a nodule of chronic pancreatitis from an adenocarcinoma remains poor.

2 EUS is also indicated in the assessment of locoregional extension of tumors judged resectionable on the basis of TDM examination. The performance of EUS seems superior to that of other imaging techniques for the diagnosis of vascular and lymph-node involvement, although recent studies report less favorable results than do studies dating from 1992 to 1994.

This chapter examines the results of ultrasonic endoscopy in the assessment of resectability of pancreatic adenocarcinoma and compares these results with those of conventional examinations, i.e., percutaneous ultrasound, TDM (scanner), MRI, and angiography.

Classification by EUS of cancers of the pancreas

An EUS examination to assess the locoregional extension of a pancreatic tumor aims to answer five questions.
1 Is there venous involvement (portal vein, superior mesenteric vein, splenic vein)?
2 Is there arterial involvement (superior mesenteric artery, celiac artery)?
3 Is there lymph-node involvement?
4 Are there signs of peritoneal carcinomatosis (surge of ascites)?
5 Are there secondary lesions on the left lobe of the liver?

The responses to these five questions enable the tumor to be classified as follows.
T1 Tumor limited to the pancreatic gland without vascular involvement.
T2 Tumor exceeding the limits of the pancreatic gland without vascular involvement.
T3 Invasive tumor with an arterial or venous vascular structure.

N0 No lymph-node involvement.

N1 Presence of lymph nodes that appear to be malignant.

M0 No distant lymph node or visceral metastasis or sign of peritoneal carcinomatosis.

M1 Distant lymph node: celiac node for tumor of the head, interaorticocaval lymph node, mediastinal lymph node.

Tumors classed as T3N0 or T3N1 must be considered nonresectable, although it is accepted that the criteria of nonresectability are very variable from one surgical team to another. This is because some teams carry out resections/reconstruction of the portal vein if it is affected, although no increased survival has been reported with this type of surgical technique.

Role of EUS in the diagnosis of pancreatic adenocarcinoma

EUS is the most appropriate exploration for the diagnosis of small tumors (< 3 cm in diameter) of the pancreas (Fig. 48.1). Its sensitivity is greater than computed tomography (CT), percutaneous ultrasound, and MRI and similar to ERCP without the invasive component. Nevertheless, the specificity of EUS for distinguishing between a chronic pancreatitis nodule and adenocarcinoma remains poor (60–75%). The major problem is the diagnosis of an adenocarcinoma that develops on chronic pancreatitis because it is very difficult to recognize with certainty the malignant character of a hypo-echoic area within chronic pancreatitis tissue. Positive diagnosis requires a biopsy specimen.

For the diagnosis of pancreatic tumors, two studies have demonstrated that EUS is superior to helical CT for small tumors measuring less than 25 mm. The first study, reported by Midwinter *et al.*, compared 58 patients who underwent helical CT and EUS. This study showed that EUS is more precise for the diagnosis and location of small-sized pancreatic tumors less than 25 mm in diameter, and that EUS provides comparable results for diagnosis of invasion of the superior mesenteric or portal veins. The second study, by Bender *et al.*, used linear EUS in 65 patients with suspected pancreatic lesions on helical CT. EUS confirmed the pancreatic lesion in 33 patients and found a normal pancreas in the other 32. When compared with the surgical findings, the specificity of EUS for the diagnosis of pancreatic cancer was significantly higher than that of helical CT (88% vs. 41%; $P < 0.005$). Finally, another study by Mertz *et al.* compared positron emission tomography (PET) for the assessment of locoregional extension of pancreatic carcinoma. Sensitivity for diagnosis of pancreatic cancer was 93% for EUS, 87% for PET, and only 53% for helical CT. EUS was more sensitive than helical CT for the diagnosis of portal invasion. Finally, PET diagnosed four metastatic localizations unrecognized with CT. These authors concluded that the EUS and PET combination was superior for the diagnosis and assessment of extension of cancer of the pancreas.

Summarizing, EUS is the best exploration for the diagnosis of small-sized pancreatic tumors; however, it is still a secondary examination after helical CT. The specificity of EUS for the diagnosis of pancreatic tumors is better than other explorations, a specificity that is further improved with the addition of guided biopsy.

Results of EUS compared with other imaging methods in the assesment of locoregional extension of cancers of the pancreas

Evaluation of T and N by EUS: data from the literature

Data in the literature show that the reliability of EUS for locoregional staging of pancreatic cancer is 80–85% for tumoral staging and 72–75% for lymph-node staging (Table 48.1). These results were reported by Rösch *et al.* in 1995 in a series of 250 patients. In all these studies, the EUS data have been compared with

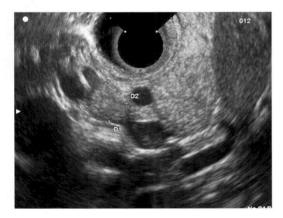

Figure 48.1 Small pancreatic adenocarcinoma of 11 mm in diameter in the body of the pancreas.

Table 48.1 Evaluation of T and N staging by endoscopic ultrasound (EUS).

| Study | No. of patients | Reliability of EUS | |
		T staging	N staging
Grimm *et al.* (1990)	26	85%	72%
Tio *et al.* (1990)	36	92%	72%
Kallimanis (1991)	32	78%	66%
Rosch (1992)	35	94%	80%
Palazzo *et al.* (1993)	38	—	74%
Wiersema (1994)	39	76%	82%
Yasuda *et al.* (1993)	29	—	66%
Giovannini (1994)	25	—	92%
Müller *et al.* (1994)	22	82%	64%
Akahoshi *et al.* (1995)	25	64%	48%
Rosch (1995)	35	69%	60%
Total		250 (80%)	327 (72%)

Table 48.2 Reliability of endoscopic ultrasound (EUS) in relation to the stage of the pancreatic lesion.

Stage	No. of patients	Correct EUS staging (%)
T1	24	80
T2	67	81
T3	75	85
N0	79	76
N1	142	81

Table 48.3 Evaluation of local extension of cancer of the pancreas with endoscopic ultrasound (EUS).

Staging	No. of patients	EUS (%)	Ultrasound (%)	TDM (%)
T staging	82	82	35	44
N staging	143	68	42	48

TDM, tomodensitometric examination.

the results of surgical exploration. Generally speaking, EUS will correctly classify a tumor of the pancreas in 80% of cases as regards the lesion itself and will correctly evaluate ganglionic involvement in 72% of cases. Moreover, the reliability of EUS does not vary according to the stage of the pancreatic lesion (Table 48.2). Finally, EUS seems to be the best examination for evaluating local extension of a cancer of the pancreas (Table 48.3).

Evaluation of vascular involvement

Invasion of the portal system (Fig. 48.2) Early studies showed an 85% reliability (Table 48.4). More recently, in 1999 Rösch reported that the reliability was close to 70–75%. The problem is the interpretation of the loss of the interface between the tumor and the wall of the portal vein: it is very difficult to determine whether the loss of this interface results from tumor invasion or is simply an inflammatory reaction.

Arterial invasion There are few studies in the literature evaluating the performance of EUS in the evaluation of arterial involvement. Only three studies have reported the results of EUS in overall figures ("vascular involvement") (Table 48.5). It would be difficult to assess the superior mesenteric artery with mechanical rotating probes. In their study of the superior mesenteric region,

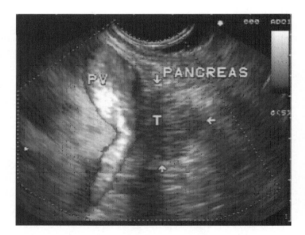

Figure 48.2 Color Doppler imaging of portal vein involvement by an adenocarcinoma of the head of the pancreas.

Rösch *et al.* were only able to visualize this area in 75% of cases. It is easier to assess this region with linear electronic probes.

Nodal invasion The last problem is that of nodal extension, particularly in cases with obstructive jaundice,

Table 48.4 Evaluation of invasion of the portal system by cancer of the pancreas with endoscopic ultrasound (EUS).

Study	No. of patients	EUS (%)	Ultrasound (%)	TDM (%)	Angiography	MRI (%)
Sugiyama (1992)	5	100	60	20	100	—
Yasuda *et al.* (1993)	37	81	—	—	—	—
Amouyal (1993)	5	80	40	80	—	—
Snady *et al.* (2000)	30	97	—	53	80	—
Rosch (1992)	40	95	55	73	85	—
Palazzo *et al.* (1993)	38	87	47	75	—	—
Giovannini (1994)	25	88	19	76	—	—
Müller *et al.* (1994)	16	88	—	88	—	63
Rosch (1995)	35	66	—	—	—	—
Akahoshi *et al.* (1995)	25	79	68	61	81	—
Total	256	85	49	69	83	63

MRI, magnetic resonance imaging; TDM, tomodensitometric examination.

Table 48.5 Evaluation of invasion of the arterial system by cancer of the pancreas with endoscopic ultrasound (EUS).

Study	No. of patients	EUS (%)	Ultrasound (%)	TDM (%)	Angiography (%)
Kobayashi *et al.* (1993)	30	73	—	—	—
Wiersema (1993)	18	80	—	—	—
Yasuda *et al.* (1993)	29	79	55	41	72

TDM, tomodensitometric examination.

where inflammatory nodes of the hepatic pedicle are frequently encountered. The problem is even more difficult when EUS is performed after insertion of a biliary stent. Of course, in the case of distant lymph nodes, as mediastinal or aorticocaval lymph nodes, an EUS-guided biopsy is mandatory to differentiate inflammatory from malignant nodes.

The development of helical CT has modified the data reported in the literature up to 1995. Legmann *et al.* compared EUS and helical CT in the assessment of resectability in 30 patients. The authors found no difference between the two methods in diagnostic sensitivity (100% vs. 92%), positive resectability (93% vs. 93%), and negative resectability (86% vs. 100%). EUS could be more informative in the diagnosis of distal nodal invasion, particularly celiac nodes for tumors of the head of the pancreas and lumboaortic nodes. Obviously, only guided biopsy can confirm tumor invasion of a lymph node.

Finally, EUS can reveal signs of peritoneal carcinomatosis, such as minimal ascites effusion around the stomach or duodenum. This sign is pathognomonic for peritoneal carcinomatosis, with a sensitivity around 85% in the absence of portal vein thrombosis. EUS also provides precise assessment of the left liver and in certain cases can show small metastasis less than 1 cm that may go unnoticed on CT.

Role of biopsy guided by EUS in solid tumors of the pancreas

The development of EUS allows a more accurate picture of the spread of pancreatic tumors. Nevertheless, EUS is not able to confirm the malignant or benign character of such pancreatic masses. The development of the linear sector-based EUS technique over the last 8 years has enabled us to perform guided biopsies of these lesions.

Equipment

Ultrasound endoscope

It is possible to perform a biopsy guided by EUS with both types of equipment (radial or linear, sector-based), although biopsy using the radial system is longer and technically more difficult and more dangerous, as it is impossible to completely follow the biopsy needle as it emerges from the operator channel and to guide it into the lesion.

Linear sector-based EUS equipment comprises a small-diameter convex electronic probe fitted onto a standard endoscope. This is a fiberoptic device with a 60° field of vision fitted with an operating channel of 2, 2.4, 2.8, 3.2, 3.7, and 3.8 mm diameter depending on the particular instrument, along which can be passed biopsy forceps, a biopsy needle, or accessories for therapeutic procedures. It is possible to carry out guided biopsies with this type of sector-based probe. This is done by following the biopsy needle at the exit of the operator channel and guiding it into the lesion. This is possible because the ultrasound beam is emitted longitudinally in the same axis as that of the endoscope and not perpendicularly as in radial ultrasound endoscopes.

There are now two series of linear electronic ultrasound endoscopes that can perform guided biopsy.

Pentax-Hitachi Several devices are available: the FG 34-X (2 mm working channel) (Fig. 48.3) and the FG 38-X (3.2 mm operating channel) are both equipped with the same ultrasound probe. The FG 36-X (2.4 mm working channel) and the EG 38UT (3.8 mm working channel) (Fig. 48.4) are also equipped with an elevator, which is very convenient for difficult EUS-guided biopsy (as in the uncinate process of the pancreas) or for therapeutic procedures (as in pancreatic pseudocyst drainage). This probe is sector-based and operates at three frequencies (5, 7.5, and 10 MHz) connected with the 6500 Hitachi-US machine. It is also possible to use a Doppler color or an angio-Doppler imager with this type of probe.

Olympus Olympus has developed two linear electronic ultrasound endoscopes: the GF UC30P (2.7 mm working channel) and the GF UCT30 (3.7 mm working channel); the latter is an interventional device and has an elevator. Both are fitted with a 7.5 and 12.5 MHz frequency probe and a Doppler color imager, although the

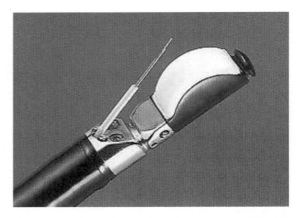

Figure 48.3 FG 34-X linear echoendoscope (Pentax-Hitachi Corporation) with a 22-gauge needle.

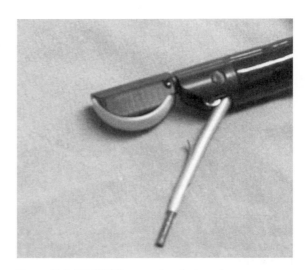

Figure 48.4 EG 38UT interventional echoendoscope (Pentax-Hitachi Corporation) with a large working channel (3.8 mm).

absence of low frequencies inhibits the penetration of the ultrasound and may render biopsies more difficult, particularly for deep-seated lesions such as some small lymph nodes.

Needle

Several types of needle of different length and caliber have been used: 25 gauge (5 cm), 22 gauge (5 cm), 22 gauge echo-tip (6 cm) (adjustable). The common problem of all these prototypes was the risk of perforation of the operating channel.

Two types of needle are now commercially available that no longer carry this risk: the Vilkmann-Hancke needle manufactured by Mediglobe Company (Gassau, Germany) and the Wilson-Cook needle. Both these needles have a Teflon-coated shaft partly made of metal. Their particular feature is a manual control screwed onto the endoscope, which has a brake preventing any manipulation of the needle when it is being inserted into the operating channel. They take 22-gauge needles of 8–12 cm in length. The advantage of the Wilson-Cook needle is that it is entirely disposable, whereas the metal-reinforced shaft and needle control of the GIP are reusable. However, after it has been used several times, the metal-reinforced channel has a tendency to get longer (the metallic spirals stretch) and cause the needle to penetrate when performing a biopsy across the wall of the digestive tract, which could lead to the needle becoming stuck in the lesion. Recently, Mediglobe have manufactured new disposable 19- and 22-gauge needles. The Wilson-Cook company offers many different type of EUS needle as different sizes (19, 22, and 25 gauge) and with different sheaths (metallic or Teflon); more recently, it has introduced a histologic needle (Quick-Core needle) that is still under evaluation.

Technique

Biopsies are performed at the end of the EUS examination, with patients lying on their left side. Neuroleptanesthesia is generally necessary. The biopsy technique is quite simple, and is performed in the following sequence.
- The lesion is positioned on the needle's exit path.
- The stylet is withdrawn and the needle is inserted into the tumor (Fig. 48.5). The operator can visualize the tip of the needle by ultrasound, enabling its correct position in the lesion to be verified.
- Aspiration is performed with the aid of a 20-mL syringe as the needle makes to-and-fro movements within the tumor. One to three passages are usually necessary in order to obtain a microbiopsy.
It is currently possible to obtain microfragments of tissue (Fig. 48.4) in about 90% of cases with the Vilkmann-Hancke type of needle, which is 22 gauge and 12 cm long. Microbiopsies are obtained in the fol-

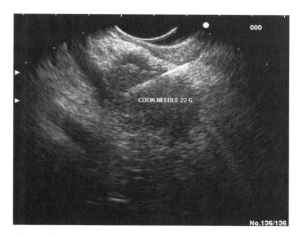

Figure 48.5 Endoscopic ultrasound-guided fine-needle aspiration of a pancreatic lesion.

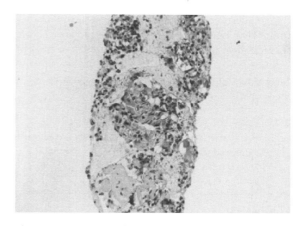

Figure 48.6 Specimen obtained from an adenocarcinoma of the pancreas using a 22-gauge needle.

lowing manner: (i) all of the sample contained within the needle is withdrawn using a foam stylet introduced into the needle (Fig. 48.6); (ii) the sample is then placed in formaldehyde or Cytolit and then completely enclosed in paraffin wax.

In contrast to American teams, we do not systematically administer an antibiotic after taking a sample. At the end of the examination, it is necessary to monitor patients for at least 3 hours. Biopsies guided by EUS can be done on an outpatient basis in the majority of cases. The main limits of the technique are size of lesion below 5 mm, depth of the lesion more than 6–7 cm compared with the probe, and a blood clotting problem (prothrombin time $< 60\%$, platelets $< 80\,000/mm^3$).

Indications and results

Data from the literature

Our experience is based on around 1500 samples. Samples have been taken from lymph nodes and mediastinal, celiac, and pelvic masses, from submucosal membrane tumors, from gastric linitis tumors with negative endoscopic biopsies, and from pancreatic tumors. The best results are obtained from lymph nodes, anastomotic recurrence of tumors, and extrinsic compressions, in addition to pancreatic tumors. In the latter, the efficacy of EUS-guided biopsy is best for lesions of small diameter (< 4 cm). This is because the larger cancers are the site of necrosis and/or of intratumoral fibrosis, both of which prevent good samples from being obtained.

If a "microbiopsy" is obtained, it enables a more accurate histologic diagnosis to be made and an accurate characterization of the tissue in about 80% of cases of diagnosis of malignancy. Furthermore, certain teams recommend the presence of an anatomic pathologist in the theater in order to ensure the high quality of the sample. No mention was found in the literature concerning the risk of spreading the cancer with this sampling technique.

The results quoted in the literature show that the overall sensitivity of the technique is 76–91%, the specificity 84–100%, and the reliability 78–94%. A prospective study investigating 457 patients from four centers (Indianapolis, Copenhagen, Marseilles, and Orange in California) has been published (Table 48.6). In the course of this study, the sensitivity of the biopsy was statistically better for lymph nodes (94%) and extraluminal tumors (86%) than for parietal lesions, i.e., submucosal tumors and large gastric folds (61%) ($P < 0.001$). On the other hand, there was no difference in the specificity for these three groups of lesions. Another multicenter study carried out by the same centers concerned EUS-guided biopsies of pancreatic tumors. This study involved 164 patients (Table 48.7); the average diameter of the lesions varied between 28.5

Table 48.6 Multicenter study involving 457 patients and 554 lesions from which biopsies were taken using sector-based endoscopic ultrasound.

Lesion	Sensitivity (%)	Specificity (%)	NPV (%)	Reliability (%)
Lymph nodes	94	95	82	94*
Pancreatic mass	86	95	67	88
Digestive tract wall	61	76	46	67*

NPV, negative predictive value.
* $P = 0.001$.

Table 48.7 Multicenter collaborative study of pancreatic tumors using endoscopic ultrasound-guided biopsy. Results from 164 patients.

	Center 1	Center 2	Center 3	Center 4
No. of lesions of the pancreas	37	44	43	40
Average diameter of tumor (mm)	41	33	32	28
Lesions visible to TDM (%)	61	52	70	48
Sensitivity (%)	62	78	94	91
Specificity (%)	78	100	100	92
Reliability (%)	67	82	95	92
Negative predictive value (%)	54	79	100	92
Cytologist present	No	No	Yes	Yes

TDM, tomodensitometric examination.

and 41.3 mm. The sensitivity, specificity, positive predictive value, and negative predictive value for the diagnosis of cancer of the pancreas were, respectively, 83%, 90%, 100%, and 80%; the diagnostic reliability was 85%.

Impact of EUS-guided biopsies on the process of diagnosis and/or therapy of a solid tumor of the pancreas

The most important question is whether performing an EUS-guided biopsy is able to modify the process of diagnosis and/or therapy. Concerning diagnosis, it seems to be accepted that EUS-guided biopsy is the least aggressive technique (five minor complications in 457 samples, three of which were directly attributable to the biopsy, i.e., two episodes of fever that responded to antibiotics and one hemorrhage during the biopsy of a pancreatic cyst). The biopsies had been done to characterize the tissue. Moreover, EUS-guided biopsies seem indispensable for pancreatic tumors, particularly those only visible to EUS. This is because the transgastric or transduodenal route of entry diminishes the risk of spread and because for tumors of the head of the pancreas the biopsy path will be operated at the time of cephalic duodenopancreactectomy.

Regarding solid pancreatic masses, what is the impact of EUS on the chosen treatment? It is probably less than that which is reported in the literature. This has to do with the low specificity of EUS images, and it is only due to guided biopsy that EUS will have a considerable impact on the treatment decision. We have carried out a prospective study on the impact of EUS-guided biopsy on patients suffering from a pancreatic mass and formed the following conclusions. EUS-guided biopsy of a solid pancreatic mass was performed on 174 patients (90 male, 84 female) of average age 66 years: 20 lesions were sited in the uncinate process, 43 in the head region, 31 in the isthmus area, 41 in the body, and 39 in the tail of the pancreas. The average diameter of the tumors was 29 mm (range 8–40 mm) and 39 patients presented with a lesion of less than 20 mm in diameter. In each lesion where biopsy was performed, one sample was taken for cytologic study and one sample for microhistologic study. The patients' dossiers were discussed by a medical team comprising gastroenterologists, surgeons, oncologists, radiologists, and specialists in radiotherapy in order to decide how the results of EUS-guided biopsy might affect the choice of treatment.

The sensitivity, specificity, and reliability of EUS-guided biopsy for the diagnosis of malignancy were, respectively, 87.2%, 100%, and 87.9%. In 143 cases, EUS-guided biopsy revealed a malignant tumor (107 adenocarcinomas, 28 neuroendocrine tumors, 7 pancreatic metastases, and 1 primitive lymphoma of the pancreas). In seven cases it revealed objects whose appearance was compatible with chronic pancreatitis and on three occasions it showed an abscess following acute pancreatitis. In 21 cases, EUS-guided biopsy did not contribute to diagnosis: 19 of these were adenocarcinomas, one a somatostatinoma, and one a pancreatic sarcoma. Of the seven investigations suggesting a chronic pancreatitis nodule, five were confirmed by surgery and two by the course of the disease (absence of change followed by regression at 24 or 36 months). The diagnosis of pancreatic abscess was confirmed by the aspiration of pus and the disappearance of the image 3 months later on a follow-up EUS. The results of EUS-guided biopsy modified or influenced treatment of the 28 neuroendocrine tumors, the seven pancreatic metastases, the three abscesses, two of seven chronic pancreatitis nodules, and 70 of 107 adenocarcinomas that were not visible on TDM examination (total 110/174, 63.2%). EUS-guided biopsy is the best technique for obtaining the histology of a pancreatic mass, with a sensitivity of 85–87%. Furthermore, it also has a considerable impact on deciding what treatment to follow, particularly in cases of adenocarcinoma not visible on TDM examination. This is particularly important because trials are being developed of preoperative radiochemotherapy for resectionable lesions.

More recently, we have published our results on 1544 patients who had EUS-guided fine-needle aspiration (FNA). The result of the biopsy was confirmed either by surgical investigation or celioscopy or by the evolution and follow-up of the patients. Complications occurred in 15 patients (0.97%), comprising nine with feverish episodes, five with acute pancreatitis, and one with bleeding. It should be noted that only one of those with pancreatitis required hospitalization of more than a week and was complicated by a pseudocyst. All the feverish episodes responded to antibiotherapy (combination of amoxicillin, clavulanic acid, and ciprofloxacin). Finally, the case of bleeding consisted of hemorrhage of the Wirsung duct after EUS-guided FNA of a pancreatic tumor; this stopped spontaneously, and had no hemodynamic consequences and did not require transfusion.

With regard to the diagnosis of malignancy, sensitivity, specificity, positive predictive value, negative predictive value, and accuracy of EUS-guided FNA were, respectively, 84.6%, 98.4%, 99.6%, 54.7%, and 86.9% for the 1544 patients. In those patients with pancreatic solid tumors ($n = 534$), cystic lesions being excluded from this study, EUS-guided FNA diagnosed adenocarcinoma in 331 cases, endocrine tumor in 76, pancreatic metastasis in 28, chronic pancreatitis nodule in 25, pancreatic abscess in 17, pancreatic sarcoma in 4, primitive pancreatic lymphoma in 5, and squamous cell carcinoma of the pancreas in 3; in 45 cases, EUS-guided FNA was not contributory. With regard to the diagnosis of these pancreatic solid tumors, the sensitivity, specificity, and accuracy of EUS-guided FNA were, respectively, 89.8%, 98.8%, and 90.1%. The 45 patients whose biopsy was not contributory were operated and the pathologic resected specimen showed adenocarcinoma in 28 cases, endocrine tumor in 3, pancreatic sarcoma in 1, and chronic pancreatitis nodule in 13.

EUS-guided FNA also modified the treatment of 242 pancreatic tumors, comprising 91 adenocarcinomas not diagnosed on CT or MRI and 151 other masses that were not adenocarcinomas (76 endocrine tumors, 28 metastases, 25 chronic pancreatitis, 17 abscess, 4 sarcomas, 5 lymphomas, and 3 squamous cell carcinomas). Overall, EUS-guided FNA modified diagnosis and therapeutic decisions in 1081 of 1544 cases (70.1%).

With regard to solid pancreatic masses, the impact of EUS on therapeutic decision-making is now well known. Nevertheless, in our series, we show that EUS is especially important because in 268 of the 534 patients presenting with a pancreatic mass it revealed histology other than adenocarcinoma (endocrine tumor, pancreatic metastasis). In particular, it allowed confirmation of the diagnosis of pancreatic cancer in 91 patients whose tumor had not been diagnosed with conventional techniques (CT, MRI).

Summary

Once the linear sector-based EUS technique has been learned, EUS-guided FNA is a simple procedure. It is currently possible to obtain material by biopsy in about 80–85% of cases, enabling the tissue to be characterized. The development of therapeutic protocols for preoperative radiochemotherapy for resectable pancreatic adenocarcinomas requires a pretreatment pancreatic biopsy to be taken. EUS with an electronic linear probe enables accurate assessment of the degree of spread to be made at the same time, together with a guided biopsy of the lesion. The technique has a sensitivity of approximately 85% and does not carry the risk of peritoneal spread described with the percutaneous route. Moreover, this biopsy enables lesions only visible to EUS to be characterized and can be used for tumors other than adenocarcinomas.

Celiac neurolysis guided by EUS

Alcohol injection of the celiac area is an effective technique for the treatment of pain due to splanchnic nerve infiltration. Until now, it was performed under X-ray or CT control. These percutaneous routes were burdened by important adverse effects (spleen injury or paraplegia due to alcohol injection at the level of Adamkiewicz's artery). EUS-guided celiac neurolysis is a simple technique and in future it will replace the percutaneous procedure under ultrasound or CT guidance.

Technique

It is advisable to first find the celiac region. The endoscope must be positioned on the small gastric curvature, between 40 and 45 cm from the dental arches. A rotation of about 90° is performed in order to show the abdominal aorta, the celiac trunk, and the superior mesenteric artery. Two ganglions are situated on both sides of the celiac trunk. The one on the right is localized 6 mm below the origin of the celiac trunk and the one on the left 9 mm below this same origin.

The needles used to perform the alcohol injection can be the same as those used for EUS-guided biopsy or can be dedicated celiac neurolysis needles (with lateral holes for right and left ganglion injection) manufactured by the Wilson-Cook company.

Two techniques have been described.
1 Once the celiac trunk has been identified, the endoscope is rotated toward the right-hand side by about 10–20° and the needle is positioned. Under EUS control, 5 mL of lidocaine (lignocaine) and then 10 mL of

pure alcohol are injected. The procedure is repeated after a rotation to the left of 10–20°. However, this technique is demanding: it is often difficult to inject the two areas of the celiac trunk correctly because the alcohol injection creates hyperechoic drops that obscure the perigastric structures.

2 It is much easier to position the needle at the origin of the celiac trunk on the aorta and to inject locally 10 mL of 1% lidocaine and then 15–20 mL of pure alcohol. The alcohol injected around the celiac trunk diffuses to the celiac nerves.

The two major indications for this technique are (i) celiac pain due to pancreatic cancers and metastastic celiac lymph nodes and (ii) chronic pancreatitis. The literature shows a significant reduction in pain in 85–90% of cases, superior to the results of percutaneous techniques. In addition, this technique is simpler, faster, and less dangerous than percutaneous techniques under CT guidance.

Results

Wiersema *et al.* have reported their experience on 45 patients with pancreatic cancer or malignant celiac nodes. After injection of 20 mL of pure alcohol, 52% of the patients did not need to increase their dose of morphine and 30% were able to significantly decrease their doses of oral morphine. Gress *et al.* published a randomized study on patients with chronic pancreatitis with incapacitating epigastric pain. The authors compared EUS-guided versus CT-guided celiac alcohol injection. The criterion of judgment was a significant decrease of pain estimated on an analog scale. In the group of patients treated under EUS guidance, 43% showed a significant reduction of pain as against only 25% in the group treated under CT control ($P = 0.008$).

Complications

Two types of complication have been described: increase in pain, and diarrhea 24–48 hours after the procedure. Two cases of retroperitoneal abscess were reported after the injection of corticosteroid instead of alcohol and bleeding due to a pseudoaneurysm created after the corticosteroid injection. It is advisable to use pure alcohol and to avoid the use of corticosteroids.

Future developments in pancreatic EUS

Recently, a new ultrasound scanner has been introduced that is capable of performing three-dimensional reconstruction. Reconstruction is very quick (< 30 s) and the images are recorded in an on-board computer (Fig. 48.7). There is very little information on the use of this technique for pancreatic cancer but our experience seems to show better definition of small tumors and better vascular staging (Fig. 48.8).

Another interesting development is the use of ultrasound contrast agents such as Levovist or Sonovue for the differentiation of chronic pancreatitis nodule and pancreatic carcinoma. The first published studies using angio-Doppler after injection of contrast agents show that chronic pancreatitis nodule, endocrine tumors, and mucinous cystadenomas increased their vascularization compared with pancreatic adenocarcinoma, in which no modification of vascularization was reported. It is possible that this technique will be very useful in cases of negative EUS-guided biopsy of a pancreatic mass.

Conclusions

EUS is the best and least invasive method for the diagnosis of small pancreatic tumors. The development of

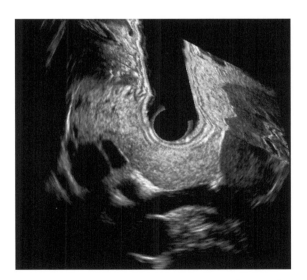

Figure 48.7 Three-dimensional reconstruction of a normal pancreas.

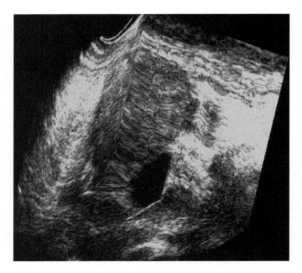

Figure 48.8 Three-dimensional reconstruction of a tumor of the body of the pancreas with portal vein involvement not seen by two-dimensional endoscopic ultrasound.

EUS-guided biopsy has increased the specificity of the technique and showed that all pancreatic masses are not *ipso facto* an adenocarcinoma (about 70% are adenocarcinomas, 30% of other histology). The role of EUS-guided biopsy will increase in the future with the development of preoperative treatment for resectable pancreatic cancer. The future development of three-dimensional EUS and the use of ultrasound contrast agents will increase the capabilities of this technique.

Recommended reading

Afify AM, Al-Khafaji BM, Klim B, Scheiman JM. EUS guided FNA of the pancreas. Diagnostic utility and accuracy. *Acta Cytol* 2003;47:341–348.

Akahoshi K, Chijiiwa Y, Nakano I *et al.* Role of endosonography in diagnosis and staging of pancreatic cancer. *Endoscopy* 1995;8:612–615.

Bender GN, Case B, Tsuchida A *et al.* Using sector endoluminal ultrasound to identify the normal pancreas when axial computed tomography is falsely positive. *Invest Radiol* 1999;34:71–74.

Bhutani M, Hoffman BJ, Van Velse A, Hawes RH. Contrast-enhanced endoscopic ultrasonography with galactose microparticles. SHU508 A (Levovist). *Endoscopy* 1997;29:635–639.

Buscail L, Pages P, Berthelemy P, Fourtanier G, Frexinos J, Escourrou J. Role of EUS in the management of pancreatic and ampullary carcinoma: a prospective study assessing resectability and prognosis. *Gastrointest Endosc* 1999;50:34–40.

Chang KJ, Katz KD, Durbin TE *et al.* Endoscopic ultrasound guided fine-needle aspiration. *Gastrointest Endosc* 1994;40:694–699.

Fritscher-Ravens A, Brand L, Knofel WT *et al.* Comparison of EUS guided FNA for focal pancreatic lesions in patients with normal parenchyma and chronic pancreatitis. *Am J Gastroenterol* 2002;97:2768–2775.

Giovannini M, Seitz JF. Endoscopic ultrasonography with a linear type echoendoscope in the evaluation of 94 patients with pancreatobiliary disease. *Endoscopy* 1994;26:579–585.

Giovannini M, Seitz JF, Monges G, Perrier H, Rabbia I. Fine needle aspiration cytology guided by endoscopic ultrasonography: results in 141 patients. *Endoscopy* 1995;27:171–177.

Giovannini M, Monges G, Bories E, Pesenti CH, Danisi C. EUS guided biopsy: results of a monocentric study of 1544 patients. *Endoscopia Digestiva* 2003;26:121–128.

Gress F, Giaccia D, Kiel J, Sherman S, Lehman G. Endoscopic ultrasound guided celiac plexus block for management of pain due to chronic pancreatitis. *Gastrointest Endosc* 1999;45:594–599.

Grimm H, Maydeo A, Sohendra N. Endoluminal ultrasound for the diagnosis and staging of pancreatic cancer. *Baillieres Clin Gastroenterol* 1990;4:869–887.

Kobayashi G, Fujita N, Noda Y *et al.* The evaluation of portal venous invasion of pancreatic cancer by endoscopic ultrasonography. *Jpn J Gastroenterol* 1993;90:49–56.

Mertz H, Sechopoulos P, Delbeke D, Steven D, Leach D. EUS, PET, and CT scanning for evaluation of pancreatic adenocarcinoma. *Gastrointest Endosc* 2000;52:367–370.

Midwinter MJ, Beveridge CJ, Wilsdon JB, Benett MK, Baudoin CJ, Charnley RM. Correlation between spiral computed tomography, endoscopic ultrasonography and findings at operation in pancreatic and ampullary tumors. *Br J Surg* 1999;86:189–193.

Müller MF, Meyenberger C, Bertschinger P *et al.* Pancreatic tumors: evaluation with endoscopic US, CT and MR imaging. *Radiology* 1994;190:745–751.

Palazzo L, Roseau G, Gayet B *et al.* Endoscopic ultrasonography in the diagnosis and the staging of pancreatic adenocarcinoma. Results of a prospective study with comparison to ultrasonography and CT scan. *Endoscopy* 1993;25:143–150.

Raut CP, Grau AM, Staerkel GA *et al.* Diagnostic accuracy of EUS guided FNA in patients with presumed pancreatic cancer. *J Gastrointest Surg* 2003;7:118–128.

Rösch T. Staging of pancreatic cancer. Analysis of literature results. *Gastrointest Endosc Clin North Am* 1995;4:735–739.

Rösch T, Dittler HJ, Lorenz R *et al*. Endsonographisches Staging des pankreaskarzinoms. *Dtsch Med Wochenschr* 1992;117:563–569.

Rösch T, Braig C, Cain T *et al*. Staging of pancreatic and ampullary carcinoma by endoscopic ultrasonography. *Gastroenterology* 1992;102:188–199.

Snady H, Bruckner H, Cooperman A, Paradiso J, Kiefer L. Survival advantage of combined chemoradiotherapy compared with resection as the initial treatment of patients with regional pancreatic carcinoma. *Cancer* 2000;89:314–327.

Tio TL, Tytgat GNJ, Cikot RJLM *et al*. Ampullopancreatic carcinoma: preoperative TNM classification with endosonography. *Radiology* 1990;175:455–461.

Ueno N, Tomiyama T , Tano S. Utility of endoscopic ultrasonography with colour Doppler function for the diagnosis of islet cell tumour. *Am J Gastroenterol* 1995;91:772–776.

Vilmann P, Hancke S. A new biopsy handle instrument for endoscopic ultrasound-guided fine needle aspiration biopsy. *Gastrointest Endosc* 1996;43:238–242.

Vilmann P, Hancke S, Henriksen FW, Jacobsen GK. Endoscopic ultrasonography with fine needle aspiration biopsy in pancreatic disease. *Endoscopy* 1993;25:523–527.

Wiersema MJ. Endosonography guided celiac plexus neurolysis. In: M Bhutani (ed.) *Interventional Endoscopic Ultrasonography*. Harwood Academic Publishers, 1999: 117–123.

Wiersema M, Chak A, Hawes RH *et al*. Evaluation of endosonography in distinguishing malignant from inflammatory pancreatic masses (abstract). *Gastrointest Endosc* 1993;39:A336.

Wiersema MJ, Kochman ML, Cramer HM, Tao LC, Wiersema LM. Endosonography-guided real-time fine-needle aspiration biopsy. *Gastrointest Endosc* 1994;40: 700–707.

Wiersema M, Vilmann P, Giovannini M, Chang KJ. Endosonography-guided fine needle aspiration biopsy: diagnosis accuracy and complication assessment. *Gastroenterology* 1997;112:1087–1095.

Williams DB, Sahai AV, Aabaken L *et al*. Endoscopic ultrasound guided fine needle aspiration biopsy: a large single centre experience. *Gut* 1999;44:720–726.

Yasuda K, Mukai H, Nakajima M *et al*. Staging of pancreatic carcinoma by endoscopic ultrasonography. *Endoscopy* 1993;25:151–155.

49 Pancreatic cancer: do we need a tissue diagnosis in order to proceed with resection?

Matthew M. Hutter and Andrew L. Warshaw

Introduction

In the past, the high mortality rate of pancreaticoduo-denectomy made surgeons reluctant to proceed without a tissue diagnosis. As recently as two decades ago, the mortality from the Whipple procedure had been as high as 20–30%. Obtaining a histologic or cytologic diagnosis before offering resection was therefore a standard part of the work-up for the management of presumed pancreatic cancer. Recent advances in medical technology and surgical techniques mandate the reevaluation of these management algorithms.

Today, mortality from pancreaticoduodenectomy is 5% or less at many high-volume centers. Pancreaticoduodenectomy is being performed safely for certain benign diseases, including polyps and chronic pancreatitis. Also, there have been significant advances in diagnostic imaging with computed tomography (CT), magnetic resonance imaging (MRI), and positron emission tomography (PET), improving our ability to characterize lesions as likely to be malignant. Advances in diagnostic procedures such as fine-needle aspiration (FNA) with CT, ultrasound, or endoscopic ultrasound (EUS), and improvements in cytologic analysis techniques have been made. Nonetheless, the overall negative predictive value of all these diagnostic modalities is only in the 90% range, which is not high enough to be certain that malignancy can be excluded.

Based on today's technologies and their limitations, potentially resectable pancreatic lesions that are highly suspicious for malignancy should be resected, even if preoperative attempts at tissue confirmation are negative. In fact, the very act of certifying the diagnosis of pancreatic cancer with a tissue specimen may destroy the potential for cure by the dissemination of cancer cells from the needle puncture site.

There are specific situations where tissue diagnosis is mandatory. With metastatic or locally advanced and unresectable disease, tissue diagnosis must be obtained to assist with counseling and with planning palliation with possible chemotherapy, radiation therapy, surgical bypass, and/or celiac block. Similarly, if neoadjuvant therapy is considered, a tissue diagnosis must be made first to justify the potentially toxic treatment. Occasionally, an alternative diagnosis calling for a very different treatment plan can be made from tissue biopsy. For example, a tissue biopsy might be recommended if there are certain radiographic or clinical characteristics that might suggest lymphoma or tuberculosis, as the treatment for these rare conditions is quite different from that for pancreatic adenocarcinoma.

The clinical situation that is hardest to differentiate from pancreatic cancer remains benign localized inflammatory lesions such as strictures in the absence of a defined mass, or focal pancreatitis. Also, chronic pancreatitis can be difficult to distinguish from malignant pancreatic disease. Elevated levels of tumor markers such as CEA or CA-19-9 might suggest malignancy; however they are not sensitive or specific enough to make a definitive diagnosis of cancer. Though attempts should be made to obtain a tissue diagnosis in these clinical scenarios, malignant disease cannot always be ruled out. Surgeons willing to proceed with resection without preoperative tissue diagnosis should be prepared to accept the occasional final diagnosis of benign disease. In our experience this is the case in less than 5%.

Advances in diagnostic imaging

Ongoing advances in diagnostic imaging are continuously increasing the sensitivity and specificity of these modalities to detect pancreatic cancer, determine the presence of metastatic disease, and ascertain resectability. The current state-of-the-art technologies include pancreatic protocol CT using helical or multislice technology with three-dimensional reconstruction and CT angiography, MRI with magnetic resonance angiography (MRA), magnetic resonance cholangiopancreatography (MRCP), and manganese administration, PET imaging and PET–CT, as well as EUS.

Pancreatic protocol CT is the diagnostic procedure of choice for assessing pancreatic masses. The study is performed with thin slices (1–1.5 mm) through the upper abdomen. Intravenous contrast is administered and images are captured during both the arterial and portal venous phase. Helical scanners are currently the norm, and have an accuracy rate of 90–95% in detecting adenocarcinoma and 70–90% for predicting resectability. Sensitivity for detecting liver metastases ranges from 38 to 73%, since subcentimeter metastases usually cannot be detected.

Newer, multislice (multidetector) CT scanners feature faster data acquisition that allows distinct multiphasic capabilities, and narrower collimation to produce exquisite detail and improvement in anatomic volume coverage to create three-dimensional reconstructed images of the arterial, venous, and biliary tree. Results with these multislice scanners will likely increase the accuracy of CT diagnosis and staging.

Magnetic resonance technology has also made dramatic advances in the diagnosis and staging of pancreatic cancer. New advances include fast breath-hold pulse sequences that increase detail by decreasing respiratory variation, gadolinium-enhanced MRI to evaluate arterial and venous patency, MRCP reconstructions that are likely to diminish the role of endoscopic retrograde cholangiopancreatography (ERCP), and manganese administration to help delineate pancreatic neoplasms since pancreatic adenocarcinomas do not take up manganese. MRI is more sensitive than helical CT for detecting small liver metastases. Compared with CT, MRI is less available, more expensive, and the acquisition and interpretation of data is more time-consuming.

Fluorodeoxyglucose (FDG)-PET is based on the principle that malignant cells selectively take up and retain the radiotracer FDG. Pancreatic cancer is therefore associated with increased glucose consumption, and is suspected if there is intense focal uptake in the pancreatic area. For pancreatic cancers less than 2 cm, PET is more sensitive than CT. For lesions greater than 4 cm, CT is superior. Overall, sensitivity and specificity of PET is 96% and 78%, slightly greater than for CT. PET also plays a role in revealing unsuspected metastatic disease to the liver, bones, lungs, and lymph nodes. PET has been shown to upstage 17% of patients who were otherwise being considered for resection based on CT and angiography. As compared with CT, PET is also thought to be more effective for differentiating pancreatic cancer from chronic inflammation. PET is also helpful in following patients who have undergone chemotherapy, radiation therapy, and/or surgical resection.

PET does not provide precise spatial or contrast resolution and the images lack anatomic detail. Therefore, PET plays no role in the determination of local invasion to the vasculature or neighboring organs. Nonetheless, PET can provide complementary information to CT, and is likely to become even more useful as PET–CT technology becomes more widely available.

EUS is a technique that has been developed in the past 10 years, and is performed with a high-frequency ultrasound probe on the end of a flexible endoscope. The degree of detail due to the proximity of the probe and the avoidance of bowel gas makes it suitable for detecting small tumors and for assessing lymph nodes and vascular invasion. As a diagnostic modality, it can at times characterize lesions that are too small to be seen on CT. Drawbacks include the limited field of view, which limits detection of liver or peritoneal metastases. As discussed later, FNA can be performed during EUS, providing accurate tissue sampling.

CT therefore remains the diagnostic and staging test of choice, with EUS, MRI, and PET playing a complementary role to CT for detecting small masses, characterizing liver lesions, and attempting to differentiate pancreatic adenocarcinoma from focal pancreatitis.

Techniques for obtaining tissue diagnosis

Tissue diagnosis can be made using either histologic or cytologic analysis. Histology requires a tissue specimen, and allows assessment of both architecture and cell morphology. Cytology is the analysis of individual cells that are exfoliated, aspirated from a fine needle, or obtained from peritoneal washings. Cytologic findings suggestive of malignancy include anisonucleosis, nuclear membrane irregularity, nuclear crowding/overlapping/three-dimensionality, and nuclear enlargement. Unfortunately, inflammation causes a reactive and regenerative process that itself leads to cellular changes that can be difficult to differentiate from malignancy, especially in well-differentiated adenocarcinoma.

In this chapter, the specific techniques available for tissue diagnosis are discussed, including their indications, sensitivity and specificity, as well as their role in the management of suspected pancreatic cancer. For any of the following methods, results are dependent on the site and characteristics of the lesion, the skill of the clinician performing the procedure, and the skill of the cytopathologist or pathologist processing and interpreting the specimen.

New developments in cytopathology may increase the sensitivity of cytologic analysis. Techniques that incorporate digital image analysis for ploidy assessment and which assess glucose 6-phosphate dehydrogenase activity show some promise. Ongoing studies looking at K-*ras* mutations are less promising. Scoring criteria appear to increase the sensitivity of cytologic analysis, especially in well-differentiated adenocarcinoma.

ERCP: aspirations, brushings, and transpapillary biopsies

Pancreatic cells can naturally exfoliate into pancreatic secretions, can be chemically stimulated to exfoliate with secretin administration, or can be mechanically exfoliated with brushings. Naturally and chemically stimulated exfoliated cells are usually destroyed by pancreatic and duodenal cytolytic enzymes, decreasing the yield from these techniques. Sensitivity of aspiration alone is 33–58%. Brush cytology can be performed using ERCP with fluoroscopic techniques, and provides a higher yield of better-preserved cells, especially for proximal lesions. Sensitivities of brush cytology range from 50 to 75%, with better results for cholangiocarcinomas compared with pancreatic carcinomas. Complications, especially pancreatitis, have been reported in 0–20%. Specificity of these exfoliative techniques is excellent, ranging from 96 to 100%. Exfoliated cells can be readily obtained at ERCP, and a positive finding is very specific for malignancy. How-

ever, the low sensitivity means that a negative result in no way rules out a malignancy.

Transpapillary biopsy at the time of ERCP can also be performed, providing tissue for histologic evaluation. Sensitivity slightly increases to 61–88%, especially when this is combined with brush cytology. The potential for complication with this more invasive approach is also higher.

As noninvasive diagnostic imaging such as CT and MRI/MRA/MRCP become more sophisticated, the role of ERCP in the management of pancreatic cancer diminishes, especially because of the potential complications of perforation, bleeding, pancreatitis, and infection of the biliary tree. ERCP may be restricted to diagnosis and therapy of biliary strictures. As the role of ERCP decreases, and as the role of EUS increases (see below), brush cytology will have less of a role in obtaining a tissue diagnosis in pancreatic cancer.

Percutaneous FNA or core needle biopsy

Percutaneous techniques for tissue diagnosis include CT-guided and ultrasound-guided FNA and core needle biopsy. As the precision of these diagnostic imaging modalities increases, so does the precision of tissue diagnosis using these techniques. Sensitivity rates of percutaneous techniques are higher than ERCP aspirations or brushings, on average in the 70–90% range, but seldom higher than 90%. Again, specificity is excellent. Sensitivity increases with the number of needle passes, as does the number of complications. Potential complications include bleeding, bile leak, abscesses, and fistulas.

Of major concern is that a percutaneous transperitoneal approach has the potential to seed the peritoneal cavity and abdominal wall with metastatic deposits. Needle-track seeding has been reported, albeit a rare finding. However, one study has shown that peritoneal washings taken from patients who appeared radiologically to be resectable were positive for malignant cells in 19% of patients who did not undergo percutaneous sampling, while in patients who had previously undergone percutaneous FNA 75% had positive peritoneal washings. Patients with positive peritoneal washings are considered to have micrometastases, and have a dismal outcome. Therefore, the very act of certifying the diagnosis of pancreatic cancer with a percutaneous tissue specimen may destroy the potential for cure. Of additional concern is that the small, early lesions are the hardest to sample, and these are the very cases for which surgical resection has the best chance of providing a cure.

The role of percutaneous FNA should therefore be restricted to confirmation of the diagnosis of pancreatic cancer when surgical resection for cure is not an option. In patients who have locally advanced disease, who have metastatic disease, or whose comorbidities preclude them from being surgical candidates, tissue diagnosis is necessary for counseling and for dictating future treatments such as chemotherapy, radiation therapy, or surgical palliation. It is also useful in ruling out metastatic disease when radiologic imaging shows a locally resectable pancreatic primary, but also shows another lesion suspicious for a metastasis. In this setting, the potential metastasis should be sampled percutaneously, not the primary. Therefore, percutaneous FNA should not be used if surgical resection is a consideration, because of the risk of a sampling error and the possibility of disseminating the cancer.

EUS with FNA

EUS is a technique that has been developed over the past 10 years, and can be used as a diagnostic imaging modality for staging as well as for localization for FNA. The degree of detail, due to the proximity of the probe and the avoidance of bowel gas, makes it suitable for detecting small tumors and assessing vascular invasion. Lymph nodes can also be characterized and sampled. EUS is best for lesions at the splenoportal junction or higher along the portal vein. The superior mesenteric vein can be distant from the probe, and poorly seen with uncinate lesions.

FNA can be performed under EUS guidance in real time, allowing accurate and confident tissue sampling. Because the probe is placed endoluminally, EUS-guided FNA has a decreased risk of seeding the peritoneal cavity, which is the major drawback of percutaneous approaches.

Sensitivity of EUS-guided FNA is 60–95%, which on average is higher than ERCP brushings and percutaneous FNA. Specificity remains quite high. Though this sensitivity is more encouraging, small resectable lesions are still not definitively excluded. A retrospective comparison at our institution of pancreatic tissue sampling by EUS, CT/ultrasound, and open surgical techniques shows nearly identical accuracy rates for all three techniques (~ 80%).

EUS is quite operator dependent, and requires a skilled endoscopist with significant experience in order to obtain reliable results. EUS is not currently widely available, and time will tell if similar results can be achieved as the technique spreads from the high-volume centers where it was developed.

EUS is therefore a promising newer modality that can detect small lesions, assess vascular invasion, and accurately sample masses and lymph nodes, and minimizes the risk of seeding the peritoneal cavity. Complication rates have been low. Sensitivity of diagnosing malignant lesions approaches the 80–90% range. However, this modality is operator dependent and is not widely available. Even with a negative study, concern about missing a small resectable tumor persists, and this concern will not be alleviated until the sensitivity approaches the high 90% range. Until such a sensitive technique is developed, surgical resection should be offered if imaging and other clinical factors suggest malignancy, even if there is no definitive tissue diagnosis.

The role of EUS is discussed in greater depth in Chapter 48.

Laparoscopy and peritoneal cytology

Pancreatic cancer frequently metastasizes via small millimeter-sized deposits in the peritoneal cavity that implant on the liver capsule, the peritoneal surfaces of the abdominal wall or diaphragm, or the omentum. The small size of these metastases prevents them from being visualized with diagnostic imaging. Staging laparoscopy can help detect these metastases, and in so doing can avoid an unnecessary abdominal exploration. Cytologic analysis of peritoneal washings can identify malignant cells even when no macrometastatic disease is evident. Malignant cells identified in the peritoneum are considered micrometastases, and the natural history of a patient with malignant cells in the peritoneum is similar to a patient with macrometastatic disease. Cytologic findings positive for malignant cells therefore contraindicate further local attempts for cure, such as resection or radiation therapy. Peritoneal washings from patients with pancreatic cancer who radiographically seem to be resectable reveal malignant cells in 8–30% of patients.

Laparoscopy with peritoneal washings should be considered prior to proceeding with pancreaticoduodenectomy. Laparoscopy has a particularly high yield for detecting small metastatic lesions in the liver or on peritoneal surfaces in patients with pancreatic adeno-carcinoma with lesions greater than 2 cm in size and which possibly involve venous structures. A positive laparoscopic finding obviously provides a tissue diagnosis in these cases. Laparoscopy also plays a role in ruling out metastatic disease in locally unresectable patients with no other evidence of metastases who might be candidates for radiation therapy (external beam or intraoperative radiation). It is far less useful for staging ampullary or duodenal cancers because of the much lower likelihood of metastases to the liver or peritoneum.

The role of laparoscopic staging and peritoneal cytology is discussed in further detail in Chapter 50.

Conclusions

In the past, the high mortality of the Whipple procedure made surgeons reluctant to proceed without a definitive tissue diagnosis. Today, with the mortality from pancreaticoduodenectomy at high-volume centers at 5% or less, this approach must be reevaluated.

There have been significant technologic advances in the diagnostic imaging modalities of CT, MRI, and PET, improving our ability to characterize lesions as likely to be malignant. Techniques of tissue diagnosis include ERCP with aspirations, brushings, and/or transpapillary biopsies; percutaneous CT- or ultrasound-guided FNA; and EUS-guided FNA. These techniques have also improved, but still do not have adequate sensitivity to rule out malignancy. The early small lesions that have the best chance for surgical cure are the hardest ones to accurately sample. Percutaneous sampling has the potential risk of seeding the peritoneum, which in essence turns a localized resectable tumor into metastatic disease.

A tissue diagnosis is necessary if neoadjuvant therapy is being considered. If palliation with chemotherapy, radiation therapy, or surgical bypass is considered, tissue confirmation must also be obtained.

Based on today's technologies and their limitations, potentially resectable pancreatic lesions that are highly suspicious for malignancy should be resected, even if preoperative attempts at tissue sampling do not demonstrate malignancy. Given the appropriate clinical scenario and corresponding diagnostic imaging, there is no need to attempt preoperative tissue confirmation since the experienced pancreatic surgeon would proceed with resection even if biopsies were negative. In fact, the very act of attempting to certify the diagnosis of pancreatic cancer with a tissue specimen may destroy the potential for cure.

Recommended reading

Abraham SC, Wilentz RE, Yeo CJ *et al.* Pancreaticoduodenectomy (Whipple resections) in patients without malignancy. Are they all "chronic pancreatitis"? *Am J Surg Pathol* 2003;27:110–120.

Kalra MK, Maher MM, Sahani DV, Digmurthy S, Saini S. Current status of imaging pancreatic diseases. *J Comput Assist Tomogr* 2002;26:661–675.

Kalra MK, Maher MM, Boland GW, Saini S, Fischman AJ. Correlation of positron emission tomography and CT in evaluating pancreatic tumors: technical and clinical implications. *Am J Roentgenol* 2003;181:387–393.

Makary MA, Warshaw AL, Centeno BA, Willett CG, Rattner DW, Fernandez-del Castillo C. Implications of peritoneal cytology for pancreatic cancer management. *Arch Surg* 1998;133:361–365.

Mallery JS, Centeno BA, Hahn PF, Chang Y, Warshaw AL, Brugge WR. Pancreatic tissue sampling guided by EUS, CT/US, and surgery: a comparison of sensitivity and specificity. *Gastrointest Endosc* 2002;56:218–224.

Warshaw AL. Implications of peritoneal cytology for staging of early pancreatic cancer. *Am J Surg* 1991;161:26–30.

Warshaw AL, Fernandez-del Castillo C. Pancreatic carcinoma. *N Engl J Med* 1992;326:455–465.

50 Staging laparoscopy and peritoneal cytology in pancreatic cancer

Ramon E. Jimenez and Carlos Fernández-del Castillo

Introduction

Staging laparoscopy has been shown to be beneficial in the evaluation of patients with pancreatic, hepatobiliary, esophageal, and gastric cancers. These tumors share a propensity to spread by exfoliation and implantation throughout the peritoneal cavity, in addition to lymphatic and hematogenous dissemination. Surgery is not offered to patients presenting with such advanced disease, because removal of their primary tumor does not improve their prognosis. Staging laparoscopy allows accurate determination of resectability without committing the patient to the morbidity of a laparotomy.

For pancreatic cancer, abdominal–pelvic computed tomography (CT) remains the primary staging modality. The "pancreatic protocol" CT offered in most institutions today consists of a triple-phase helical scan with thin-sectioning through the pancreatic parenchyma. This CT study provides exquisite detail of the anatomy of the pancreatic tumor and its relationship to important surrounding structures such as blood vessels. Additionally, it is very sensitive in demonstrating metastatic disease in the liver and elsewhere in the peritoneal cavity. The current resolution of "pancreatic protocol" CT has virtually eliminated the use of invasive angiography in the work-up of patients with pancreatic cancer. Despite these important refinements in imaging technology, the sensitivity of CT is poor for lesions less than 1 cm in size such as peritoneal implants.

Laparoscopy provides valuable complementary data to that of CT. It can detect lesions beyond the resolution of CT and help clarify equivocal radiographic findings. Laparoscopy may also detect micrometastatic disease in the form of positive peritoneal cytology. Patients with negative findings on CT and laparoscopy minimize their chance of undergoing a nontherapeutic laparotomy. For patients with unresectable disease, laparoscopy allows procurement of tissue for pathologic and genetic analysis that can expedite the initiation of nonsurgical therapy in the form of chemotherapy or radiation. Therefore, an accurate preoperative staging protocol for pancreatic malignancy must include a diagnostic laparoscopy.

This chapter provides a review of our experience and that of others in the use of laparoscopy for the staging of pancreatic cancer.

Indications

The findings on abdominal CT primarily determine which patients with suspected pancreatic cancer should proceed to staging laparoscopy. Patients with clearly demonstrable metastasis to sites such as the liver, peritoneum, or lung should not undergo laparoscopy. If tissue diagnosis is required, percutaneous needle biopsy with radiologic guidance or endoscopic biopsy may be employed with high success rates.

The principal candidates for staging laparoscopy are those patients with no evidence of distant metastasis on CT. Laparoscopy is particularly valuable for tumors of the body and tail of the pancreas. Because of their lack of symptomatology, these tumors are often of large size at presentation and have a high risk of occult metastasis. Most patients with tumors in the head of the pancreas should also undergo staging laparoscopy. At Massachusetts General Hospital (MGH), patients with tumors in the head of the gland measuring less than 2 cm are rarely found to have metastasis at laparoscopy. In many of these patients laparoscopy can be avoided.

Staging laparoscopy is also helpful for patients with locally advanced disease. These patients are deemed unresectable by virtue of encasement of the superior mesenteric artery, celiac axis, and/or portal vein on CT. In these patients, staging laparoscopy is done to determine their candidacy for radiotherapy. Radiotherapy is offered only to those with locally advanced disease and no peritoneal metastases. Some of these patients can show dramatic tumor responses to neoadjuvant treatment, and may potentially be downstaged to resectability.

Technique

Laparoscopic examination is most commonly performed under general anesthesia. Following establishment of pneumoperitoneum, a 10-mm trocar is inserted through a small infraumbilical incision. The 30° angled telescope is introduced through this trocar, and examination begins by inspection of the lower abdomen and pelvis. The lower abdomen is a frequent site of peritoneal metastasis in pancreatic cancer, and laparoscopic visualization of this area is often superior to laparotomy. Free fluid is aspirated and saved for cytology. The laparoscope is then rotated for examination of the upper quadrants. Inspection begins by assessment of the omentum and the subdiaphragmatic spaces. The liver surface is then meticulously evaluated by a combination of visualization and palpation with a blunt forceps or suction tip. The falciform ligament and umbilical fissure are then carefully inspected for metastatic implants. Insertion of a second 5-mm trocar in the right upper quadrant is often necessary for adequate evaluation of the undersurface of the liver. A rod, suction tip, or liver retractor inserted through this second trocar site is used to elevate the liver for inspection of the gallbladder fossa and liver hilum.

If peritoneal washings are desired, they are collected before further dissection or biopsy to prevent sample contamination. Biopsy of peritoneal or omental nodules can be taken using cup-biopsy forceps inserted through the second trocar site. Access to lesions in the pelvic peritoneum may require insertion of a third 5-mm trocar in the lower midline. Implants in the liver are most easily biopsied using the Tru-Cut needle

inserted directly through the abdominal wall or through the second trocar site. Enlarged lymph nodes may also be sampled by fine-needle aspiration.

An extensive evaluation of the pancreas is possible during staging laparoscopy. Division of the gastrohepatic omentum permits examination of the caudate lobe of the liver, the vena cava, and the celiac axis. Visualization of the body and tail of the gland can be performed by entering the lesser sac through the gastrocolic omentum. Most recently, development of ultrasonography probes adaptable to laparoscopic equipment have led to application of this technology in the staging of pancreatic cancer. Laparoscopic ultrasonography can locate deep liver metastasis not detectable by simple surface inspection. The primary tumor can be evaluated for size and extension into the stomach, colon, or retroperitoneum. Ultrasonography can also provide impressive information regarding vascular invasion and lymphadenopathy, particularly with respect to the celiac axis, superior mesenteric vessels, and portal vein.

Palliative procedures can be performed at the time of laparoscopic staging if the primary tumor is found to be unresectable. Laparoscopic cholecystojejunostomy and gastrojejunostomy have been described in the literature.

Laparoscopic detection of metastatic disease

Some of the largest recent series of staging laparoscopies for potentially resectable pancreatic cancer are included in Table 50.1. All series include patients evaluated during the 1990s, when high-quality CT scanners were widely accessible. All patients included in Table 50.1 had preoperative CT that did not demonstrate metastatic disease. The prevalence of liver and peritoneal metastases detected in these patients by simple laparoscopy is approximately 25%. In other words, these results illustrate that one-quarter of patients had false-negative CT examinations. In our experience, peritoneal or liver implants are twice as common in tumors located in the body or tail of the pancreas (39%) than in cancers of the head of the gland (17%). This observation probably reflects the relative delay in diagnosis of tumors of the distal pancreas, which remain asymptomatic in the absence of jaundice.

Other techniques have been combined with

Table 50.1 Laparoscopic detection of intraabdominal metastasis in pancreatic cancer.

Series	No. of patients	Gross metastases	Additional staging technique	Unresectable*
Bemelman *et al.* (1995)	72	10 (14)	Ultrasound	16 (22)
John *et al.* (1995)	40†	14 (35)	Ultrasound	23 (58)
Fernandez-del Castillo *et al.* (1995)	114	27 (24)	Peritoneal cytology	33 (29)
Conlon *et al.* (1996)	108†	28 (26)	Dissection	41 (38)
Minnard *et al.* (1998)	90	19 (21)	Dissection and ultrasound	49 (54)
Jimenez *et al.* (2000)	125	30 (24)	Peritoneal cytology	42 (34)
Vollmer *et al.* (2002)	84	18 (21)	Ultrasound	26 (31)

* As determined by laparoscopic staging procedure.
† Includes a small number of patients with nonpancreatic periampullary malignancies.
Numbers in parentheses represent percentages.

laparoscopy to enhance the sensitivity of the staging procedure. The group at MGH routinely collects peritoneal washings for cytology at the time of laparoscopy (discussed below). The series by John *et al.* evaluated the use of laparoscopic ultrasound during staging laparoscopy, and showed that ultrasound increased their yield of unresectable cases from 35 to 58%. Similar findings are reported by Minnard *et al.* at Memorial Sloan-Kettering Cancer Center (MSKCC). Conlon *et al.*, also at MSKCC, made use of laparoscopic dissection to gain access to the lesser sac and evaluate the celiac axis and superior mesenteric vessels. When compared with simple laparoscopy, detection of unresectable disease increased from 26 to 38% using this technique. In general, most of the new information gained by laparoscopic ultrasonography or extended dissection pertains to vascular invasion at the celiac axis, portal vein, or superior mesenteric vessels. In our estimation, satisfactory resolution of these structures is obtained by CT, and available data from these studies do not justify a more time-consuming and risky laparoscopic staging protocol.

A final evaluation of laparoscopy in the staging of pancreatic cancer must include an assessment of the specificity and sensitivity of the procedure. The specificity of staging laparoscopy is 100% because diagnosis of metastatic carcinoma is always based on tissue diagnosis and not on visual impression alone. The sensitivity of the procedure can be calculated by analyzing the laparotomy findings of those patients explored shortly after staging laparoscopy. These data are listed in Table 50.2 and show that sensitivity estimates range

Table 50.2 Resectability after staging laparoscopy.

Series	Sensitivity (%)	Resectability rate*
Bemelman *et al.* (1995)	76	27/35 (77)
John *et al.* (1995)	88	11/12 (92)
Fernandez-del Castillo *et al.* (1995)	94	30/40 (75)
Conlon *et al.* (1996)	88	61/67 (91)
Minnard *et al.* (1998)	100	39/40 (98)
Jimenez *et al.* (2000)	98	23/30 (77)
Vollmer *et al.* (2002)	88	47/60 (78)

* In patients explored with intent to resect.
Numbers in parentheses represent percentages.

from 88 to 98%. It seems surprising to find that sensitivity was not significantly improved by the use of additional laparoscopic techniques such as ultrasound or extended dissection.

Peritoneal cytology

Peritoneal washings are easily collected at the time of laparoscopy. It is important to perform peritoneal lavage prior to dissection or biopsy to prevent sample contamination. Procurement of peritoneal washings involves instillation of 400 mL of 0.9% normal saline into the subhepatic space and dispersion by abdominal agitation or manipulation of the operating table. The

421

Table 50.3 Peritoneal cytology in pancreatic cancer.

Series	No. of patients	Positive cytology	With gross metastases*
Martin & Goellner (1986)	23	5 (22)	3 (60)
Warshaw *et al.* (1991)	40	12 (30)	2 (17)
Lei *et al.* (1994)	36	3 (8)	3 (100)
Leach *et al.* (1995)	60	4 (7)	0 (0)
Fernandez-del Castillo *et al.* (1995)	94	16 (17)	10 (63)
Merchant *et al.* (1999)	228	34 (15)	26 (76)
Jimenez *et al.* (2000)	117	24 (21)	12 (50)

* Detected by laparoscopy.
Numbers in parentheses represent percentages.

fluid is then aspirated under direct vision and collected for cytologic evaluation. Samples are routinely analyzed by cytomorphologic criteria. When confusion arises due to inflammatory or reactive mesothelial cells, application of immunohistochemistry may aid identification of malignant cells. If used routinely, immunohistochemistry can increase tumor cell detection when compared with cytomorphologic criteria alone.

Table 50.3 summarizes published data on peritoneal cytology in pancreatic cancer. All series involve potentially resectable patients except those by Martin *et al.* and Lei *et al.* The data reveal that malignant cells can be found in 7–30% of peritoneal washings taken from pancreatic cancer patients. The institutional experience at MGH includes 251 patients, in whom cytology was positive in 21% of cases. Table 50.3 demonstrates that 50–60% of positive samples are associated with metastatic disease detected at laparoscopy. Our data reveal that positive cytology occurs in 45% of patients with visible metastases, but in only 14% of those without.

Several studies have evaluated the significance of positive peritoneal cytology in the absence of gross metastasis for pancreatic cancer patients. Most studies confirm that positive cytology is an indicator of unresectable aggressive disease characterized by early metastasis and short survival. In fact, no difference in survival exists between patients with gross metastasis detected at laparoscopy and those with positive cytology but no visible metastatic disease. We advocate classification of patients with positive peritoneal cytology as M1 in the TNM system, as is the case for gastric, ovarian, and endometrial cancers. These patients would therefore not derive further benefit from surgical resection or radiation therapy. The combination of peritoneal cytology and laparoscopy has increased our detection of metastatic disease during staging from 24 to 31% (Table 50.1).

Differences in staging algorithms

In the USA, most of the literature on the topic of staging laparoscopy for pancreatic cancer comes from MGH or MSKCC. Significant differences in the staging protocol exist between these two centers.

At MGH, staging laparoscopy with peritoneal cytology is performed in a brief outpatient session prior to the planned pancreatic resection. The laparoscopy procedure is kept as simple as possible, consisting mostly of visual inspection of the parietal and visceral peritoneum, collection of peritoneal cytology, and biopsy of suspicious sites. This operation rarely takes longer than 30 min. No extensive laparoscopic dissection of the lesser sac or the celiac axis is done because of the potential for bleeding complications. Laparoscopic ultrasound of the liver is used infrequently because it adds minimal new information to pancreas protocol CT. The delay between the staging procedure and the planned pancreatic resection allows for review of the peritoneal cytology data, which are considered in the final determination of resectability. The simplicity of this staging algorithm supports its use by the general surgeon in the community hospital setting to screen for patients who may benefit from transfer to tertiary referral centers for treatment.

In contrast, the group at MSKCC advocates a complex staging protocol consisting of laparoscopic dissection of the lesser omentum and exploration of the lesser sac, with biopsy of suspicious implants and lymph nodes near major vessels. Laparoscopic ultrasound of the liver, portal vein, superior mesenteric vessels, and celiac axis is also performed in a majority of patients. While peritoneal cytology is often collected, results are not used in determining resectability. Rather, peritoneal cytology data help to determine which patients may benefit from adjuvant chemotherapy. A negative staging laparoscopy (negative frozen sections and no encasement of the celiac axis or superior mesenteric artery) is followed by pancreatic resection in the same operating room session. The level of laparoscopic expertise required by the staging protocol at MSKCC supports early referral of patients with suspected pancreatic cancer to specialized pancreatic surgery centers for staging as well as treatment.

Despite differences in the details of the staging laparoscopy itself, published resectability and survival rates for pancreatic adenocarcinoma remain remarkably similar between MGH and MSKCC. It appears reasonable to suggest that the simpler protocol endorsed by MGH is less technically demanding for the surgeon, less risky to the patient, and more efficient for the hospital.

Patient management after staging laparoscopy

Accurate selection of patients for resection is one of the main goals of staging laparoscopy. Most of the published series provide data on resectability rates after negative laparoscopy, and use this information to assess the success of their staging protocol. Table 50.2 includes published resectability rates for patients explored with intent to resect. More than three-quarters of patients deemed resectable after staging laparoscopy can be successfully resected. As expected, resectability rates are slightly higher after more exhaustive laparoscopic evaluations, such as those by Conlon *et al.* and John *et al.* Overall, the resectability rates in Table 50.2 are significantly higher than those reported without the use of staging laparoscopy.

Staging laparoscopy allows optimization of resources and avoidance of unnecessary surgery in pancreatic cancer. At MGH, greater than 90% of patients with laparoscopically detected metastases did not undergo further surgery. This experience is confirmed by Espat *et al.*

from MSKCC. Almost all patients with symptomatic malignant biliary obstruction have been successfully treated by endoscopic or percutaneous palliation techniques. The introduction of endoscopic intestinal stents has allowed outpatient, minimally invasive treatment of gastric outlet obstruction for many patients.

Current trends for aggressive neoadjuvant treament with combinations of radiotherapy and chemotherapy underscore the importance of excluding metastatic disease. The morbidity, cost, and time commitment required by these new treatment modalities are not negligible, and patient selection is as important as for surgical resection. Most neoadjuvant treatment protocols include a staging laparoscopy before the onset of treatment. Patients demonstrating good response to chemoradiation on CT may undergo a second staging laparotomy to reassess their candidacy for resection.

Future directions

Laparoscopy is an integral part of the current staging protocol for pancreatic cancer. However, despite current efforts to select the best patients for surgical treatment, 5-year survival rates after resection for cure remain low at 15–20%. Clearly, new staging strategies are needed to improve on these results. Further additions to the current laparoscopic staging procedure are unlikely to contribute to improving patient survival.

We need to look at other diagnostic modalities to help in patient selection for treatment. As an example, positron emission tomography (PET) has been shown to be helpful in identifying patients with cystic tumors of the pancreas who may benefit from surgery. In these patients, PET has been shown to detect cysts carrying premalignant or malignant changes. Some cystic tumors of the pancreas are now followed expectantly with serial PET, allowing some patients to safely avoid surgery.

Ultimately, an accurate staging algorithm will need to consider tumor biology in its most basic form: genetics. More and more tumors today are being studied by genetic array analysis. Patterns of genetic abnormalities are starting to be recognized that determine a tumor's response to radiation or chemotherapy. In the future, this technology will hopefully provide a fingerprint for tumors that will allow customization of therapy to individual patients.

Recommended reading

Bemelman WA, de Wit LT, van Delden OM *et al*. Diagnostic laparoscopy combined with laparoscopic ultrasonography in staging of cancer of the pancreatic head region. *Br J Surg* 1995;82:820–824.

Conlon KC, Dougherty E, Klimstra DS *et al*. The value of minimal access surgery in the staging of patients with potentially resectable peripancreatic malignancy. *Ann Surg* 1996; 223:134–140.

Espat NJ, Brennan MF, Conlon KC. Patients with laparoscopically staged unresectable pancreatic adenocarcinoma do not require subsequent surgical biliary or gastric bypass. *J Am Coll Surg* 1999;188:649–655.

Fernandez-del Castillo C, Rattner DW, Warshaw AL. Further experience with laparoscopy and peritoneal cytology in the staging of pancreatic cancer. *Br J Surg* 1995;82:1127–1129.

Jimenez RE, Warshaw AL, Rattner DW *et al*. Impact of laparoscopic staging in the treatment of pancreatic cancer. *Arch Surg* 2000;135:409–414.

John TG, Greig JD, Carter DC, Garden OJ. Carcinoma of the pancreatic head and periampullary region. Tumor staging with laparoscopy and laparoscopic ultrasonography. *Ann Surg* 1995;221:156–164.

Leach SD, Rose JA, Lowy AM *et al*. Significance of peritoneal cytology in patients with potentially resectable adenocarcinoma of the pancreatic head. *Surgery* 1995;118:472–478.

Lei S, Kini J, Kim K, Howard JM. Pancreatic cancer. Cytologic study of peritoneal washings. *Arch Surg* 1994; 129:639–642.

Martin JKJ, Goellner JR. Abdominal fluid cytology in patients with gastrointestinal malignant lesions. *Mayo Clin Proc* 1986;61:467–471.

Merchant NB, Conlon KC, Saigo P *et al*. Positive peritoneal cytology predicts unresectability of pancreatic adenocarcinoma. *J Am Coll Surg* 1999;188:421–426.

Minnard EA, Conlon KC, Hoos A *et al*. Laparoscopic ultrasound enhances standard laparoscopy in the staging of pancreatic cancer. *Ann Surg* 1998;228:182–187.

Vollmer CM, Drebin JA, Middleton WD *et al*. Utility of staging laparoscopy in subsets of peripancreatic and biliary malignancies. *Ann Surg* 2002;235:1–7.

Warshaw AL. Implications of peritoneal cytology for staging of early pancreatic cancer. *Am J Surg* 1991;161:26–29.

51 Management of pain in pancreatic cancer: an algorithm for clinical routine

Åke Andrén-Sandberg

The World Health Organization (WHO) has designated pain relief, and palliative care, as a priority in its global program for cancer control. Although it is possible to offer adequate pain control to more than 90% of cancer patients, the reality may be very different because of lack of knowledge and skills, lack of empathy, and failing attitude. With regard to pancreatic cancer, too little interest has been shown in the care of these patients. The considerable psychosocial and lifestyle consequences of uncontrolled pain are often overlooked and it should be underlined that pain always has an important emotional component. Pain is therefore devastating not only for the patient but also for the family and for all those caring for the patient, and all possible efforts should be made to eliminate the pain. Despite the publication and widespread distribution of guidelines for pain management, many patients with pancreatic cancer receive inadequate analgesia.

When discussing pain it must be stressed that there is no better treatment than resection of the tumor; if this is possible technically and biologically, it should always have the highest priority. The discussion below is therefore confined to the cases where resection is not performed, irrespective of cause.

Pain as part of a symptom complex

The symptom given most attention in pancreatic cancer patients is pain, although jaundice, gastric outlet obstruction, and weight loss are also described in detail in the literature. However, there are also other symptoms that deserve special attention, such as gastrointestinal bleeding with and without anemia, anorexia/cachexia and dysphagia, nausea and vomiting, dehydration and dryness in the oral cavity, fatigue, depression, anxiety, insomnia, ascites, hypostatic edema, venous thromboembolism, recurrent infections, diarrhea/constipation, postoperative sequelae including fistulas, and endocrine and exocrine insufficiency (diabetes and steatorrhea). Patients with pancreatic cancer also suffer "social complications," such as economic problems, feelings of dependence on relatives and others, unwillingness to appear in public due to extreme weight loss, unwillingness to discuss their own health status in public, inability to carry out those activities formerly associated with their professional and social lives, sexual inability, and the urgent need of toilets. The patient's relatives also have different views on how the care and nursing should best be provided. First and foremost, however, there is always the need for hope; if patients have no hope that the future holds something worth living for, they will give up the struggle to remain alive.

Even though pain may be the main symptom, it should be understood that there is always something "worse," which implies that even if the pain is treated successfully, there will still be other "new" symptoms that deserve attention. Therefore, it is important to have a holistic view about pain treatment, even for those with the special task of treating the specific symptom "pain."

Prevalence of pain in pancreatic cancer

More than 50% of all patients with exocrine pancreatic cancer have pain as an initial symptom and practically all will suffer significant pain at some stage before they succumb to the disease (Table 51.1). Pain occurs in at least 85% of patients with advanced disease (Table 51.1) and is related to shortened survival, especially if opioids are being administered (Table 51.2). For some patients with the disease, the pain is so severe that all waking hours are devoted to its control, leading to a very poor quality of life. Empirically it is obvious that patients with pancreatic cancer are one of the cancer groups with the most severe pain problems.

Origin of the pain in pancreatic cancer

Pancreatic cancer pain can be subdivided into somatic, visceral, and neuropathic in origin. *Somatic pain* occurs as a result of the activation of nociceptors in cuta-neous and deep tissues. Somatic pain is typically constant and well localized and is frequently described as aching, throbbing, or gnawing. Both bone metastasis and mucosal injury produce somatic pain. *Visceral pain* originates from injury to sympathetically innervated organs. Mechanisms of visceral pain include necrosis, ischemia of visceral muscles, serosal or mucosal irritation by analgesic substances, or abnormal distension or contraction of smooth muscle walls within a hollow viscus. The pain is characterized as either dull, deep, and aching or paroxysmal and colicky. *Neuropathic pain* refers to pain syndromes that occur as a result of nerve injury. Neuropathic pain can occur following surgery or radiation therapy. In addition, certain chemotherapeutic agents (e.g., taxanes, vincristine, vinblastine, cisplatin) can produce neuropathic pain. The pain is characterized by burning, tingling, and numbing sensations.

From an anatomic point of view, pancreatic cancer pain may result from intrapancreatic and peripancreatic inflammatory processes, an obstructed main pancreatic duct, as well as perineural invasion of the tumor. It is possible that recurrent ischemia of the parenchyma and intrapancreatic causes such as acute pseudocysts and extrapancreatic causes such as common bile duct or duodenal stenosis cause pain. The relative contribution of inflammation, obstruction, neuritis, and scarring to the pathogenesis of pain is still unclear and may vary from patient to patient.

Obstruction of the pancreatic duct system was for a

Table 51.1 Sixty-six consecutive patients operated on for pancreatic cancer with pancreatectomy in Lund, Sweden, 1995–98.

Pain first symptom	37%
Pain at diagnosis	58%
Not requiring medicine	37%
Requiring nonopioids	16%
Requiring opioids	5%
Pain requiring analgesics at recurrence	88%
Pain requiring analgesics 1 month before death	98%

Table 51.2 Prospective registration of pain at diagnosis in 160 consecutive, nonradically operated patients with pancreatic cancer in Scandinavia, 1995–98.

Visual analog scale	Percent	Patients on morphine (percent of total)	Median survival (days)	Median survival on morphine (days)
0	27	6	280	222
1	14	3	263	171
2	14	2	223	178
3	2	—	238	—
4	8	2	167	113
5	15	7	138	111
6	10	5	101	62
7	5	—	97	—
8	5	—	63	—
9	—	—	—	—
10	—	—	—	—

long time seen as the major factor in the pathogenesis of chronic pancreatitis and has also been proposed as a cause of pain in pancreatic cancer. However, the relationship between morphologic changes, ductal pressures, and pain has repeatedly been shown to be very variable, and other factors must be implicated. An increased intracystic pressure may be assumed when a pseudocyst communicates with a stenotic duct. On the other hand, the same anatomic abnormalities sometimes relate to a painless course. Although data indicate that increased intraductal or parenchymal pressure is associated with pain in pancreatic cancer, the pathomechanism by which increased pressure causes pain is not clear.

A more recent pain concept in pancreatic cancer regards direct alterations of pancreatic nerves as one of the major pathophysiologic events in pain generation. It has been reported that phenotypic modification of primary sensory neurons may play a role in the production of persistent pain. Autodigestion with tissue necrosis and both pancreatic and peripancreatic inflammation in the earlier stages change the focal release and uptake of mediators in peptidergic nerves and could be an important cause of pain. Pancreatic nerves are preferentially retained while exocrine pancreatic parenchyma atrophies and degenerates and is replaced by fibrosis. Moreover, in pancreatic cancer, compared with normal pancreas, the number and diameter of pancreatic nerves are significantly increased and analysis of neuroplasticity markers provides evidence that the nerves actively grow. This leads to differential expression of neuropeptides, such as substance P and vasoactive intestinal peptide (VIP), in the chronically irritated pancreas. In addition, electron microscopic examination has revealed that the perineurium of theses nerves is partially destroyed, indicating loss of the barrier between nerve fibers and bioactive material in the perineural space. Bockman *et al.* have put forward a concept they call "pancreatitis-associated neuritis," which implies a comparative increase in the number of sensory nerves in inflammatory pancreatic tissue together with round cell infiltration and a striking disintegration of the perineurium. The loss of function of the perineural barrier may allow an influx of inflammatory mediators or active pancreatic enzymes that could act directly on the nerve cells. It can be speculated that these two mechanisms, increased pancreatic tissue pressure and neuritis, could work together. High tissue fluid pressure would then facilitate influx of pain mediators into the nerves and result in more long-standing pain.

There is also evidence that pancreatic ischemia may occur in an experimental model of chronic pancreatitis, and possibly pancreatic cancer, leading to decreased pancreatic blood flow, ischemia, and local depression of parenchymal pH. During ischemia xanthine oxidase becomes activated, which leads to the generation of toxic oxygen metabolites that may contribute to pain in chronic pancreatitis. However, the xanthine oxidase inhibitor allopurinol did not reduce pain in a randomized, two-period, crossover clinical trial.

Characteristics of pancreatic cancer pain

The characteristic pattern of pain in pancreatic cancer is that of a dull ache in the mid-epigastrium that radiates to the back, especially if the body and tail of the pancreas are involved. Pain is usually accentuated at night and may be spasmodic. This symptom is not something usually associated with a visceral solid carcinoma. The pain is typically more severe in the supine position and improves when the patient leans forward.

The pain progresses over time and never leaves the patient totally, usually not even with treatment. Compared with the pain of chronic pancreatitis, which may have the same distribution, there is less fluctuation in intensity from day to day and there is less influence of eating and drinking.

When the cause of the pain is explained to the patient, there is also another obvious difference between patients with pancreatic cancer and those with chronic pancreatitis. The first group is usually very reluctant to take analgesics for the pain, whereas the second group usually needs no persuasion to take drugs but rather has a tendency to use excessively strong analgesics from the start. This is very rarely a problem with pancreatic cancer patients.

Sometimes, patients with pancreatic cancer initially describe the pain as a tiredness in the back, making it impossible to work and relax. Later on, they find it difficult to sit and stand without having severe fatigue of the mid-back, which is then impossible to differentiate from pain. At this stage the patients are often restless and seem to continuously move in their search for a position that relieves the fatigue and pain. In later stages, patients tend to lie on the bed and to move as little as possible, which further decreases their muscle strength, making movements more difficult.

An algorithm for pain management in pancreatic cancer

There are several algorithms for the management of pain in pancreatic cancer, most of them with unique positive aspects. However, and unfortunately, most of them focus only on pharmacologic treatment. The most important part of the WHO "analgesic ladder," and the reason for its success, is probably the efficient use of oral opioids for moderate to severe pain, while making it clear that this treatment is very effective and that dependence problems are negligible. However, this does not mean that alternative analgesics should not be used. For example, acetaminophen (paracetamol) is a potent and cheap analgesic with very few adverse effects and has a central effect like morphine but without the latter's drug-abuse problems.

An algorithm is presented here in which pharmacologic treatment is but *one* part of the management of pain in pancreatic cancer. It can be used in association with literature more concerned with the details of drugs and how to use them optimally (Fig. 51.1).

Is the diagnosis of pancreatic cancer correct?

When a patient with pancreatic pain for the first time needs treatment, it is obligatory to critically review the evidence for the diagnosis: does this patient really have pancreatic cancer? In the past, patients have all too often been given the diagnosis of pancreatic cancer when follow-up has shown that the true disease has been, for example chronic pancreatitis. This may be a grave misdiagnosis, as the cancer patient can be expected to have increasing pain and there is little purpose in limiting analgesic use unless the patient is pain-free, whereas patients with chronic pancreatitis may respond better to alternative therapies.

Also, patients with other types of cancer might benefit from other types of treatment. An example of this is endocrine pancreatic cancer, for which there is an arsenal of treatment options, analgesics being only one but probably not the first choice. There are also lymphomas and sarcomas and other rare tumors of the pancreas where good alternative treatment options are available. Once again, if the pancreatic cancer can be resected, this is almost always the best choice.

Is the pain due to the cancer or to concomitant diseases?

It should be emphasized that not all the symptoms in patients with pancreatic cancer are due to the cancer. Especially common are gallstone disease and peptic ulcers in the stomach and duodenum. Ileus and subileus due to causes other than pancreatic cancer (or peritoneal carcinomatosis) are found occasionally. If in these cases the pain is treated strictly according to the WHO cancer analgesic ladder, there is a severe risk that the patient will be harmed, and indeed may not be well treated regarding the pain. If possible it is always better to treat the cause of the pain rather than the symptom of pain itself.

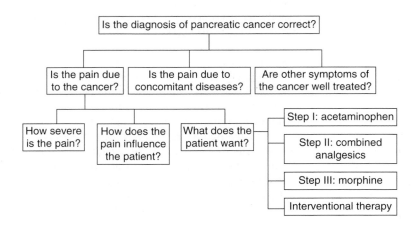

Figure 51.1 Algorithm for management of pancreatic cancer pain.

Are other symptoms of the cancer well treated?

There are many symptoms of pancreatic cancer that influence the experience of pain. For example, tired patients have more pain; depressed patients cannot participate in treatments as well as they should; patients with great weight loss experience more pain; ascites, constipation, and pneumonia may generate pain themselves. Moreover, some pharmacologic agents may produce discomfort or pain, for example opioid-induced constipation and nonsteroidal anti-inflammatory drug (NSAID)-induced peptic ulcer.

Therefore, it is important to understand that the pain must be treated as part of a symptom complex rather than *the* symptom. Patients themselves frequently remark on this: "Doctor, if I could only sleep better/have less nausea/did not have this swollen abdomen, I could stand the pain better." Thus nutrition support and therapy for insomnia and the like may also be important in pain management.

How severe is the pain?

Unfortunately, it is a common experience that the language of patients and the language of those who care for them may differ in ways that lead to troublesome misunderstandings. Patients not only use words that overrate the pain but also use words that make caregivers think there is less pain than that actually experienced. The solution to the problem of the description of pain intensity attempts to avoid the use of words like "severe" and "terrible" and instead applies a standardized scale.

The standard measurement of pain intensity today is the 10-cm visual analog scale (VAS). The 0–10 numeric rating scale (NRS) is also often used, but it should be understood from a scientific point of view that there are some small but consistent differences between a VAS and an NRS. All the commonly used scales are considered to be reliable and have been shown to give rather similar results as regards construct validity. However, one special problem in pancreatic cancer is that patients, and healthcare providers including doctors, find it difficult to understand VAS and NRS when discussing a variable pain over time. It must also be understood that any given change in NRS or VAS score has no intrinsic meaning. On the other hand, there is almost always good agreement between pain scores derived from VAS and similar scales and those derived from categoric pain relief scales and graphic rating scales. Elderly individuals with chronic pain find scoring on the VAS more difficult than younger patients. Also, simple interest in the measurement of pain may influence the outcome of the patient's pain score. A discrepancy between physician perception and patient report of pain intensity has been shown to be a predictor of inadequate pain management.

How does the pain influence the patient and what does the patient want?

The International Association for the Study of Pain defines pain as "an unpleasant sensory and emotional experience associated with actual or potential tissue damage or described in terms of such damage." The important part in this context is "emotional experience," which means that even though pain intensity might be standardized, not all patients demand the same treatment for the same pain intensity.

There are patients who are so afraid of a potentially increasing pain that they want analgesics "in case it gets worse," whereas others do not want any analgesic drugs until it is "really needed." The solution to this problem may be to watch their behavior: if patients are unable to do what they want due to the pain, then caregivers should act; conversely, if patients continue with their normal way of life despite the pain, it might be wise to wait until they ask for help.

If patients have a desire to work or do something else that is important to them, they probably have greater overall ability and greater capacity to cope with the pain. On the other hand, if nothing is important, it is likely that the patient will suffer more pain.

The analgesic ladder

Step 1 (Fig. 51.2)

Nutritional support is one of the most important parts of the first step in pain management. Weight loss typically correlates with inability to tolerate pain and increases the depression and fatigue that make the pain unbearable. Nutritional support must be individualized. For some patients it may be enough to provide the food they like, while others need liquid food, some need a better social environment in which to eat, and yet others require special liquid formula diets. Often the addition of pancreatic enzymes improves the absorption of ingested food and it should at least be tried.

Is the diagnosis correct?

Can the cancer be removed?

Treat concomitant diseases: gallstones, peptic ulcer, ileus, etc.

Concomitant cancer symptoms: nausea, emesis, obstipation, weight loss, depression, etc.

Nutritional support including vitamins, trace elements, energy, and water

Pancreatic enzymes

Become acquainted with the language of the patient, the reactions, and the expectations. Is the patient afraid?

Investigate social support network and supporter's network

Make the patient understand that we *know* how to treat cancer pain

Document the decisions of pain treatment (make sure that all involved agree, including patient and relatives)

Acetaminophen 1 g four times daily (not on demand)

Figure 51.2 The analgesic ladder: step 1.

Acetaminophen + NSAID (not acetylsalicylic acid and dextropropoxyphene)

NSAIDs + ω-fatty acids?

Codeine

Other nonopioid analgesic drugs

Grade of anxiety: benzodiazepines, SSRIs

Make sure the patient sleeps well

Figure 51.3 The analgesic ladder: step 2. NSAID, nonsteroidal antiinflammatory drug; SSRIs, selective serotonin reuptake inhibitors.

Patients must understand that the enzymes should be taken with meals, and the effect should be evaluated after 10–14 days. If there are questionable effects, the enzymes should be withdrawn and the effects evaluated once more.

It is also important to become acquainted with the way patients react and their expectations. Is the patient afraid and how are relations with the relatives? Did the relationship with the relatives change after the illness was detected? These and similar questions can help in the care of the patient. Social support is often worth much more than any drug, and if there is a long disease process it may also be important to investigate the supporter's network: how long can they stand the extraordinary pressure? Can they be supported mentally and physically?

It is also important to make patients understand that care-givers *know* how to treat cancer pain. If they are assured that pain relief can be provided, then it is easier for them to tolerate pain at the borderline of what needs to be treated. It is important that everybody involved in nursing the patient should know what measures have been taken, and this should include the patient and the relatives. This means that all decisions concerning care must be documented.

When pharmacologic measures are required, acetaminophen 1 g four times daily is the drug of choice.

There is overwhelming scientific evidence that this drug should be the basis of all pain treatment in pancreatic cancer and that it should be given regularly and not on demand.

Step 2 (Fig. 51.3)

If acetaminophen is not enough to eliminate the pain, it may be combined with NSAIDs. This combination frequently has a combined effect that is significantly better than either drug given alone. The doses used may be the same as those usually given to patients with joint pain for example. It is possible that the antiinflammatory effect is just as important as the analgesic effect, and there are indications that patients with high levels of cytokines and C-reactive protein suffer less anorexia, which may also potentiate the analgesic effect. There are also indications that this can be further potentiated by ω-fatty acids, which are without adverse effects. Acetylsalicylic acid and dextropropoxyphene are just as good as acetaminophen from an analgesic point of view, but in clinical practice have been shown to have substantial adverse effects (bleeding tendency and liver toxicity, respectively) and should therefore not be used routinely. If further potentiation is needed, codeine and other nonopioid analgesic drugs can be used, but always in combination with acetaminophen. Codeine may be considered an opioid drug but can be included in this concept.

If these measures are insufficient, other drugs should be considered. Neuroleptics may be used to potentiate the other drugs, although some patients become drowsy, with little pain relief, and may experience dysphoria. If there is some degree of anxiety, benzodiazepines are a better choice. The modern selective serotonin reuptake inhibitors (SSRIs) can also be used successfully in some patients, but never on a routine basis: some sadness is a natural and realistic reaction to the disease, and only if there are signs of medically defined depression should SSRIs be recommended.

It is important to make sure the patient sleeps well. However, many of these patients have too little to do during the daytime and will therefore not be tired at night, especially if they also sleep during the day. Therefore activation during the day may be the best way to treat insomnia at night. A short nap at noon is not a problem, but the patient must then be active during the afternoon. Only when all these measures have been tried should sleeping pills be used.

Step 3 (Fig. 51.4)
As a "pure" analgesic drug there is nothing better than morphine or its derivatives. However, whether hydromorphone, fentanyl, oxycodone, or some other drug should be given instead of morphine mostly depends on the experience of the doctor. There is little indication that any one of these drugs is significantly better than another. Therefore it is a good rule of thumb to use few opioids but to be well acquainted with the one usually used.

The half-life of morphine is 2–4 hours, while its clinically relevant pain-relieving effects usually last 3–5 hours. In renal failure, the metabolites can accumulate in the body, and thus patients with reduced kidney function must be observed more closely after receiving repeated doses of morphine. There is wide individual variation in plasma opioid concentrations, but no sim-

---

Morphine
  10 mg as often as patient needed (tablets if patient not
    vomiting)
  When steady state: long-acting twice daily
  Transcutaneously delivered drugs more expensive but
    good for patients with stable level of pain

Go to step 4 if excessive adverse effects, such as:
  Rapidly increasing demand
  Inability to cooperate with pain treatment
  Akathisia
  Decreasing effect (tachyphylaxis)
  Severe obstipation
  Drowsiness to apathy, inability to resume activities of
    daily life

Figure 51.4 The analgesic ladder: step 3.

ple correlation between opioid and metabolite concentrations and pain relief has been found, although there is a report of a tendency toward greater stable phase morphine concentrations in cancer patients with optimal pain control.

Besides the peroral route, which is the route of choice ordinarily, there are several other ways to administer opioids: sublingual, subcutaneous, intravenous, epidural/intrathecal, transdermal, and rectal, but not intramuscular as this can be painful, particularly for debilitated patients with wasted muscles. All the different routes have their special advantages and disadvantages.

If morphine is used, it is wise to start with 10 mg on demand, i.e., when the patient asks for it (tablets if patient not vomiting, otherwise rectal administration). This course of action not only allows patients to become pain-free but also helps to reassure them that the use of morphine can always lead to freedom from pain: it is just a question of dosage. When a steady dosage of morphine has been achieved, it will be easier for the patient to use long-acting formulas twice daily. This means that the patient receives the same amount of morphine but on a fixed schedule and not on demand. If needed (i.e., for "breakthrough" pain), ordinary morphine tablets (10 mg) are used as a complement. If this supplement is used regularly, the dosage of the long-acting drug is increased. However, it should be emphasized to the patient that long-acting drugs do not reach a steady state until after 5 days, and sometimes not until after 10 days. Thus the dosage should not be changed more often than once a week; usually it is changed once a month.

Transcutaneously delivered drugs are more expensive but have some advantages for patients who are experiencing a stable level of pain. Firstly, the patient does not have to think about medication more than once every third day and does not need to worry about missed doses. From the doctor's point of view one can expect total compliance. On the negative side, there are some patients who experience less effect with the transcutaneous route, probably because of individual skin properties and blood circulation. Also, the dosage can be changed only in rather large steps and it is impractical to change the dosage more than once every 6 or 9 days.

Sedation and nausea occur particularly when starting the drug, although this is usually temporary but may recur with dose increases. Nausea can be avoided by using a centrally acting antiemetic prophylactically. Sedation is usually unavoidable but short-lived (48–72 hours) among patients starting off on low doses.

There is no clinically relevant ceiling in analgesia: doses of oral morphine may be varied 1000-fold or more in order to achieve the same end point of pain relief. A change of opioid may be tried if pain relief with one opioid is inadequate or unacceptable adverse effects occur, especially when pain management requires increasing dose escalation. It cannot be overemphasized that pain is multifactorial and that successful treatment depends on comprehensive evaluation. For the suffering patient it is important that the pain be treated quickly when needed, which indicates the use of an opioid with a rather short half-life. Once stable, sustained-release formulations reduce dose frequency to once or twice daily. Breakthrough pain is controlled with extra doses of the unmodified drug (calculated as one-sixth of the total 24-hour opioid dose requirement). Drugs with a very short half-life (e.g., pethidine) are unsuitable because of the need for more frequent repeat dosing, which is inconvenient and may cause build-up of toxic metabolites. Drugs with inherently long half-lives (e.g., methadone) may be difficult to titrate safely in unstable pain. Many patients with pancreatic cancer are elderly and have concurrent medical conditions, both of which may influence the pharmacokinetics of opioids. Renal impairment is most important as it affects clearance of many opioids. There is a recommendation that conventional dose intervals should be increased by about 50% at moderately reduced renal clearance. Concurrent drug therapy can also alter opioid pharmacokinetics.

Generally, at least 90% of pancreatic cancer patients with pain will be effectively treated by steps 1–3. However, if opioids have excessive adverse effects, step 4 may be tried. Such adverse effects may include not only rapidly increasing demand for drug and inability to cooperate with pain treatment, but also akathisia and tachyphylaxis (decreasing effect). One of the most troublesome adverse effects for many patients is obstipation. This is due to the direct effects of opioids on gut motility, but also to low intake of food and water and an overly sedentary lifestyle. Because this is so common, all patients given opioids on a regular basis should receive prophylaxis against obstipation, such as lactulose once daily.

Some patients experience drowsiness approaching apathy and feel unable to resume activities of daily life

Subcutaneous/intravenous infusion pump (morphine/ fentanyl)
Attack the celiac plexus
  Resection or block at laparostomy
  Block at angiography
  Block at ultrasonography, computed tomography, endoscopic ultrasound, or fluoroscopy
Thoracoscopic splanchnicectomy
Epidural block (morphine/bupivacaine)
Transcutaneous nerve stimulation
Chordotomy

Figure 51.5 The analgesic ladder: step 4.

and so on. When it is obvious that the patient feels that life is of very limited value, alternatives should be considered. There is no evidence that the use of high-dose opiates in the palliative chronic setting leads to a dangerous level of respiratory depression, not even among patients with respiratory impairment.

Step 4 (Fig. 51.5)
For some patients subcutaneous or intravenous infusion pumps administering morphine and fentanyl have good effects. An advantage is that patients can to some degree increase the dosage on demand, usually with an upper limit to prevent a suddenly confused patient self-administering an overdose. Often the patient can include the procedure in their daily lives, but for some it is not acceptable to be dependent on mechanical devices. Old people especially dislike it, as they have difficulties learning how to handle the devices.

Epidural block with morphine and bupivacaine provides the required pain relief but there is an increased risk of adverse effects, such as intraspinal infections, pneumonia, urinary infections, and gastrointestinal disturbances. Also, the patient needs qualified medical attention on a 24-hour basis.

The nerves in the pancreas comprise sympathetic, parasympathetic, sensory, and motor fibers. The sensory fibers mediating pain are conducted toward the central nervous system, without synapsing, via the celiac plexus and the splanchinc nerves to the thoracic spinal cord. From a theoretic point of view, the pain can be inhibited by cutting the nerve fibers anywhere along this path.

Celiac plexus block is a neurolytic block of the celiac plexus. For a long time, a block using 50% alcohol was the most common and best-described therapy for the specific back pain in patients with pancreatic carcinoma, a good result being expected in the majority of cases. It can be performed intraoperatively or by a percutaneous approach, from the back or from the abdomen. The percutaneous route can be guided by the bony landmarks, by fluoroscopy, by angiography, or by ultrasonography, computed tomography, or magnetic resonance imaging. The choice between the different methods cannot be determined from the results of randomized studies, probably due to large differences in skill of the performers of different approaches but also to the different traditions underlying those skills. However, randomized trials show a clear advantage for patients treated with celiac plexus block during surgery compared with untreated patients. One problem is that tumor masses may displace the celiac plexus, and when using the classical method guided by bony landmarks the success rate varies from 33 to 94%. The limited use of the technique is due to its short duration (usually a mean of about 3 months in successful cases), its dependence on individual skill, and the effectiveness of the pharmacologic alternatives.

Thoracoscopic splanchnicectomy has been used since the mid-1990s. It is a safe and easy procedure that undoubtedly helps some patients with severe pain. However, the method's place in the algorithm of pain management in pancreatic cancer is still not settled due to lack of appropriate data on effectiveness, which in turn may be due to attempts to treat not only patients with localized painful disease but also those with pain emanating from ingrowth into the abdominal wall, sensory pain afferents from which do not travel through the splanchnic nerves.

Whether drainage of a pretumoral dilatated pancreatic duct provides pain relief in pancreatic cancer is not documented. There are also single reports of transcutaneous nerve stimulation, intrapleural block, and chordotomy. These types of procedures should only be used in specialist centers with both sufficient experience and the ability to evaluate each method.

Evaluation of treatment options

Patients with established pancreatic cancer do not present uniformly with regard to stage of the disease (early or late), extrapancreatic secondary symptomatology, or morphologic features. This also influences the pattern of pain and the outcome of attempts to manage not only the symptoms but the patient as a whole. The major goal of new treatment modalities must be improvement of the patient's quality of life, which has many dimensions.

To compare the efficacy of different treatments, it is necessary to have a baseline inventory of the patient's general health status. However, even in the most recent literature there is no consensus on a standard method for assessing pain relief and improved quality of life. In the absence of such a standard method, it is recommended that the European Organisation for Research and Treatment of Cancer (EORTC) QLQ-30 is used. This questionnaire consists of a core of 30 generally applicable items and includes scales on physical functioning; role of functioning; cognitive, emotional, and social functioning; pain; fatigue; and nausea and vomiting. This may be used together with its pancreas-specific part, PAN26, which includes scales on pancreatic pain, digestive function, bowel habit, body image, satisfaction with care, and sexuality.

Summary and options for the future

The principal prerequisite for treating pain optimally in patients with pancreatic cancer is good personal contact with the patient on a regular basis, so that doctor and patient can try to agree to cooperate. This may be hard if the patient is frightened of the disease. However, if the patient has confidence in the doctor's management, he or she will be able to withstand more pain without escalating analgesic use, and the treatment can be seen from a long-term and holistic perspective. Therefore, continuity of the patient–doctor relationship is of the utmost importance in these patients. An established relationship between the patient and the doctor, whether surgeon, oncologist, general practitioner, or gastroenterologist, helps evaluation of each attempt to optimize treatment. Pharmacologic treatment of pain is of the utmost importance in patients with pancreatic cancer, but it is not the only option and it should be seen as *one* option that is strengthened by others.

Recommended reading

Aaronson NK, Ahmedzai S, Bergman B *et al.* The European

Organisation for Research and Treatment of Cancer QLQ-C30: a quality-of-life instrument for use in international clinical trials in oncology. *J Natl Cancer Inst* 1993;85:365–376.

Andrén-Sandberg Å. Pain relief in pancreatic disease (editorial). *Br J Surg* 1997;84:1041–1042.

Bockman DE, Büchler M, Malfertheiner P, Beger H. Analysis of nerves in chronic pancreatitis. *Gastroenterology* 1988;94:1459–1469.

Fitzsimmons D, Johnson CD, George S *et al*. Development of a disease specific quality of life (QoL) questionnaire module to supplement the EORTC core cancer QoL questionnaire, the QLQ-C30 in patients with pancreatic cancer. *Eur J Cancer* 1999;35:939–941.

Grahm AL, Andrén-Sandberg Å. Prospective evaluation of pain in exocrine pancreatic cancer. *Digestion* 1997;58:572–579.

Ihse I, Zoucas E, Gyllstedt E, Lillo-Gil R, Andrén-Sandberg Å. Bilateral thoracoscopic splanchnicectomy: effects on pancreatic pain and function. *Ann Surg* 1999;230:785–791.

Ischia S, Ischia A, Polati E, Finco G. Three posterior percutaneous celiac plexus block techniques. A prospective, randomised study in 61 patients with pancreatic cancer pain. *Anesthesiology* 1992;76:534–540.

52

What is the optimal surgical treatment for resectable pancreatic cancer?

Beat M. Künzli, Helmut Friess, and Markus W. Büchler

Introduction

Pancreatic cancer is still a devastating disease that is presently the fourth or fifth leading cause of cancer-related death in Western countries, with a poor prognosis even after tumor resection. Approximately 150 000 people worldwide and 40 000 people in Europe die each year of pancreatic cancer, making it one of the five leading causes of death associated with cancer and one of the most aggressive human tumors. An overall 5-year survival of less than 1% is frequently reported and little progress has been achieved in the last decades. It is still a challenging task to diagnose pancreatic cancer in early tumor stages, the chance of cure being higher the lower the disease stage. However, the overall resectability rate of pancreatic cancer is only 10–15%, although rates ranging from 0.4 to 33% are reported. On the other hand, rapid tumor progression and poor responsiveness to chemotherapy, radiotherapy, immunotherapy, and antihormonal treatment contribute to the poor prognosis. These facts together result in low tumor resectability rates after diagnosis, early tumor recurrence after resection, and poor overall survival rates. The survival rates are not at all satisfactory and reach a median of only 10–18 months. In the last decade surgical outcomes have improved, mostly because of better perioperative treatment. Begg *et al.* and Birkmeyer *et al.* demonstrate that operation-related morbidity and mortality has significantly decreased in centers with high patient load. This critical aspect of the value of centralization on the outcome of pancreatic surgery in high-volume institutions has been demonstrated in several studies. The current mortality rate following pancreatic resection is below 5% in specialized

surgical centers and thereby significantly lower than in units with a low frequency of pancreatic surgery. Pancreatic anastomosis was long considered to be the critical step and represented the main cause of morbidity and death in pancreatic surgery. To reduce morbidity, the concept of secretory inhibition of the pancreas by octreotide was investigated in large, randomized, placebo-controlled, multicenter trials and by meta-analysis, which demonstrated the effectiveness of octreotide with regard to postoperative complications and costs. These nonsurgical improvements combined with better surgical quality and postoperative care in high-volume centers have improved postoperative patient outcome. These parameters are also contributing to the improvement of postoperative quality of life. Unfortunately, they have not yet improved the curability rate of patients suffering from pancreatic cancer.

What procedures are presently available for resectable pancreatic cancer?

Classical Kausch–Whipple procedure

Pancreaticoduodenectomy, as described by Allen O. Whipple in 1935, is still the standard operation for pancreatic head carcinoma, as well as for ampullary and distal bile duct cancer. In the years preceding 1935, most surgeons avoided pancreatic resection and favored the use of gastroenterostomy to reconstruct food passage in patients with pancreatic malignancies because of fear of resection-related postoperative complications (e.g., anastomotic leakage). Although Walter Kausch had already reported the first successful duodenopancreatectomy in 1912, this procedure was not immediately accepted by surgeons due to high mortality. For the next two decades after Kausch's report, surgeons were hesitant to employ duodenopancreatectomy as the treatment of choice in patients with pancreatic head tumors. Interest in pancreatic resections was renewed, however, when Allen O. Whipple reported three successful duodenopancreatectomies in 1935. The procedure became to be known and standardized as the Whipple procedure in honor of this surgeon who performed 37 pancreatic resections in his lifetime.

Approximately 60–70% of all pancreatic cancers are located in the head of the pancreas and the Kausch–Whipple resection is considered the operation of choice for these particular patients. A survey of surgeons in the USA revealed that two-thirds of the resections for pancreatic head cancer were performed by the Kausch–Whipple method.

The procedure consists of complete resection of the pancreatic head (transection of the pancreas above the portal vein/superior mesenteric vein), duodenum, distal part of the stomach, common bile duct, and gallbladder. The ligamentum of Treitz is divided and the first part of the jejunum is also dissected and resected. To achieve tumor-free margins it may be necessary to resect the mentericoportal vein and/or accessory organ structures. Dissection and removal of the lymph-node stations with the standard, radical, and extended radical procedures is discussed later (Fig. 52.1).

Pylorus-preserving Whipple operation

An organ-preserving alternative to the classical Kausch–Whipple procedure is known as the pylorus-preserving Whipple. This operation was originally performed by Kenneth Watson in 1942, an English surgeon who used this particular procedure on a patient with ampullary cancer. However, 33 years before this Walter Kausch had performed a pylorus-preserving pancreatic head resection, although he did not take advantage of the preserved pylorus and performed a gastrojejunostomy instead of a duodeno (pyloro)jejunostomy for food passage. Watson found it advantageous to preserve the integrity of the stomach since the incidence of postoperative jejunal ulcerations was less than in patients who underwent partial gastrectomy. Nevertheless, nearly 40 years later, in 1978, the publication of Traverso and Longmire reintroduced the pylorus-preserving pancreatic head resection to the surgical world. Their arguments were similar to those of Watson, reasoning that the preservation of the stomach leads not only to less postoperative ulcer complications but also reduces the adverse effects of the gastroenterostomy. In the following years, more and more surgeons switched to the pylorus-preserving Whipple for the treatment of pancreatic head cancer and tumors of the periampullary region, even though use of the pylorus-preserving Whipple was contested at the beginning (Fig. 52.2).

Depending on the extent of lymphadenectomy, three different radical approaches are described here inde-

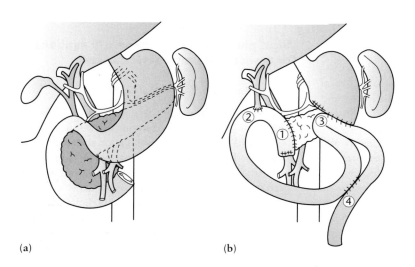

(a)   (b)

Figure 52.1 Classical Whipple operation. (a) Normal situs before the operation. (b) Pancreatic head resection has been performed with the following anastomoses: 1, pancreatojejunostomy; 2, choledochojejunostomy; 3, gastrojejunostomy; 4, Braun'sche anastomosis.

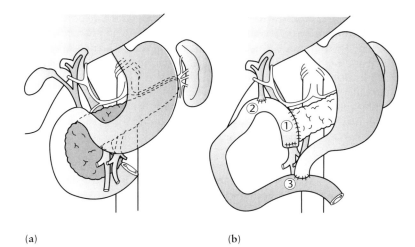

Figure 52.2 Pylorus-preserving Whipple operation. (a) Normal situs before the operation. (b) Pancreatic head resection has been performed with the following anastomoses: 1, pancreatojejunostomy; 2, choledochojejunostomy; 3, gastrojejunostomy.

(a)　　　　　　　　　　　　　　　　**(b)**

pendently to demonstrate whether the pylorus is preserved or not (classical Kausch–Whipple or pylorus-preserving Whipple): standard, radical, and extended radical pancreatoduodenectomy.

1 Standard pancreatoduodenectomy: encompasses regional lymphadenectomy around the duodenum and resected pancreas.

2 Radical pancreatoduodenectomy: encompasses regional lymphadenectomy plus skeletonization of the hepatic arteries, the superior mesenteric artery between aorta and the inferior pancreaticoduodenal and celiac trunk, and dissection of the anterolateral aspect of the aorta and vena cava including Gerota's fascia.

3 Extended radical pancreatoduodenectomy: encompasses radical lymphadenectomy plus clearance of the anterior aorta between the diaphragmatic hiatus (around the celiac trunk) and the origin of the common iliac arteries.

Pancreatic left resection

The standard surgical therapy for pancreatic cancer left lateral of the portal vein (pancreatic corpus and/or tail) is the pancreatic left resection with splenectomy (also named distal pancreatectomy). Left resections that reach this imaginary orientation mark of the portal vein are described as classical left resections; more right lateral resections are described as extended left resections. Subtotal pancreatic left resection of up to 95% of the pancreatic parenchyma is named Child's operation.

Carcinomas of the pancreatic corpus and tail are more infrequent and are often diagnosed in advanced disease. Pancreatic left resection comprises removal of the pancreatic corpus and tail together with the peripancreatic lymph nodes and the spleen in order to achieve sufficiently radical surgery. The choice of resection margin is dependent on the progression and location of the tumor. Closure of the pancreatic stump can be performed in two principal ways: blind closure of the stump or pancreaticointestinal anastomosis (with the jejunum/stomach).

Depending on the extent of lymphadenectomy, two different procedures are identified: standard and radical.

1 Standard left resection: encompasses regional lymphadenectomy, including lymph-node groups at the celiac trunk, hilum of the spleen, splenic artery, and inferior border of the body and tail of the pancreas.

2 Radical left resection: encompasses regional lymphadenectomy plus lymphadenectomy along the hepatic artery and of the anterolateral aspect of the aorta and vena cava including Gerota's fascia.

Adenocarcinomas of the pancreatic corpus and tail are often diagnosed when the tumor is no longer locally resectable or when distant metastases (most frequently in the liver) are present. Therefore, the median survival time of patients with pancreatic corpus and tail carcinomas is generally shorter compared with those with pancreatic head carcinomas. Extended radical operations are possible and increase the resectability rate. Japanese studies provide evidence that extended resections can improve the curative (R0) resection rate.

437

Konoshi *et al.* demonstrated that resection of the truncus celiacus with a partial reconstruction of the hepatic artery and portal vein is a more radical operation for pancreatic body and tail carcinomas. A monocentric study by Sohn *et al.*, including 616 patients with resected adenocarcinoma of the pancreas, underlines the above-mentioned aspects. Of the 616 patients, 526 (85%) underwent pancreaticoduodenectomy for adenocarcinoma of the head, neck, or uncinate process of the pancreas, 52 (9%) underwent distal pancreatectomy/left resection for adenocarcinoma of the body or tail, and 38 (6%) underwent total pancreatectomy for adenocarcinoma involving the whole gland. Patients undergoing left pancreatic resection for left-sided tumors had larger tumors but less frequent lymph-node metastases and fewer poorly differentiated tumors as compared with those undergoing pancreaticoduodenectomy for right-sided cancer. The survival of the entire group was 63% at 1 year and 17% at 5 years, with a median survival of 17 months. For right-sided lesions the 1-year and 5-year survival rates were 64% and 17% respectively compared with 50% and 15% for left-sided lesions. Why left-sided tumors have a worse prognosis in this study, even though the included left-sided pancreatic carcinomas had fewer lymph-node metastases, is not evident. However, in left-sided tumors the diameter of the tumor seems to be more important for prognosis than lymph-node status. Without question, the completeness of resection and the biological characteristics, including tumor size and its ability to metastasize in surrounding tissue, are important prognostic indicators.

In another study enroling 590 patients with pancreatic corpus and tail carcinoma, only patients with lymph node-negative tumors with a diameter below 4 cm and without distant metastases showed a survival benefit. Patients with distant metastases independent of the surgical procedure (resection, bypass, or exploration) showed an average survival time of only 3.4 months. If lymph-node involvement was present, there was no difference in survival time between resected tumors and palliative surgical procedures. Patients without metastases and negative lymph nodes showed 1-year and 3-year survival rates of 38% and 12% respectively after resection. However, the resectability rate achieved only 10%, which is, in comparison with other studies, much lower. Although the long-term survival data in patients with left-sided pancreatic carcinoma are still unsatisfactory, no other therapy

achieves better survival rates or disease-free intervals than resection. Early establishment of the diagnosis and early and more aggressive surgery might improve the rate of resection and thereby the prognosis.

Total pancreatectomy

The first total pancreatectomy was performed by Ross in 1954 and reported in the same year by Porter. In 1960, Howard reported a perioperative mortality rate of 37% for total pancreatectomy, which was the main reason why this particular procedure was not accepted by most surgeons at that time. However, because the classical Whipple procedure could not fulfill initial expectations, based on the high perioperative mortality, total pancreatectomy was for a short time considered the appropriate procedure to improve short- and long-term survival of patients with pancreatic cancer. Total pancreatectomy combines the standard pancreatoduodenectomy (Whipple procedure) with a pancreatic left resection including a splenectomy. The entire pancreas with all lymph nodes along the left gastric artery, the splenic artery, and the celiac trunk are removed. Reconstruction is by an end-to-side hepaticojejunostomy and a gastroenterostomy. Initially, total pancreatectomy seemed to have several advantages compared with the Whipple operation. Some authors described that multicentric tumors often appear in the entire pancreas and therefore the removal of the whole organ (total pancreatectomy) is necessary. Moreover, pancreatic anastomosis, which had a high rate of complications at the time, could be avoided. As a result, perioperative morbidity and mortality could be potentially diminished when performing a total pancreatectomy. People also believed that a more radical procedure would improve the postoperative survival time. These are some of the reasons why total pancreatectomy was chosen by many surgeons and was considered an appropriate procedure in patients with pancreatic cancer. However, total pancreatectomy has many disadvantages that cannot offset the described advantages. Perioperative mortality and long-term survival proved to be the same as in the Whipple procedure. A major disadvantage of total pancreatectomy is the deterioration of the metabolic condition and the presence of insulin-dependent diabetes mellitus, with difficulties in handling blood sugar levels. Furthermore, in the long term total pancreatectomy is associated with an increased incidence of liver diseases and osteopenia. However, the death of patients with uncontrollable diabetes mellitus and impaired quality of life is the reason why total pancreatectomy was not accepted as a standard operation in pancreatic cancer patients. These disadvantages, together with the fact that a safe pancreatic anastomosis can nowadays be safely performed in experienced hands, led to the conclusion that total pancreatectomy is not justified as a routine procedure for pancreatic cancer and should be restricted to only a few indications: when the tumor is expanding over the whole pancreas, where several multilocular tumors are present in the pancreas, or where pancreatic anastomosis is technically not performable.

Controversies in pancreatic cancer surgery

Cancer of the head of the pancreas: what is the adequate operation?

More than 60% of all pancreatic cancers appear in the head of the pancreas. In these cases, pancreatoduodenectomy (classical Kausch–Whipple or pyloruspreserving Whipple) is considered the operation of choice. However, the question which type of Whipple operation is best is still controversial.

Several randomized controlled studies have been performed that compared the classical Kausch–Whipple with pylorus-preserving Whipple operation. Lin *et al.* demonstrated in a study with 15 patients who had undergone classical Kausch–Whipple procedure and 16 patients with pylorus-preserving Whipple that both procedures are comparable with regard to operation time and postoperative morbidity and mortality rates. Only delayed gastric emptying was reported more frequently (but was not statistically significant) in the group of patients with pylorus-preserving Whipple. Wenger *et al.* examined 24 patients with the classical Kausch–Whipple and 34 patients with pyloruspreserving Whipple operation. This study also did not reveal any difference in operation-related morbidity and mortality. However, the classical Whipple procedure needed a longer operation time and resulted in a reduced quality of life compared with the pyloruspreserving Whipple. The study that enrolled the largest patient population so far was published by Seiler *et al.* This compared 51 patients with classical Kausch–Whipple procedure and 42 patients with pyloruspreserving Whipple. Mortality was again comparable in the two groups, as well as the occurrence of delayed gastric emptying. The classical Kausch–Whipple procedure showed a prolonged operation time and was associated with a higher perioperative morbidity. Apart from this, it should be emphasized that in this study both procedures showed no difference in quality of life and long-term survival.

Taken together, the data show that the pyloruspreserving Whipple procedure is as effective as the classical Kausch–Whipple procedure without any difference in postoperative morbidity and quality of life. Therefore, the pylorus-preserving Whipple is becoming more accepted and more frequently performed because this procedure preserves the organ and requires less operation time. However, more randomized controlled studies with larger patient groups are needed to prove the definite advantages and disadvantages of both procedures for pancreatic cancer surgery.

Anastomosis of the pancreas: which type of drainage should be performed?

An area of continuing controversy is which technique is best for fashioning the pancreatic anastomosis. Some surgeons insert the stump of the pancreas into the stomach (pancreatogastrostomy), whereas most surgeons prefer to perform a pancreatojejunostomy. Neither technique has shown clear superiority to the other; rather, it is the experience and technical skills of the surgeon that result in uneventful anastomotic healing.

In our department, the pancreatic stump is anastomosed with the jejunum as described previously, i.e., a two-layer single-stitch pancreaticojejunostomy (5/0 PDS outer suture rows: seromuscular on to the pancreatic capsule/parenchyma; inner suture rows: mucosa to duct mucosa of the pancreatic duct) (Fig. 52.3). From November 1993 to May 1999, in 331 consecutive operations for patients undergoing pancreatic head resections (133 pylorus-preserving Whipple and 83 classical Kausch–Whipple procedures), the pancreatic fistula rate was 0% for the classical Kausch–Whipple and 3% in the pylorus-preserving Whipple. These data clearly demonstrate that a pancreatojejunostomy performed by experienced hands and in a center with a high patient load can be a safe operative procedure. Although such low fistula rates have not been reported after pancreatogastrostomy, the surgeon has to decide which procedure works out best in his hands. Pancreatogastrostomy might be a suitable method

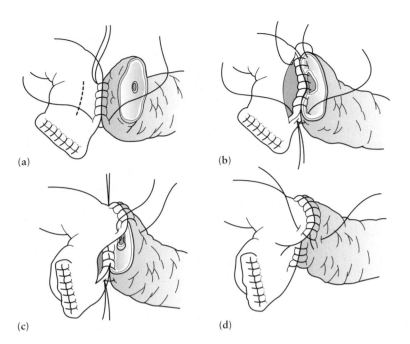

(a)

(b)

(c)

(d)

Figure 52.3 Technique of pancreatojejunostomy. A two-layer single-stitch pancreaticojejunostomy is performed: (a, d) 5/0 PDS outer suture rows: seromuscular on to the pancreatic capsule/parenchyma; (b, c) inner suture rows: mucosa to duct mucosa of the pancreatic.

in small surgical centers with a low caseload of pancreatic resections because this technique may simplify the anastomotic technique and help to reduce pancreatic fistula and subsequent postoperative complications and deaths related to partial pancreatoduodenectomy.

Left-sided pancreatic resections are usually performed without anastomosis, although in some cases a pancreaticointestinal anastomosis has to be considered. Perioperative and postoperative administration of octreotide (a synthetic somatostatin analog that inhibits exocrine pancreatic secretion) can also reduce resection-related postoperative morbidity.

Extent of lymphadenectomy: does more extended lymphadenectomy improve the prognosis?

Despite the progress made in pancreatic surgery, the long-term survival of patients with pancreatic cancer is still unsatisfactory. At the time of diagnosis, about 80% of patients have lymph-node and/or distant metastases. Most of the resected patients develop local recurrence and/or distant metastases after resection. Therefore, we have to ask whether more radical surgery could im-

prove the long-term outcome of patients with pancreatic cancer.

Japanese surgeons have developed the technique of extended lymphadenectomy for pancreatic cancer, which is based on the principle of regional lymphadenectomy. Depending on tumor location and the surgical technique, this procedure includes excision of all lymph-node stations around the aorta, vena cava, superior and inferior mesenteric artery, splenic artery, and celiac trunk. Many variations of extended lymphadenectomy are described, mainly by Japanese surgeons. However, only one prospective, randomized, controlled trial comprising a limited number of patients has been performed to judge whether extended lymph-node dissection is of any survival benefit.

Pedrazzoli *et al.* examined 81 patients undergoing pancreaticoduodenal resection for a potentially curable ductal adenocarcinoma of the head of the pancreas. Using a multicenter approach, a total of 40 patients were randomized to the standard lymphadenectomy group and 41 to the extended lymphadenectomy group. Standard lymphadenectomy included removal of the anterior and posterior pancreatoduodenal, pyloric and biliary duct, superior and inferior pancreatic head and pancreatic body lymph nodes. In addition to the above, extended lymphadenectomy included the removal of lymph nodes from the hepatic hilum and along the aorta from the diaphragmatic hiatus to the inferior mesenteric artery and laterally to both renal hila, with circumferential clearance to the origin of the celiac trunk and superior mesenteric artery. Transfusion requirements, postoperative morbidity and mortality rates, and overall survival did not differ between the two lymphadenectomy groups. Only when subgroups of patients were analyzed (not planned when the study was designed) was there a significantly ($P < 0.05$) longer survival rate in lymph node-positive patients after extended (18 months) compared with standard lymphadenectomy (11 months). Nevertheless, the survival curves in node-negative patients did not differ according to the magnitude of lymphadenectomy. The conclusion of this study is simple: the addition of extended lymphadenectomy and retroperitoneal soft-tissue clearance to pancreaticoduodenectomy does not significantly increase morbidity and mortality rates but, in general, does not influence long-term survival rate.

Johns Hopkins University has also investigated the influence of the extent of lymphadenectomy in a study with 294 patients, 146 receiving standard and 148 radical lymphadenectomy. All patients in the radical group underwent distal gastric resection, whereas 86% of the patients in the standard group underwent pylorus preservation. The mean operative time in the radical group was 6.4 hours compared with 5.9 hours in the standard group. There were no significant differences between the two groups with respect to intraoperative blood loss, transfusion requirements, location of the tumor, mean tumor size, positive lymph-node status, or positive margin status on final permanent sections. The overall complication rates were 29% for the standard group compared with 43% for the radical group, with patients in the radical group having significantly higher rates of early delayed gastric emptying and pancreatic fistula and a significantly longer mean postoperative hospital stay. What was most interesting in this trial was that there was absolutely no difference in long-term survival between the two lymphadenectomy groups.

Taken together, all the data fail to demonstrate a survival benefit of distal gastrectomy and/or extended lymphadenectomy compared with standard resection in patients with pancreatic cancer.

Perspectives: multimodality treatment and modern strategies with pancreatic resection

There is no doubt that surgical resection, as compared with nonresection, offers significantly longer median survival times and a fairly good chance for cure, if the tumor is resectable. However, even though small tumors (< 3 cm in diameter) have a significantly better prognosis than larger tumors after resection, they nevertheless have high recurrence rates and only limited survival rates. Since resection alone may not result in disease control, several adjuvant therapies, such as radiotherapy and chemotherapy, have been tested to improve the surgical outcome after resection of pancreatic cancer.

The Gastrointestinal Tumor Study Group (GITSG) trial suggested that adjuvant postoperative radiochemotherapy (40 Gy radiotherapy combined with fluorouracil and then weekly fluorouracil for 2 years) improves the short- and long-term prognosis of patients with R0-resected pancreatic cancer. The median survival time of 20 months versus 11 months and 5-year survival rates of 20% versus 5%, respectively, were significantly longer in 21 patients receiving radiochemotherapy compared with 22 nontreated patients. However, the results of the European Organization for Research and Treatment of Cancer (EORTC) Gastrointestinal Tract Cancer Cooperative Group trial, in which 114 patients with pancreatic cancer were randomized (60 for treatment, 54 for observation) using the same protocol as in the GITSG study, contradicted that study by suggesting that radiochemotherapy does not prolong survival in resected patients with pancreatic cancer (17.1 months in treated vs. 12.6 months in nontreated patients and 2-year survival rate of 51% vs. 41% respectively; $P > 0.05$). In February 1994 the European Study Group of Pancreatic Cancer (ESPAC) initiated a randomized adjuvant study with a 2×2 factorial design to compare postoperative radiochemotherapy, six cycles of chemotherapy (5-fluorouracil plus folinic acid), and a combination of postoperative radiochemotherapy followed by six cycles of chemotherapy with no adjuvant treatment (observation arm) in patients with R0 or R1 resected pancreatic cancer. Radiotherapy was given as external beam radiotherapy following recovery from surgery, with 5-fluorouracil given as a radiosensitizing agent. A course of 40 Gy using megavoltage equipment was given in two split courses of 20 Gy in two 2-week periods with a 2-week rest period in between. On each of the first 3 days of each 20-Gy segment of radiation therapy, 5-fluorouracil 500 mg/m^2 body surface area was administered intravenously as a bolus. Systemic chemotherapy with folinic acid was given as an intravenous bolus injection of 20 mg/m^2, followed by 5-fluorouracil as an intravenous bolus injection of 425 mg/m^2. Chemotherapy was given for five consecutive days every 28 days for six cycles for a total of 28 weeks.

At a median follow-up of 10 months, 227 patients (42%) were alive. Overall results showed no benefit of chemoradiation (median survival 15.5 months in 175 patients with chemoradiation vs. 16.1 months in 178 patients without, $P = 0.24$). However, there was strong evidence of a survival benefit of chemotherapy (median survival 19.7 months in 238 patients with chemotherapy vs. 14.0 months in 235 patients without, $P = 0.0005$). The effect was reduced when taking into account whether patients also received chemoradiotherapy ($P = 0.001$), indicating that chemoradiotherapy may reduce the overall survival benefit of chemotherapy. A recent analysis of the ESPAC-1 data with a median follow-up of 24 months confirmed the previous findings, indicating that adjuvant chemotherapy with 5-fluorouracil and folinic acid is of benefit in resected pancreatic cancer (data not published, but presented at the EPC meeting in Liverpool, June 2003).

Since recurrence of resected pancreatic cancer occurs in the pancreatic bed (retropancreatic space) and in the liver, the combination of radical tumor resection with regional adjuvant chemotherapy and intraoperative radiotherapy might be a logical consequence for survival improvement. Using this concept, a 5-year survival rate of 32% was reported. Presently the concept of adjuvant regional chemotherapy is being tested in a prospective randomized trial by ESPAC (ESPAC-2). Furthermore, new trials testing gemcitabine in an adjuvant setting are also presently running (e.g., ESPAC-3).

Discussion

Elective pancreatic resections have developed into safe surgical procedures and current mortality rates in specialized centers have decreased to 2–5%. Several concepts to increase the safety of pancreatic surgery have been adopted into clinical routine. Among these are the formation of pancreatic centers with high caseload, standardized perioperative management including secretory inhibition of the pancreas, and various methods to increase the safety of pancreatic resection and the formation of a proper pancreaticointestinal anastomosis. Centralization as a concept for reducing postoperative morbidity and mortality has been demonstrated in many surgical areas including pancreas surgery and may be more important in improving postoperative outcomes than differences in surgical technique.

The pylorus-preserving Whipple operation represents one of the most significant recent advances in pancreatic cancer surgery. It is as radical as the classical Kausch–Whipple operation and is associated with a decrease in operation time and reduced blood loss since gastric resection is omitted. Furthermore, access to the biliary anastomosis may be more easily accomplished for postoperative endoscopic investigations than after the classical Kausch–Whipple procedure. The perioperative morbidity and mortality of the pylorus-preserving Whipple procedure seems to be lower or at least similar to that of the classical Kausch–Whipple operation. In addition, preservation of the pylorus seems to result in improved postoperative weight gain and improved quality of life compared with the classical Kausch–Whipple procedure. All these arguments lead to the conclusion that the pylorus-preserving Whipple should be favored over the classical Kausch–Whipple whenever the tumor can safely be R0-resected, because it preserves gastric integrity. In relation to postoperative gastrointestinal function, there are no data showing that one operative procedure is superior to another. However, the pylorus-preserving Whipple tends to show a lower postoperative complication rate in relation to the upper gastrointestinal tract. Based on prospective randomized trials, the pylorus-preserving Whipple should be the surgical procedure of choice for pancreatic, especially periampullary, tumors.

Until now, there have been very few prospective, randomized, controlled trials that could provide unbiased answers to these important questions. This is also the main reason why there is no conclusive evidence-based statement about which surgical procedure is best for pancreatic neoplasms in relation to radical surgery, long-term survival, postoperative mortality and morbidity, quality of life after surgery, intraoperative blood loss, and operation time. The data available today are based mostly on retrospective analysis or prospective studies with low patient numbers on the one hand and mostly monocentric studies on the other. Unbiased, controlled, and prospective randomized trials, with large numbers of patients and, whenever possible, a multicenter design, are urgently needed. These types of studies would have the potential to reveal whether today's proposed strategies for the therapy of patients with pancreatic cancer are based on real evidence or whether they can only be reproduced in single centers under controlled circumstances. The future of pancreatic cancer treatment is dependent on the achievements of multicenter, randomized, controlled trials, which will complement the development of newer therapeutic approaches emerging from molecular research.

Conclusion

Treatment of pancreatic cancer has made progress in the past few years. Pancreatic tumors can today be safely resected with a low risk of postoperative morbidity and mortality. Although surgery is safe in centers with high caseload, there are still controversies regarding extent of local resection (classical Kausch–Whipple vs. pylorus-preserving Whipple), extent of lymph-node resection, and type of pancreaticointestinal reconstruction. Large multicenter studies are needed to end the debate regarding these surgical aspects and to further improve the outcome in patients with pancreatic cancer.

The initiation of ESPAC has provided fundamental progress in the treatment of pancreatic cancer. The ESPAC-1 study provides, for the first time, solid statistical power (almost 600 patients) that adjuvant chemotherapy (5-fluorouracil plus folinic acid) prolongs survival following pancreatic cancer resection. ESPAC-3, which is presently running, will provide data about whether gemcitabine treatment has any advantage over 5-fluorouracil plus folinic acid.

The prognosis of resectable pancreatic cancer has improved, although further progress is still needed in the coming years.

Recommended reading

Büchler M, Friess H, Klempa I et al. The role of octreotide in the prevention of postoperative complications following pancreatic resection. Am J Surg 1992;163:125–131.

Lin PW, Lin YJ. Prospective randomized comparison between pylorus-preserving and standard pancreaticoduodenectomy. Br J Surg 1999;86:603.

Neoptolemos JP, Russell RCG, Bramhall S, Theis B. Low mortality following resection for pancreatic and periampullary tumours in 1026 patients: UK survey of specialist pancreatic units. UK Pancreatic Cancer Group. Br J Surg 1997;84:1370–1376.

Neoptolemos JP, Stocken DD, Dunn JA et al. Influence of resection margins on survival for patients with pancreatic cancer treated by adjuvant chemoradiation and/or chemotherapy in the ESPAC-1 randomized controlled trial. Ann Surg 2001;234:758–768.

Neoptolemos JP, Dunn JA, Stocken DD et al. Adjuvant chemoradiotherapy and chemotherapy in resectable pancreatic cancer: a randomised controlled trial. Lancet 2001;358:1576–85.

Seiler CA, Wagner M, Schaller B, Sadowski C, Kulli C, Büchler MW. Randomized prospective trial of pylorus-preserving vs. classical duodenopancreatectomy: initial clinical results. J Gastrointest Surg 2000;4:443–452.

Yeo CJ, Cameron JL, Sohn TA et al. Six hundred fifty consecutive pancreaticoduodenectomies in the 1990s: pathology, complications, and outcomes. Ann Surg 1997;226:248–257.

Yeo CJ, Cameron JL, Lillemoe KD et al. Does prophylactic octreotide decrease the rates of pancreatic fistula and other complications after pancreaticoduodenectomy? Results of a prospective randomized placebo-controlled trial. Ann Surg 2000;232:419–429.

Yeo CJ, Cameron JL, Lillemoe KD et al. Pancreaticoduodenectomy with or without distal gastrectomy and extended retroperitoneal lymphadenectomy for periampullary adenocarcinoma, part 2: randomized controlled trial evaluating survival, morbidity and mortality. Ann Surg 2002;236:355–365.

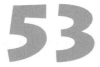

53 Adjuvant and neoadjuvant treatment of resectable pancreatic cancer: what is worth attempting?

Michael G.T. Raraty, Paula Ghaneh, and John P. Neoptolemos

Introduction

Pancreatic cancer has historically been classed as a tumor that is largely resistant to chemotherapy due to its aggressive biological phenotype, and in which surgery conveys the only hope of cure. It is also a tumor that tends to present late, and therefore resection rates of only 4% have been reported in general surgical practice, although these have improved to 10–15% in specialist pancreatic units. After successful surgery the prognosis is still relatively poor (median and 5-year survivals of around 13–15 months and 15–20% respectively) but is far superior in specialist centers. Attempts at more radical pancreatic resections and extended lymphadenectomy, although feasible without excessive morbidity and mortality, have failed to produce any convincing improvement in survival. Over the last few years, therefore, efforts have been directed toward the development of adjuvant and neoadjuvant therapies in an attempt to improve outcome.

Adjuvant systemic chemotherapy

There are very few studies published on adjuvant chemotherapy alone in pancreatic cancer. Most published series also include chemoradiotherapy as part of the regimen, and data on the efficacy of chemotherapy alone are scarce. The few published studies are summarized in Table 53.1. Splinter *et al.* in the early 1980s treated 16 patients with five courses of 5-fluorouracil (5-FU), Adriamycin, and mitomycin C (FAM) and compared them with a historical control group of 36 patients. The FAM regimen was poorly tolerated and

half of the treatment group received no more than 60% of the predetermined chemotherapy dose. There was no benefit from adjuvant chemotherapy, with similar 3-year actuarial survival rates of 24% and 28% for the treatment and control groups respectively. The first prospective, randomized, controlled trial was performed by Bakkevold *et al.* in 1993, in which 47 patients with resected pancreatic ductal adenocarcinoma (including 14 with ampullary tumors) were randomized to either postoperative combination chemotherapy of 5-FU, doxorubicin, and mitomycin C every 3 weeks or surgery only. Although a statistically significant improvement was seen in median survival from 11 months to 23 months with chemotherapy, no improvement in long-term 3- and 5-year survival rates was seen. Toxicity resulted in one death, secondary to septicemia, and multiple hospital admissions. Unfortunately, due to the inclusion of ampullary carcinomas, it is difficult to draw conclusions on this study in relation to pancreatic cancer alone. In 1994 Baumel *et al.* reported a survey of 787 patients who had undergone pancreatic resection, 43 of whom received adjuvant chemotherapy. No survival benefit was demonstrated, although this was a retrospective report with no standardization of chemotherapy regimens and therefore the results must be interpreted as such.

The European Study Group for Pancreatic Cancer (ESPAC) in the ESPAC-1 trial randomized 550 patients to adjuvant chemotherapy, chemoradiotherapy, and surgery alone (in a 2 × 2 factorial design or to a single randomization) in centers across 11 European countries. The chemotherapy regimen comprised intravenous bolus 5-FU (425 mg/m^2) and folinic acid (20 mg/m^2) and was given on 5 days out of 28 days for

Table 53.1 Adjuvant systemic chemotherapy for pancreatic ductal adenocarcinoma.

Series	Year	Number of cases	Regimen	Median survival (months)	Actuarial survival (%)			
					1 year	2 years	3 years	5 years
Splinter *et al.*	1989	36	—				28	
		16	FAM				24	
Bakkevold *et al.**	1993	31 (24 PDAC)	—	11	45		30	8
		30 (23 PDAC)	FAM	23	70		27	4
Baumel *et al.*	1994	527	—	12.4				
		43	Various	11.5				
Neoptolemos *et al.**	2001–2004	237	—	14.8		28.7		9.9
		244	5-FU/FA	21.6		43.3		23.3
Takada *et al.**	2002	77 PDAC	—	} ~12†				18
		81 PDAC	MMC/5-FU					11.5

FA, folinic acid; FAM, 5-fluorouracil, doxorubicin, and mitomycin C; 5-FU, 5-fluorouracil; MMC, mitomycin C; PDAC, pancreatic ductal adenocarcinoma.
* Randomized controlled trial.
† Data extrapolated from graph.

six cycles. The median survival was 21.6 months for chemotherapy versus 14.8 months for no chemotherapy. Even after stratification for resection margin involvement, lymph-node involvement, and tumor grade and size, the survival benefit was still maintained. Serious toxic effects (grade 3 or 4) were reported in 46 of 244 patients allocated to chemotherapy (19%), but there were only three treatment-associated deaths, one for each treatment group. The same survival benefits for chemotherapy were observed irrespective of the extent of resection or the development of postoperative surgical complications. Tumor recurrence was reported in 122 of 178 patients randomized to chemotherapy (69%) and in 132 of 165 patients randomized to no chemotherapy (80%). Median time to recurrence was 15.6 months and 8.8 months respectively ($P < 0.001$). Overall, the ESPAC-1 study showed a reduction in the hazard ratio (HR) of 36% in favor of adjuvant chemotherapy (HR 0.64, confidence interval (CI) 0.52–0.78).

Since ESPAC-1 demonstrated a significant survival advantage for adjuvant chemotherapy in preliminary results, although not significant when analyzed by the 2×2 factorial design, it was deemed necessary to maintain the observation arm in the ESPAC-3 adjuvant trial. The design of this trial originally involved the random-

ization of 990 patients into three arms following resection: an observation arm and two arms comparing 5-FU and folinic acid as in ESPAC-1 with gemcitabine (Cancer Research UK). However, with the publication of more mature follow-up results from ESPAC-1 demonstrating such a definite survival advantage for adjuvant chemotherapy, the observation arm has been dropped for pancreatic adenocarcinoma (although it still remains for the smaller groups of ampullary carcinoma and intrapancreatic bile duct tumors). Over 250 patients have already been recruited to ESPAC-3.

The latest randomized adjuvant trial comes from Japan and evaluated 5-FU and mitomycin C in resected pancreaticobiliary carcinomas. Over 6 years, 508 patients were randomized, of whom 173 had pancreatic ductal adenocarcinomas. There were 89 patients admitted to the chemotherapy arm and 84 to the control arm, of whom 45 and 47 respectively underwent curative resections. The chemotherapy group received rapid-infusion mitomycin C on the day of surgery, slow-infusion 5-FU for 5 days in weeks 1 and 3, followed by oral 5-FU. The median survival was approximately 12 months in both the chemotherapy and control groups, with no significant difference in 5-year survival (11.5% and 18% respectively). The overall survival in both groups was very low, possibly due to the unpredictable absorption and resultant poor efficacy of orally administered 5-FU (which was the mainstay of chemotherapy).

Adjuvant regional chemotherapy

In an attempt to maximize the given chemotherapeutic dose while reducing the systemic effects, there has been increasing interest in regional administration of chemotherapy. The published studies have been small but have produced encouraging results and are listed in Table 53.2. Different therapeutic regimens have been tried using selective arterial and/or venous delivery. Ishikawa *et al.* delivered postoperative hepatic perfusion of 5-FU, via catheters placed in both the hepatic artery and portal vein, in 27 patients. This perfusion was undertaken for 28–35 days. There were no treatment-related complications in the 20 patients who survived surgery. A 3-year survival rate of 54% was achieved, with mortality from hepatic metastases at a mere 8%. This was compared with historical controls and found

to be significantly better. The group of Hans Beger carried out several studies using regional adjuvant chemotherapy of 5-FU, mitoxantrone, folinic acid, and cisplatin. Initially 20 patients (18 with pancreatic ductal adenocarcinoma, 2 with cystadenoma) underwent this regimen infused via the celiac axis. A median survival of 21 months was achieved compared with 9.3 months for historical controls. This study was further updated and 24 patients had a median survival of 23 months and a 4-year survival of 54% with this regional perfusion. Regional adjuvant therapy shows some promise but further trials are required to support these initial data in the form of randomized controlled trials.

Adjuvant chemoradiotherapy

Adjuvant external beam radiotherapy (EBRT) with chemoradiotherapy has been used in a number of non-randomized studies mainly in the USA (Table 53.3), which although generally well tolerated has not been

Table 53.2 Adjuvant regional chemotherapy for pancreatic ductal adenocarcinoma.

Series	Year	Number of cases	Regimen	Median survival (months)	Actuarial survival (%)			
					1 year	3 years	4 years	5 years
Ishikawa *et al.*	1994–97	67	—		62	35		25
		27	HAI + HPVI		92	51		41
Gansauge *et al.* *	1996	18	CAI	17.8				
Link *et al.* *	1997	29	—	9.3				
		20 (18 PDAC)	CAI	21				
Beger *et al.* *	1999	?	—	10.5			9.5	
		24	CAI	23			54	
Ozaki *et al.*	2000	27†	IORT + HPVI or HAI	31.1				31
		19‡	IORT + HPVI or HAI	36	95	50		28
Papachristou *et al.*	2003	31 (27 PDAC)	CAI	21				

CAI, celiac artery infusion; HAI, hepatic arterial infusion; HPVI, hepatic portal vein infusion; IORT, intraoperative radiotherapy; PDAC, pancreatic ductal adenocarcinoma.
* Refer to the same series, but with increasing numbers of cases.
† 27/30 patients, excluding three with metastasis to liver, peritoneum, or lung.
‡ 19/30 patients with regional lymph-node metastases.

Table 53.3 Adjuvant chemoradiotherapy for pancreatic ductal adenocarcinoma.

Series	Year	Number of cases	EBRT (Gy)	IORT (Gy)	Median survival (months)	Actuarial survival (%)			
						1 year	2 years	3 years	5 years
Willett et al.	1993	16 (nm)	40–50		21				29
		23 (pm)	40–50		11				0
Johnstone et al.	1993	26	45–55	20	18				
Zerbi et al.	1994	43		12.5–20	19	71		7	
		47			12	49		10	
Di Carlo et al.	1997	27			14				
		27		12.5–20	17				
Dobelbower et al.	1997	14			6.5	15		0	0
		6		10–20	9	50		35	33
		14	50–67		14.5	64		28	0
		10	27–54	10–25	18	70		10	0
Farrell et al.	1997	14	60	12–15	16	62		22	15
Hishinuma et al.	1998	34	n = 24	n = 13 EBRT + IORT	13	59			19
Klinkenbijl et al. (EORTC)*	1999	54 PDAC			12.6				
		60 PDAC	40		17.1				
Mehta et al.	2000	52 PDAC	45–54 (PVI 5-FU)	n = 8	32		62	39	
		17 PDAC	Not specified (bolus 5-FU)		12				
Lee et al.	2000	22						47	
		13	49					81	
Kokubo et al.	2000	34 PDAC†		25	15		25		
		18 PDAC†	45–55		17		24		
Alfieri et al.	2001	20	n = 26	n = 21	10.8				6
		26			14.3				16
Allen et al.	2002	29 PDAC	42 (with gemcitabine)		16.2				
Neoptolemos et al.*	2004	178 PDAC	40		15.5		27.7		10.3
		180 PDAC			16.7		37.9		19.5

EBRT, external beam radiotherapy; 5-FU, 5-fluorouracil; IORT, intraoperative radiotherapy; nm, negative resection margin; pm, positive resection margin; PDAC, pancreatic ductal adenocarcinoma; PVI, protracted venous infusion.
* Randomized controlled trial.
† All had negative resection margins (R0) and some had regional chemotherapy.

clearly shown to offer a survival advantage over either no adjuvant treatment or chemotherapy alone. A multicenter randomized phase III trial organized by the European Organisation for Research and Treatment of Cancer (EORTC) compared chemoradiotherapy with surgery alone in 218 patients following potentially curative surgery for pancreatic or ampullary cancers; 110 patients were randomized to receive 40 Gy EBRT with concomitant continuous infusion of 5-FU (but this was only actually given to 93 patients). There were 114 patients with pancreatic ductal adenocarcinoma, comprising 54 in the observation group and 60 in the treatment group. The apparent improvement in survival in the latter treatment group (median survival 17.1 months vs. 12.6 months for observation) was not statistically significant. The trial was compromised by the fact that it was probably underpowered and around 20% of patients with pancreatic ductal adenocarcinoma did not receive the assigned treatment. Unlike the Gastrointestinal Tumor Study Group (GITSG) adjuvant trial (see below), there was no maintenance treatment with 5-FU. In addition, there was incomplete knowledge about resection margin status because the posterior resection margin was not assessed. It was concluded that adjuvant chemoradiotherapy was safe and well tolerated but that there was no survival benefit. This conclusion is supported by the overall results of the ESPAC-1 trial, with a median survival of 15.5 months in the 175 patients who received chemoradiation compared with 16.7 months in the 180 patients who did not. Again, there was no survival benefit conferred by adjuvant chemoradiation in those patients with histologically positive resection margins (R1). The HR actually shows a 23% benefit in favor of no chemoradiotherapy, although the 95% CIs for this estimation cross unity (HR 1.23, CI 0.98–1.54).

One nonrandomized study of particular interest is by Mehta and colleagues from Stanford who treated 52 patients between 1994 and 1999. The tumor bed and regional nodes were irradiated with a dose of 45 Gy in 1.8-Gy fractions followed by a boost to the tumor bed in the 35% of patients with a positive resection margin (total dose 54 Gy). Concomitant portal venous infusion of 5-FU (200–250 mg/m^2 per day, 7 days per week) was given during the entire radiotherapy course. A remarkable median survival of 32 months was achieved. Certainly these results are far superior to other studies that have used concomitant bolus 5-FU or even continuous-infusion 5-FU.

Allen *et al.* from the University of Michigan undertook a phase I study to determine the maximum tolerated dose of EBRT (with a conformal technique) in combination with full-dose gemcitabine (1000 mg/m^2 weekly for 3 weeks) in patients with a positive resection margin ($n = 9$), positive nodes ($n = 27$), or both ($n = 7$). The starting EBRT dose was 24 Gy in 1.6-Gy fractions and escalation was achieved by increasing the fraction size in 0.2-Gy increments, keeping the duration at 3 weeks. Twenty-five patients completed the protocol therapy, and at the final EBRT dose of 42 Gy two out of two patients experienced gastrointestinal dose-limiting toxicity. The median survival was 16.2 (95% CI 12.3, 19.9) months.

Adjuvant chemoradiotherapy with maintenance chemotherapy

The regimen originally adopted by GITSG for patients with advanced pancreatic cancer was used in the adjuvant setting for a randomized trial in the 1970s (Table 53.4); 43 patients, all with clear resection margins (R0), were randomized to either surgery alone or surgery combined with 40 Gy radiotherapy (with 5-FU radiosensitization) and weekly 5-FU for 2 years or until relapse. The median survival in the treated group was 20 months compared with 11 months in the surgery only group and the 2-year survival rates were 42% and 15% respectively. To increase numbers in the treatment group, a further 30 patients were added to the adjuvant therapy arm and the outcome modified to a median survival of 18 months and a 2-year survival of 46%. Unfortunately, the number of patients was still too small for convincing conclusions to be drawn and it was uncertain whether any benefit was wholly due to the combination, the chemotherapy alone, or the radiotherapy alone. Despite these caveats, variations of this combination protocol were widely adopted, especially in the USA (Table 53.4).

Yeo *et al.* from Johns Hopkins reported a retrospective analysis of three different regimens in selected patients who had undergone pancreatoduodenectomy. Patients received one of (a) 40–45 Gy EBRT plus follow-on bolus 5-FU for 4 months; (b) 50–57 Gy EBRT plus hepatic radiation plus continuous-infusion 5-FU/folinic acid for 4 months; or (c) no adjuvant treatment. Group (a) had a significantly better median survival (21 months) and 2-year survival (44%) when compared with the control group (13.5 months and

Table 53.4 Combination adjuvant chemoradiotherapy with follow-on chemotherapy for pancreatic ductal adenocarcinoma.

Series	Year	Number of cases	Radiotherapy (Gy)	Chemotherapy	Median survival (months)	Actuarial survival (%)			
						1 year	2 years	3 years	5 years
Kalser et al.*	1985	21	EBRT 40	5-FU	20	67	42	24	18
		22			11	50	15	7	8
GITSG	1987	30	EBRT 40	5-FU	18		46		
Conlon et al.	1996	56	EBRT 45	5-FU	20		35		
Yeo et al.	1997	99	EBRT 40–45	5-FU	21		44		
		21	EBRT 50–57	5-FU + FA	17.5		22		
		53			13.5		30		
UKPACA	1998	34	EBRT 40	5-FU	13	56	38	29	15
Abrams et al.	1999	23	EBRT	5-FU + FA	15.9				
Paulino et al.	1999	30	EBRT	5-FU	26				
		8	EBRT	5-FU	5.5				
Andre et al.	2000	10	EBRT	5-FU + FA + Cis	17				
Nukui et al.	2000	16	EBRT 40	5-FU			54		
		17	EBRT 45–54	5-FU + Cis + IFN-α			84		
Sohn et al.	2000	333	EBRT 40–50	5-FU (mostly; also FA, MMC, dipyridamole)	19	71			20
		119			11	48			9
Chakravarthy et al.	2000	29	EBRT 50	5-FU, FA, MMC, dipyridamole	16	52			
Kachnic et al.	2001	9	EBRT 40–50.4	Gemcitabine	16	78	39	39	
Van Laetham et al.	2003	22	EBRT 40	Gemcitabine	15				

Cis, cisplatin; EBRT, external bean radiotherapy; FA, folinic acid; 5-FU, 5-fluorouracil; IFN-α, interferon-α; MMC, mitomycin C.
* Randomized controlled trial.

449

30% respectively). However, there was no significant difference between groups (b) and (c), questioning the value of adjuvant treatment *per se* because of patient selection. The same group treated 23 patients with continuous infusion of 5-FU and folinic acid during radiation for 5 days per week, and then 1 month later four cycles of the same chemotherapy regimen for 2 weeks out of every four. Patients were given either "low-dose" radiotherapy (comprising 23.4 Gy to the whole liver, 50.4 Gy to regional nodes, and 50.4 Gy to the tumor bed) or "high-dose" radiotherapy (comprising 27.0 Gy to the whole liver, 54.0 Gy to regional nodes, and 57.6 Gy to the tumor bed). The overall median survival was 15.9 months, with little difference in median survival between the "low-dose" and "high-dose" groups (14.4 vs. 16.9 months respectively). The Johns Hopkins group also treated 29 patients with split-course locoregional EBRT and concurrent 5-FU, folinic acid, dipyridamole, and mitomycin C. The EBRT consisted of split-course 50 Gy over 20 fractions with a 2-week planned rest after the first 10 fractions (25 Gy). Every 4 weeks the patients received bolus 5-FU (400 mg/m^2) and folinic acid (20 mg/m^2) on days 1–3, dipyridamole (75 mg p.o., four times daily) on days 0–3 and every 8 weeks, and mitomycin C (10 mg/m^2, maximum 20 mg) on day 1 during EBRT. This was followed by four cycles of the same chemotherapy as adjuvant therapy 1 month following the completion of EBRT. The median survival was 16 months and the 1-year survival was 58%. Altogether between 1984 and 1999 the Johns Hopkins team treated 333 patients selected from a consecutive series of 616 patients who had had resection for pancreatic ductal adenocarcinoma with adjuvant chemoradiotherapy and maintenance chemotherapy. Even given the biased treatment sample, the median survival was 19 months, the 1-year survival was 71%, and the 5-year survival was 20%.

The UKPACA-1 trial utilized the same adjuvant regimen as in the GITSG trial in 34 patients with pancreatic ductal adenocarcinoma and six with ampullary carcinoma. The median survival rate for patients with pancreatic ductal adenocarcinoma was 13.2 months and the 5-year survival was 15%. Survival in patients with clear lymph nodes was 60% at 2 years compared with 18% in those with positive lymph nodes at the time of resection. There were no treatment-related deaths and no hospitalizations due to this regimen even with a prolonged course of postoperative chemotherapy that laid the basis of the ESPAC trials in Europe.

The RTOG adjuvant phase III study #97-04 recruited over 500 patients to receive a 3-week course of chemotherapy, then chemoradiotherapy, and then a final 3-month course of chemotherapy. Patients were randomized to one of two adjuvant pre-chemoradiotherapy chemotherapy regimens (continuous-infusion 5-FU 250 mg/m^2 daily for 3 weeks vs. gemcitabine 1000 mg/m^2 daily once weekly for 3 weeks) and parallel post-chemoradiotherapy chemotherapy (two 4-week cycles of continuous-infusion 5-FU 250 mg/m^2 daily for 3 weeks each followed by 2 weeks' rest for 3 months vs. three cycles of gemcitabine 1000 mg/m^2 daily once weekly followed by 1 week's rest for 3 weeks also for 3 months). Both groups received identical chemoradiotherapy starting 1–2 weeks after completion of pre-chemoradiotherapy chemotherapy and then no later than 13 weeks after resection [50.4 Gy per 5.5 weeks at 1.8 Gy per fraction (field reduction at 45 Gy) and continuous-infusion 5-FU 250 mg/m^2 daily during EBRT]. The survival results from this trial will be of enormous importance for comparing survival achieved with other large adjuvant therapy trials.

Neoadjuvant therapy

Proponents of neoadjuvant therapy for pancreatic cancer point out that a significant proportion of patients are not considered for adjuvant treatment because of postoperative complications, which occur in 30–45% of patients. Neoadjuvant therapy may also be given in the hope of being able to downstage locally advanced tumors and achieve an enhanced resection rate.

There have been no large randomized controlled studies on the use of neoadjuvant therapy in pancreatic cancer (Table 53.5). The total number of patients that have actually had resection following neoadjuvant therapy is rather small. The series shown in Table 53.5 also include patients that have been "counted twice" as the initial series are expanded, such as that from the M.D. Anderson group. The quoted resection rates vary considerably, from 45 to 100% in patients with tumors initially deemed "resectable" and from 20 to 64% in those with "unresectable" tumors. The median survival rates in general range from 16 to 21 months, which is comparable with both adjuvant systemic chemotherapy and regional chemotherapy.

Specific comment is necessary on two studies with

Table 53.5 Neoadjuvant therapy for pancreatic ductal adenocarcinoma.

Series	Year	Number of cases	Neoadjuvant regimen	Pretreatment assessment of (un)resectability	Number resected (%)	Median survival (months)	Actuarial survival (%) 3 years	4 years	5 years
Ishikawa et al.	1994	23	EBRT	Both	17 (74)				22
Coia et al.	1994	27	EBRT + 5-FU/MMC	Both	13 (48)	16	43		
Staley et al.	1996	39	EBRT + IORT + 5-FU	Resectable	39 (100)	19		19	
Spitz et al.	1997	91	EBRT + 5-FU	Resectable	41 (51)	19.2			
Hoffman et al.	1998	53	EBRT + 5-FU/MMC	Resectable	24 (45)	15.7			
White et al.	1999	25	EBRT + 5-FU/MMC/Cis	Unresectable	5 (20)				
Wanebo et al.	2000	14	EBRT + 5-FU/Cis	Unresectable	9 (64)				
Snady et al.	2000	68	EBRT + 5-FU/Cis/Strep	Unresectable	20 (29)	32	32		
					48 not resected	21	13		
		(91)*	(± adjuvant chemotherapy ± EBRT)	Resectable	(63 with adjuvant treatment)	16	13		
					(28 no adjuvant treatment)	11	11		
Mehta et al.	2001	15	EBRT + 5-FU	Unresectable	9 (60)	30			
Breslin et al.	2001	(132)	EBRT + 5-FU/Pac/Gem	Resectable	132 (not applicable)	21			

C; Cis, cisplatin; EBRT, external beam radiotherapy; 5-FU, 5-fluorouracil; Gem, gemcitabine; IORT, intraoperative radiotherapy; MMC, mitomycin; Pac, paclitaxel; Strep, streptozotocin.
* All these patients had resection and none had neoadjuvant treatment, but some had adjuvant treatment.

451

exceptional median survival rates of 31 and 32 months respectively. Snady *et al.* reported a median survival of 32 months in 20 (29%) patients who had resection from an original group of 68 patients treated first with simultaneous split-course EBRT plus 5-FU, streptozotocin, and cisplatin (RT-FSP; 0% mortality rate < 30 days). The median survival of the whole group was 23.6 months and 32 months in the 20 patients who also had resection. During the same period another group of 91 patients initially underwent resection (5% mortality rate < 30 days), of which 63 (69%) received adjuvant chemotherapy with or without EBRT. The median survival in this latter group was 14.0 months ($P = 0.006$ compared with RT-FSP group). Median survival in patients who had resection and adjuvant treatment was 16 months compared with 11 months in those who did not have adjuvant therapy after resection ($P = 0.025$). In contrast, the M.D. Anderson group in their (non-randomized) studies have not shown a significant difference in survival between those patients who received neoadjuvant compared with adjuvant treatment. Mehta *et al.* have recently reported a median survival of 30 months with neoadjuvant treatment but only in nine selected patients.

All of the aforementioned studies suffer to a greater or lesser extent from a number of confounding factors. A specialist pancreatic cancer surgery team can often resect what is considered by another team to be "unresectable locally advanced disease." For example, the Johns Hopkins group was able to resect 52 (67%) of 78 patients operated upon elsewhere and thought to have had unresectable diseases. Patients with intrapancreatic bile duct cancers and/or ampullary cancers, who have much better survival figures than those with pancreatic ductal adenocarcinoma, are not always excluded from neoadjuvant series. Indeed the distinction between intrapancreatic bile duct adenocarcinoma and pancreatic ductal adenocarcinoma cannot be made except on the resected specimen. A tumor in the head of the pancreas is almost invariably affected by EBRT to the extent that often the tissue of origin of the adenocarcinoma cannot be determined. Following neoadjuvant therapy, the tumor undergoes restaging (usually several months after the initial diagnosis) and patients who have developed interval metastases are excluded. Thus the group of patients who eventually go on to resection are a biased population with a better prognosis than the group as a whole. Finally, subgroup analysis of selected patients from single institutions is subject to

significant statistical error, especially with the small numbers quoted. Thus in the absence of randomized studies the role of neoadjuvant treatment for pancreatic cancer can only be regarded as experimental.

Conclusions

The relative lack of high-quality randomized trials in the treatment of pancreatic cancer is alarming but this situation is now beginning to change. There is little evidence to support the use of intraoperative radiotherapy either alone or in combination in pancreatic ductal adenocarcinoma. In the absence of controlled trials the roles of regional chemotherapy and neoadjuvant treatment are not yet defined but perhaps have a place in selected cases. The best evidence so far suggests that adjuvant chemotherapy is probably of benefit after resection of pancreatic cancer. The current standard treatment regimen is 5-FU/folinic acid, although this may be superseded or complemented by gemcitabine pending the results of currently ongoing clinical trials such as ESPAC-3. There is evidence from the ESPAC-1 trial that EBRT given before maintenance chemotherapy may even have a detrimental effect on the response to chemotherapy.

The three largest randomized controlled trials of adjuvant treatment of pancreatic cancer are consistent with each other and swamp the previous very small GITSG trial. Despite this there is still healthy criticism of the ESPAC-1 trial and continued support for adjuvant chemoradiotherapy. The retrospective and small prospective studies from the Johns Hopkins (among others) are mentioned as support for continuing the use of adjuvant chemoradiotherapy. Despite the selection bias, the median survival of patients with pancreas cancer treated at the Johns Hopkins with a combination of chemoradiotherapy and maintenance chemotherapy was no better than that of patients randomized to chemotherapy in the ESPAC-1 study (19.0 vs. 21.6 months respectively). It is argued that neither of the two European trials of adjuvant chemoradiotherapy used sufficient radiation yet this dose was identical to that given in the GITSG study. Since the ESPAC-1 trial was initiated, conformal beam radiotherapy, which enables more radiation to be delivered to targeted areas in the abdomen, has been introduced. Even so the median survival rates using conformal EBRT with more intensive radiation and chemotherapy regimens have for example produced median survival rates of only 14.4, 16.0, and 16.9 months. The survival rates using these intensive combination regimens are consistent with a median survival of 15.5 months in the 178 patients treated with split-course chemoradiotherapy in the ESPAC-1 trial and 17.1 months in the 60 patients treated in the same way in the EORTC trial. Indeed a remarkably good survival rate was achieved in the control arm of the ESPAC-1 trial, with a median of 16.7 months in the 180 patients not given chemoradiotherapy. The survival results of combination regimens using other approaches including intraoperative radiotherapy (Table 53.3) and neoadjuvant chemoradiotherapy (Table 53.5) are also comparable to the survival achieved by the chemotherapy arm of ESPAC-1. Adjuvant and neoadjuvant chemoradiotherapy exposes the patient to an extra burden of treatment and related toxicity and their use can only be justified if survival is shown to be prolonged. This is of great importance given the limited life expectancy of patients with pancreatic cancer undergoing resection.

Many other approaches and agents are at differing stages of development, but some of these are almost certain to find a place in the adjuvant setting in due course. However, participation in major trials is a necessary prerequisite for such progress. While the proliferation of phase I and phase II studies is most welcome, clinical practice should be developed around the consolidated results of phase III studies. With this in mind we can conclude that there is now considerable scope for optimism in the treatment of pancreatic cancer.

Recommended reading

Abrams RA, Grochow LB, Chakravathy A et al. Intensified adjuvant therapy for pancreatic and periampullary adenocarcinoma: survival results and observations regarding patterns of failure, radiotherapy dose and CA19–9 levels. Int J Radiat Oncol Biol Phys 1999;44:1039–1046.

Allen AM, Zalupski MM, Eckhauser FE et al. A phase I trial of radiation (RT) dose escalation with concurrent full dose gemcitabine (GEM) following resection of pancreatic cancer. Proc Am Soc Clin Oncol 2002;21:138 (abstract 549).

Bakkevold KE, Arnesjo B, Dahl O et al. Adjuvant combination chemotherapy (AMF) following radical resection of carcinoma of the pancreas and papilla of Vater: results of a controlled, prospective, randomised multicentre study. Eur J Cancer 1993;29A:698–703.

Baumel H, Huguier M, Manderscheid JC et al. Results of re-section for cancer of the exocrine pancreas: a study from the French Association of Surgery. Br J Surg 1994;81:102–107.

Beger H, Gansauge F, Büchler MW et al. Intraarterial adjuvant chemotherapy after pancreaticoduodenectomy for pancreatic cancer: significant reduction in occurrence of liver metastasis. World J Surg 1999;23:946–949.

Breslin TM, Hess KR, Harbison DB et al. Neoadjuvant chemoradiotherapy for adenocarcinoma of the pancreas: treatment variables and survival duration. Ann Surg Oncol 2001;8:123–132.

Chakravarthy A, Abrams RA, Yeo CJ et al. Intensified adjuvant combined modality therapy for resected periampullary adenocarcinoma: acceptable toxicity and suggestion of improved 1-year disease-free survival. Int J Radiat Oncol Biol Phys 2000;48:1089–1096.

Coia L, Hoffman J, Scher R et al. Preoperative chemoradiation for adenocarcinoma of the pancreas and duodenum. Int J Radiat Oncol Biol Phys 1994;30:161–167.

Douglass HO Jr. Further evidence of effective adjuvant combined radiation and chemotherapy following curative resection of pancreatic cancer. Gastrointestinal Tumor Study Group. Cancer 1987;59:2006–2010.

Ishikawa O, Ohigashi H, Sasaki Y et al. Regional chemotherapy to prevent hepatic metastasis after resection of pancreatic cancer. Hepatogastroenterology 1997;44:1541–1546.

Ishikawa O, Ohhigashi H, Imaoka S et al. Extended pancreatectomy and liver perfusion chemotherapy for resectable adenocarcinoma of the pancreas. Digestion 1999;60(Suppl 1):135–138.

Kachnic LA, Shaw JE, Manning MA et al. Gemcitabine following radiotherapy with concurrent 5-fluorouracil for nonmetastatic adenocarcinoma of the pancreas. Int J Cancer 2001;96:132–139.

Klinkenbijl JH, Jeekel J, Sahmoud T et al. Adjuvant radiotherapy and 5-fluorouracil after curative resection of cancer of the pancreas and periampullary region: phase III trial of the EORTC gastrointestinal tract cancer cooperative group. Ann Surg 1999;230:776–782; discussion 782–784.

Mehta VK, Fisher GA, Ford JM et al. Adjuvant radiotherapy and concomitant 5-fluorouracil by protracted venous infusion for resected pancreatic cancer. Int J Radiat Oncol Biol Phys 2000;48:1483–1487.

Neoptolemos JP, Baker P, Spooner D et al. Adjuvant radiotherapy and follow-on chemotherapy in patients with pancreatic cancer. Results of the UK Pancreatic Cancer Group Study (UKPACA-1). GI Cancer 1998;2:235–245.

Neoptolemos JP, Dunn JA, Stocken DD et al. Adjuvant chemoradiotherapy and chemotherapy in resectable pancreatic cancer: a randomised controlled trial. Lancet 2001;358:1576–1585.

Neoptolemos J, Cunningham D, Freiss H et al. Adjuvant therapy in pancreatic cancer: historical and current perspectives. Ann Oncol 2003;14:675–692.

Neoptolemos JP, Stocken DD, Freiss H *et al.* The final results of the European Study Group for Pancreatic Cancer randomized controlled trial of adjuvant chemoradiotherapy and chemotherapy in patients with resectable pancreatic cancer. *N Engl J Med* 2004;350:1200–1210.

Raraty MGT, Magee CJ, Ghaneh P *et al.* New techniques and agents in the adjuvant therapy of pancreatic cancer. *Acta Oncol* 2002;41:582–595.

Shore S, Raraty MGT, Ghaneh P *et al.* Chemotherapy for pancreatic cancer. *Aliment Pharmacol Ther* 2003;18:1049–1069.

Snady H, Bruckner H, Cooperman A *et al.* Survival advantage of combined chemoradiotherapy compared with resection as the initial treatment of patients with regional pancreatic carcinoma. An outcomes trial. *Cancer* 2000;89:314–327.

Spitz FR, Abbruzzese JL, Lee JE *et al.* Preoperative and postoperative chemoradiation strategies in patients treated with pancreaticoduodenectomy for adenocarcinoma of the pancreas. *J Clin Oncol* 1997;15:928–937.

Splinter TA, Obertop H, Kok TC *et al.* Adjuvant chemotherapy after resection of adenocarcinoma of the periampullary region and the head of the pancreas. A non-randomized pilot study. *J Cancer Res Clin Oncol* 1989;115:200–202.

Takada A, Amano H, Yasuda H *et al.* Is postoperative adjuvant chemotherapy useful for gallbladder carcinoma? A phase III multicentre prospective randomised controlled trial in patients with resected pancreaticobiliary carcinoma. *Cancer* 2002;95:1685–1695.

Yeo CJ, Abrams RA, Grochow LB *et al.* Pancreaticoduodenectomy for pancreatic adenocarcinoma: postoperative adjuvant chemoradiation improves survival. A prospective, single-institution experience. *Ann Surg* 1997;225:621–633; discussion 633–636.

54 The role of endoscopy in the management of unresectable pancreatic cancer

Richard A. Kozarek

Background

Approximately 25 000 cases of pancreatic carcinoma are diagnosed in the USA yearly. Despite tumor downstaging with chemoradiation in some high-volume centers, most series suggest that only 20–30% of these patients prove resectable and the majority of the latter have a mean survival of less than 2 years. Endoscopic interaction in the setting of malignant obstructive jaundice does not occur in a vacuum. From a diagnostic standpoint, noninvasive abdominal imaging procedures including ultrasonography, computed tomography (CT), magnetic resonance imaging (MRI), and positron emission tomography (PET) are both competing and complementary technologies, one or more of which is invariably used in lieu of, or in conjunction with, endoscopic retrograde cholangiopancreatography (ERCP). In addition, invasive studies, including ultrasound- or CT-directed biopsy or fine-needle aspiration (FNA), endoscopic ultrasound (EUS), diagnostic laparoscopy, or even exploratory laparotomy, may be required for tissue diagnosis prior to or after ERCP. This is particularly apropos as most series suggest that only 40–50% of pancreatic cancers are positively diagnosed using ERCP despite use of brush cytology, intraductal biopsy, or transductal FNA. Finally, it is unusual to perform diagnostic ERCP in patients with possible malignant obstructive jaundice without obtaining such tumor markers as carcinoembryonic antigen (CEA) or CA-19-9 in advance.

From a therapeutic standpoint, surgery has been the traditional palliative modality in nonresectable patients, either hepaticojejunostomy for malignant obstructive jaundice or gastrojejunostomy for gastric outlet obstruction, or a combination of the two. While open surgery is still used palliatively in patients explored for potential cure but found to be unresectable, laparoscopic biliary bypass or gastrojejunostomy are being done with increasing frequency. Percutaneous transhepatic biliary drainage procedures are also still variably utilized for malignant obstructive jaundice in the setting of unresectable pancreatic malignancy, contingent upon institutional expertise and the success of endoscopic biliary decompression. In most centers, however, percutaneous transhepatic biliary drainage has been supplanted by ERCP.

Endoscopic palliation in pancreatic cancer includes plastic or metallic prosthesis insertion for malignant obstructive jaundice and self-expandable metal stent (SEMS) placement for gastric outlet obstruction. Less commonly, pancreatic duct stents have been endoscopically inserted for obstructive pancreatitis and, less commonly still, endotherapy may be used to palliate gastrointestinal bleeding associated with neoplasia (esophagogastric varices in the setting of portal vein thrombosis/tumor erosion into the duodenal C-loop). The latter are temporizing measures often applied in the preterminal state. Table 54.1 summarizes the palliative modalities that can be applied endoscopically to treat the consequences of pancreatic cancer.

Palliation of biliary obstruction

Following pancreas protocol CT and possibly EUS to define signs of unresectability for cure (liver metastases, malignant ascites, multiple large lymph nodes, vascular invasion, tumors > 5 cm in size), most patients with ob-

455

Table 54.1 Endoscopic treatment of pancreatic cancer.

Obstructive jaundice
    Plastic prostheses
    Self-expandable metal stent (SEMS)
Gastric outlet obstruction
    ± Balloon dilation
    ± Thermal ablation, e.g., laser, argon plasma coagulation
      SEMS
Gastrointestinal bleeding
    ± Variceal banding/sclerosis
    ± Thermal therapy

structive jaundice as a consequence of pancreatic malignancy undergo ERCP as the next step, not only to obtain a tissue diagnosis but also in an attempt to relieve biliary obstruction.

Plastic prostheses (Fig. 54.1)

Since the initial description by Soehendra *et al.* in 1980, there have been numerous prospective and retrospective series documenting efficacy of plastic or Teflon stents in the relief of malignant obstructive jaundice. The advantages of plastic prostheses include up-front prosthesis cost, relative placement ease, and the fact that stent insertion does not preclude resection in patients studied and decompressed preoperatively.

Technically, the procedure requires an adequately se-dated patient, usually with intravenous narcotics, ben-zodiazepines, or propofol, prophylactic antibiotics, and a team consisting of an endoscopist, experienced nursing staff, and fluoroscopist. Prosthesis insertion presupposes adequate cholangiography, free access into the biliary tree, usually with some form of hydrophilic guidewire, and accurate measurement of stricture length (Fig. 54.2). After access has been achieved, sphincterotomy may or may not be required. The stenosis may require either catheter or balloon di-lation, and contingent upon a previous tissue diagnosis from a pre-ERCP biopsy or FNA, stricture sampling with brush cytology, needle aspirate, or directed biopsy should be considered. Prostheses selected are usually 10–11.5 Fr, 2–3 cm longer than the stricture to be stented, and are usually pushed into place over a guide-wire and stiffening catheter. Proper placement presup-poses free flow of bile through the stent once the guidewire and stiffening catheter have been withdrawn.

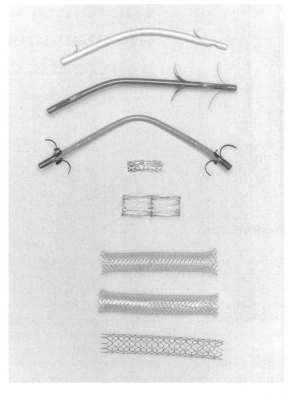

Figure 54.1 Various plastic, Teflon, and composite conventional prostheses (*top*) as well as some of the commercially available self-expandable metal stents (SEMS) (*bottom*) that have been used to treat malignant obstructive jaundice.

Self-expandable metal stent (Fig. 54.1)

A variety of SEMS are currently available to treat ma-lignant biliary obstruction. Summarized in Table 54.2, these devices differ in design, including the type, gauge, and weave of the interlocking wires used to fabricate the stent. Moreover, the delivery systems used to insert the stent are also variable and range from withdrawal of a constraining sheath or release of tripwires to allow a memory metal to reexpand to its original shape. In contrast to plastic prostheses, which often require catheter or balloon dilation for placement, the small diameter of the delivery systems (7–8 Fr) usually allows SEMS insertion without predilation (Fig. 54.3). How-ever, the prostheses themselves do have other inherent risks, and stent foreshortening at time of delivery

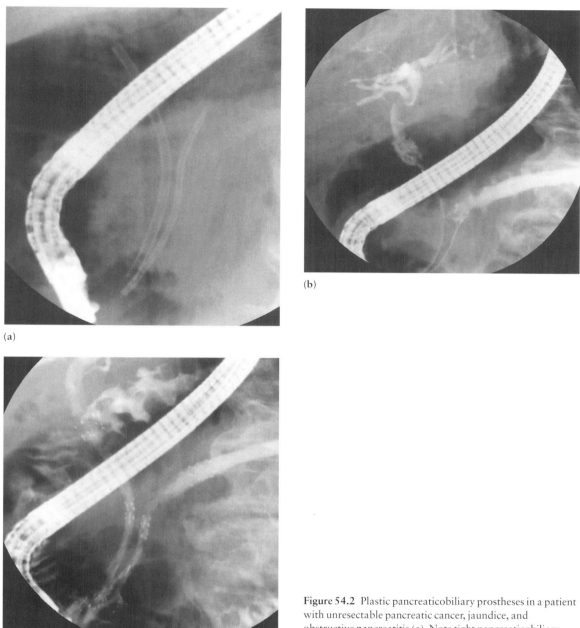

(a)

(b)

(c)

Figure 54.2 Plastic pancreaticobiliary prostheses in a patient with unresectable pancreatic cancer, jaundice, and obstructive pancreatitis (a). Note tight pancreaticobiliary strictures (b) subsequently treated with dual Diamond stents (c).

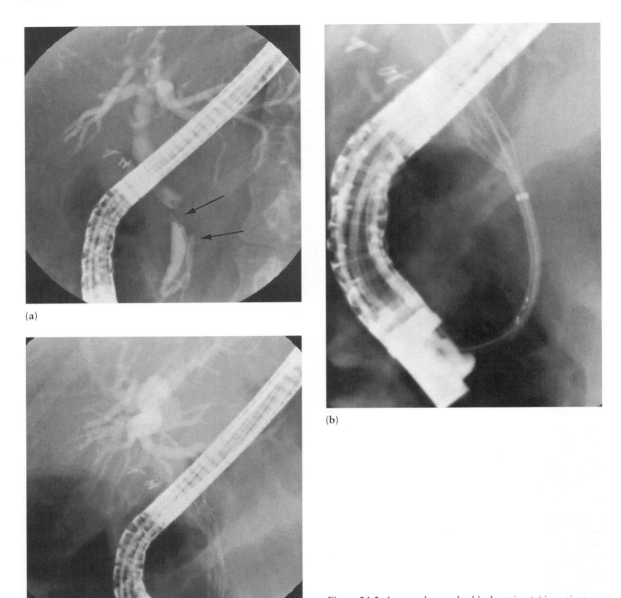

(a)

(b)

(c)

Figure 54.3 Arrows denote double duct sign (a) in patient treated with endoscopic self-expandable metal stent insertion (b, c).

Table 54.2 Commercially available self-expandable biliary stents for malignant obstructive jaundice.

	Wallstent	Endocoil	Diamond	Spiral Z	Za	Zilver	Luminex
Design	Mesh	Spiral coil	Mesh	Mesh	Mesh	Mesh	Mesh
Material	Stainless steel	Nitinol	Nitinol	Stainless steel	Nitinol	Nitinol	Nitinol
Length (cm)	4, 6, 8, 10	6, 7.5	4, 6, 8	5.7, 7.5	4, 6, 8	4, 6, 8	6, 8
Diameter (mm)	8, 10	6, 8	10	10	10	6, 8, 10	10
Stent foreshortening	Yes	Yes	Yes	No	No	No	No
Introducer diameter (Fr)	7, 7.5	8, 10	9	8.5	8.5	7.5	7.5

makes malplacement a potential problem and may require insertion of a second SEMS. Moreover, release of SEMS that have an excessive intraduodenal length may cause contralateral duodenal wall ulceration and contained or free perforation. Like conventional prostheses, delivery does not imply functional result, and free flow of bile with or without concomitant contrast injection through the stent is required to assure neoluminal patency.

Results

Most of the series looking at palliation of biliary obstruction by plastic prostheses are old. Nagger *et al.* performed a metaanalysis on nine studies comprising 856 patients, demonstrating successful stent placement and jaundice relief in 90%. Median survival in this analysis approximated 5 months. Additional series have prospectively randomized either endoscopic or percutaneous drainage with surgical bypass of the biliary tree in patients with unresectable distal bile duct or pancreatic malignancies. Of the five studies published to date, there was no significant advantage of either method with regard to treatment success, complications, 30-day mortality, or median survival (mean 3–6 months). What was significant, however, was the risk of stent occlusion with recurrent obstructive jaundice and cholangitis, as well as an increased risk of gastric outlet obstruction in stented patients in contrast to those who underwent combined biliary and gastric bypass surgically. This has to be contrasted with resource utilization, as our center has previously documented that from diagnosis to death, patients treated medically with conventional stent placement utilize less than 50% of the dollars spent for surgically bypassed patients. Although there have been multiple attempts to improve the long-term patency of plastic prostheses,

i.e., larger prosthesis diameter, addition of ursodeoxycholic acid or oral or stent-impregnated antibiotics, change of stent materials (e.g., Vivithane, Teflon, silver coated, or hydrophilic polymer), or modification of stent design (e.g., elimination of proximal and distal side holes), all studies to date suggest progressive luminal occlusion by the development of bacterial biofilms.

SEMS were developed partly to minimize the 30–80% occlusion rate noted with plastic prostheses. Despite the paucity of controlled trials that have randomized unresectable pancreatic cancer patients with jaundice to SEMS or surgery, there have been at least five randomized trials comparing SEMS with plastic prostheses. All have demonstrated a statistically significant duration of stent patency (10–12 months vs. 3–4 months) and dysfunction rate from placement to death. Median survival, in turn, is unchanged and usually ranges from 3 to 6 months. Virtually all these studies have been done with the biliary Wallstent (Boston Scientific, Natick, MA), and despite one randomized prospective study demonstrating comparable patency between Spiral Z (Wilson-Cook, Inc., Winston-Salem, NC) and Wallstent there is no guarantee that these data can be generalized to the multitude of other SEMS currently flooding the market. As such, wide-mesh prostheses are more likely to allow tumor ingrowth; thicker wires seem to elicit more granulation tissue, the primary cause of SEMS dysfunction, and recurrent jaundice; and SEMS that generate minimal expansile force can occlude by virtue of inadequate expansion. Because the studies are inadequate, data that covered SEMS have prolonged patency compared with uncovered prostheses are unconvincing, partly because of development of lithogenic bile with an incompetent biliary sphincter and partly because of mucosal hyperplasia at the proximal uncovered portion of the prosthesis.

459

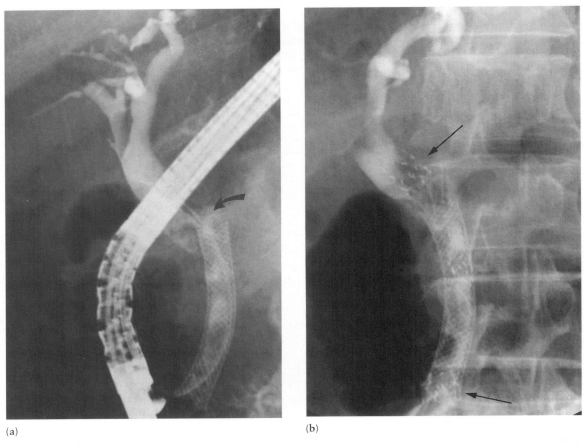

(a)   (b)

Figure 54.4 Arrow denotes locally perforated Wallstent (a) treated with insertion of a second self-expandable metal stent (arrows) (b).

Occasionally, SEMS may also become dysfunctional by virtue of local bile duct perforation at the proximal stent margin. This occurs most commonly with Wall-stents, in which the exposed stent wires erode through an acutely strictured bile duct (Fig. 54.4).

Despite an incomplete database and the problems outlined above, data are reasonably clear that SEMS insertion is cost-effective for the treatment of malignant obstructive jaundice in the setting of unresectable pancreatic cancer despite a 20–30-fold cost increment of SEMS compared with plastic prostheses. This cost-efficacy is related to both prolonged SEMS patency as well as incremental costs associated with need for repeated ERCP in patients who obstruct polyethylene prostheses.

Palliation of pancreatic duct obstruction
(Fig. 54.2)

Until recently, most of the pain associated with ductular adenocarcinoma was thought to be related to perineural encasement by tumor or invasion of contiguous organs. This belief changed when steatorrhea associated with ductal obstruction was treated by pancreatic stent placement in lieu of enzyme supplementation.

This practice was associated with postprandial pain reduction in a subset of patients as well as with improvement in the incidence of obstructive pancreatitis in some patients with pancreatic malignancy. Despite its variable application, risks, including procedurally related pancreatitis and stent occlusion with subsequent pancreatic sepsis or obstructive pancreatitis, have relegated this to an investigational procedure in most centers. Even more investigational are recent descriptions of endoscopically facilitated photodynamic therapy or intraluminal brachytherapy to treat unresectable pancreaticobiliary malignancies.

Palliation of gastric outlet obstruction

Historically, prospective studies have suggested that 5–30% of patients who underwent biliary bypass for unresectable pancreatic cancer developed gastric outlet obstruction. As a consequence, many surgeons began to routinely add gastrojejunostomy at the time of cholecystojejunostomy or hepaticojejunostomy. Gastric outlet obstruction is also noted with comparable frequency in pancreatic cancer patients palliated with endoscopically placed biliary stents. In the preterminal state, treatment may consist of comfort care or diverting percutaneous endoscopic gastrostomy in conjunction with feeding percutaneous endoscopic jejunostomy. Good-risk patients required palliative surgical bypass.

With the introduction of through-the-scope hydrostatic balloons, one could transiently improve the postprandial pain, reflux, nausea, and vomiting associated with partial outlet obstruction. However, it took the development of endoscopically placed enteral SEMS for there to be a viable option to surgery for high-grade gastric outlet obstruction. Technically, enteral SEMS are usually placed after initial insertion of a biliary SEMS, as access to the pancreaticobiliary tree is dramatically limited by a metal mesh stent that blocks the papilla. In the USA currently only the Enteral Wallstent (Boston Scientific, Natick, MA) has been released for relief of malignant gastric outlet obstruction. Following delineation of stricture length with an upper gastrointestinal series or contrast injected through an ERCP catheter, a stent 3–4 cm longer in length is selected for placement. As current prostheses are either 6 or 9 cm in length and 18–22 mm in diameter after release, the longer prosthesis is preferable in all but very short stenoses. The stent delivery system requires use of a therapeutic gastroscope or duodenoscope for placement and insertion itself presupposes passage of the delivery system over a stiff or hydrophilic guidewire. The prosthesis is delivered by pulling back the restraining sheath, which releases the SEMS. Like those used in the biliary tree, the latter foreshortens by approximately one-third of its constrained length, mostly from the distal end, and occasionally balloon dilation of the prosthesis is required for full stent expansion (Fig. 54.5). Most commonly, however, SEMS will fully expand on their own over the first 24–48 hours after insertion. Up to one-third of patients may require a second Wallstent at time of SEMS placement, either because of the length of the stricture or because an acutely angulated segment of bowel proximally or distally precludes proper prosthesis functioning.

Results

There are now multiple series attesting to the feasibility and results associated with SEMS insertion for gastric outlet obstruction, although there are no prospective randomized trials comparing this treatment with surgery. Instead, there are single-center and multicenter series such as a recent report by Nassif *et al*. This trial documented successful placement in 60 of 63 patients (95%) with no procedural mortality and a median survival of 7 weeks (range 1–64 weeks). There were no complications in 44 (70%) of the patients from time of placement to death, whereas 30% of patients had significant problems, including two duodenal perforations treated surgically, four prosthesis migrations, and 13 stent obstructions. In turn, Wong *et al*. retrospectively reviewed 250 patients with pancreatic cancer, 10% of whom developed gastric outlet obstruction. Two-thirds of these were bypassed or underwent palliative resection and one-third underwent SEMS placement. Median survival in the surgical group was 64 days compared with 110.5 days in the stented group. Median postoperative stay for surgically treated patients was 15 days compared with 4 days for the stented group, and 30-day mortality was 17.6% and 0% respectively. It is data such as these, as well as the delayed gastric emptying noted in up to half of surgically bypassed patients, that has led to a dramatic change in practice patterns in many medical centers when treating patients with unresectable malignant gastric outlet obstruction.

461

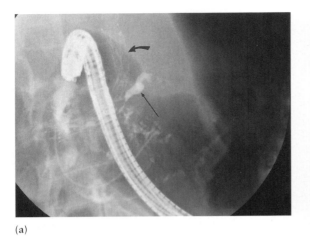

(a)

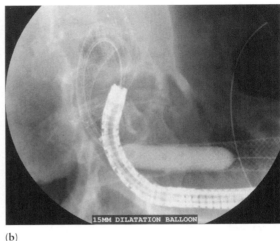

(b)

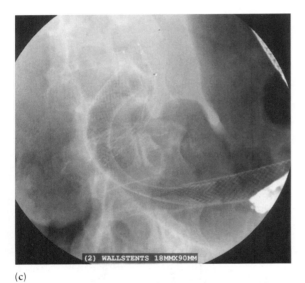

(c)

Figure 54.5 Small arrow depicts obstructed pancreatic duct, large arrow self-expandable metal stent in patient with pancreatic cancer and gastric outlet obstruction (a). Obstruction was treated with two interlocking Enteral Wallstents (b, c).

Palliation of associated gastrointestinal bleeding

Pancreatic head tumors not infrequently invade the portal vein causing portal vein thrombosis, while those in the body and tail can be associated with splenic vein thrombosis. This can cause esophagogastric and gastric varices respectively. Bleeding can occasionally occur in this setting, with need for sclerotherapy or variceal banding. In my experience, however, this is often a preterminal event and even if bleeding can be locally controlled, demise from other causes (sepsis, liver failure) is often imminent.

Bleeding from a pseudoaneurysm that communicates with the pancreaticobiliary tree may present as hemocholedochus or hemopancreaticus respectively.

Endoscopy may be useful in diagnosis but therapy requires surgical resection of the tumor, if possible. Usually, however, these conditions are approached by angiographic embolization.

Finally, direct tumor invasion is often associated with chronic tumor or duodenal C-loop oozing. Endotherapy is often unsatisfactory and repetitive but thermal modalities including heater probe, bipolar cautery, neodymium YAG laser, and argon plasma coagulation have all been used, as has injection with epinephrine (adrenaline), sclerosants, or absolute alcohol.

Conclusions

Endoscopic palliation in pancreatic cancer is imperfect. Nevertheless, it affords results comparable to surgical bypass in unresectable jaundiced patients at approximately 50% of the resources expended from time of diagnosis to death. SEMS placement for gastric outlet obstruction has expanded therapeutic options in a situation previously approached only surgically for fit patients or treated with comfort care measures for individuals with significant comorbid or far-advanced disease.

Decompression of the pancreatic duct is a therapy in evolution but seems to make sense in patients with obstructive pancreatitis or those who develop significant postprandial pain. In contrast, treatment of cancer-associated bleeding remains suboptimal and usually occurs in the setting of aggressive or far-advanced disease.

Recommended reading

Brandabur JJ, Kozarek RA, Ryan JA Jr et al. Nonoperative versus operative treatment of obstructive jaundice in pancreatic cancer: cost and survival analysis. Am J Gastroenterol 1988;83:1132–1139.

Bruha R, Petryl J, Kubecova M et al. Intraluminal brachytherapy and self expandable stents in nonresectable biliary malignancies: the question of long-term palliation. Hepatogastroenterology 2001;48:631–637.

Costamagna G, Gabbrielli A, Mutigani M et al. Treatment of "obstructive pain" by endoscopic drainage in patients with pancreatic head carcinoma. Gastrointest Endosc 1993;39: 774–777.

DeBellis M, Sherman S, Fogel EL et al. Tissue sampling at ERCP in suspected malignant biliary strictures (part 1). Gastrointest Endosc 2002;56:552–561.

DeBellis M, Sherman S, Fogel EL et al. Tissue sampling at ERCP in suspected malignant biliary strictures (part 2). Gastrointest Endosc 2002;56:720–730.

Ferlitsch A, Oesterreicher C, Dumonceau JM et al. Diamond stents for palliation of malignant bile duct obstruction: a prospective multicenter evaluation. Endoscopy 2001;33: 645–650.

Fogel EL, Sherman S, Park S-H et al. Therapeutic biliary endoscopy. Endoscopy 2003;35:156–163.

Hawes RH. Diagnostic and therapeutic uses of ERCP in pancreatic and biliary tract malignancies. Gastrointest Endosc 2002;56:5201–5205.

Kaassis M, Boyer J, Dumas R et al. Plastic or metal stents for malignant stricture of the common bile duct? Results of a randomized prospective study. Gastrointest Endosc 2003; 57:178–182.

Kim HS, Lee DK, Kim HG et al. Features of malignant biliary obstruction affecting the patency of metallic stents: a multicenter study. Gastrointest Endosc 2002;55:359–365.

Kozarek RA. Endoscopic maneuvers for diagnosis and palliative treatment of pancreatic cancer. In: LW Traverso (ed.) Pancreatic Cancer. New York: Lippincott Raven, 1997: 13–26.

Mergener K, Kozarek RA. Pancreatic endotherapy 2002. Endoscopy 2003;35:48–54.

Nagger E, Krag E, Matzen P. Endoscopically inserted biliary endoprosthesis in malignant obstructive jaundice: a survey of the literature. Liver 1990;10:321–324.

Nakamura T, Hiral R, Kitagawa M et al. Treatment of common bile duct obstruction by pancreatic cancer using various stents: single center experience. Cardiovasc Intervent Radiol 2002;25:373–380.

Nassif T, Prat F, Medari B et al. Endoscopic palliation of malignant gastric outlet obstruction using self-expandable metallic stents: results of a multicenter study. Endoscopy 2003;35:483–489.

Pinol V, Castells JM, Bordas JM et al. Percutaneous self-expanding metal stents versus endoscopic polyethylene endoprostheses for treating malignant biliary obstruction: randomized clinical trial. Radiology 2002;225:27–34.

Reknimitr R, Fogel EL, Kalay CL et al. Microbiology of bile in patients with cholangitis or cholestasis with and without plastic biliary endoprosthesis. Gastrointest Endosc 2002; 56:885–889.

Rey JF, Dumas R, Canard JM et al. Guidelines of the French Society of Digestive Endoscopy: biliary stenting. Endoscopy 2002;34:169–173.

Rösch T, Meining A, Frümergen S et al. A prospective comparison of the diagnostic accuracy of ERCP, MRCP, CT, and EUS in biliary strictures. Gastrointest Endosc 2002; 55:870–876.

Shah RJ, Howell DA, Desilets DJ et al. Multicenter randomized trial of the spiral Z-stent compared with the Wallstent for malignant biliary obstruction. *Gastrointest Endosc* 2003;57:830–836.

Strasberg SM. ERCP and surgical intervention in pancreatic and biliary malignancies. *Gastrointest Endosc* 2002;36(6 Suppl):S213–S217.

Van Berkel AM, Brando MJ, Bergman JJGHM *et al*. A prospective randomized study of hydrophilic polymer-coated polyurethane versus polyethylene stents in distal malignant biliary obstruction. *Endoscopy* 2003;35:478–482.

Van Wagensveld BA, Coene PPLO, Van Galik TM *et al*. Outcome of palliative biliary and gastric bypass surgery for pancreatic head carcinoma in 126 patients. *Br J Surg* 1997;84:1402–1406.

Wong YT, Brams DM, Munson L *et al*. Gastric outlet obstruction secondary to pancreatic cancer. *Surg Endosc* 2002;16:310–312.

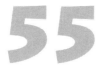

Palliative chemotherapy and/or radiotherapy for pancreatic cancer: what can be expected?

Matthias Löhr and Frederik Wenz

Treatment of patients with pancreatic cancer has always been a challenge due to the short natural course of the disease and our inability to extend this substantially at the present time. This chapter addresses conventional chemotherapy, radiotherapy, and combinations thereof; novel treatments are discussed in the following chapter. In line with the focus of this book, only drugs in clinical studies are mentioned and discussed. The most important thing we can do for these patients is to be there and to offer what is called "best supportive care," which should adequately address the two major issues, pain and appetite/weight loss, as well as any anxiety that may be associated with pancreatic cancer.

Palliative chemotherapy

Single-agent chemotherapy

Until recently 5-fluorouracil (5-FU) has been the most commonly used chemotherapeutic agent for pancreatic cancer either alone or in combination with other agents. However, in 1997 gemcitabine was brought on to the market and has rapidly become the chemotherapeutic treatment of choice for pancreatic cancer. Gemcitabine is a deoxycytidine analog (difluorodeoxycytidine; dFdC) that is phosphorylated intracellularly by deoxycytidine kinase to its active form, difluorodeoxycytidine triphosphate (dFdCTP). DNA synthesis is inhibited if dFdCTP is incorporated into nascent DNA strands instead of dCTP. Interestingly, insertion of dFdCTP into DNA allows the further insertion of an additional base pair before DNA polymerase is inhibited and this "masked termination" makes DNA repair more difficult.

Gemcitabine also has self-potentiating activity in that it (i) stimulates the activity of intracellular deoxycytidine kinase, thereby increasing its own concentration in treated cells; (ii) inhibits the activity of ribonucleotide reductase, thus reducing the intracellular pool of deoxynucleoside triphosphates including dCTP; and (iii) inhibits the activity of deoxycytidine monophosphate deaminase, the enzyme involved in gemcitabine degradation.

Gemcitabine has also gained fame for being the first chemotherapeutic agent to be approved that has a primary end point of clinical benefit (reduction of pain, improvement in performance status, weight gain) rather than the conventional end point of response as measured by tumor response, survival, and time to disease progression. After promising results were obtained in early trials, a multicenter phase III study comparing 63 patients receiving gemcitabine with 63 patients receiving 5-FU was performed. Although over 70% of the patients entering the trial had Stage IV disease, patients receiving gemcitabine showed a statistically significant advantage in median survival (5.7 months) compared with those treated with 5-FU (4.4 months), leading to a 1-year survival probability of 18% for gemcitabine-treated patients compared with 2% for 5-FU-treated patients. However, irrespective of the treatment received, none of the patients in this study survived beyond 19 months. As mentioned above, clinical benefit was taken as the primary end point of this phase III study. The primary end point was achieved by almost 24% of the patients treated with gemcitabine whereas only 5% of the patients receiving 5-FU experienced a clinical benefit. Gemcitabine has also been shown in a phase II clinical trial to have an effect in patients previously treated with 5-FU but who did not respond to treatment.

Gemcitabine is generally a well-tolerated chemotherapeutic agent, with less than 10% of patients discontinuing therapy. The most commonly reported adverse effects have been neutropenia, fever, nausea and vomiting, as well as abnormalities in liver function. Minimal and reversible hair loss has been experienced by 15% of patients treated with gemcitabine.

Even though gemcitabine has been widely accepted as a benchmark by the clinical oncologist for pancreatic cancer, it should be noted that the best combination treatments still only result in median survival of under a year. The overall response rate from several thousand patients treated is about 15%. Despite novel developments in the administration of the drug ("fixed-dose rate"), the search is on for novel and sometimes unconventional alternatives that may, either singly or in combination with gemcitabine, 5-FU, or other agents, significantly increase median survival of patients with pancreatic cancer.

Combination chemotherapy

The combination of gemcitabine with other chemotherapeutic agents may be expected to increase both the median survival time and clinical benefit response. A phase II study combining gemcitabine with 5-FU in 54 patients resulted in a median survival time of 7 months and a clinical benefit response of 51%. A median survival of 10.4 months was obtained in another study where the dose of 5-FU was kept constant and escalating doses of gemcitabine were given. The combination of gemcitabine with an orally administered 5-FU compound (capecitabine) in a phase II study did not result in prolonged survival of the patients.

Within a large phase III study, more than 300 patients with advanced pancreatic cancer were treated with either gemcitabine alone or gemcitabine plus oxaliplatin (GEMOX). Preliminary data presented at ASCO 2003 showed a significant advantage of the GEMOX scheme in response rate and progression-free survival. This study is ongoing. The combination of gemcitabine with the original platinum compound cisplatin did not demonstrate a significant advantage over the single gemcitabine treatment. Nevertheless, several large phase III clinical studies are ongoing, both in the USA (Gastrointestinal Tumor Study Group, GITSG) and in Europe (EORTC).

It is the clinical experience that some patients will respond to chemotherapy for some time (progression-free survival) before the tumor starts to grow again. While in other diseases such as breast cancer and colorectal cancer second-line regimens are standard, this has not been studied in pancreatic cancer. Therefore, trials addressing this issue are of utmost importance. At the moment, there is an ongoing study examining the benefit of combination chemotherapy (oxaliplatin, 5-FU, folinic acid) versus best supportive care, including erythropoietin.

In summary, gemcitabine monotherapy has become the benchmark for palliative chemotherapy of inoperable pancreatic carcinoma. So far, combinational regimens have not provided a breakthrough but there is an incremental extension of the overall survival with some of the drugs, such as oxaliplatin. Second-line therapy will eventually be offered to those who responded intitially and are in good general condition.

Novel agents and enzymes

Matrix metalloprotease inhibitors

Membrane type 1 matrix metalloprotease (MT1-MMP) is an enzyme that plays a major role in the remodeling of the extracellular matrix (ECM). It cleaves ECM components such as fibronectin and type 1 collagen and activates other ECM remodeling enzymes such as progelatinase A and procollagenase 3. MT1-MMP is overexpressed both in the stromal cells surrounding malignant tumors and in invasive tumor cells, where it may play an important role in tumor metastasis. Thus this enzyme represents a legitimate target for potential antitumor therapies. A matrix metalloprotease inhibitor called marimastat has been tested in phase I/II clinical trials in pancreatic cancer patients. Unfortunately, although the initial results suggested a clinical effect, lack of efficacy was reported for marimastat in a phase IIb/III multicenter trial as a monotherapeutic agent for pancreatic cancer. A phase III multicenter trial investigating the efficacy of marimastat in combination with gemcitabine in a large placebo-controlled study also failed to show either a significant increase in survival or a clinical benefit response compared with gemcitabine alone, although the manageable tolerability of marimastat and its ease of administration may be advantageous.

Antitopoisomerases

During the replication of DNA, the enzyme topoisomerase causes DNA nicking and unwinding. After replication, the nicked DNA is then religated and rewound by this enzyme. Antitopoisomerases prevent DNA ligation after replication by interfering with the topoisomerase enzyme and thus disrupt DNA synthesis. Antitopoisomerases have been shown to be nontoxic in nude mice even at high doses and give good activity against transplanted xenogenic tumors. Topoisomerase inhibitors such as irinotecan and the semisynthetic camptothecin analog topotecan, also known as Hycamtin, are often used in the treatment of colorectal and ovarian cancer.

Topoisomerase inhibitors such as irinotecan, topotecan, rubitecan, and DX-8951f have been extensively tested in clinical trials for pancreatic cancer. Generally, these drugs seem to be particularly effective in combination with classic chemotherapeutic agents such as gemcitabine, docetaxel, or 5-FU, although the best results obtained to date still only seem to give median survival times of around 6 months. The main adverse effect associated with these drugs is diarrhea and while there is some evidence for potential resistance mechanisms, the clinical trials so far have not yet generated any data in this regard.

Irinotecan was approved for recurrent colorectal cancer in the USA in 1996 and has undergone extensive testing for its efficacy against a variety of solid tumors since. Two early phase II studies in which irinotecan was used alone demonstrated objective response rates of around 10% for patients with advanced pancreatic cancer. These studies provided the basis for both phase I and phase II studies that compared the effects of gemcitabine alone to a combination therapy with irinotecan. Of the 45 patients treated with both agents, nine had an objective response with a median survival of 6 months. These findings have led to a phase III trial currently underway, as well as a phase II trial evaluating a combination of docetaxel with irinotecan.

The results from a phase I clinical trial in which topotecan was given in combination with gemcitabine has been published. In this dose-finding study, gemcitabine (400–1000 mg/m^2) was given intravenously over 30 min followed by a 15-min infusion of topotecan (0.75–2.5 mg/m^2) weekly for three consecutive weeks in a 4-week treatment cycle; 38 patients with advanced refractory solid tumors, including pancreatic cancer, and good performance status were treated. The major dose-limiting toxicity in this study was found to be myelosuppression. Partial responses were observed in two patients (one with pancreatic carcinoma). Disease stabilization occurred in five patients (three with pancreatic carcinoma, one with rectal carcinoma, and one with metastatic carcinoma of an unknown primary site). Gemcitabine 1000 mg/m^2 and topotecan 2.5 mg/m^2 were the maximum tolerated doses for this combination.

Rubitecan or RFS2000 has been tested in a phase II clinical trial for pancreatic cancer. Of the 60 patients that completed a minimal 2-month treatment period with the orally administered topoisomerase inhibitor, 19 patients (31.7%) responded to treatment (one patient surviving 4 years), a further 19 patients (31.7%) exhibited stable disease, whereas the remaining 22 (36.6%) were nonresponders. These studies have been extended to pivotal phase III multicenter studies, including 50 centers in the USA, comparing rubitecan with either the most appropriate treatment or with gemcitabine.

Another topoisomerase I inhibitor, DX-8951f, has completed phase I evaluation and shows activity against a wide range of tumor types. DX-8951f may be of particular interest since it may overcome the usual mechanism by which cells acquire resistance to camptothecin analogs by reducing intracellular drug accumulation. A phase II study has been completed using DX-8951f for patients with advanced and metastatic pancreatic cancer. In this trial, the median survival for the 39 patients enrolled was 5.5 months, with a 1-year survival of 27%. These figures increased considerably to 10.6 months and 35% if only the 19 patients who had not received prior chemotherapy were considered. These results have led to a phase III trial comparing DX-8951f plus gemcitabine with gemcitabine alone.

Nucleoside analogs

Troxacitabine (also known as BCH-4556, Troxatyl, SPD 758) is a dioxolane nucleoside analog of cytidine. Incorporation of this analog during DNA replication results in termination of DNA synthesis and inhibition of DNA polymerase. In contrast to other cytidine analogs used in cancer gene therapy, troxacitabine cannot be degraded by cellular cytidine deaminases. After good preclinical data in pancreatic human tumor xenograft models and encouraging results from a phase I trial, a phase II clinical trial involving about 250 patients with a number of different types of solid tumor, including pancreatic cancer, has been initiated and is ongoing.

Carbohydrates

Carbohydrates play an important and often underestimated role in tumor biology, for example expression of the galectin-3 receptor is correlated with metastatic spread in preclinical animal models. Carbohydrates such as the pectin derivative GBC-590 have been shown to bind the galectin-3 receptor, thereby reducing metastatic potential as well as causing direct shrinkage of tumors in preclinical models. Based upon encouraging results obtained from a phase I trial in which the dose-limiting toxicity of GBC-590 was determined, a phase II clinical trial is ongoing where patients with refractory or relapsing carcinoma are treated with GBC-590. Preliminary results from this trial were presented at ASCO 2001 but have subsequently not been published as a full paper. Treatment consisted of GBC-590 20 mg/m^2 given intravenously over 3 hours twice weekly. Toxicity was minimal, the most common adverse effect being progressive fatigue. The preliminary conclusion of this study was that although GBC-590 is a well-tolerated agent at the dose used, it did not show antitumor efficacy at this dose in pancreatic adenocarcinoma.

Acylfulvenes

Chemically modified versions of toxins naturally produced by the sesquiterpene mushroom *Omphalotus illudens* are called acylfulvenes. One of these, hydoxymethylacylfulvene (HMAF or irofulven) is a potent antiproliferative agent. Irofulven alkylates cellular nucleophiles to form adducts with proteins, DNA, and RNA. It induces single-strand DNA breaks that cause the cells to arrest at the S-phase of the cell cycle, thereby resulting in cell death by a caspase-dependent apoptotic pathway. This antitumor activity is specific and not dependent on the status of the tumor-suppressor proteins p21 and p53 in the tumor cell. The interaction of irofulven with so many cellular targets may account for its potent antitumor activities. Irofulven has shown efficacy against a number of different xenograft tumor models established by injection of various human tumor cells. Even tumors previously shown to be refractory to other antitumor agents have responded to treatment with irofulven. Use of an agent that affects proteins, RNA, and DNA may be expected to elicit unacceptable adverse effects. However, the re-

sults of a phase I clinical trial with this agent showed that irofulven dose levels could be attained that were consistent with those that demonstrated a significant antitumor response in animal models. Moreover, the adverse effects observed in the phase I trial also paralleled those in animals, with the primary dose-limiting effect being bone marrow suppression. A phase II clinical trial involving patients who had failed treatment with gemcitabine revealed that 8 of 22 patients (36%) treated with irofulven were alive at 6 months and two of the patients had greater than 50% shrinkage of the measurable tumor. A pivotal phase III trial for patients with gemcitabine-refractory pancreatic cancer was initiated in February 2001 and is ongoing. Other studies in which irofulven is combined with gemcitabine or other agents are also planned. The US Food and Drug Administration has granted Fast Track designation for the use of irofulven in patients with gemcitabine-refractory pancreatic cancer.

Kinase inhibitors

Based on our current understanding of the tumor biology of pancreatic carcinoma (see Chapter 56), it seemed natural to explore the therapeutic effect of a variety of inhibitors of pivotal enzymes. One target is farnesyltransferase, the key enzyme activating the *ras* oncogene. While a phase I study demonstrated safety, a recently published phase II clinical trial using the R11577 compound resulted in a median survival of 20 weeks, similar to the natural course or gemcitabine monotherapy. However, several other compounds are currently being investigated in ongoing clinical studies. Similar results were obtained with a tyrosine kinase inhibitor, raltitrexed (Tomudex), in combination with gemcitabine during a phase II study, showing a median survival in 25 patients of 200 days (7.3 months).

Palliative radiotherapy

Combined radiochemotherapy for locally advanced disease

About 25% of all pancreatic cancer patients present with locally advanced, inoperable, but not metastasized tumor. Untreated, these patients have a median survival time of about 3 months and most patients suffer from local symptoms, e.g., back pain due to infiltration of the celiac plexus or the vertebral column, or from obstruction of the bowel.

A series of prospective randomized studies, including the hallmark study from GITSG, defined combined radiochemotherapy using 5-FU as the standard of care for these patients in the early 1980s. The median survival time of about 8–9 months was superior to the results from radiotherapy alone. Escalating the radiation dose to 60 Gy compared with 40 Gy had no measurable effect using these irradiation techniques. However, due to the comparatively high rate of acute gastrointestinal adverse effects, the question was raised whether this toxic treatment was justified in patients with a limited lifespan.

Since then, several newer drugs like gemcitabine or paclitaxel have shown considerable antitumor efficacy in pancreas cancer. Several promising phase II studies with considerable numbers of selected patients have reached median survival times of up to 11 months, suggesting superiority compared with historical radiochemotherapy trials. In contrast, the published results of the subsequent larger phase III trials including unselected patients were rather disappointing, with a median survival in the range of 6 months and only 15% of patients surviving 1 year. Complete and partial responses have been reported in only about 11% of the cases.

Over the last two decades, there has been significant progress in treatment planning and delivery of radiation therapy in parallel with the advances in chemotherapy. In addition, refined noninvasive staging methods (e.g., high-resolution ultrasound and magnetic resonance imaging) enable reliable detection of metastases and exclusion of these patients from aggressive therapies.

The main progress in radiation oncology relevant to the treatment of locally advanced pancreatic cancer is the advent of treatment planning based on three-dimensional computed tomography (CT) and conformal delivery to reduce the irradiated volume of normal tissue. This is especially significant for the small bowel because nausea and vomiting as well as late intestinal damage are the major limitations of radiotherapy of organs in the upper abdomen. Compared with the standard of care 20 years ago (i.e., X-ray simulator planned administration of opposing anteroposterior portals), the volume of small bowel in the high dose volume is reduced by about 50% simply by using a four-field box technique. Furthermore, the radiation dose to the kidney, especially relevant when radiotherapy is combined with chemotherapy, can be markedly reduced, decreas-

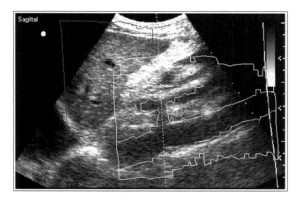

Figure 55.1 Pancreas and celiac trunk located using a stereotactic ultrasound device (BAT, Nomos Corp.) before each daily dose of radiation, increasing the precision of dose application and reducing the dose to healthy structures.

ing the probability of late delayed radiation damage. Using modern radiotherapy techniques, doses up to 72 Gy can be given to the pancreas with a low risk of acute and late radiation-induced toxicity, as has been shown in a prospective phase II study from Japan that yielded a median survival of 11 months and a 1-year survival of 39%.

Using these conformal radiotherapy techniques, doses of 50 Gy and more can be safely delivered in combination with chemotherapy. A recent phase III study demonstrated a median survival of 13 months and 1-year survival of 53% with radiation and 5-FU. The patients in the control arm received best supportive care and survived a median of 6.4 months.

Inoperable, locally advanced tumors of the pancreas are ideal targets for future developments in image-guided radiotherapy, e.g., using ultrasound (Fig. 55.1) and/or CT, and combination therapy. Continuous-infusion 5-FU, gemcitabine, paclitaxel, oxaliplatin, and cisplatin all act as potent radiosensitizers and show considerable activity in this disease entity. It appears obvious from the literature that patients in good overall condition without distant metastases benefit from the addition of radiotherapy to chemotherapy.

Palliative radiotherapy for metastatic or recurrent disease

The majority of patients with pancreatic cancer suffer from distant metastases either at initial diagnosis or later during their lifespan. Radiotherapy is an effective method for alleviating symptoms from circumscribed metastases like liver, lung, or bone metastases. In addition, local recurrences or progressive disease can cause severe symptoms secondary to infiltration of the celiac plexus or bowel structures. Palliative radiotherapy is usually given in 10–15 fractions over 2–3 weeks in an outpatient setting and is a very cost-effective treatment modality.

Liver and lung metastases

Local treatment options for visceral metastases of gastrointestinal tumors were neglected for many years. Experience from pediatric oncology, where patients with oligometastases are often treated aggressively with curative attempt, has spurred recent interest in local ablative treatment of solitary or oligometastases, especially in the liver and lung. A series of studies demonstrated that local treatment of metastases especially from colorectal cancer can result in 5-year survival rates of more than 25%.

A noninvasive treatment option for visceral metastases is a novel method called stereotactic radioablation or extracranial radiosurgery (Fig. 55.2). Radiosurgery techniques, i.e., the focal application of a single high dose of radiation (> 20 Gy) in a stereotactic setup, have been technically transferred from the brain to extracranial body sites. The patient is immobilized using alpha cradles or vacuum pillows. After CT-based radiotherapy treatment planning, 10–15 focused, individually collimated treatment portals are used to irradiate the metastasis in a single setting within less than 60 min. Local control rates of 80–90% can be achieved using this method, comparable to other local ablative therapy options.

Local recurrence/progression

The uncontrolled local progression of an inoperable or recurrent pancreatic tumor is often accompanied by severe symptoms, mainly caused by infiltration or compression of the celiac plexus and/or compression of parts of the bowel. Palliative radiotherapy can reduce the pain secondary to infiltration of the nerval plexus when drugs fail. The mechanism of pain reduction is comparable to the effects radiotherapy induces in the case of bone metastases. Even a minor shrinkage of the tumor reduces the compression of the nerve roots. Lymphocytes, which constitute a considerable part of the macroscopic tumor volume and the peritumoral in-

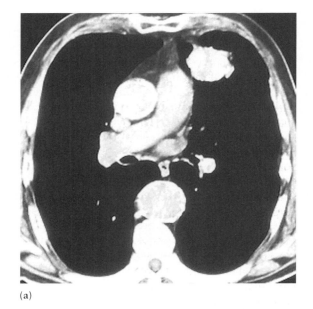

(a)

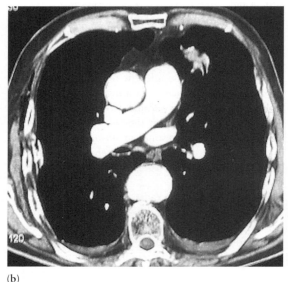

(b)

Figure 55.2 CT images of a lung metastasis (a) before and (b) 1 year after radiosurgery with locally applied dose of 20 Gy.

flammation, are very sensitive to radiation-induced cell killing. Lymphocytes are among the few cell types undergoing rapid apoptosis after exposure to radiation and therefore symptomatic response may be seen as early as within hours to a few days after therapy.

Conclusions

What can be expected from palliative chemotherapy alone or in combination with radiotherapy? Firstly, treatment of pancreatic cancer must not be more severe than the disease itself; this is mandatory and one of the rules in clinical oncology. This principle is generally fulfilled by the quasi-standard gemcitabine monotherapy. However, with response rates oscillating around 15%, this does not qualify under strict oncologic guidelines as a standard therapy. Combination chemotherapy, especially with oxaliplatin, seems to be more efficient but is also accompanied by increased adverse effects, thus infringing the quality of life of the patient. Nevertheless, with novel substances being entered into clinical trials, there may be some progress. The combination of conventional chemotherapy with other principles, e.g., enzyme inhibitors or antibodies, is suggestive and promising, especially because of the few adverse effects reported to date. The combination of chemotherapy with radiation seems to offer substantial benefit for patients with locally advanced disease or local recurrence. Due to the new technical developments in this field, we may expect considerable progress here in the next few years.

Recommended reading

Alberts SR, Townley PM, Goldberg RM *et al*. Gemcitabine and oxaliplatin for metastatic pancreatic adenocarcinoma: a North Central Cancer Treatment Group phase II study. *Ann Oncol* 2003;14:580–585.

Ashamalla H, Zaki B, Mokhtar B *et al*. Hyperfractionated radiotherapy and paclitaxel for locally advanced/unresectable pancreatic cancer. *Int J Radiat Oncol Biol Phys* 2003;55:679–687.

Atkins JH, Gershell LJ. Selective anticancer drugs. From the analyst's couch. *Nat Rev Cancer* 2002;1:645–646.

Cohen SJ, Ho L, Ranganathan S *et al*. Phase II and pharmacodynamic study of the farnesyltransferase inhibitor R115777 as initial therapy in patients with metastatic pancreatic adenocarcinoma. *J Clin Oncol* 2003;21:1301–1306.

El-Rayes BF, Zalupski MM, Shields AF *et al*. Phase II study of gemcitabine, cisplatin, and infusional fluorouracil in advanced pancreatic cancer. *J Clin Oncol* 2003;21:2920–2925.

Haller DG. New perspectives in the management of pancreas cancer. *Semin Oncol* 2003;30(Suppl 11):3–10.

Kralidis E, Aebi S, Friess H, Buchler MW, Borner MM. Activity of raltitrexed and gemcitabine in advanced pancreatic cancer. *Ann Oncol* 2003;14:574–579.

Kurtz JE, Negrier S, Husseini F *et al*. A phase II study of docetaxel–irinotecan combination in advanced pancreatic cancer. *Hepatogastroenterology* 2003;50:567–570.

McKenna S, Eatock M. The medical management of pancreatic cancer: a review. *Oncologist* 2003;8:149–160.

Wenz F, Tiefenbacher U, Fuss M, Lohr F. Should patients with locally advanced, non-metastatic carcinoma of the pancreas be irradiated? *Pancreatology* 2003;3:359–366.

56 Novel treatments and gene therapy in pancreatic cancer

Matthias Löhr and Nicholas R. Lemoine

This chapter provides some insight into recent developments in novel approaches to the treatment of pancreatic carcinoma besides conventional chemotherapy and also covers the growing field of gene therapy for pancreatic cancer. While there is tremendous progress being made in the laboratory, the focus is on substances and concepts that have reached the clinic, albeit in experimental settings (phase I/II studies). There is no doubt that some of the strategies studied in the laboratory, such as expression of dominant-negative receptors or targeting p53-deficient tumor cells, may eventually make it to early clinical studies.

Immunologic strategies

Monoclonal antibodies

Monoclonal antibodies have been approved and are already used in the clinic to treat HER2-expressing breast cancers (Herceptin) and CD20-expressing non-Hodgkin's lymphomas (Rituxan; generic name rituximab). Binding of the monoclonal antibody to the target tumor-associated protein results in recruitment of the body's natural defenses, which attack and kill the marked B cells. A humanized monoclonal antibody directed against carcinoembryonic antigen (CEA), expressed on many tumors including those of the pancreas (30%), recently received orphan drug status from the US Food and Drug Administration (FDA) for the treatment of pancreatic cancer and is currently being evaluated in phase I clinical trials.

SB408075 is a humanized monoclonal antibody that recognizes C242, an epitope on the glycoprotein Lewis

A, found on more than 90% of pancreatic cancers as well as on other carcinomas. This monoclonal antibody has been attached to the chemotherapeutic antimicrotubule agent maytansine. Evidence for antitumor activity was observed in several patients after administration of SB408075 to 37 patients suffering from pancreatic or colorectal cancer or certain non-small-cell cancers. In a second approach, also targeting C242, the staphylococcal enterotoxin A has been coupled to the Fab fragment of the C242 antibody. Staphylococcal enterotoxin A is a strong superantigen that binds to both the T-cell receptor and the major histocompatibility complex (MHC) II, resulting in more than 10% of all T cells being stimulated to produce cytokines. The combination of specific antibody response and the cytokine release from stimulated T cells is expected to give strong antitumor activity. The results of a phase I trial at the San Antonio Cancer Institute showed unexpected severe toxicity resulting in termination of this study.

The epidermal growth factor receptor (EGFR) is often expressed on the surface of a number of human tumor cells, including 30–50% of all pancreatic cancers, and this expression is associated with a poor prognosis. A monoclonal antibody called Erbitux or IMC-C225, directed against EGFR, blocks the ability of EGF to initiate receptor activation and thus growth signaling to the tumor. Erbitux has been tested in combination with gemcitabine in a phase II trial involving patients with EGFR-positive tumors. The response rate was 12%, with a 1-year survival rate of 32.5%. Currently, there are some randomized phase II studies ongoing or just closed using Erbitux in combination with conventional chemotherapy.

Herceptin, the above-mentioned antibody against the second EGFR (HER2/neu), has also been investigated in combination with gemcitabine in a clinical phase I study. Although only 21% of the tumors were HER2-positive, the response rate was 24%, the median survival 7.5 months, and 1-year survival 24% (of 32 patients).

Immunomodulation

The immune response modifier Virulizin is derived from bovine bile. This agent recruits both monocytes and macrophages as well as stimulating tumor necrosis factor-α production from tumor cells and promoting the apoptosis (programmed cell death) of tumor cells, though the exact mechanism of action of Virulizin is not fully understood and is the subject of ongoing research. The median survival time recorded in a small trial of Virulizin at the University of Nebraska Medical Center was 6.7 months, with 11 of 19 patients still alive after 6 months and one patient surviving 2 years. Furthermore, in contrast with other chemotherapeutic agents and biological response modifiers, the maximum tolerated dose has yet to be reached in clinical studies. This lack of toxicity may (i) provide patients receiving Virulizin with a better quality of life compared with those receiving classical chemotherapeutic agents and (ii) allow its use in combination therapies with such chemotherapeutics without additional adverse effects. In a phase II clinical trial involving 22 patients with measurable biopsy-proven pancreatic cancer, 6 of 17 evaluable patients demonstrated stable disease but none of the 17 patients showed evidence of tumor regression. Recently, a phase III trial was initiated aimed at enrolling 350 patients with advanced (unresectable, recurrent, or metastatic) pancreatic cancer with a view to submitting an investigative new drug at the completion of the study. These patients will be randomized to receive treatment with either gemcitabine or gemcitabine plus Virulizin. Those patients who fail to respond, or become refractory, to gemcitabine will then be treated with 5-fluorouracil (5-FU) either alone or in combination with Virulizin.

Therapeutic vaccines

A therapeutic vaccine is able to reverse the effects of an ongoing and established disease process and, as such, is conceptually different to the more well-known and widely used prophylactic vaccines. Most tumor cell-specific vaccines being developed are therapeutic in that the intention is to direct the immune system against an already established tumor rather than protecting the individual from future tumors, although if efficacious therapeutic vaccines can be produced, they may also be useful in the long term in a prophylactic setting as has recently been proven for cervical cancer.

Around 90% of pancreatic cancer patients have activating mutations in the K-*ras* oncogene, which makes it a potential target for therapy. One approach is to inhibit the cascade leading to the activation of Ras protein via the enzyme farnesyltransferase (see Chapter 55). Another is vaccination. In such an approach, autologous antigen-presenting cells are either loaded with synthetic Ras peptides, carrying identical mutations to those found in the patient, or are transduced and then reinfused into the patient. In a peptide loading study, a peptide-specific immune response was detected in two of five treated patients. The investigators hope to be able to boost the immune response to the tumor using multiple vaccinations according to this method. However, this has not been published so far. Another study using synthetic Ras mutant peptides plus granulocyte–macrophage colony-stimulating factor (GM-CSF) as an immunobooster resulted in a significant immune response in 58% of the patients. Those who responded are reported to have a longer survival (148 vs. 61 days).

The hormone human chorionic gonadotropin (hCG) plays a role in promoting the growth of a number of different tumor cells. It also promotes angiogenesis and thus encourages the formation and establishment of metastases. Peptides derived from hCG have been used to create a therapeutic cancer vaccine known as Avicine. Avicine has been used to treat a variety of solid tumors including pancreatic cancer. A multicenter phase II clinical trial of Avicine in patients with advanced pancreatic cancer was initiated in June 1999 and compares the efficacy of Avicine alone with the potential synergistic effects of gemcitabine. The 1-year survival data for patients receiving Avicine alone were found to be similar to those reported for gemcitabine. However, patients had no significant vaccine-related adverse effects, in contrast to gemcitabine-associated adverse effects. Interestingly, the 1-year survival for the patient group treated with both Avicine and gemcitabine was significantly better than either treatment alone. The trial is still ongoing but of the patients treated so far, one has shown survival for 22 months. As well as survival, the study included as end points (i) specific antibody responses to the vaccine and (ii) influence of chemotherapy on antibody response. Patients treated with chemotherapy and vaccine together had nearly equivalent antibody responses to vaccination, indicating that gemcitabine had little or no impact on the ability of pancreatic cancer patients to respond to a new immune challenge.

The hormone gastrin, like hCG, also stimulates the growth of many gastrointestinal tract cancers. Consequently, a therapeutic vaccine consisting of the aminoterminal portion of the hormone linked to a diphtheria toxoid was produced. This vaccine is expected to raise antibodies that block the interaction of the amino terminus of gastrin with its receptor. The results from two phase II trials have been encouraging, with one study reporting 46% and 82% of patients producing antibodies to gastrin when given low and high doses of vaccine, respectively. The median survival calculated for all patients was 187 days; when limited to patients showing antigastrin antibodies, it was 217 days compared with 130 days for patients given best supportive care. In the second study, patients received only the higher dose of the vaccine and the median survival was 297 days. Over one-third of these patients gained weight. A pivotal phase III trial with this therapeutic vaccine alone or in combination with gemcitabine was started in 2000 but stalled by the company and the FDA for reasons yet to be unraveled.

Heat-shock proteins (HSPs) act as intracellular policemen or chaperones, keeping other proteins in the right places and in the correct conformation in cells. As a result of this function they are intimately associated with a large number of cellular proteins and recently have been shown to be involved in the process of antigen presentation. Purification of HSPs results in the copurification of various peptides. If these HSP–peptide complexes are purified from tumor cells, they should carry tumor-specific peptides and thus can be used as a tumor-specific vaccine. Such autologous HSP–peptide complexes (HSPPC-96) prepared from patients with pancreatic cancer as patient-specific tumor vaccines were studied in a phase I clinical trial. The HSP–peptide vaccine was applied to each patient more than once. To date, one of the five vaccinated patients has shown a significant CD8$^+$ T-cell-mediated antitumor response. Like the immune stimulatory

approach, for example with GM-CSF (see below), this method is laborious, since a treatment has to be prepared for each individual patient and this depends on access to high-tech facilities [good manufacturing practice (GMP)].

GM-CSF transfected allogeneic tumor cells

A popular strategy for the immune therapy of a wide variety of tumors is stimulation of the patient's own immune system. This approach makes the assumption that the immune system is failing to recognize the tumor as foreign. The immune system may be alerted to recognize and destroy tumor cells if it is primed with tumor cells that have been genetically modified to express a potent immunostimulatory cytokine. GM-CSF is one such candidate cytokine. It plays a central role in the recruitment and differentiation of the cells required for efficient presentation of antigens to other cells of the immune system, thereby generating an efficient immune response. In this approach, a vaccine (called GAX) is produced based on the patient's own tumor cells. The cells are obtained from a biopsy and grown in cell culture, modified by transduction with a retroviral vector carrying the GM-CSF gene, lethally irradiated, and reintroduced into the patient, a so-called *ex vivo* approach. Researchers at Johns Hopkins University Medical Center in Baltimore have taken this kind of approach to modify allogeneic pancreas carcinoma cells. The results of this phase I trial indicated both antitumor immune responses and prolonged, ongoing, disease-free survival for as long as 4 years, albeit in a subset of patients. A phase II trial has recently been published in which the efficacy of GVAX was evaluated in up to 60 patients who had undergone surgical resection of their tumor. GVAX was given in combination with surgical resection and followed by standard adjuvant radiation and chemotherapy. Although disease-free survival was within the range of 10–15 months, there was a subset of patients in whom no recurrence has been recorded to date.

Although there are a large number of immune stimulatory molecules to choose from, only single- or two-component systems have been used for immunotherapy in a number of tumors. Since the immune system relies on a series of signals that have to be given in a coordinated fashion, this approach may be insufficient.

Gene therapy

Antisense nucleic acid strategies

Many antisense-based approaches to therapy target and bind to mRNAs encoding proteins that are necessary for maintenance of tumorigenesis. The Ras family of proteins, which are involved in signal transduction, represent one such target. Activating mutations at codon 12 (by far the most common in this disease) as well as at codons 13 and 61 subvert the normal regulation of these proteins so that they become constitutively active, driving cells into inappropriate cell divisions. The validity of these proteins as key players directly involved in the transformation process and the maintenance of tumorigenicity is supported by substantial evidence.

One potent, chemically synthesized, selective antisense inhibitor of H-*ras* gene expression, ISIS 2503, has been designed to bind specifically only the mRNA for the H-*ras* protein, and has no effect on the other members of the *ras* gene family. ISIS 2503 therefore has the potential to achieve a much higher level of specificity for its gene target than is possible with traditional drugs. Prolonged and stable disease was observed in a phase I clinical trial involving four patients, including one with pancreatic cancer. However, 75–90% of human pancreatic tumors carry a mutated K-*ras* gene, whereas H-*ras* has not been reported to be activated in this disease. Indeed, antisense K-*ras* has been shown to inhibit pancreatic tumor dissemination in the murine peritoneal cavity. Thus it would be advantageous to test an antisense drug directed against K-*ras* in pancreatic cancer therapy.

ISIS 5132 is a similar antisense drug that binds to an mRNA encoding another oncogenic protein, the human c-*raf* kinase, another protein involved in signal transduction. Raf kinases are downstream of Ras in the signal transduction cascade and should affect tumors with *raf* mutations as well as those with activated *ras*. Antisense *raf* has been shown to have an antitumor effect in a lung carcinoma model in nude mice and has been used in a clinical trial for advanced solid cancers. A liposomal formulation of a nuclease-sensitive, end-modified, antisense *raf* oligonucleotide has been shown clinically to have some potential as a tumor radiosensitizer. However, results presented at the 2000 ASCO and AACR/NCI/EORTC meetings have only described one case of stable disease in a patient with pancreatic cancer in a trial combining ISIS 5132 with 5-FU and leucovorin.

While promising data have been obtained for this type of approach in the treatment of a variety of cancers, there are problems with the dosing of these agents. Another point of concern is that although antisense oligonucleotides are designed to be targeted, the actual degree of targeting is difficult to ascertain, as is the true mechanism by which they may exert potential anti-tumor effects.

Classical gene therapy with suicide gene strategies

The use of suicide genes in combination with prodrugs, also know as genetic prodrug activation therapy or gene-directed enzyme prodrug therapy, is a popular strategy as a potential cancer therapy. The most commonly used system is the thymidine kinase gene from herpes simplex virus (HSV-tk) that converts the prodrug ganciclovir into a phosphorylated form that is incorporated into newly synthesized DNA, causing chain termination and cell death. A bystander effect can be observed using this system, i.e., not all cells have to produce HSV-tk in order to be killed. In studies employing xenografted pancreatic tumor cells in nude mice as a model system, the HSV-tk gene was delivered using adenoviral or retroviral vectors as gene transfer vehicles. The gene encoding cytosine deaminase (CD) also has been used as a suicide gene. The product of this gene deaminates the prodrug 5-fluorocytosine (5-FC) to form cytotoxic 5-FU. Pancreatic cancer-derived cell lines modified to express CD showed sensitivity to 5-FC treatment, and in immunocompetent animal models the immune system seems to be activated by the resultant cell death, potentiating the effects of the CD/5-FC treatment.

Another gene that has been exploited as conferring drug-mediated suicide is the nitroreductase gene from *Escherichia coli*. The enzyme this gene encodes can convert the prodrug CB1954 to a potent DNA alkylating agent. As with the above suicide genes, animal studies have been intriguingly promising. In this respect it should be mentioned that clinical application of any of the nonreplicating gene transfer systems currently available is unlikely to result in 100% gene transfer efficacy. Moreover, this classical suicide gene therapy approach has not been used in clinical studies until now. However, a clinical trial has recently been approved in the UK for the intraarterial delivery of Metxia (Oxford

Biomedica), a retroviral delivery vehicle carrying cytochrome P450 (CYP2B6) combined with the prodrug cyclophosphamide for patients with advanced pancreatic cancer.

Cell-based gene therapy

The chemotherapeutic agent ifosfamide is often used to treat a number of different tumors. There is some evidence for a therapeutic effect in patients with pancreatic cancer, although this is controversial and the concentrations required are so high that they result in debilitating adverse effects that preclude its routine use. Ifosfamide itself is not toxic until it is metabolized into the 4-hydroxyifosfamide form by liver cytochrome P450 enzymes such as the 2B1 isoform (CYP2B1). The 4-hydoxyifosfamide form spontaneously decays to phosphoramide mustard and acrolein, which alkylate DNA and protein respectively. Cells such as tumor cells that are dividing are then eliminated, whereas nondividing cells are not harmed. Since the half-life of these active compounds in plasma is in the order of a few minutes, ifosfamide must be administered systemically at relatively high and thus poorly tolerated doses in order to achieve a therapeutic effect in pancreatic adenocarcinoma after liver activation. Use of the ifosfamide-activating cytochrome P450 enzymes has been made in two ways. Initially, CYP2B1 was transfected into tumor cells prior to establishing a tumor in nude mice. In this setting, an excellent killing of cells carrying the transgene plus a substantial bystander effect could be demonstrated. Another approach used a cell line transfected with CYP2B1 and further microencapsulated. This system also was very successful in killing pancreatic cancer cells and tumors in the nude mouse. For the clinical setting, this concept of cell-based gene therapy has been developed for intraarterial use in patients with advanced pancreatic cancer. A phase I/II study has been completed demonstrating stable disease in 12 of 14 patients and a partial response in 2 of 14 patients treated with the microencapsulated CYP2B1-transfected cells (trademarked as CapCell) and low-dose ifosfamide administered systemically. Further, the patients did not experience any adverse effects from the chemotherapy. Survival was almost doubled compared with a control group (44 vs. 22 weeks). The treatment also resulted in clinical benefit according to the established criteria. A phase II study started but had to be paused due to problems in upscaling the production of CapCell.

Tumor suppressor replacement therapy

Targeting tumor-suppressor gene pathways is an attractive therapeutic strategy in cancer. Since the first clinical trial took place in 1996, at least 20 other trials have investigated the possibility of restoring *p53* function, either alone or in combination with chemotherapy, but with limited success. Other recent clinical trials have sought to harness abnormalities in the *p53* pathway to permit tumor-selective replication of adenoviral vectors such as *dl*1520 (Onyx-015). Other tumor-suppressor genes, such as *Rb* and *PTEN*, are potential targets for future gene therapy.

After the promise of the first clinical trial of *p53* gene replacement in nonsmall-cell lung carcinoma, those published in the past 2 years have been somewhat disappointing. In patients with locally advanced bladder cancer treated with intravesical adenoviral p53, only two of seven (29%) tumors demonstrated *p53* transgene expression, with no detectable changes in the expression of either $p21^{Waf1/Cip1}$ or *Bax*. In a phase I recurrent glioma trial, 12 patients received intratumoral adenoviral *p53* at doses between 3×10^{10} and 3×10^{12} particles, followed by tumor resection, at which time more adenoviral *p53* was injected into the tumor bed. Before treatment, only one of eight tumors was *p53* positive, whereas 10 of 12 showed nuclear *p53* staining after injection and seven of eight showed positive staining for $p21^{Waf1/Cip1}$. However, the zone of transfected cells extended no more than 8 mm from the injection site and the median overall survival for the whole cohort was only 43 weeks.

In nonsmall-cell lung cancer, intratumoral injection of 7.5×10^{12} particles of adenoviral *p53* every 21 or 28 days produced transgene expression in 17 of 25 (68%) tumors. Patients also received chemotherapy (either carboplatin/paclitaxel or cisplatin/vinorelbine), but the frequency of overall tumor response was the same in adenoviral *p53*-injected lesions and noninjected comparator lesions (52% vs. 48% respectively).

The extensive experience of *p53* gene therapy in ovarian cancer culminated in a phase III trial in which women with *p53* null or *p53* mutant tumors were randomized to chemotherapy alone or chemotherapy plus intraperitoneal adenoviral *p53* following optimum debulking primary surgery. However, the first interim analysis indicated that not only did adenoviral *p53* fail to improve effectiveness but it was also associated with increased toxicity. As a result, the study has been abandoned. A recent preclinical study in a gastric xenograft model showed enhanced efficacy of a binary adenoviral vector system expressing the proapoptotic gene *Bax* together with *p53* in clearing intraperitoneal disease.

Rb is the tumor-suppressor gene target for transforming viral proteins such as human papillomavirus (HPV) E7 and adenovirus E1A. The pathway has many components that are potential targets for therapy. Rather surprisingly, there have been many fewer studies on replacement of Rb family members than p53. Early reports suggested that the ability of Rb expression alone to inhibit tumor cell growth is variable and that Rb expression may, paradoxically, inhibit p53-induced apoptosis. Rb phosphorylation mutants and truncated variants may have enhanced tumor-suppressor function compared with the wild-type protein. One such derivative is Rb94, a splice variant initiated from a second AUG codon in the Rb mRNA and which lacks the N-terminal 112 amino acids of the full-length protein. There is evidence that Rb94 has a longer half-life than Rb itself and remains in the hypophosphorylated form for extended periods. Two recent reports suggest that adenovirus-mediated Rb94 gene transfer can induce apoptosis in models of head and neck and bladder cancers, with minimal effects on nonimmortalized normal cells. In addition to caspase-mediated apoptosis, Rb94 appeared to induce cell-cycle blockade at G2/M (rather than G1) and also rapid telomere erosion with ensuing chromosomal instability. Although it had previously been reported that full-length Rb could inhibit telomerase, the cell-cycle findings are novel and as yet unexplained.

Another Rb variant, Rb56, is also a C-terminal derivative. It contains the regions necessary for E2F binding and may be capable of inhibiting E2F-mediated transcription more efficiently than full-length Rb. Recent work on Rb56 has demonstrated the ability of a fusion protein, consisting of Rb56 and the DP-1 binding domains of E2F, to induce cell-cycle arrest in vascular smooth muscle cells and inhibit smooth muscle cell hyperplasia in response to intimal injury. Taken together, these reports suggest that Rb mutants and splice variants may be more potent tumor suppressors than Rb. Data on the potential of the other two members of the Rb family, p107 and p130, in gene therapy are very limited, but retrovirus-mediated transfer of the p130 gene can suppress the growth of lung carcinoma cells *in vitro* and *in vivo*.

Oncolytic viruses

Since adenoviruses destroy infected cells after replication by lysis and since the majority of pancreatic tumor cells carry mutations in the *p53* gene, this appears to represent a good opportunity for a therapeutic approach toward tumor selective killing. After encouraging results were obtained using nude mice xenografted with human tumor cell lines derived from cervical, laryngeal, or colorectal carcinomas, a number of human clinical trials with the Onyx-015 virus were initiated. These trials generally demonstrated that no serious adverse effects were associated with the treatment. The results of two phase I trials for pancreatic cancer failed to show evidence for replication or regression after direct intratumoral injection (computed tomography or endoscopic ultrasound), even though initial results were reported as encouraging. All the patients had tumor progression and died.

Following on from *dl*1520, a second generation of selectively replicating adenoviral vectors has now been developed. The viruses nearest to clinical trial specifically target Rb function. The adenoviral E1A protein contains two conserved regions, CR-1 (amino acids 30–60) and CR-2 (amino acids 120–127), the latter critical for binding to and inactivating Rb and whose deletion prevents formation of E1A–Rb complexes. Two similar mutants have been described recently: *dl*922/947 is deleted in amino acids 122–129, whereas Δ24 is deleted in amino acids 121–128. Both have been assessed in *in vitro* and *in vivo* models of cancer and *dl*922/947 is capable of replicating with much greater efficiency within a panel of tumor cell lines (including pancreatic cancer) than *dl*1520, with minimal S-phase induction in quiescent nonimmortalized cells. Most recently, Δ24 has been modified further to include an RGD-4C peptide into the adenoviral fiber, which permits infection of cells independently of the normal coxsackie adenovirus receptor that is frequently expressed at very low levels on tumor cells. Δ24-RGD is capable of lysing carcinoma cells *in vitro*, as well as extending the survival of mice bearing tumor xenografts. Of note, Δ24-RGD appeared to have a significantly greater cytopathic effect than Δ24 and its replication on normal human cells was at least three log scales lower than a wild-type adenovirus. Clinical trials of both Δ24-RGD and *dl*922/947 are imminent.

Further adenoviral mutants also explore targeting of the Rb pathway. Ar6pAE2fF and Onyx-411 both have an E2F promoter in place of the adenoviral E1A promoter. In addition, Onyx-411 has a second E2F promoter to drive expression of the E4 region and is also deleted in the E1A CR-2 region, like *dl*922/947. The rationale behind these modifications is that the E2F promoter is selectively activated in the presence of a defective Rb pathway and E4 gene products, especially E4 orf4/6, cooperate with E1A and E1B proteins to create a cellular environment that permits efficient expression of viral genes and thus productive viral infection. Both Ar6pAE2fF and Onyx-411 demonstrate tumor-specific replication with minimal effect on normal cells, including proliferating epithelial cells, and both were more potent and tumor-selective than *dl*1520.

In order to enhance the efficacy of the treatment, virus application has been combined with cisplatin and 5-FU in a phase II trial for head and neck cancer and resulted in a synergistic effect. Such a combination therapy could also be used for pancreatic cancer. Although the reasons for the observed synergistic effect are not known, the mechanisms of tumor cell destruction are independent and thus no cross-resistance is expected; indeed cells resistant to chemotherapy are apparently generally more responsive to virus infection.

Conclusions

Although the outlook for the pancreatic cancer patient is still bleak, there are a few rays of sunshine on the horizon, some of which may translate into efficacious therapies. It is most probable that the ability to extend life expectancy well past the 1-year mark will come from the judicious combination of some of the new therapies mentioned above with existing therapies. Indeed the way forward for these interesting modalities appears, in the first instance, to be their combination in new clinical trials with gemcitabine.

Recommended reading

Adjei AA. Blocking oncogenic Ras signaling for cancer therapy. *J Natl Cancer Inst* 2001;93:1062–1074.

Bauerschmitz GJ, Lam JT, Kanerva A *et al*. Treatment of ovarian cancer with a tropism modified oncolytic adenovirus. *Cancer Res* 2002;62:1266–1270.

Branton PE, Roopchand DE. The role of adenovirus E4orf4 protein in viral replication and cell killing. *Oncogene* 2001;20:7855–7865.

Fueyo J, Gomez-Manzano C, Alemany R *et al*. A mutant oncolytic adenovirus targeting the Rb pathway produces anti-glioma effect *in vivo*. *Oncogene* 2000;19:2–12.

Günzburg WH, Löhr M, Salmons B. Novel treatments and therapies in development for pancreatic cancer. *Expert Opin Invest Drugs* 2002;11:769–786.

Hawkins LK, Lemoine NR, Kirn D. Oncolytic biotherapy: a novel therapeutic platform. *Lancet Oncol* 2002;3:17–26.

Heise C *et al*. An adenovirus E1A mutant that demonstrates potent and selective systemic anti-tumoral efficacy. *Nat Med* 2000;6:1134–1139.

Jakubczak JL, Ryan P, Gorziglia M *et al*. An oncolytic adenovirus selective for retinoblastoma tumor suppressor protein pathway-defective tumors: dependence on E1A, the E2F-1 promoter, and viral replication for selectivity and efficacy. *Cancer Res* 2003;63:1490–1499.

Johnson L, Shen A, Boyle L *et al*. Selectively replicating adenoviruses targeting deregulated E2F activity are potent, systemic antitumor agents. *Cancer Cell* 2002;1:325–337.

Kasid U, Dritschilo A. RAF antisense oligonucleotide as a tumor radiosensitizer. *Oncogene* 2003;22:5876–5884.

Löhr M, Hoffmeyer A, Kröger J *et al*. Microencapsulated cell-mediated treatment of inoperable pancreatic carcinoma. *Lancet* 2001;357:1591–1592.

Mulvihill S, Warren R, Venook A *et al*. Safety and feasibility of injection with an E1B-55 kDa gene-deleted, replication-selective adenovirus (ONYX-015) into primary carcinomas of the pancreas: a phase I trial. *Gene Ther* 2001;8:308–315.

Parr M, Manome Y, Tanaka T *et al*. Tumor selective expression *in vivo* mediated by an E2F-responsive adenoviral vector. *Nat Med* 1997;3:1145–1149.

Rosenberg L, Lipsett M. Biotherapeutic approaches to pancreatic cancer. *Expert Opin Biol Ther* 2003;3:319–337.

Tseng JF, Mulligan RC. Gene therapy for pancreatic cancer. *Surg Oncol Clin North Am* 2002;11:537–569.

Spectrum and classification of cystic tumors of the pancreas

Markus Kosmahl and Günter Klöppel

Introduction

Cystic tumors of the pancreas are uncommon compared with ductal adenocarcinoma. However, they are of importance because nowadays most of the cystic lesions and neoplasms of the pancreas are curable, regardless of their pathology and biology.

Until the end of the 1970s the spectrum of cystic diseases of the pancreas was relatively narrow and consisted mainly of serous and mucinous neoplasms. In the 1980s, the development and widespread use of new imaging techniques led to the discovery and delineation of new categories of cystic and pseudocystic tumors, such as intraductal papillary mucinous neoplasms (also known as mucinous tumors, mucinous ductal ectasia, or intraductal papillary and mucin-hypersecreting tumors) and solid and pseudopapillary neoplasms (also known as solid and cystic tumors). In the past 10 years, improvements in imaging techniques and their systematic application in patients suffering from unexplained abdominal symptoms has led to a further increase in the number of resected cystic lesions. This in turn advanced our knowledge about these lesions. New entities (such as macrocystic serous cystadenoma, serous oligocystic and ill-demarcated tumor, solid variant of serous cystadenoma, intraductal papillary oncocytic neoplasm, mucinous nonneoplastic cyst, and acinar cell cystadenoma) have been described and the pathogenesis, morphology, and biology of the previously known entities studied in more detail.

Except that they are rare, little is known about the incidence of pancreatic lesions and neoplasms with a cystic appearance and their relative frequency. This is due to the fact that most series come from referral centers and are therefore biased with regard to the proportional distribution of the various tumor types to each other and in comparison with solid tumors. This is also true of our series of 418 cases (unpublished observations). In this series, solid pseudopapillary neoplasms with cystic changes (21.2%), intraductal papillary mucinous neoplasms (18.3%), serous cystic neoplasms (11%), mucinous cystic neoplasms (7.6%), and ductal adenocarcinomas with cystic changes (7.6%) were most frequent. The remaining uncommon cystic tumors included such lesions as lymphoepithelial cysts, cystic endocrine tumors, and cystic nonepithelial neoplasms. Pseudocysts accounted for 16.1%. In a series from the Memorial Sloan-Kettering Center in New York, the most common cystic tumors were microcystic serous cystadenomas (35.8%), intraductal papillary mucinous neoplasms (30.6%), solid pseudopapillary tumors (11.9%), mucinous cystic neoplasms (9.7%), and cystic ductal adenocarcinomas (3.7%).

Classification of cystic lesions and neoplasms of the pancreas

Throughout this chapter the term "cystic lesion" is used to designate any nonneoplastic tumorous change, whereas the term "cystic tumor" denotes any cystic lump regardless of whether it is neoplastic. The oldest classification systems for pancreatic cystic tumors are those by Yamane and Wegelin, both published in 1921, which distinguished congenital cysts, retention cysts, pseudocysts, and cystadenomas. This classification was adopted almost unchanged in the different *Atlas of Tumor Pathology* fascicles on pancreatic tumors that appeared over the years. However, our understanding of cystic pancreatic tumors has increased notably and several new entities, mentioned in the introduction to this chapter, have been described in recent years. The classification we use in this chapter considers the histopathologic features and biology of all cystic tumors of the pancreas known so far. We distinguish four groups: nonneoplastic epithelial tumors, nonneoplastic nonepithelial tumors, neoplastic epithelial tumors, and neoplastic nonepithelial tumors. The largest and most important group, the neoplastic epithelial tumors, also contains the most frequent cystic tumors, such as intraductal papillary mucinous neoplasm (IPMN), mucinous cystic neoplasm (MCN), serous cystic neoplasm (SCN), solid pseudopapillary neoplasm (SPN), ductal adenocarcinoma with cystic features (DAC), and cystic endocrine tumors. We subdivide this group, according to the WHO classification, into benign, borderline, and malignant tumors, a classification that reflects the biology of these tumors. Table 57.1 shows the detailed classification system.

Intraductal papillary mucinous neoplasm

Among the uncommon exocrine tumors of the pancreas, IPMNs have received increasing attention in recent years because of their clinical picture, favorable prognosis, unclear nature, and their obscure relationship to DAC. Although the diagnosis of IPMNs has improved considerably during the past years because the disease is better recognized, the nature of these neoplasms, their pathogenesis, and their relationship to DAC have remained obscure. Recent studies, however, seem to throw some light on these issues.

IPMNs are characterized by intraductal proliferation of mucin-producing cells, which are arranged in papillary patterns. In many IPMNs hypersecretion of mucin leads to cystic dilatation of the involved ducts (Fig. 57.1). In a few IPMNs, focal or diffuse intraductal papillary growth causes duct dilatation. The cytologic atypia in IPMNs ranges from minimal to severe; consequently they can be divided into adenomas, borderline tumors, and intraductal carcinomas. In addition, intestinal, pancreatobiliary, and oncocytic differentiation may be distinguished. Although these neoplasms are usually slow-growing tumors, approximately 30% may eventually become invasive and metastasize. IPMNs are most frequently localized in the main duct

Table 57.1 Classification of cystic neoplasms and nonneoplastic lesions of the pancreas.

Neoplastic epithelial tumors
Benign
Intraductal papillary mucinous adenoma
Mucinous cystic adenoma
Serous microcystic adenoma
Serous oligocystic ill-demarcated adenoma
Solid serous adenoma
Von Hippel–Lindau associated cystic neoplasm
Acinar cell cystadenoma
Benign neuroendocrine tumor, cystic
Cystic teratoma (dermoid cyst)
Accessory-splenic epidermoid cyst
Lymphoepithelial cyst

Borderline
Intraductal papillary mucinous neoplasm, borderline
Mucinous cystic neoplasm, borderline

Malignant
Intraductal papillary mucinous carcinoma, invasive or noninvasive
Mucinous cystic carcinoma, invasive or noninvasive
Ductal adenocarcinoma, cystic
Serous cystadenocarcinoma
Acinar cell carcinoma, cystic
Pancreatoblastoma, cystic
Solid pseudopapillary neoplasm
Low-grade malignant neuroendocrine tumor, cystic
Cystic metastatic epithelial neoplasm
Rare cystic epithelial neoplasms (e.g., paraganglioma)

Neoplastic nonepithelial tumors
Benign
Lymphangioma, cystic
Other rare nonepithelial neoplasms (e.g., schwannoma)

Malignant
Rare nonepithelial neoplasms (e.g., sarcomas)

Nonneoplastic epithelial tumors
Retention cyst
Mucinous nonneoplastic cyst
Enterogeneous cyst
Paraduodenal wall cyst
Endometrial cyst
Congenital cyst (e.g., intrapancreatic choledochal cyst)
Cystic hamartoma

Nonneoplastic nonepithelial tumors
Pseudocyst
Parasitic cyst

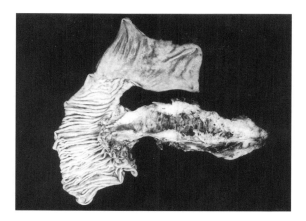

Figure 57.1 Intraductal papillary mucinous carcinoma in a 47-year-old man: Whipple resection specimen with polypoid proliferations in the main pancreatic duct.

Table 57.2 Clinicopathologic features of intraductal papillary mucinous neoplasms of the pancreas.

Ratio of men to women: 1.5 : 1
Age range: 35–85 (mean 64) years
Localization: 74% in the head region
Morphology: intraductal papillary growth and mucin production
Prognosis: favorable in at least 70% of patients

of the head region of the pancreas. Those IPMNs that arise from secondary ducts seem to have an even better prognosis than IPMNs of the main duct.

IPMNs were thought to be very rare, accounting for 1% or less of pancreatic exocrine tumors. However, in recent years better recognition of this neoplasm has led to an increase in its incidence. In our series of exocrine pancreatic tumors, the incidence of IPMNs is approximately 3%, and among the cystic neoplasms IPMNs account for 18.3%. IPMNs occur slightly more frequently in men than in women and the age range is 37–80 with a mean of 64 years (Table 57.2). Symptoms of acute and/or chronic pancreatitis are most common, but IPMNs may also be detected incidentally. Recently, it was reported that a number of patients with IPMN showed an increased rate of extrapancreatic malignancies.

The cause and pathogenesis of IPMN are obscure, but it is interesting to note that in IPMNs associated with invasive carcinoma the invasive component shows either a tubular or a mucinous pattern. The tubular invasion pattern resembles DAC, while the mucinous pattern shows the features of colloid (mucinous noncystic) carcinoma. Moreover, those IPMNs with a tubular, DAC-like invasion pattern exhibit a pancreatobiliary cell type, whereas IPMNs with the muconodular invasion pattern show a gastrointestinal cell phenotype.

Recent studies in which the mucin production in IPMNs was typed have shown that IPMNs with a gastrointestinal phenotype produce MUC2 but not MUC1, whereas IPMNs that show a pancreatobiliary phenotype lack MUC2 expression but may stain for MUC1. In addition to these distinct types of IPMNs, a third type that coexpresses MUC1 and MUC2 was distinguished. This type included the recently described oncocytic subtype of IPMN. From these studies it appears that IPMNs form a heterogeneous group of neoplasms that can be divided into at least three types on the basis of their mucin immunophenotype: a common MUC2$^+$ gastrointestinal type and two less frequent forms, either MUC2$^-$/MUC1$^+$ pancreatobiliary or MUC1$^+$/MUC2$^+$ oncocytic types. Although the common MUC2$^+$ gastrointestinal IPMNs form one group together with MUC2$^+$ colloid (mucinous noncystic) carcinoma and may be considered to be the precursor of this carcinoma, MUC2$^-$/MUC1$^+$ pancreatobiliary IPMNs appear to have a close relationship to DACs. The third IPMN type, the oncocytic type, may represent a group of its own. The molecular mechanisms involved in the altered regulation of *MUC* genes in IPMNs are not yet known, but they may be related to a different cell lineage-associated tumorigenesis in these neoplasms. It also appears that the various types of IPMNs also differ in prognosis, since MUC2$^+$ IPMNs obviously fare better than the other IPMNs. Recently, IPMNs were observed in two patients with Peutz–Jeghers syndrome.

Mucinous cystic neoplasm

MCNs of the pancreas afflict women almost exclusively, involve predominantly the body–tail of the pancreas, do not communicate with the ductal system, and may be unilocular or multilocular (Table 57.3). Since

481

Table 57.3 Clinicopathologic features of mucinous cystic neoplasms.

Ratio of women to men: 9 : 1
Age range: 23–78 (mean 47) years
Localization: > 90% in the body–tail region
Morphology: mucinous cyst without duct communication
Prognosis: excellent after complete resection

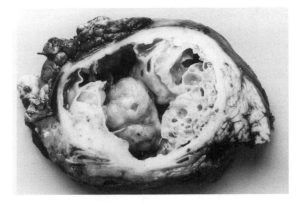

Figure 57.2 Mucinous cystic adenoma in a 42-year-old woman: the multicystic tumor is well demarcated.

the seminal paper by Compagno and Oertel in 1978, there has been a debate about the prognosis and origin of these neoplasms. Two recent studies seem to have settled the first issue. On the second, a hypothesis has been advanced.

More than 90% of MCNs occur in the body and tail of the pancreas, where they form large round cystic tumors (Fig. 57.2) showing a unilocular or multilocular cut surface and diameters between 2.7 and 23 cm. Multilocularity, localization in the head region, and presence of papillary projections and stromal nodules all correlate with an associated invasive component. The cystic spaces are lined by mucin-producing epithelial cells that are supported by an ovarian-like stroma which may be focally hyalinized. MCNs composed of cells exhibiting only minimal atypia are adenomas, whereas those with moderate or even severe atypia are borderline tumors and carcinomas respectively.

Invasive MCNs show the pattern of either a DAC or an undifferentiated carcinoma with osteoclast-like giant cells. The stroma may also contain sarcomatous nodules.

MCNs comprise approximately 1% in our series of pancreatic exocrine tumors and among the cystic neoplasms they account for approximately 7.6%. The higher frequencies that have been reported in some previous studies are probably due to the fact that IPMNs and MCNs were not clearly distinguished from each other or were still interpreted as a single entity. The clear differentiation of MCNs from IPMNs also revealed that MCNs are extremely rare in men. The age at diagnosis ranges from 23 to 78 years, though patients with invasive carcinoma are often older than 50 years (Table 57.3). More than 60% of the patients experience abdominal discomfort or pain or present with a palpable tumor. In the remaining patients the tumor is an incidental finding. The cyst fluid is usually rich in carcinoembryonic antigen (CEA) and CA-19-9 and contains columnar cells.

The prognosis of MCNs has been found to be excellent if the tumors are completely resected, and this can be achieved today in more than 90% of cases. Two recent studies based on extensive tumor sampling have shown that recurrence and tumor-related death were features of deeply invasive MCNs only.

MCNs of the pancreas resemble the same tumor category in the ovary. Like ovarian MCNs, the epithelial cells of pancreatic MCNs show gastroenteropancreatic differentiation and the stromal cells may express estrogen and progesterone receptors as well as inhibin, which has been recommended as a marker of certain ovarian neoplasms including MCN. Because of this similarity between pancreatic and ovarian MCNs, the "genital ridge hypothesis" has been advanced, which infers that cellular stromal elements from the genital ridge may associate with the dorsal pancreatic anlage, or rarely the ventral anlage, and might thus later give rise to an MCN.

The differential diagnosis of MCNs is with IPMNs especially. IPMNs, in contrast to MCNs, communicate with the duct system, are mainly localized in the pancreatic head, and occur more often in men than in women. Immunocytochemically, noninvasive MCNs are negative for MUC1 or MUC2 (except for single MUC2-positive goblet cells). Only in cases with an invasive component was MUC1 expression observed.

Serous cystic neoplasms: serous microcystic adenoma, serous oligocystic and ill-demarcated adenoma, and von Hippel–Lindau associated cystic neoplasm

Serous microcystic adenoma (SMA), serous oligocystic and ill-demarcated adenoma (SOIA), and von Hippel–Lindau associated cystic neoplasm (VHL-CN) are composed of the same cell type. This cell is characterized by glycogen-rich cytoplasm and a ductal immunoprofile. However, despite these cytologic similarities, the three types of SCN differ in their localization in the pancreas, gross appearance, gender distribution, and genetic alterations, suggesting that they represent different entities (Table 57.4). The role of the solid variant of serous cystic adenoma and of serous cystadenocarcinoma in the spectrum of SCNs is not yet clear, mainly owing to the small number of cases that have been reported so far.

In our series, SMAs equal MCNs in frequency (5.7% vs. 7.6% of cases). If SOIAs and VHL-CNs are added, the group of SCNs accounts for approximately 11% of all pancreatic cystic lesions and neoplasms. Most common are SMAs, which make up 50% of all SCNs. They present as single, well-circumscribed, slightly bosselated round tumors, with diameters ranging from 2.5 to

16 cm. Their cut surface shows numerous small (honeycomb-like) cysts arranged around a (para)central stellate scar (Fig. 57.3), which may contain calcifications. About two-thirds of SMAs occur in the body–tail region and almost all in women. They are usually found incidentally. SOIAs, which account for 35% of SCNs, are composed of few relatively large cysts (for which reason they have also been described as macrocystic serous adenoma), lack the stellate scar and round shape, and occur predominantly in the head of the pancreas, where they may obstruct the common bile duct and cause jaundice. They show no sex predilection. In patients with VHL, the SCNs arise at multiple sites and in advanced stages of the disease they may merge and involve the entire pancreas. Because VHL-CNs affect the pancreas diffusely, they differ markedly from the gross features of both SMAs and SOIAs. Biologically, it is also important to note that patients with VHL, like those with SOIA but in contrast to those with SMA, are not predominantly female. This suggests that SMAs differ in their pathogenesis from VHL-CNs and SOIAs. Recently reported molecular data support this assumption. While VHL-CNs were found to be characterized by both loss of heterozygosity (LOH) at chromosome 3p (which contains the *VHL* gene) and a germline mutation of the *VHL* gene, only 40% of SMAs had LOH at chromosome 3p and of these tumors only two (22%) exhibited a somatic *VHL* gene mutation. Interestingly, more than 50% of SMAs showed LOH at 10q. It appears therefore that alterations of the *VHL* gene are of minor importance in SMAs, while gene changes at 10q may play a major role. Whether the *VHL* gene is involved in the pathogenesis of SOIAs remains to be

Table 57.4 Clinicopathologic features of serous cystic tumors of the pancreas.

Serous microcystic adenoma
Ratio of women to men: 9 : 1
Age range: 45–91 (mean 71) years
Localization: more than 75% in body–tail region, stellate scar
Prognosis: good

Serous oligocystic adenoma
Women and men alike
Age range: 38–85 (mean 63) years
Localization: head region (60%)
Prognosis: good

Von Hippel–Lindau associated cystic neoplasm
Women and men alike
Age range: 30–70 (mean 42) years
Localization: diffuse involvement
Prognosis: good

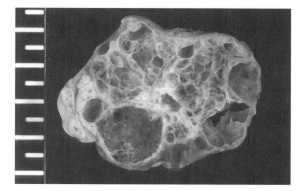

Figure 57.3 Serous microcystic adenoma in a 69-year-old woman: well-demarcated multicystic tumor with central scar.

483

elucidated. The same also holds for the extremely rare serous cystadenocarcinoma.

The differential diagnosis of SMAs is primarily with multiloculated MCNs, although their honeycomb appearance and stellate scar distinguish them quite clearly. SOIAs are more difficult to differentiate from other cystic lesions because of their variegated gross appearance. Recently we found that inhibin is expressed in the epithelial cells of all types of SCNs, but not in the epithelial lining of MCNs (unpublished observation). In MCNs inhibin only occurs in stromal cells, making inhibin a good marker for use in differentiating SCNs from MCNs.

Solid pseudopapillary neoplasm

SPNs are round tumors whose diameters may range from 2 to 17 cm. They are found in any region of the pancreas or loosely attached to it. The cut surface typically shows friable tan-colored tumor tissue, the center of which is undergoing hemorrhagic cystic degeneration, thereby forming irregular bloody cavities (Fig. 57.4). Usually SPNs appear to be demarcated by a pseudocapsule in which calcifications may occur. Histologically, there are three main features. First, solid areas merge with pseudopapillary, hemorrhagic, and pseudocystic structures. Second, the tumor tissue shows a delicate microvasculature that forms pseudorosettes or may be accompanied by hyalinized or myxoid stroma. The third feature concerns the tumor cell itself. It is unique because it does not resemble any of the known cell types in the pancreas. It shows eosinophilic or foamy cytoplasm (often containing PAS-positive globules) and a hybrid immunophenotype combining mesenchymal (vimentin, α_1-antitrypsin), endocrine (neuron-specific enolase, synaptophysin, progesterone receptor), and epithelial (cytokeratin) differentiation.

Once thought to be very rare, SPNs have distinctly increased in frequency as they came to be better recognized, and in our series they account for approximately 6% of all exocrine pancreatic tumors. If only cystic tumors are considered, SPNs (with cystic changes) are the most common type (21.2%). They occur predominantly in young women (15–35 years of age), but may occasionally be encountered in older women and also in men (Table 57.5). Many SPNs are detected incidentally. However, the patients may also present with sudden pain (because of bleeding into the tumor) or symptoms related to compression of adjacent organs.

In 90% of the patients the prognosis of SPN is excellent. In the remaining patients, metastases (peritoneum, liver) are present at the time of diagnosis or occur later after removal of the primary. Even if metastases have developed, many of them are amenable to resection, usually resulting in long-term survival of the affected patients. There are still no prognostic factors that could help in the distinction between SPNs with or without malignant potential. It is therefore necessary to treat all SPNs by complete surgical resection.

The pathogenesis of SPN is obscure. Because of its complex and hybrid immunoprofile, the cellular phenotype is not consistent with any of the known pancreatic cell types. In view of their striking female preponderance and the known close approximation of the genital ridges to the pancreatic anlage during embryogenesis, it has been hypothesized that SPNs, like MCNs, might derive from genital ridges/ovarian anlage-related cells, which were attached to the

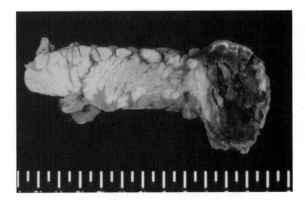

Figure 57.4 Solid pseudopapillary neoplasm in a 42-year-old woman: pseudocystic and partly hemorrhagic tumor in the tail of the pancreas.

Table 57.5 Clinicopathologic features of solid pseudopapillary neoplasms.

Ratio of women to men: 9:1
Age range: 11–73 (mean 30) years
Localization: no preference
Morphology: hemorrhagic pseudocyst in tumor
Prognosis: rarely malignant (5–10%)

pancreatic tissue during early embryogenesis. Recently it was found that most SPNs show nuclear expression of β-catenin, associated with mutations in exon 3 of the β-catenin gene.

The differential diagnosis of cystic SPNs includes pseudocysts and cystic forms of endocrine tumors of the pancreas. Apart from the typical histologic features of SPNs, the expression of such markers as vimentin and neuron-specific enolase in the absence of chromogranin A and the very faint expression of cytokeratin and synaptophysin distinguish this most enigmatic neoplasm of the pancreas from all other tumors.

Ductal adenocarcinoma and variants with cystic features

DACs and variants thereof showing cystic features are relatively frequent. In our series of cystic tumors they account for 7.6%. Three pathologic mechanisms may explain the development of cystic changes in these primarily solid neoplasms. Well-differentiated DACs may show ectatic duct-like structures that acquire a microcystic, grossly visible appearance. However, the cysts are usually no larger than 0.5 cm. The second mechanism by which DACs and their variants can become cystic is central tumor necrosis. This may occur in large tumors and especially in poorly differentiated or undifferentiated sarcomatoid carcinomas. Finally, DACs may obstruct not only the main pancreatic duct but also single secondary ducts, thereby producing small nonneoplastic retention cysts. While in the first and third cases the cystic changes are so subtle that they are usually not revealed by imaging techniques, central tumor necrosis may produce a radiographically visible cystic cavity.

Uncommon cystic neoplasms and lesions

Among the uncommon cystic tumors of the pancreas are a variety of neoplastic and nonneoplastic changes. The neoplasms include such tumors as cystic acinar cell carcinomas, cystic endocrine tumors, cystic metastases (i.e., from renal cell carcinoma), dermoid cysts, and a number of cystic nonepithelial tumors. The rare benign cystic changes include lymphoepithelial cysts, paraampullary duodenal wall cysts usually associated with duodenal wall pancreatitis (also called groove pancre-

atitis), ciliated foregut cysts, enteric duplication cysts, dermoid cysts, multicystic hamartoma, congenital cysts, endometrial cysts, parasitic cysts, and the recently briefly mentioned mucinous nonneoplastic cyst and acinar cell cystadenoma. Although the prognosis of cystic epithelial neoplasms depends on the malignant potential of the respective type of tumor, the prognosis of nonneoplastic cystic lesions is good.

Pseudocysts

The frequent pancreatitis-associated pseudocyst belongs to the nonneoplastic/nonepithelial group, indicating that it takes a benign course. A pseudocyst presents as a grossly visible and well-demarcated cystic lesion, which contains necrotic–hemorrhagic material and/or turbid fluid rich in pancreatic enzymes. The cystic contents are enclosed by a wall of inflammatory and fibrous tissue devoid of an epithelial cell lining. Pseudocysts usually occur attached to the pancreas and are a sequela of extensive confluent autodigestive tissue necrosis caused by alcoholic, biliary, or traumatic acute pancreatitis.

Pseudocysts are thought to be the most common type of cystic lesion of the pancreas, with an estimated relative frequency of 75%. In our series, pseudocysts account for only 16.1% of the cases, most likely because this is a series from a referral center, which accumulates more tumors than pseudocyst cases. The correct prevalence figures may therefore be higher than 16.1% but probably also lower than 75%, since the latter figure was generated at a time when only large cystic lesions in the pancreas were detected with certainty.

Pseudocysts develop as a consequence of an episode of severe acute pancreatitis, usually in the setting of alcoholic pancreatitis. Most of the patients are men in the age range 31–62 years (Table 57.6). If children and

Table 57.6 Clinicopathologic features of pancreatitis-associated pseudocysts in the pancreas.

Ratio of men to women: 3 : 1
Age range: 31–62 years
Localization: extrapancreatic > intrapancreatic
Morphology: no epithelial lining, hemorrhagic debris
Pathogenesis: caused by severe episodes of acute pancreatitis

adolescents are affected by pseudocysts, these are caused by hereditary or traumatic pancreatitis.

The most common differential diagnosis of pseudocyst is with IPMN, MCN, and SPN, because the gross appearance of the latter may be similar to that of pseudocysts. Histologically and cytologically, however, pseudocysts differ from the cystic neoplasms in that they lack any epithelial lining but display hemorrhagic debris and inflammatory cells. Moreover, pseudocysts contain pancreatic enzymes, such as amylase and lipase, and lack elevated levels of CEA and CA-19-9.

Recommended reading

Abraham SC, Klimstra DS, Wilentz RE *et al.* Solid-pseudopapillary tumors of the pancreas are genetically distinct from pancreatic ductal adenocarcinomas and almost always harbor β-catenin mutations. *Am J Pathol* 2002;160:1361–1369.

Adsay NV, Klimstra DS. *Cystic Lesions of the Pancreas.* Philadelphia: Saunders, 2000.

Adsay NV, Longnecker DS, Klimstra DS. Pancreatic tumors with cystic dilatation of the ducts: intraductal papillary mucinous neoplasms and intraductal oncocytic papillary neoplasms. *Semin Diagn Pathol* 2000;17:16–30.

Adsay NV, Pierson C, Sarkar F *et al.* Colloid (mucinous noncystic) carcinoma of the pancreas. *Am J Surg Pathol* 2001;25:26–42.

Adsay NV, Merati K, Andea A *et al.* The dichotomy in the preinvasive neoplasia to invasive carcinoma sequence in the pancreas: differential expression of MUC1 and MUC2 supports the existence of two separate pathways of carcinogenesis. *Mod Pathol* 2002;15:1087–1095.

Adsay NV, Hasteh F, Cheng JD *et al.* Lymphoepithelial cysts of the pancreas: a report of 12 cases and a review of the literature. *Mod Pathol* 2002;15:492–501.

Capella C, Solcia E, Klöppel G, Hruban RH. Serous cystic neoplasms of the pancreas. In: SR Hamilton, LA Aaltonen (eds) *Pathology and Genetics of Tumours of the Digestive System. WHO Classification of Tumours.* Lyon: IARC Press, 2000:231–233.

Kimura W, Makuuchi M, Kuroda A. Characteristics and treatment of mucin-producing tumor of the pancreas. *Hepatogastroenterology* 1998;45:2001–2008.

Klöppel G. Clinicopathologic view of intraductal papillary-mucinous tumor of the pancreas. *Hepatogastroenterology* 1998;45:1981–1985.

Klöppel G. Pseudocysts and other non-neoplastic cysts of the pancreas. *Semin Diagn Pathol* 2000;17:7–15.

Klöppel G, Hruban RH, Longnecker DS, Adler G, Kern SE,

Partanen TJ. Ductal adenocarcinoma of the pancreas. In: SR Hamilton, LA Aaltonen (eds) *Pathology and Genetics of Tumours of the Digestive System. WHO Classification of Tumours.* Lyon: IARC Press, 2000:221–230.

Klöppel G, Lüttges J, Klimstra D, Hruban R, Kern S, Adler G. Solid-pseudopapillary neoplasm. In: SR Hamilton, LA Aaltonen (eds) *Pathology and Genetics of Tumours of the Digestive System. WHO Classification of Tumours.* Lyon: IARC Press, 2000:246–248.

Kosmahl M, Seada LS, Jänig U, Harms D, Klöppel G. Solid-pseudopapillary tumor of the pancreas: its origin revisited. *Virchows Arch* 2000;436:473–480.

Longnecker DS, Adler G, Hruban RH, Klöppel G. Intraductal papillary-mucinous neoplasms of the pancreas. In: SR Hamilton, LA Aaltonen (eds) *Pathology and Genetics of Tumours of the Digestive System. WHO Classification of Tumours.* Lyon: IARC Press, 2000:237–240.

Lüttges J, Zamboni G, Longnecker D, Klöppel G. The immunohistochemical mucin expression pattern distinguishes different types of intraductal papillary mucinous neoplasms of the pancreas and determines their relationship to mucinous noncystic carcinoma and ductal adenocarcinoma. *Am J Surg Pathol* 2001;25:942–948.

Lüttges J, Feyerabend B, Buchelt T, Pacena M, Klöppel G. The mucin profile of noninvasive and invasive mucinous cystic neoplasms of the pancreas. *Am J Surg Pathol* 2002;26:466–471.

Mohr VH, Vortmeyer AO, Zhuang Z *et al.* Histopathology and molecular genetics of multiple cysts and microcystic (serous) adenomas of the pancreas in von Hippel–Lindau patients. *Am J Pathol* 2000;157:1615–1621.

Moore PS, Zamboni G, Brighenti A *et al.* Molecular characterization of pancreatic serous microcystic adenomas. Evidence for a tumor suppressor gene on chromosome 10q. *Am J Pathol* 2001;158:317–321.

Nakamura A, Horinouchi M, Goto M *et al.* New classification of pancreatic intraductal papillary-mucinous tumour by mucin expression: its relationship with potential for malignancy. *J Pathol* 2002;197:201–210.

Rattner DW, Fernandez-del Castillo C, Warshaw AL. Cystic pancreatic neoplasms. *Ann Oncol* 1999;10(Suppl):S104–S106.

Sugiyama M, Atomi Y. Extrapancreatic neoplasms occur with unusual frequency in patients with intraductal papillary mucinous tumors of the pancreas. *Am J Gastroenterol* 1999;94:470–473.

Terris B, Ponsot T, Paye F *et al.* Intraductal papillary mucinous tumors of the pancreas confined to secondary ducts show less aggressive pathologic features as compared with those involving the main pancreatic duct. *Am J Surg Pathol* 2000;24:1372–1377.

Wilentz RE, Albores-Saavedra J, Zahurak M *et al.* Pathologic examination accurately predicts prognosis in mucinous cystic neoplasms of the pancreas. *Am J Surg Pathol* 1999; 23:1320–1327.

Wilentz RE, Albores-Saavedra J, Hruban RH. Mucinous cystic neoplasms of the pancreas. *Semin Diagn Pathol* 2000;17:31–42.

Zamboni G, Scarpa A, Bogina G *et al*. Mucinous cystic tumors of the pancreas. Clinicopathological features, prognosis and relationship to other mucinous cystic tumors. *Am J Surg Pathol* 1999;23:410–422.

Zamboni G, Klöppel G, Hruban RH, Longnecker DS, Adler G. Mucinous cystic neoplasms of the pancreas. In: SR Hamilton, LA Aaltonen (eds) *Pathology and Genetics of Tumours of the Digestive System. WHO Classification of Tumours*. Lyon: IARC Press, 2000:234–236.

Zamboni G, Terris B, Scarpa A *et al*. Acinar cell cystadenoma of the pancreas. A new entity? *Am J Surg Pathol* 2002;26:698–704.

58 Diagnosis and differential diagnosis of pancreatic cystic tumors

Roberto Salvia, Isabella Frigerio, Claudio Bassi, Massimo Falconi, and Paolo Pederzoli

Introduction

The identification of cystic tumors of the pancreas has become clearer only in the past few years. Since first identified by Becourt in 1930, the major unsolved issue has been a definitive preoperative diagnosis. This clinical problem is obviously due to the fact that different cystic neoplasms require different treatment. The initial differentiation of pancreatic cystic lesions is between cystic tumors and nonneoplastic cystic lesions: this is based on the presence or absence of an epithelial lining inside the cystic wall and permits the exclusion of all simple cysts and pseudocysts. Once an epithelial lining is detected, its characteristics define different kinds of tumors.

This chapter attempts to resolve the diagnostic problems and doubts that always affect clinicians and surgeons in the management of pancreatic cystic tumors.

Classification

Our understanding of pancreatic cystic tumors is based on the WHO classification of tumors (Table 58.1).

Laboratory findings

There is no reliable serum tumor marker that can diagnose serous cystic tumor (SCT) and spare some patients unnecessary operations. Nonetheless, positive carcinoembryonic antigen (CEA) serum marker status and/or the presence of more than two positive serum markers (CEA, CA-19-9, CA-125) indicates the presence of a mucinous cystic tumor (MCT) and can prevent delay in diagnosis. Positive CEA or presence of more than two markers suggests a definitely or potentially malignant tumor and can prevent delay in diagnosis.

Serous cystic tumors

Women in their fifties seem to be the population more affected by SCTs. Any portion of the pancreatic gland can be affected by SCTs but they are more frequently detected in the pancreatic head. At histology, SCTs take the form of multiple cysts lined with cuboid flat epithelium with clear cytoplasm rich in glycogen. Based on morphologic aspects these tumors can be divided into three types: microcystic, macrocystic or oligocystic (< 3% of cases), and mixed (micro-macrocystic).

Serous cystic adenoma

Clinical findings
Serous cystic adenomas (SCAs) are mostly asymptomatic and are often detected incidentally during radiologic investigations for symptoms that may not be related to the pancreas (Fig. 58.1). When present, the most common clinical complaint is some degree of abdominal discomfort or pain. Weight loss, palpable mass, jaundice, and obstruction of the upper gastrointestinal tract are very rare and may correlate with extensive growth of the lesion. Once detected, accurate characterization of a pancreatic mass as an SCA is of primary importance since this tumor, unlike the other cystic tumors of the pancreas, is benign and therefore a

Table 58.1 Histologic classification of pancreatic cystic tumors.

Serous cystic tumors
    Serous cystadenoma
    Serous cystadenocarcinoma
Mucinous cystic tumors
    Mucinous cystadenoma
    Mucinous cystadenoma with moderate dysplasia
    Mucinous cystadenocarcinoma
      Not infiltrating
      Infiltrating
Intraductal papillary mucinous adenoma
Intraductal papillary mucinous tumors with moderate dysplasia
Intraductal papillary mucinous carcinoma
    Not infiltrating
    Infiltrating

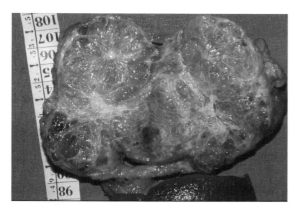

Figure 58.1 Macroscopic view of a serous cystic adenoma (microcystic pattern).

conservative approach should be the treatment of choice whenever possible. Despite the fact that symptoms are not helpful for diagnosis, overall they can guide the identification of a benign or malignant neoplasm. Suspicion of SCA should also arise in the presence of Von Hippel–Lindau syndrome, a genetic condition associated in 15% of cases with SCA.

Radiology

Ultrasound is usually the first step in diagnosis, and as a result of its widespread use in clinical practice it has significantly increased the number of incidental observations of SCA. The diagnosis is easily made when ultrasound shows a mass with multilobulated borders, no posterior acoustic enhancement, and an internal "honeycomb" architecture due to the presence of multiple septae that delimit small (< 2 cm diameter) cystic spaces. In 10–30% of cases, there can be calcifications within the septae and, even less frequently, a central calcified scar. The microcystic appearance is also seen in SCA associated with von Hippel–Lindau syndrome, although in these cases the tumor is multicentric or diffusely involves the whole gland. There are two circumstances where ultrasound may fail to recognize a microcystic SCA: in the presence of a sponge-like mass where the multiplicity of small cysts and thick fibrous stroma produce the false impression that the tumor is solid; and in the case of a mixed tumor when the macrocystic component conceals the microcystic with the misdiagnosis of a macrocystic mass. The macrocystic type is easily detectable even when the size is small. The aspect is of a sharply marginated, hypoechoic mass; there might be sparse, thin, central septae and in this case the differential diagnosis from the other cystic mass is very difficult. In the mixed SCA, together with the microcysts, larger (> 2 cm) cystic spaces can be found at the periphery of the lesions resulting in a mixed pattern. The macrocyst can grow up to 8–10 cm, making it difficult to recognize the true nature of the tumor. The false-negative rate is low and is due to tumor location (tail) or patient characteristics (obesity, meteorism).

The appearance of SCA on computed tomography (CT) depends on two factors: macroscopic features and timing of data acquisition. Microcystic tumors appear as an unenhanced mass affecting or deforming the profile of the gland. The density is homogeneous or slightly superior to that of water, isodense in respect to the parenchyma. When calcifications are present the location is always quite central, punctate, or globular, as opposed to the lamellar calcifications seen in MCTs. Usually a central fibrous scar is visible in the larger masses since it forms later. Maximal visualization of septae, as well as the honeycomb appearance, occurs in the pancreatic parenchymal phase. The presence of central calcification in conjunction with scars or septae definitively characterizes a cystic mass as an SCA. In the mixed forms peripheral macrocysts are even more easily recognizable than by ultrasound, thus making the diagnosis easier. In the delayed phase of contrast injection, recognition of septae is very difficult because of their resemblance to intracystic liquid. Macrocystic patterns are indistinguishable from other macrocystic masses of the pancreas (e.g., MCTs).

Magnetic resonance imaging (MRI) is assuming an important role in the work-up of these tumors due to the accurate information it provides about the structure of the lesion, in particular the presence of septae. In the microcystic pattern, MRI is able to demonstrate even a small amount of fluid within the dense septae of a "sponge-like" mass but has the disadvantage that it is insensitive to calcifications. In macro-microcystic cases the two components are easily recognizable. The technique of magnetic resonance cholangiopancreatography (MRCP) provides even better evaluation of the spatial relationship between the mass and the biliary or pancreatic duct and thus can be used to discriminate the diagnosis with intraductal papillary mucinous neoplasm (IPMN), particularly when the tumor is located on the head or in the uncinate process of the gland. MRCP should be carried out routinely in the staging of these tumors since it helps to distinguish microcystic SCA from intraductal tumor of the peripheral branches, which has a septate appearance. The absence of communication with the Wirsung duct confirms the diagnosis of SCA. MRI investigation of oligocystic forms is nonspecific and does not lead to a definitive differential diagnosis from mucinous forms.

Serous cystic adenocarcinoma

Serous cystic adenocarcinoma is a malignant form of SCT, all cases being described as microcystic forms. We concur that SCT should be basically considered a benign lesion and, if no complications or diagnostic doubts occur, conservative treatment and follow-up is the chosen policy.

Differential diagnosis

The finding of a mass with the described features in the pancreatic head of a female patient with no dilation of the duct, a normal parenchyma, and calcification leads to a definitive diagnosis of SCT. The diagnosis can be considered definite when the lesion shows a mixed aspect with macrocysts in the periphery of a microcystic nucleus. Despite the microcystic aspect, the diagnosis is less certain when the cystic mass is located in the uncinate process of a male patient and associated with main duct dilation: in this event, in order to make the dif-

ferential diagnosis with IPMN of branch ducts, it is mandatory to demonstrate the relationship between the mass and the duct of Wirsung. MRCP is useful for this purpose, but in those cases where the lesion is very close to the main duct endoscopic retrograde cholangiopancreatography (ERCP) is necessary. For different reasons, as we previously stressed, a mass can appear as a solid lesion therefore leading to misdiagnosis with other bright enhanced solid lesions, such as nonfunctioning neuroendocrine tumors. In these cases MRI will be able to detect the microcystic aspect.

Since accurate radiologic characterization of macrocystic SCT is not possible using ultrasound, CT, or MRI, endoscopic ultrasound seems to be the only technique able to supply further information.

Mucinous cystic tumors

Epidemiology
MCTs occur exclusively in women. These neoplasms are preferentially located in the body and tail and are characterized by unilocular/multilocular cysts that do not communicate with the ductal system. The tumor is encapsulated and lined by columnar mucin-producing cells overlying an ovarian-type stroma, thus explaining the exclusive incidence in a female population. The patient age range is huge, with an average that seems to depend on the degree of malignancy of the neoplasm: patients with malignant MCT appear to be older, suggesting a time-related degeneration from benign lesions. Early diagnosis of malignant transformation of MCT is essential since the prognosis, once the malignant form occurs, is the same as for ductal adenocarcinoma, whereas in the *in situ* forms surgery could be curative.

MCT is, at best, a premalignant lesion and it is therefore important to distinguish it from other cystic lesions of the pancreas. Pathologically, all the different degrees of malignant transformation can be detected at the same time in the same lesion. This has a great relevance, suggesting an adenoma–carcinoma sequence.

Clinical findings
Once again symptoms are few, nonspecific, and do not help in the diagnostic process. Abdominal discomfort or pain is the most frequent in both benign and malignant lesions and, even if present, it is unusual

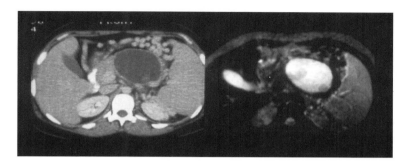

Figure 58.2 Mucinous cystic tumor of the pancreatic tail with radiologic features suggesting malignancy: thick wall, papillary growth on the posterior wall, and collateral vessels from vascular compression/infiltration (computed tomography and magnetic resonance respectively).

for patients to complain about pancreatic-specific pain (radiation to the flanks); even early symptoms might not be of concern. However, nonspecific symptoms can also suggest malignant forms: weight loss, anorexia, and obstructive jaundice are common in malignancies.

Radiology

Radiologic investigations describe two patterns of MCT: macrocystic multilocular and macrocystic unilocular. The macrocystic multilocular pattern is not pathognomonic but is frequently located in the body–tail of the gland, appearing on ultrasound images as a sharply defined mass surrounded by a variably thickened wall. Thin septae delimit cystic spaces and calcifications are a common finding. On CT, the pre-contrast phase can easily detect calcifications. The density of the content depends on the amount of mucin or fluid–fluid level from underlying bleeding. This pattern is clearly demonstrated by contrast medium: walls and septae display lower enhancement compared with the surrounding pancreatic parenchyma because of the fibrous composition and minimal vascularization. The outer wall and septa have similar thickness. The macrocystic unilocular pattern is less specific and simulates any kind of pancreatic cystic mass on both ultrasound and CT. As a consequence, differentiation cannot be made easily in cases with unique cysts having a thin wall, no calcifications, and no parietal nodules.

From the radiologic point of view, thickened wall, presence of papillary proliferations arising from the wall or septae, evidence of peripheral calcifications, as well as invasion of surrounding vascular structure are considered the best signs of malignancy (Fig. 58.2). The diagnosis will be clearer if extracapsular extension of the lesion is detected on contrast-enhanced CT. When

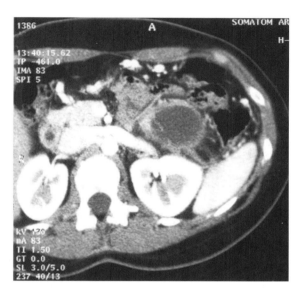

Figure 58.3 Computed tomography of a mucinous cystic tumor of the pancreatic tail showing intratumoral septae.

thick walls, thick septae, and calcifications are simultaneously present, the probability of malignancy is 95%. When fewer than three signs are present, the probability of malignancy declines, being zero when there are no calcifications, no septae, and the wall is thin. Because calcifications cannot be detected by MRI, CT is the primary imaging modality for these patients (Figs 58.3 & 58.4).

The predominant fluid content of these masses renders MCT brighter on T2-weighted MRI. The presence, features, and distribution of internal septae are better seen with these techniques. T2-weighted images are optimal for the study of the Wirsung duct. When the mass clearly appears to be isolated from it, thereby

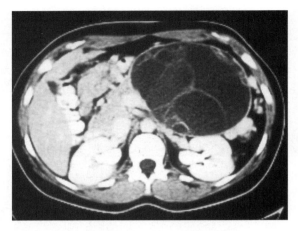

Figure 58.4 Computed tomography of a mucinous cystic tumor of the body–tail of the pancreas showing thin septae.

excluding the possibility of an intraductal tumor, no further examination with MRCP is required.

Differential diagnosis

The macrocystic multilocular pattern is considered typical but not pathognomonic. Oligocystic SCT, solid pseudopapillary tumors (cystic variant), and cystic endocrine tumors have identical appearance. In these cases, clinical history and laboratory data are essential for diagnosis. Oligocystic SCT is almost never preoperatively differentiated from benign MCT.

In neuroendocrine and pseudopapillary tumors, the cystic component is due to previous necrosis and intra-tumoral bleeding. In the former the clinical syndrome might help in diagnosis; in the latter MRI will enhance the different appearance of fluid content.

Pseudocysts make the diagnosis difficult, mainly with the macrocystic unilocular pattern. MCT should be suspected if there is no history of severe acute pancreatitis that might explain the presence of a cystic lesion as a pseudocyst.

Intraductal papillary mucinous tumors

IPMNs of the pancreas are a relatively new entity among mucinous cystic tumors. Described for the first time in 1982 as neoplasms with mucin hyper-production, dilatation of the duct of Wirsung, and protruding papilla (the Ohashi triad), there has been a true epidemiologic "explosion" in recent years. The disease originates in the epithelium of the pancreatic ducts, all the biological stages (i.e., from slight dyspla-sia to carcinoma) being simultaneously present within the same lesion. Currently, most agree that evolution toward the carcinoma stage is slow but probably inexorable.

Initially, the main clinical problem was to recognize IPMN and to differentiate it from chronic pancreatitis. The majority of undiagnosed IPMNs are, in fact, wrongly interpreted as chronic pancreatitis. Increased awareness of these tumors has decreased the number of incorrect diagnoses. Nowadays, preoperative recogni-tion of the histologic grading of these tumors is desirable. The need for this is related to a series of considerations concerning patients and disease: the only option for treatment is partial or total surgical re-section although this option applies to patients who are generally elderly (65–70 years old) with comorbidity. However, patients with malignant tumor benefit from surgery and resection, whereas patients harboring a be-nign tumor should be strictly followed up.

Diagnosis and the evaluation of clinical/radiologic data for preoperative staging are the main goals in the assessment of IPMNs.

Epidemiology

Men and women, equally distributed, in their sixties and seventies represent the population affected by this tumor, a feature useful for distinguishing IPMN from chronic pancreatitis (marked male predominance and average age of 42). In our experience alcohol and tobacco intake are also important.

Clinical findings

Unlike the other cystic tumors, recurrent pain is com-mon and described as pancreatitis-like. The painful symptomatology is generally continuous, related to meals, and localized in the upper area of the abdomen, radiating to the back. However, in our experience an episode of acute pancreatitis severe enough to poten-tially develop a pseudocyst has occurred in less than 2% of all IPMNs observed. Another frequent symptom is weight loss, which is found in 42% of our patients. Weight loss might be caused by two different phys-iopathologic mechanisms related to the stage of the dis-ease. In the early phases, hyperproduction of mucin obstructs normal pancreatic secretion, causing the pain related to meals. Thus patients stop eating in order to avoid pain, as happens in those with chronic pancreatitis. In more advanced stages, the weight loss is more likely due to the production of neoplastic factors responsible for cachexia. Asthenia was more frequent in those patients with advanced disease ($P < 0.05$). The sudden onset of diabetes almost always leads to the suspicion of ductal adenocarcinoma; 11% of patients suffering from IPMN have diabetes. In our experience, the recent onset of diabetes or its worsening within a year more frequently occurred in patients with advanced tumors ($P < 0.005$). The symptom, when present, therefore has a double significance: suspicion of the neoplasm and tumor malignancy. Jaundice, like diabetes, plays an important role, being a typical symptom of pancreatic head disease. Jaundice is a sign of the tumor in its advanced stages. In conclusion, incidental diagnosis of IPMN occurs only in 30–35% of cases, while the majority are symptomatic.

Radiology

The widespread use of ultrasound and CT and the greater familiarity with the typical findings are the most important reasons why these lesions are more frequently recognized. The imaging findings depend on whether the tumor is located in the main duct or in the collateral duct or both (Figs 58.5–58.7).

Ultrasound detection of a dilated main duct in the absence of an obstructing mass or a history that explains a postinflammatory stenosis should arouse suspicion of segmental IPMN. In the diffuse form, the whole duct is dilated to different degrees and, unlike the segmental forms, it is common to find ectasia of the duct, typically in the head. In this case it is not always easy to establish whether the whole duct is affected or if the cephalic tract neoplasm is associated with dilation of the upstream duct because of the obstruction. Parenchymal atrophy is usually proportional to ductal dilation. It is not always possible to distinguish whether echogenic spots within the ducts are due to mucin plugs or papillary proliferation. IPMN of collateral ducts is easier to identify because of its location mainly in the head or uncinate process. The lesion, with honeycomb microcystic or unilocular/multilocular macrocystic architecture, never appears as a solid mass. Ultrasound fails to identify the communication of cystic lesions with the pancreatic ducts.

CT has significantly improved the recognition of IPMN. With noncontrast images it is possible to identify the ectasia and, by distending the duodenal lumen with water, to recognize the protruding papilla. Calcifications can be due to associated chronic pancreatitis or, when centrally located in the duct, to deposits of calcium within the mucin. When the lesion originates in collateral branches, it is recognizable whenever it

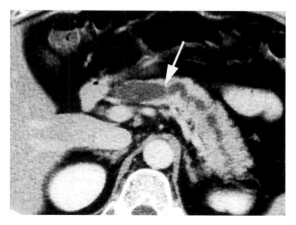

Figure 58.5 Computed tomography of a diffuse intraductal papillary mucinous tumor of the main duct.

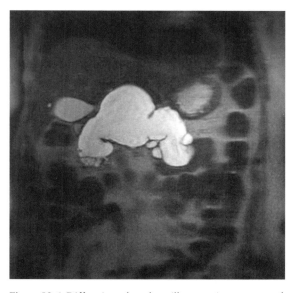

Figure 58.6 Diffuse intraductal papillary mucinous tumor of the main duct with massive dilation of the duct of Wirsung Colangio–Wirsung magnetic resonance image.

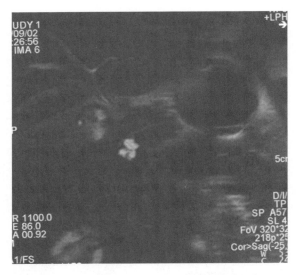

Figure 58.7 Magnetic resonance image of a peripheral-branch intraductal papillary mucinous tumor of the uncinate process.

ly this information was achievable only with ERCP. Nowadays, the thin sections obtained by both CT and MRI allow the communication to be recognized. In particular, MRCP with intravenous injection of secretin is very sensitive. The thick mucin can obstruct the small collateral ducts, and therefore the contrast medium cannot spread into the most peripheral branches to allow visualization of the cystic dilation.

In the forms involving both the main duct and collateral branches, the true site of origin cannot be discerned. Ultrasound can distinguish the main duct from secondary branches but more often there may be one large mass that occupies the whole pancreatic head. Dilation of the bile duct is the result of this mass effect. CT documents the multiple ductal ectasia associated with dilation of the main duct. Mucin deposit is always seen in the advanced forms. Despite their large size, multiple lesions sometimes have thin walls that protrude toward the peritoneal cavity, with the appearance of ascites.

Differential diagnosis

Demographic data (sex, age) and lifestyle may contribute to the differential diagnosis between IPMN and chronic pancreatitis, whereas once the diagnosis is made the presence of jaundice and diabetes are suggestive of malignancy. Although IPMNs of the main duct can simulate chronic pancreatitis, tumors involving the secondary ducts ("side branch" IPMNs) must be differentiated from other cystic tumors.

The differential diagnosis between branch side IPMNs and SCA is difficult and particularly important since the latter is almost always benign. SCA is more common in females (female to male ratio 6.7 : 1), with an average age of 51.8 years, 10 years younger than for IPMN. The tumor is mainly located in the head of the pancreas. In our experience, about 45% of SCAs were located within the head and the pancreatic neck, 27% in the body, and 28% in the tail. The demographic characteristics, case history, and lifestyle do not lead to differentiation between the two types of tumor. The presence of symptoms, mainly jaundice, diabetes and "pancreatitis-like" pain, may indicate IPMN since almost all SCAs (75%) are discovered incidentally.

The differences in clinical presentation between IPMN and MCT are less important, because the potential malignancy of all these forms always indicates surgical treatment. MCT occurs almost exclusively in

produces a localized mass. On contrast-enhanced images the central lesion is better outlined against the contrast-enhanced parenchyma. In the lumen of the duct it is possible to recognize mucin or papillary proliferations because of their higher density. Malignant degeneration must be considered whenever significant ductal dilation with normal or increased parenchymal thickness is present. This suspicion is also supported by the presence of papillary proliferations. Even in advanced stages of malignancy, the cystic component is always recognizable, allowing differentiation from ductal adenocarcinoma. Coexisting cystic ectasia of the collateral ducts and a protruding papilla make the diagnosis of diffuse forms easier. In segmental forms, CT is nonspecific. If the pattern is of a cystic mass, most commonly in the tail, a communication with the pancreatic duct should confirm the diagnosis.

Frequently, but not always, IPMN of collateral ducts has a unifocal character. When multiple lesions are present, they can involve the whole gland. Assessment of wall and septal thickness is a useful indicator of malignancy, but it should be stressed that a thin wall does not rule out a malignant form.

Demonstration of a communication with the main duct is mandatory for a precise diagnosis. Until recent-

women of around 45 years of age. The average age is higher when the neoplasm exhibits malignant behavior. The topography of the neoplasm can be useful for differential diagnosis, since IPMN is usually located in the uncinate process whereas 93% of MCTs involve the body–tail. Moreover, it is necessary to point out that IPMN is almost always symptomatic, mimicking chronic pancreatitis, whereas MCT is almost always asymptomatic. At imaging, the radiologist should be aware of all appropriate history and clinical information.

Recommended reading

Bassi C, Salvia R, Gumbs AA, Butturini G, Falconi M, Pederzoli P. The value of standard serum tumor markers in differentiating mucinous from serous cystic tumors of the pancreas: CEA, Ca 19-9, Ca 125, Ca 15-3. *Langenbecks Arch Surg* 2002;387:281–285.

Bassi C, Salvia R, Molinari E, Biasiutti C, Falconi M, Pederzoli P. Management of 100 consecutive cases of pancreatic serous cystadenoma: wait for symptoms and see at imaging or vice versa? *World J Surg* 2003;27:319–323.

Brat DJ, Lillemoe KD, Yeo CJ, Warfield PB, Hruban RH. Progression of pancreatic intraductal neoplasias to infiltrating adenocarcinoma of the pancreas. *Am J Surg Pathol* 1998;22:163–169.

Buetow PC, Rao P, Thompson LD. From the archives of the AFIP. Mucinous cystic neoplasms of the pancreas: radiologic–pathologic correlation. *Radiographics* 1998; 18:433–449.

Carbognin G. *Serous Cystic Tumors*. New York: Springer-Verlag, 2003.

Eriguchi N, Aoyagi S, Nakayama T *et al*. Serous cystadenocarcinoma of the pancreas with liver metastases. *J Hepatobiliary Pancreat Surg* 1998;5:467–470.

Falconi M, Salvia R, Bassi C, Zamboni G, Talamini G, Pederzoli P. Clinicopathological features and treatment of intraductal papillary mucinous tumour of the pancreas. *Br J Surg* 2001;88:376–381.

Fukukura Y, Fujiyoshi F, Sasaki M, Inoue H, Yonezawa S, Nakajo M. Intraductal papillary mucinous tumors of the pancreas: thin-section helical CT findings. *Am J Roentgenol* 2000;174:441–447.

Furukawa T, Takahashi T, Kobari M, Matsuno S. The mucus-hypersecreting tumor of the pancreas. Development and extension visualized by three-dimensional computerized mapping. *Cancer* 1992;70:1505–1513.

Klöppel GSE, Longnecker DS, Capella C, Sobin LH. Histological typing of tumours of the exocrine pancreas. In: *World Health Organization International Histological Classification of Tumours*. Berlin: Springer-Verlag, 1996.

Koito K, Namieno T, Ichimura T *et al*. Mucin-producing pancreatic tumors: comparison of MR cholangiopancreatography with endoscopic retrograde cholangiopancreatography. *Radiology* 1998;208:231–237.

Longnecker DS. Observations on the etiology and pathogenesis of intraductal papillary-mucinous neoplasms of the pancreas. *Hepatogastroenterology* 1998;45:1973–1980.

Navarro F, Michel J, Bauret P *et al*. Management of intraductal papillary mucinous tumours of the pancreas. *Eur J Surg* 1999;165:43–48.

Neumann HP, Dinkel E, Brambs H *et al*. Pancreatic lesions in the von Hippel–Lindau syndrome. *Gastroenterology* 1991;101:465–471.

Nishihara K, Kawabata A, Ueno T, Miyahara M, Hamanaka Y, Suzuki T. The differential diagnosis of pancreatic cysts by MR imaging. *Hepatogastroenterology* 1996;43:714–720.

Ohashi K, Murakami Y, Murayama M *et al*. Four cases of mucus secreting pancreatic cancer. *Prog Dig Endosc* 1982;20:348–351.

Procacci C. Intraductal papillary mucinous tumors: imaging. In: Procacci C, Megibow AJ, eds. *Imaging of the Pancreas*. New York: Springer-Verlag, 2003:97–137.

Procacci C, Graziani R, Bicego E *et al*. Intraductal mucin-producing tumors of the pancreas: imaging findings. *Radiology* 1996;198:249–257.

Procacci C, Graziani R, Bicego E *et al*. Serous cystadenoma of the pancreas: report of 30 cases with emphasis on the imaging findings. *J Comput Assist Tomogr* 1997;21:373–382.

Procacci C, Biasiutti C, Carbognin G *et al*. Characterization of cystic tumors of the pancreas: CT accuracy. *J Comput Assist Tomogr* 1999;23:906–912.

Rivera JA, Fernandez-del Castillo C, Pins M *et al*. Pancreatic mucinous ductal ectasia and intraductal papillary neoplasms. A single malignant clinicopathologic entity. *Ann Surg* 1997;225:637–644; discussion 644–646.

Salvia R. Intraductal cystic tumors: clinical manifestations and therapeutic management. In: Procacci C, Megibow AJ, eds. *Imaging of the Pancreas*. New York: Springer-Verlag, 2003.

Sperti C, Cappellazzo F, Pasquali C *et al*. Cystic neoplasms of the pancreas: problems in differential diagnosis. *Am Surg* 1993;59:740–745.

Sugiyama M, Atomi Y. Intraductal papillary mucinous tumors of the pancreas: imaging studies and treatment strategies. *Ann Surg* 1998;228:685–691.

Traverso LW, Peralta EA, Ryan JA Jr, Kozarek RA. Intraductal neoplasms of the pancreas. *Am J Surg* 1998;175:426–432.

Warshaw AL. Mucinous cystic tumors and mucinous ductal

ectasia of the pancreas. *Gastrointest Endosc* 1991;37: 199–201.

Widmaier U, Mattfeldt T, Siech M, Beger HG. Serous cystade-nocarcinoma of the pancreas. *Int J Pancreatol* 1996;20: 135–139.

Zamboni G, Scarpa A, Bogina G *et al*. Mucinous cystic tumors of the pancreas: clinicopathological features, prognosis, and relationship to other mucinous cystic tumors. *Am J Surg Pathol* 1999;23:410–422.

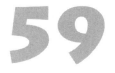

The role of endoscopic ultrasonography in the diagnosis and management of cystic tumors of the pancreas

Enrique Vazquez-Sequeiros and Julio Iglesias-García

Introduction

Pancreatic cysts may be classified as benign lesions or as malignant lesions or lesions with malignant potential. It is important to accurately differentiate those cysts that have a potential for degeneration from those that do not, as treatment decision and patient prognosis depends on the nature of the lesion. Differential diagnosis is usually based on a combination of clinical symptoms, laboratory data, and imaging studies such as transabdominal ultrasound, computed tomography (CT), and magnetic resonance imaging (MRI), sometimes complemented with biopsy sampling and cyst aspiration for fluid analysis. However, in certain cases, the limited resolution of these imaging tests may preclude adequate imaging of small pancreatic cystic lesions or prevent differentiation of a macrocystic mucinous tumor from a benign inflammatory pseudocyst. The image resolution provided by current endoscopic ultrasound (EUS) processors, which is higher than that of conventional imaging techniques, has permitted the targeting of tiny cystic lesions of the pancreas that are often too small to be identified by these complementary imaging techniques or too well encased by surrounding vascular structures to allow percutaneous biopsy methods. For these reasons, EUS and EUS-guided fine-needle aspiration (FNA) have acquired in recent years a prominent role in the evaluation of patients with known or suspected pancreatic cystic lesions.

Equipment

Current echoendoscopes consist of a conventional endoscope provided with an oblique forward viewing fiber or video optic system, and a high-frequency ultrasound transducer located at the tip of the scope. High-resolution images of the gut wall and surrounding organs, including the pancreas, may be obtained with the echoendoscope.

Two different types of dedicated instrument are currently employed for EUS examinations. The most commonly used is the radial echoendoscope (mechanical Olympus GIF-UM 160: 5–20 MHz, 360° image; electronic Pentax EG-3630UR: 5–10 MHz, 270° image), which provides a transverse image perpendicular to the longitudinal axis of the endoscope. The ultrasound transducer operates at different frequencies and can be switched remotely from one frequency to another during the examination, modifying the depth of penetration and the degree of definition (e.g., higher ultrasound frequencies provide higher image resolution but lower penetration than the lower frequencies). The curved linear electronic array echoendoscope (Pentax EG-3630U, EG-3830UT, FG-34/36/38X: 5–10 MHz; Olympus GF-UC30P, GF-UCT160-OL5: 7.5 MHz) provides a sagittal scan parallel to the longitudinal axis of the endoscope, allowing one to biopsy lesions under real-time EUS guidance. Doppler and color Doppler are also available and may be employed to identify vascular structures. At present, different types of needles are available for EUS FNA. The most commonly used in clinical practice are made by Wilson-Cook (Echotip EUSN-1, Echotip EUSN-19T, Quick-Core EUSN1-19QC: 19–22 gauge), GIP-Mediglobe (Sonotip: 19–22 gauge), and Olympus (NA-10J-1: 19 gauge).

Technique

The EUS examination typically commences with use of the radial echoendoscope to identify the lesion and characterize its location, morphology (presence of septa, solid component, debris), and size and to establish a diagnosis of suspicion. When clinically indicated, the cystic lesion of the pancreas is sampled and aspirated fluid sent for analysis. EUS-guided cyst aspiration is performed by gradually advancing the needle to the center of the cyst. Traversal of the muscularis propria and the cyst wall may sometimes be difficult and occasionally a swift jabbing motion is necessary to accomplish this. When the needle has entered the lesion, the needle stylet is removed and negative pressure is applied to aspirate the cyst fluid. Occasionally, the aspirated fluid can be quite viscous (mucinous tumors and chronic pseudocysts) and it may take some time to completely drain the material.

Although infrequent, infection of the cyst, hemorrhage, or pancreatitis related to EUS FNA may occur. To minimize the risk of infection, most experts recommend making a single needle pass into the cyst in order to drain the cyst dry and to administer prophylactic antibiotics for a few days. To avoid accidental vessel puncture and bleeding, the use of Doppler is advised; to prevent pancreatitis, care should be taken to avoid traversing normal pancreatic parenchyma during cyst aspiration.

Pancreatic cystic lesions

The evaluation of cystic lesions of the pancreas is complicated due to the wide spectrum of pathologies that may present in this way and to the difficulty of differentiating lesions that are malignant or have a malignant potential (mucinous-type tumors) from those that have no malignant potential (e.g., serous cystadenomas, pseudocysts) (Table 59.1). As previously mentioned, the treatment decision differs depending on the histology of the tumor. Mucinous cystadenomas should be resected by surgery, as some reports have suggested that approximately 20% of surgical specimens have malignant degeneration. The prognosis in patients with mucinous cystadenomas is impaired, with a 5-year survival rate of 30–64% according to literature reports. In contrast, serous cystadenomas have a much better

Table 59.1 Benign and malignant pancreatic cystic lesions.

Benign/no malignant potential
Inflammatory (pseudocyst)
Serous cystadenoma (microcystic)
Lymphangioma
Hemangioma
Cystic teratoma
Paraganglioma

Malignant/malignant potential
Mucinous cystadenoma
Mucinous cystadenocarcinoma
Intraductal papillary mucinous tumor
Cystic islet-cell tumor

prognosis and rarely degenerate. For this reason surgical resection is only recommended if symptoms due to obstruction of the duodenum are present. Inflammatory pseudocysts arise in patients with a background of acute or chronic pancreatitis, and in most cases resolve with conservative measures. However, those pseudocysts that cause abdominal pain or duodenal obstruction or present signs of infection should be drained by radiologic, endoscopic, or surgical means.

Although ultrasound, CT, and MRI may identify cystic lesions of the pancreas, in many cases it is not possible to determine the nature of the lesion using these imaging techniques. In these cases, the higher resolution of current EUS scopes (as low as 0.07 mm) may help obtain the correct diagnosis. The precise images provided by EUS allow the identification of certain morphologic features that are of great assistance in the differential diagnosis of these lesions, e.g., septation, thickness and presence of irregularities in the septum, intramural internal projections, debris in the cyst fluid, communication with the main pancreatic duct, size of the cyst (microcystic vs. macrocystic lesions), presence of a central scar (microcystic adenoma). The accuracy of EUS in the diagnosis of these patients appears to be high, with most studies reporting more than 80% accuracy. EUS can also help differentiation if the cystic lesion identified by other imaging tests (i) arises in an extrapancreatic location (mesentery, kidney), (ii) represents a dilated pancreatic or bile duct imaged in cross-section, or (iii) denotes a fluid-filled diverticulum in the duodenum mimicking a cystic lesion of the pancreas.

The following sections present the results of EUS and EUS FNA of the most common pancreatic cystic lesions.

Serous-type tumor (serous cystadenoma)

The endosonographic appearance of this type of lesion is characterized by the presence of a cluster of small cysts (< 1 cm) separated by a thin wall that adopt a honeycomb pattern distribution (microcystic lesion) (Fig. 59.1a). Occasionally, a characteristic central scar or calcification may be present in the center of the lesion. Typically, microcystic adenomas do not invade the pancreatic duct. The fluid aspirated from the cyst should not be viscous and may exhibit glycogen-staining cells, which are diagnostic of serous cystadenoma. Cytologic analysis of the aspirated fluid has shown to be of little help in diagnosing this pathology (accuracy < 50%).

Mucinous-type tumors

Mucinous cystadenoma and cystadenocarcinoma

Contrary to serous-type lesions, mucinous cystadenomas typically adopt a macrocystic pattern (cysts > 1 cm in diameter) (Fig. 59.1b). More commonly, these types of lesions are unilocular, but sometimes thin septations may be observed inside the cyst. The presence of a solid component in the cystic lesion or a focal thickening in the cyst wall should raise concerns regarding malignant degeneration. Infiltration of the pancreatic duct may be observed in patients with mucinous cystadenocarcinoma.

The aspirate from these cysts is typically a dense mucoid fluid, and may sometimes require large needles to be aspirated. Needling of the cyst wall and/or any solid component of the lesion is advised in order to improve the yield of cytology. Cytologic analysis of the aspirated fluid may show columnar epithelial cells and mucin in approximately 48% of cases. This finding is diagnostic of mucinous cystadenoma. Malignant epithelial cells may be seen in the aspirate when malignant degeneration (cystadenocarcinoma) is present.

Intraductal papillary mucinous tumor

Intraductal papillary mucinous tumor (IPMT) is a rela-

tively rare tumor that originates in the pancreatic duct, producing a diffusely dilated duct with mucus inside, papillary projections, and sometimes a solid mass component. Intraductal ultrasound has been recently shown to be a useful tool for diagnosing this type of lesion and determining its extension. On certain occasions, IPMT may present as a cystic lesion (macrocystic or microcystic) in the pancreas. When IPMT is suspected, both the pancreatic duct and the cyst should be aspirated and the fluid obtained sent for cytology. Cytologic findings are similar to those observed in mucinous cystadenomas.

Inflammatory pseudocyst

These lesions may be unilocular or multilocular. Chronic pseudocysts typically show complex septations, a thick wall adherent to the gastric or duodenal wall, and solid material inside the cyst (debris and necrotic tissue) (Fig. 59.1c). Aspirated fluid tends to be dark and shows inflammatory cells under the microscope. Amylase levels in cyst fluid tend to be elevated in this type of patient, while tumor markers are within the range of normal values.

Pancreatic fluid analysis

As previously mentioned, EUS FNA allows aspiration of fluid from the cyst (Fig. 59.2). However, the usefulness of pancreatic fluid analysis is controversial. Although some studies provide data supporting this practice, others have not been able to reproduce the same positive results.

Apart from cytology, several markers have been employed to study the nature of pancreatic cysts (Table 59.2). Fluid aspirate viscosity is elevated in mucinous tumors but not in inflammatory cysts or serous cystadenoma. Amylase levels are elevated in the cyst fluid in those lesions communicating with the pancreatic duct, such as pseudocysts (very high levels of amylase) or side-branch IPMT. Several studies have shown carcinoembryonic antigen (CEA) and CA-72-4 to be elevated in the cyst aspirate of mucinous tumors but not in inflammatory or serous cysts (CA-72-4: sensitivity 87.5%, specificity 94%). CA-19-9 has been found elevated in both benign and malignant lesions and does not appear to be useful in the evaluation of these

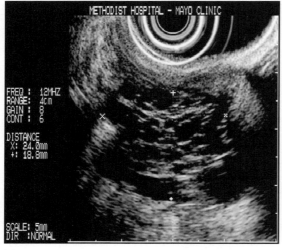

(a)

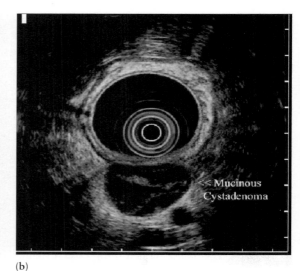

(b)

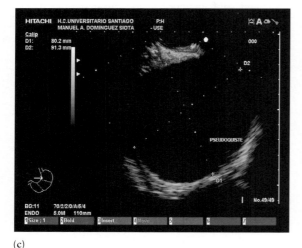

(c)

Figure 59.1 (a) Serous cystadenoma: a microcystic tumor of the pancreas (cysts < 10 mm in diameter). The lesion measures 18 × 24 mm and presents the characteristic central scar (arrowheads). (b) Mucinous cystadenoma: pancreatic cyst that shows longitudinal septae dividing the cyst cavity (arrowheads). The endosonographic appearence of the lesion is consistent with a macrocystic tumor of the pancreas (cysts > 10 mm in diameter). In this particular case it was confirmed by surgery to be a mucinous cystadenoma. (c) Inflammatory pseudocyst: a large cyst is observed in the pancreatic gland (80 × 91 mm) in a patient with a recent episode of acute pancreatitis. The cyst presents thin walls, is not septated, and shows echogenic material inside (debris) (arrowheads). These findings are suggestive of an inflammatory pseudocyst in the acute/subacute phase.

patients. Although one small study showed that K-*ras* mutations were absent in all cases of serous cystadenoma and present in all cases of cystadenocarcinoma, the role of K-*ras* mutation detection in these patients is still under evaluation.

EUS-guided celiac plexus block

Patients with pancreatic neoplasms frequently seek relief from pain related to their pancreatic disease. When analgesic medication is no longer effective for pain

control in these patients, celiac plexus block (CPB) should be considered. Patients with advanced pancreatic cystic tumors may benefit from CPB. The celiac ganglia are located at the level where the celiac artery leaves the aorta, which is easily visualized with EUS due to its proximity to the posterior gastric wall. This proximity allows a needle to be inserted into the celiac ganglia under EUS guidance and alcohol to be injected in order to achieve chemical neurolysis of the celiac plexus. Wiersema and Gunaratnam performed EUS CPB for palliation of pancreatic cancer pain in 58 patients, showing a significant improvement in pain

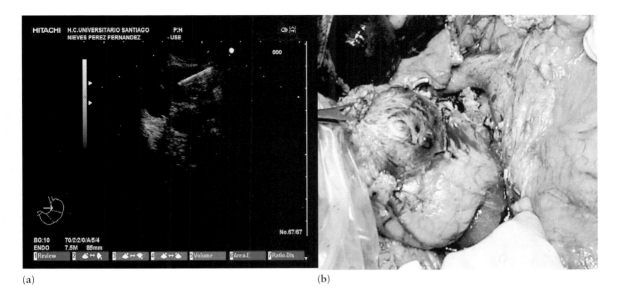

(a)   **(b)**

Figure 59.2 Endoscopic ultrasound (EUS) fine-needle aspiration of a pancreatic cystic lesion and surgical resection of the lesion. (a) A cystic lesion is identified in the pancreas by EUS. Under EUS guidance, a 22 gauge fine needle is advanced into the cyst and fluid is aspirated for analysis. (b) Macroscopic appearance of the pancreatic cyst at surgery. Surgical pathology established a definitive diagnosis of serous cystadenoma.

Table 59.2 Laboratory findings in pancreas cyst aspirate.

Diagnosis	Viscosity	Amylase	CA-72-4	CEA	CA-15-3	CA-19-9
Pseudocyst	Low	High	Low	Low	Low	Variable
Serous cystadenoma	Low	Variable	Low	Low	Low	Variable
Mucinous cystadenoma	Often high	Variable	High	High	High	Variable
Mucinous cystadenocarcinoma	High	Variable	High	High	High	Variable

CEA, carcinoembryonic antigen.

scores in 78% of patients at 2 weeks after the procedure. This improvement in patient symptoms persisted for at least 24 weeks (6 months), independent of adjuvant therapy or concomitant analgesics administered. No major complications were registered in this study.

Summary

EUS is a very useful technique for detecting the presence of a pancreatic cystic lesion and for characterizing its nature. EUS FNA permits cyst aspiration and fluid analysis that may provide a definitive diagnosis of the nature of the lesion. Table 59.3 is a summary of the most characteristic clinical, endosonographic, and laboratory findings observed in patients with pancreatic cystic lesions.

Acknowledgments

Special thanks to Michael J. Levy MD and the Mayo Clinic, Rochester, MN, for their generous contribution with pictures from their personal archives.

Table 59.3 Summary of clinical, endosonographic, and laboratory findings in pancreatic cystic lesions.

	Mucinous cyst	Serous cyst	Pseudocyst
Patient demographics	Woman, 40–50 years	> 60 years	Any age group
Patient history	Pancreatitis (±)	Incidental finding	Pancreatitis (+)
Cyst structure	Unilocular (thin septa)	Multilocular Multiseptated	Unilocular (thick septa)
Cyst size	Macrocystic (> 1 cm)	Microcystic (< 1 cm)	Macrocystic (> 1 cm)
Cyst wall	Thin	Thin	Thin (acute) Thick (chronic)
Solid component in cyst	±	–	±
Cyst communicates with MPD	±	–	+
Cyst content	Mucoid (↑ viscosity)	Serous (↓ viscosity)	Turbid (↑↓ viscosity)
Mucin stain in cyst fluid	++	–	–
Amylase in cyst fluid	±	–	++++
CEA in cyst fluid	++	±	±
CA-72-4 in cyst fluid	++	±	±
CA-19-9 in cyst fluid	±	±	±

CEA, carcinoembryonic antigen; MPD, main pancreatic duct.

Recommended reading

Bartsch D, Bastian D, Barth P et al. K-ras oncogene mutations indicate malignancy in cystic tumors of the pancreas. Ann Surg 1998;228:79–86.

Breslin N, Wallace MB. Diagnosis and fine needle aspiration of pancreatic pseudocysts: the role of endoscopic ultrasound. Gastrointest Endosc Clin North Am 2002;12: 781–790.

Brugge WR. The role of EUS in the diagnosis of cystic lesions of the pancreas. Gastrointest Endosc 2000;52:S18–S22.

Gunaratnam NT, Sarma AV, Norton ID, Wiersema MJ. Endosonography guided celiac plexus neurolysis (EUS CPN) for pancreatic cancer (PCA) pain: indications, efficacy, complications and patient outcomes. Gastrointest Endosc 2001;54:316–324.

Hammel P, Voitot H, Vilgrain V, Levy P, Ruszniewski P, Bernades P. Diagnostic value of CA 72-4 and carcinoembryogenic antigen determination in the fluid of pancreatic cystic lesions. Eur J Gastroenterol Hepatol 1998;10:345–348.

Hara T, Yamaguchi T, Ishihara T et al. Diagnosis and patient management of intraductal papillary mucinous tumor of the pancreas by using peroral pancreatoscopy and intra-ductal ultrasonography. Gastroenterology 2002;122:34–43.

Kawano T, Oshima M, Endo M. Endoscopic ultrasonographic diagnosis. Stomach Intestine 1995;30:365–371.

Koito K, Namieno T, Nagakawa N, Morita K. Solitary cystic tumors of the pancreas: EUS pathologic correlation. Gastrointest Endosc 1997;45:268–276.

Mallery S, Quirk D, Lewandrowski K, Centeno B, Warshaw A, Brugge WR. EUS-guided FNA with cyst fluid analysis in pancreatic cystic lesions. Gastrointest Endosc 1998;47: AB149.

Menzel J, Domschke W. Gastrointestinal miniprobe sonography: the current status. Am J Gastrenterol 2000;95:605–616.

Michael H, Gress F. Diagnosis of cystic neoplasms with endoscopic ultrasound. Gastrointest Endosc Clin North Am 2002;12:719–733.

Procacci C, Biasutti C, Carbognin G et al. Characterization of cystic tumors of the pancreas: CT accuracy. J Comput Assist Tomogr 1999;23:906–912.

Sand JA, Hyoty MJK, Mattila J, Dagorn JC, Norback IH. Clinical assessment compared with cyst fluid analysis in the differential diagnosis of cystic lesions in the pancreas. Surgery 1996;119:275–280.

Sarr MG, Carpenter HA, Prabhakar LP *et al.* Clinical and pathologic correlation of 84 mucinous cystic neoplasms of the pancreas: can one reliably differentiate benign from malignant (or premalignant) neoplasms? *Ann Surg* 2000; 231:205–212.

Sedlack R, Affi A, Vazquez-Sequeiros E, Norton ID, Clain JE, Wiersema MJ. Utility of EUS in the evaluation of cystic pancreatic lesions. *Gastrointest Endosc* 2002;56:543–547.

Siech M, Tripp K, Schmidt-Rohlfing B *et al.* Cystic tumours of the pancreas: diagnostic accuracy, pathologic observations and surgical consequences. *Langenbecks Arch Surg* 1998; 383:56–61.

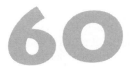

Therapeutic approach to cystic tumors

Laureano Fernández-Cruz, Isidro Martínez, Rosa Gelabert, Gleydson Cesar-Borges, Emiliano Astudillo, and Salvador Navarro

Introduction

In the last few years, cystic neoplasms of the pancreas have been diagnosed much more frequently and the treatment varies with the type of neoplasm. In patients with serous cystic neoplasms, resection should probably be reserved for mass-related symptoms or when differentiation from mucinous cystic neoplasms cannot be made confidently. However, mucinous cystic neoplasms of the pancreas should be considered premalignant or overtly malignant and, whenever safe, resected. For cystic neoplasms in the body or tail of the pancreas, a classical distal pancreatectomy with splenectomy may be the best treatment. Nevertheless, splenic preservation has been described in conjunction with distal pancreatectomy. Warshaw describes a technique of distal pancreatectomy with splenic preservation in which splenic vessels are ligated but the short gastric and left gastroepiploic vessels are preserved. Others have described the technique of preserving both the splenic artery and vein. Both strategies work and each has its place.

Laparoscopic pancreatic procedures are still at the stage of evaluation with regard to their indications and the technical variations used. Laparoscopic pancreatic surgery is currently used for staging malignant pancreatic tumors, for occasional management of inflammatory disorders of the pancreas, and for the resection of benign pancreatic tumors.

The use of laparoscopic ultrasonography and the advent of technologic refinements in laparoscopic instruments have led some groups, including our own, to explore the role of laparoscopic surgery in patients with cystic neoplasms of the pancreas. This chapter evaluates the feasibility and outcome of laparoscopic spleen-preserving distal pancreatectomy (LapSPDP) in patients with cystic neoplasms of the pancreas and provides information on the indications and limitations of the procedure.

Patients and methods

In January 1999 a prospective study was initiated using the laparoscopic approach in patients with cystic neoplasms of the pancreas. The group included 19 patients, 17 women and 2 men, with a mean age of 55 (range 34–70) years. Abdominal or back pain was the most common complaint. The tumors were characterized by computed tomography (CT). The average size was 5.2 cm (range 4–8 cm) and they were located in the body–tail of the pancreas.

In all patients a LapSPDP was planned. In a subgroup of 11 consecutive patients, splenic vessel preservation was performed; in this subgroup, the mean tumor size was 5.3 cm. In another subgroup of eight consecutive patients a LapSPDP without splenic vessel preservation, following Warshaw's technique, was performed. In this latter group, the spleen was kept vascularized by preserving the short gastric vessels and the left gastroepiploic vessels. In this subgroup of patients the mean tumor size was 5.1 cm.

Laparoscopic surgery

In our approach, the patient is placed in the half-lateral position with the left side up. The surgeon and assistant

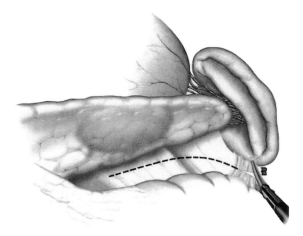

Figure 60.1 The splenocolic ligament is divided using the Harmonic Scalpel. The splenic flexure of the colon is mobilized downward.

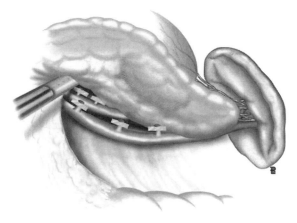

Figure 60.2 A tunnel is created between the splenic vessels and the pancreas.

stand on the left side of the patient and the camera person and scrub nurse on the opposite side. Four 10–12 mm trocars are inserted in the abdominal wall 3–4 cm above the umbilicus, on the xiphoid area, subcostal on the midaxillary line, and subcostal to the midclavicular line. Two monitors are used. Carbon dioxide pneumoperitoneum is used. Abdominal pressure is monitored and maintained at less than 14 mmHg. A 30° scope is used. The liver is explored visually and by laparoscopic ultrasonography (7.5 MHz probe, 10 mm diameter; B-K Medical, Gentolfe, Denmark).

The first step is to section the lienorenal ligament and dissect the subjacent fascia lateral to the spleen. The splenocolic ligament is divided using the harmonic scalpel (Fig. 60.1). The splenic flexure of the colon is mobilized downward. The gastrocolic omentum is widely opened up to the level of the mesenteric vessels, and the body–tail of the pancreas is then visualized. The anterior aspect of the pancreas is exposed by dividing the adhesions between the posterior surface of the stomach and the pancreas. Care must be taken to preserve the short gastric and left gastroepiploic vessels. The inferior border of the pancreas is dissected and the body and tail of the pancreas are completely detached from the retroperitoneum. This mobilization of the left pancreas allows visualization of the posterior wall of the gland, where the splenic vein is easily identified (Fig. 60.2). The splenic vein is pushed away from the poster-

ior pancreatic wall with gentle blunt dissection. Visual magnification through the laparoscope permits excellent control of the small pancreatic veins, which are coagulated using the LigaSure device, the harmonic scalpel, or clipped with titanium clips. A tunnel is created between the splenic vein and the pancreas. The splenic artery is identified through this space using careful blunt dissection with a curve dissector. The pancreas is then transected with a 30-mm endoscopic linear stapler. Usually two stapler applications are necessary. The tail of the pancreas is then grasped and retracted anteriorly with a 5-mm forceps, and traction is applied to expose the small branches of the splenic artery and vein, which are coagulated using the LigaSure device (Fig. 60.3). The dissection is continued laterally to the splenic hilum. All specimens are extracted within an endoscopic plastic bag.

The technique of SPDP without splenic vessel preservation follows the same surgical steps as described above until the plane behind the neck–body of the pancreas and in front of the superior mesenteric and portal veins. At this point the splenic vein is divided between clips. The use of laparoscopic ultrasonography demarcates the line of pancreatic transection 2 cm away from the tumor. After pancreatic transection the splenic artery is divided between clips. The left pancreas is then lifted up and mobilized posteriorly with the splenic artery and vein. The latter are clipped

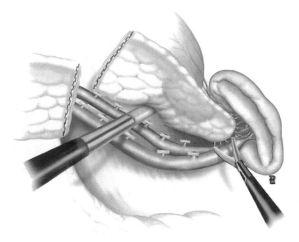

Figure 60.3 The pancreas is transected with a 30-mm endoscopic linear stapler. The head of the pancreas is retracted anteriorly and traction is applied to explore the small connections of the splenic artery and vein, which are coagulated with the LigaSure device.

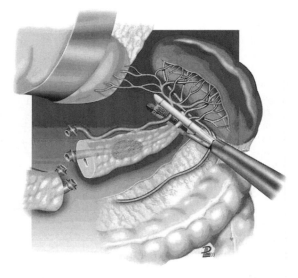

Figure 60.4 Laparoscopic spleen-preserving distal pancreatectomy without splenic vessel preservation. The spleen is kept vascularized by the short gastric and left gastroepiploic vessels.

and divided as they emerge from the pancreatic tail to enter the hilum of the spleen. The spleen is kept vascularized solely from the short gastric and left gastroepiploic vessels (Fig. 60.4). All specimens are extracted in an endoscopic plastic bag. A silicon drain is left in the pancreatic bed close to the pancreatic stump.

Evaluation criteria included operative factors, such as estimated blood loss, operative time, and intraoperative complications, and postoperative factors such as length of hospital stay and postoperative complications, with a specific focus on pancreatic leak, intraabdominal abscess, splenic complications, and other major infectious complications (i.e., pneumonia, wound infection). Postoperative pancreatic leaks were defined as a drain amylase level (measured after the third postoperative day) more than three times the upper limit of the normal serum amylase level in the absence of clinical sequelae. A clinical leak was defined as a biochemical leak in the presence of clinical sequelae such as fever or elevated white blood cell count, intraabdominal abscess, or the need for percutaneous drainage or reoperation.

Color Doppler ultrasound was performed with a Toshiba Powervision or a Sequoia (Acuson, Siemens) with a multifrequency 2–4 MHz transducer. Color Doppler studies were carried out in the postoperative period in all patients undergoing LapSPDP without splenic vessel preservation and when clinically indicated (i.e., unexplained fever, abdominal pain, or elevated white cell count). The color Doppler study included a complete abdominal examination: liver, bile ducts, portal vein patency, kidneys, pancreatic area, spleen, and search for intraabdominal fluid collections. Spleen evaluation included size, echostructure, and presence of fluid collections, which were evaluated by real-time ultrasonography. The Doppler study (pulsed and color) was done at hilar and parenchymal levels, just at the point at which the branches enter into the spleen. The arterial waveform was quantified by the resistive index (RI), where RI = (peak systolic velocity – end-diastolic velocity)/peak systolic velocity. Doppler parameters were adjusted to optimize the detection of low blood flow velocities.

Statistical analysis was performed using the Sigma Plot software package for Windows (SPSS Inc., Chicago, IL). Data were expressed as mean ± SD. The Kruskal–Wallis test and Student's t test were applicable. A P value less than 0.05 was considered significant.

Table 60.1 Laparoscopic spleen-preserving distal pancreatectomy with and without splenic vessel preservation.

	Splenic vessel preservation	Without splenic vessel preservation	P
Patients (n)	11	8	NS
Mean tumor size (cm)	5.3	5.1	NS
Patients with intraoperative complications (bleeding)	5	0	NS
Mean operative time (min)	222.7 ± 65.2	165 ± 16.9	0.002
Mean blood loss (mL)	495.5 ± 228.5	275 ± 84.5	0.017
Postoperative complications			
Pancreas related	2	1	NS
Spleen related	1	2	NS
Mean hospital stay (days)	5.45	5.63	NS

NS, not significant.

Results

In the subgroup of 11 patients undergoing LapSPDP with preservation of splenic vessels, splenic vessel preservation was feasible in six patients; however, five patients suffered intraoperative bleeding, at the time of pancreatic transection in two patients and during dissection of the splenic vessels when separating the tumor from the pancreas in three patients. As a result, in three patients the splenic artery was ligated using four clips and then divided so that two clips were left in the remnant, although the splenic vein remained intact. In one patient the splenic vessels were divided using endoscopic staplers. In another patient, with a tumor 8 cm in diameter, following stapling of the splenic vessels the procedure was converted to a hand-assisted technique and *en bloc* resection that included the spleen because the tumor was densely adherent to the splenic hilum. The mean operative time of the whole group with splenic vessel preservation was 222.7 ± 65.2 min (range 180–400 min) and intraoperative blood loss 495 ± 228.5 mL (range 200–850 mL). No patient required blood transfusion. In the subgroup of eight patients undergoing LapSPDP without splenic vessel preservation following Warshaw's technique, the mean operative time was 165 ± 16.9 min (range 150–190 min) and the mean blood loss 275 ± 84.5 mL (range 200–450 mL) (Table 60.1). No patient required blood transfusion. A comparative study between the two subgroups showed that the mean operative time was significantly shorter (P = 0.002) and mean blood loss significantly lower (P = 0.017) in the subgroup with LapSPDP using Warshaw's technique.

Overall postoperative complications (31.6%) were observed in six patients following LapSPDP. Pancreatic fistulas of low volume (< 100 mL) and a drain amylase greater than 5000 U/L developed postoperatively in two patients after LapSPDP with splenic vessel preservation and in one patient after LapSPDP without splenic vessel preservation, but without clinical symptomatology. These patients had a hospital stay of 5 days but were discharged home with the drain *in situ* based on persistent drain output. The drain was discontinued 2 weeks after surgery.

Evaluation of the vascularity of the spleen by Doppler showed an RI between 0.44 and 0.52 in the patients undergoing LapSPDP without splenic vessel preservation. Splenic complications occurred in three patients (RI 0.44, 0.46, and 0.48 respectively). One patient, in whom splenic vessel division was performed for intraoperative bleeding, was discharged 5 days after surgery; however, 2 days later he presented with fever (38°C) and clinical sepsis. The patient was rehospitalized and splenectomy was performed for massive necrosis of the spleen. Two other patients who underwent LapSPDP without splenic vessel preservation presented early in the postoperative period with pain in the left upper quadrant of the abdomen. Color Doppler ultrasound showed a focal splenic infarct of 3 and 4 cm respectively. Both patients were treated with antibiotics to prevent abscess formation in the splenic infarct.

The mean length of postoperative hospital stay was 5.7 days (range 5–8 days). In patients who had an uncomplicated course, the mean hospital stay was 5 days, whereas patients with complications had a mean hospital stay of 6.6 days; this difference was statistically significant ($P = 0.01$). There were no late postoperative complications and no deaths within 30 days of operation. The majority of patients returned to previous activities 3 weeks after the operation. The final pathology report showed mucinous cystadenoma in 17 patients, mucinous cystic tumor bordeline in one patient, and mucinous cystadenocarcinoma in another patient. The mean follow-up was 22 months (range 6–42 months). No tumor recurrences were observed.

Discussion

The use of laparoscopy for managing benign pancreatic tumors has still not been defined. With the introduction of each new laparoscopic technique, there have been predictable cycles characterized by an introductory phase (in which the surgical technique is developed), a definition phase (with exploration of technical variations and classification of the operative indications), and an educational phase. The definition phase is currently underway for laparoscopic pancreatic surgery. Laparoscopic pancreatic surgery must be considered an advanced laparoscopic procedure and should be performed only in institutions with expertise in pancreatic surgery by a team with advanced laparoscopic skills. Most published reports on laparoscopic pancreatic surgery resections are on single cases or limited series of patients. Moreover, the follow-up is short, so little is known about the long-term results. Three factors should be considered when formulating the indications for this new procedure: the proper patient, the proper procedure, and proper performance.

Proper patient

The apropriate treatment for cystic neoplasms of the pancreas varies considerably based on the specific type of neoplasm. Serous cystadenoma of the pancreas affects predominantly women with an average age of 50 (range 35–84) years. Most patients experience vague abdominal pain and symptoms seemingly related to the mass effect of the tumor. Serous cystade-

noma can often be distinguished quite reliably by their characteristics: multiple small (< 2 cm) cystic areas, often resembling a honeycomb both grossly and on imaging. Occasionally they have a starburst appearance, with a centrally located calcified scar. These neoplasms are universally benign, although there have been occasional cases with histologically documented malignant serous cystadenocarcinomas. Surgical treatment is indicated in symptomatic patients. Mucinous cystic neoplasms are the most frequently encountered cystic tumors of the pancreas, accounting for 45% of cases. These neoplasms predominate in women with an average age of 53 (range 19–82) years. The most common symptoms seem to be related to a local mass effect. These neoplasms, more common in the body or tail of the pancreas (70%), are composed of cystic areas filled with viscous mucous material, and the cyst walls are dense and fibrous with occasional calcification. Pathognomonic findings on CT include the presence of thin or thick papillary fronds or septae on the individual cysts. A detailed clinicopathologic correlation has been proposed by Sarr *et al.*, which separates these tumors into three groups:

1 mucinous cystadenomas, comprising 65% of mucinous tumors;
2 proliferative cystic mucinous neoplasms (30% of mucinous neoplasms) composed of varying degrees of atypia, dysplasia, and even changes of carcinoma *in situ* but without tissue invasion;
3 mucinous cystadenocarcinomas (< 10% of all mucinous cystic neoplasms) with frank stromal invasion beyond the epithelium.

The latter group behaves like ductal adenocarcinoma of the pancreas. However, according to the Mayo Clinic experience, there were no recurrences in patients with either cystadenoma or proliferative mucinous cystic neoplasms on follow-up of up to 30 years. However, two recent series of mucinous cystic neoplasms describe invasive carcinoma in 36% (47/130) and 29% (16/56).

We believe that serous cystadenomas and mucinous cystic neoplasms are suitable for the laparoscopic approach based on the frequent location of these tumors in the body and tail of the pancreas and the high frecuency of these neoplasms being benign or premalignant lesions. The laparoscopic approach is probably unsuitable for large tumors with evidence of malignancy.

Proper procedure

The aim here is to reproduce the technique used for open pancreatic surgery and the application of the principles of oncologic surgery. Enucleation or pancreatic resection has been advocated in open surgery of these tumors. Enucleation of pancreatic cystic tumors offers the possibility of complete tumor removal without loss of pancreatic parenchyma, possible diabetes, and splenectomy. Enucleation can be safely performed laparoscopically and has been proposed as the technique of choice in patients with insulinoma. However, enucleation appears to be a debatable procedure in patients with cystic neoplasms of the pancreas. Tumor enucleation does not address the malignant potential of these tumors and should be used (in selected cases) with caution to avoid inadequate tumor margins. In addition, the incidence of pancreatic fistulas after tumor enucleation was reported to be 30–50%, leading to long hospital stay (19.5 days in the Johns Hopkins' series).

In the literature, when the tumor was located in the body or tail of the pancreas, the technique most frequently used was distal pancreatectomy with *en bloc* resection that included the spleen. Talamini *et al.* reported that 74% of patients with mucinous cystadenomas undergoing distal pancreatectomy had splenectomy. One late septic death occurred in this group. Nevertheless, distal pancreatectomy with splenic preservation has been advocated by a number of others. The question of spleen-preserving distal pancreatectomy is controversial. Recently, Lillemoe *et al.* have reported the largest single-institution experience with distal pancreatectomy (235 patients) for a variety of pancreatic disorders, including chronic pancreatitis and benign and malignant pancreatic tumors; only 16% of patients had splenic preservation. In another series of 71 patients reported by Fernández-del Castillo *et al.*, the incidence of spleen preservation was 20%. It might be suspected that for patients in whom distal pancreatectomy is considered appropriate, simultaneous splenectomy is routine because of its technical simplicity. However, since it became apparent that the incidence of sepsis after splenectomy is about 0.28–1.9%, with a mortality rate of 2.2%, the significance of spleen preservation has come to be widely recognized.

Published data from two retrospective reviews comparing patients who had surgery mainly for trauma or pancreatitis, undergoing distal pancreatectomy with and without splenectomy, showed no differences in complication rates between groups, the reports concluding that splenectomy should not be a routine part of distal pancreatic resection. On the other hand, Benoist *et al.* analyzed 40 patients undergoing distal pancreatectomy for indications other than chronic pancreatitis; 15 patients underwent distal pancreatectomy with spleen conservation and 25 had splenectomy. Pancreatic left resection with splenectomy turned out to have a lower morbidity rate, as pancreatic complications such as fistula or subphrenic abscess occurred more frequently in patients after spleen-conserving surgery. More recently, Shoup *et al.* reported the series from the Memorial Sloan-Kettering Cancer Center including 211 patients undergoing distal pancreatectomy. Splenectomy was performed in 79 patients (63%) and splenic preservation in 46 (37%). The most common histopathologic conditions were neuroendocrine tumors (*n* = 45) and benign cystic tumors (*n* = 44). Perioperative complications occurred in 49% following splenectomy and in 39% following splenic preservation. Perioperative infectious complications and severe complications were significantly higher in the splenectomy group (28% and 11%) compared with the splenic preservation group (9% and 2%). Length of hospital stay was 9 days following splenectomy and 7 days following splenic preservation.

We encourage laparoscopic spleen-preserving pancreatectomy in order to prevent the potential long- and short-term complications associated with splenectomy. The question is whether it should be performed with or without splenic vessel preservation. The latter technique, in which the short gastric and gastroepiploic arteries are the only blood suply to the spleen, was described by Warshaw. Splenomegaly is a contraindication for this method of spleen conservation because the increased mass is insufficiently nourished by the short gastric vessels. There is no doubt that by preserving the splenic artery and vein, the blood supply to the spleen is well maintained and the danger of splenic necrosis and abscess formation is reduced. On the other hand, distal pancreatectomy with conservation of the splenic artery and vein is both time- and labor-consuming. Dissecting the splenic vessels from the pancreas may be difficult to perform in the presence of tumors distorting and compressing the course of the vessels.

In this report we conducted a prospective study to evaluate the feasibility and outcome of LapSPDP with and without splenic vessel preservation. In this series the mean tumor diameter was 5.2 cm. Splenic vessel preservation was performed in 11 patients. Only in six of these patients (54.5%) was the spleen preserved with an intact splenic artery and vein. In the remainder, intraoperative bleeding due to injury of splenic vessels required the sacrifice of the splenic artery (but the splenic vein remained intact) or the splenic artery and vein, and the spleen was kept vascularized by the short gastric and left gastroepiploic vessels. Our results indicate that preservation of the splenic vessels is not always possible when dealing with large tumors. In another eight consecutive patients, the splenic artery and vein were secured by clips and the short gastric and gastroepiploic collaterals were preserved to nourish the spleen. The comparison between the groups undergoing splenic vessel preservation and Warshaw's technique demonstrates a statistically significant difference in the parameters of operative time and intraoperative blood loss in favor of division of the splenic vessels.

In all circumstances, we advocate LapSPDP that preserves the short gastric and gastroepiploic vessels, and thus where it is necessary to remove the splenic artery and vein the spleen will be kept vascularized. Furthermore, Warshaw's technique is less technically demanding than the dissection and conservation of the splenic artery and vein. In answer to the question of whether to conserve the splenic vessels, we believe, in accordance with Warshaw, "if the goal is to save the spleen, having options allows the surgeons to match the tactics to the terrain."

Proper performance

The aims of minimally invasive surgery are not only to minimize parietal damage but also to diminish the incidence of postoperative complications. In this report the overall complication rate was 31.6%, which includes pancreatic leaks as well as splenic complications.

In patients undergoing open surgery, significant morbidity follows distal pancreatic resection. In the literature, pancreas-related complications ranged from 5 to 26%. In the published reports there is a lack of consensus regarding the optimal method of pancreatic stump closure and the contribution of spleen salvage on the development of pancreatic leak. Also, the role for routine use of somatostatin analogs after elective left pancreatectomy remains unclear. In our current series, 3 of 19 patients (15.7%) after laparoscopic pancreatic re-

section (mechanical stapling) developed a low-volume pancreatic fistula without clinical symptomatology, classified as a biochemical leak. Patients with this complication were managed as outpatients until the drainage decreased and the drain was discontinued. In a recent report, the incidence of pancreatic leak was reduced significantly when the pancreatic duct was identified, dissected, and ligated during open left pancreatectomy. This technical approach could be incorporated after laparoscopic mechanical stapling of the parenchyma. This technical refinement may result in a reduction of the rate of postoperative pancreatic leaks.

Spleen salvage was possible in the majority of patients. Only in one patient was hand-assisted laparoscopic distal pancreatectomy with *en bloc* resection of the spleen thought to be necessary because of the close relation of the tumor (8 cm diameter) to the splenic hilum. Splenic complications were observed in 3 of 18 patients (16.6%) after LapSPDP, and interestingly this complication was only observed in patients undergoing Warshaw's technique. One explanation could be that after division of the splenic vessels in cases of inadvertent injury to the gastroepiploic vessels during dissection of the inferior margin of the tail of the pancreas, the organ receives blood directly from the short gastric vessels, and in the absence of vascular communication between superior and inferior splenic lobes, splenic infarct results. This complication may be suspected clinically with the presence of fever and left upper abdominal pain. Color Doppler ultrasonography will show the area of infarct. Abscess formation can be prevented with antibiotic administration. A more serious complication is massive necrosis of the organ with local infection that requires splenectomy. Shein *et al.* reported that splenectomy had to be performed 24 hours after Warshaw's technique because of necrosis of the spleen. However, the reduction of blood supply leading to splenic necrosis may take days, as happened in our patient, who was discharged 5 days after operation but rehospitalized 2 days later with clinical sepsis, splenectomy being performed through a left subcostal incision. It might be that the splenic complications following Warshaw's technique are not the result of failure of the technique but a failure of proper performance of the method as it was originally described, i.e., preservation of all the vascular collaterals to nourish the spleen.

Our study suggests that patients undergoing spleen-preserving distal pancreatectomy using Warshaw's technique should be followed carefully from the immediate postoperative period with color Doppler ultrasonography in order to detect morphologic changes in the spleen, so that when focal splenic infarct is identified prompt treatment with antibiotics prevents splenic abscess. It is noteworthy that after LapSPDP without splenic vessel preservation the RI at the splenic hilum was in the range 0.48–0.52, lower than that reported in healthy controls (0.53–0.56). This finding could be attributed to the small caliber of the collateral vessels nourishing the spleen. Similar low-resistance arterial waveforms (< 0.50) are observed in liver transplant patients with hepatic artery thrombosis in whom collateral arterial vessels are newly formed or in patients with hepatic artery stenosis.

In this study the mean hospital stay of the whole group was 5.7 days. This is a notable reduction of the postoperative length of stay in comparison with the largest single-institution experience with distal pancreatectomy (mean stay 15 days). A recent report from the Massachusetts General Hospital demonstrated that the length of stay after distal pancreatectomy decreased from 9 to 7 days.

Conclusions

Laparoscopic distal pancreatectomy is feasible, with an acceptable complication rate in patients with cystic neoplasms of the pancreas. Laparoscopic ultrasound should be routinely used to achieve an adequate margin. Spleen salvage is possible in 94.7% of cases during pancreatic resection with or without splenic vessel preservation. Warshaw's technique is faster and less technically demanding than splenic vessel preservation but associated splenic complications are usually managed conservatively. Color Doppler ultrasonography is mandatory in the immediate postoperative period in cases of division of the splenic vessels in order to detect splenic abnormalities. The advantages of the laparoscopic approach are reasonably short hospital stay and an early return to previous activities. A cosmetic advantage is also clear because of the absence of long abdominal incisions. Surgical cure can be achieved in most patients with cystic neoplasms of the pancreas, with complete relief of symptoms. No tumor recurrences were observed but the follow-up is relatively short.

Recommended reading

Balcom JH, Rattner DW, Warshaw AL, Chang Y, Fernández-del Castillo C. Ten year experience with 733 pancreatic resections. Changing indications, older patients, and decreasing length of hospitalization. *Arch. Surg* 2001;136: 391–398.

Benoist S, Dugué L, Sauvanet A *et al*. Is there a role of preservation of the spleen in distal pancreatectomy? *J Am Coll Surg* 1999;188:255–260.

Bilimoria MM, Cormier JN, Mun Y, Lee JE, Evans DB, Pisters PWT. Pancreatic leak after pancreatectomy is reduced following main pancreatic duct ligation. *Br J Surg* 2003;90: 190–196.

Cuschieri A. Laparoscopic surgery of the pancreas. *J R Coll Surg Edinb* 1994;39:178–184.

Fabre JM, Dulucq JL, Vacher C, Lemoine MC, Wintringer P, Nocca D. Is laparoscopic left pancreatic resection justified? *Surg Endosc* 2002;19:507–510.

Fernández-Cruz L, Sáenz A, Astudillo E, Pantoja JP, Uzcátegui E, Navarro S. Laparoscopic pancreatic surgery in patients with chronic pancreatitis. *Surg Endosc* 2002;16:996–1003.

Fernández-Cruz L, Sáenz A, Astudillo E *et al*. Outcome of laparoscopic pancreatic surgery: endocrine and non endocrine tumors. *World J Surg* 2002;26:1057–1065.

Fernández-del Castillo C, Rattner DW, Warshaw L. Standards for pancreatic resection in the 1990s. *Arch Surg* 1995;130: 295–300.

Gagner M, Pomp A. Laparoscopic pancreatic resection. Is it worthwhile? *J Gastrointest Surg* 1997;1:20–26.

Kimura W, Inoue T, Futawake N, Shiukai H, Hau I, Muto T. Spleen-preserving distal pancreatectomy with conservation of the splenic artery and vein. *Surgery* 1996;120:885–890.

Klinger PJ, Hinder RA, Menke DM. Hand-assisted laparoscopic distal pancreatectomy for pancreatic cystoadenoma. *Surg Laparosc Endosc* 1998;8:180–184.

Lillemoe KD, Kaushal S, Cameron JL, Sohn TA, Pitt HA, Yeo CJ. Distal pancreatectomy: indications and outcomes in 235 patients. *Ann Surg* 1999;229:693–700.

Ohwada S, Ogawa T, Tanahashi Y *et al*. Fibrin glue sandwich prevents pancreatic fistula following distal pancreatectomy. *World J Surg* 1998;22:494–498.

Park AE, Heniford BT. Therapeutic laparoscopy of the pancreas. *Ann Surg* 2002;236:149–158.

Park A, Schwartz R, Tandan V, Anvari M. Laparoscopic pancreatic surgery. *Am J Surg* 1999;177:158–163.

Sarr M, Carpenter H, Prabhakar L. Clinical and pathological correlation of 84 mucinous cystic neoplasms of the pancreas. *Ann Surg* 2000;231:205–212.

Sarr MG, Murr M, Smyrk TC *et al*. Primary cystic neoplasms of the pancreas. Neoplasic disorders of emerging importance. Current state of the art and unanswered questions. *J Gastrointest Surg* 2003;7:417–428.

Shoup M, Brennan MF, McWhite K, Leung DHY, Klimstra D, Conlon KC. The value of splenic preservation with distal pancreatectomy. *Arch Surg* 2002;137:164–168.

Talamini M, Moesinger R, Yeo CH. Cystadenoma of the pancreas: is enucleation an adequate operation? *Ann Surg* 1998;227:896–903.

Vezakis A, Davides D, Larvin M. Laparoscopic surgery combined with preservation of the spleen for distal pancreatic tumors. *Surg Endosc* 1999;13:26–29.

Warshaw L. Conservation of the spleen with distal pancreatectomy. *Arch Surg* 1998;123:550–553.

Watanabe Y, Motomichi S, Kikkawa H *et al*. Spleen-preserving laparoscopic distal pancreatectomy for cystic adenoma. *Hepatogastroenterology* 2002;49:148–152.

Index

Note: page numbers in *italics* refer to figures, those in **bold** refer to tables.

517